Principles and Practice of Panoramic Radiology

INCLUDING INTRAORAL RADIOGRAPHIC INTERPRETATION

OLAF E. LANGLAND, D.D.S., M.S., F.A.C.D.

Diplomate, American Board of Oral and Maxillofacial Radiology; Professor and Director of the Division of Oral and Maxillofacial Radiology, Department of Dental Diagnostic Science, The University of Texas Health Science Center at San Antonio, San Antonio, Texas

ROBERT P. LANGLAIS, B.A., D.D.S., M.S.

Diplomate, American Board of Oral and Maxillofacial Radiology; Diplomate, American Board of Oral Medicine; Associate Professor and Director of the Graduate Program in Dental Diagnostic Science, Department of Dental Diagnostic Science, The University of Texas Health Science Center at San Antonio, San Antonio, Texas

CHARLES R. MORRIS, D.D.S., F.A.C.D.

Diplomate, American Board of Oral and Maxillofacial Surgery; Professor and Chairman, Department of Dental Diagnostic Science, The University of Texas Health Science Center at San Antonio, San Antonio, Texas

1982 W. B. SAUNDERS COMPANY

Philadelphia/London/Toronto/Mexico City/Rio de Janeiro/Sydney/Tokyo

W. B. Saunders Company: West Washington Square
Philadelphia, PA 19105

1 St. Anne's Road
Eastbourne, East Sussex BN21 3UN, England

1 Goldthorne Avenue
Toronto, Ontario M8Z 5T9, Canada

Apartado 26370—Cedro 512
Mexico 4, D.F., Mexico

Rua Coronel Cabrita, 8
Sao Cristovao Caixa Postal 21176
Rio de Janeiro, Brazil

9 Waltham Street
Artarmon, N.S.W. 2064, Australia

Ichibancho, Central Bldg., 22-1 Ichibancho
Chiyoda-Ku, Tokyo 102, Japan

Library of Congress Cataloging in Publication Data

Langland, Olaf E.

Principles and practice of panoramic radiology.

1. Teeth—Radiography. 2. Jaws—Radiography. 3. Radiography, Panoramic. I. Langlais, Robert P. II. Morris, Charles R. (Charles Robert), 1924– . III. Title. [DNLM: 1. Radiography, Panoramic. WN 230 L282p]

RK309.L357 617.6′07572 81-50623

ISBN 0-7216-5612-9 AACR2

Front cover illustration: A panoramic image of clinical anatomy by Carolyn Wittlif. (Courtesy of the authors)

Principles and Practice of Panoramic Radiology ISBN 0-7216-5612-9

Last digit is the print number: 9 8 7 6 5 4 3 2 1

To our wives,

Ruth

Denyse

Evelyn

Contributors

STEVEN L. BRICKER, D.D.S., M.S.

Associate Professor, Department of Dental Diagnostic Science, The University of Texas Health Science Center at San Antonio, San Antonio, Texas

MICHAEL D. CALLIHAN, D.D.S., M.S., Dip.A.B.O.P.

Captain, United States Department of the Navy; Chief, Division of Hard Tissue, Oral Pathology, Armed Forces Institute of Pathology, Washington, D.C.

A. PETER FORTIER, B.S., D.D.S., M.Ed.

Professor, Department of Oral Diagnosis/Medicine/Radiology, Louisiana State University School of Dentistry, New Orleans, Louisiana

BIRGIT JUNFIN GLASS, B.S., D.D.S., M.S.

Assistant Professor, Department of Dental Diagnostic Science, The University of Texas Health Science Center at San Antonio, San Antonio, Texas

WILLIAM D. McDAVID, Ph.D.

Assistant Professor, Department of Dental Diagnostic Science, The University of Texas Health Science Center at San Antonio, San Antonio, Texas

CHRISTOFFEL J. NORTJÉ, B.Ch.D., Ph.D.

Professor and Head, Department of Dento, Maxillo, and Facial Roentgenology, Faculty of Dentistry, University of Stellenbosch, Tygerberg, Republic of South Africa

GUS C. PAPPAS, D.D.S.

Professor Emeritus, School of Dentistry, Ohio State University, Columbus, Ohio

CARLOS PORTALES, D.D.S.

Chief, Oral Surgery, Santa Rosa Hospital; Clinical Assistant Professor, Department of Oral Surgery, The University of Texas Health Science Center at San Antonio, San Antonio, Texas

JOHN W. PREECE, D.D.S., M.S.D.

Professor, Dental Diagnostic Science Department; The University of Texas Health Science Center at San Antonio, San Antonio, Texas

FRANK C. SAMMIS, JR., D.D.S., Dip.A.B.O.M.S.

Clinical Professor, Department of Oral Surgery, The University of Texas Health Science Center at San Antonio, San Antonio, Texas

DOUG W. STONEMAN, D.D.S., F.R.C.D.(C)

Professor and Chairman, Department of Oral Radiology, Faculty of Dentistry, University of Toronto, Toronto, Ontario, Canada

GUNILLA TRONJE, D.D.S., Ph.D.

Associate Professor, Department of Oral Radiology, School of Dentistry, Karolinska Institutet, University of Stockholm, Stockholm, Sweden

ULF E. WELANDER, D.D.S., Ph.D.

Professor and Chairman, Department of Oral Radiology, School of Dentistry, University of Umeå, Umeå, Sweden

Foreword

As co-holder of a U.S. patent, along with John W. Kumpula, for the first commercially successful dental panoramic x-ray machine produced in the United States, I am pleased to provide the foreword to this text by Drs. Langland, Langlais, and Morris covering the use and operation of such machines and the interpretation of the resulting panoramic projections.

As part of this foreword, I would like to caution the user that the panoramic dental x ray is not, nor was it designed to be, a substitute for intraoral films; rather, it is a device suited to the mass screening of large numbers of people such as may be found at military induction centers or large clinical operations such as those at dental schools.

The apparatus cannot be counted on to disclose very small interproximal carious lesions or minimal periodontal involvement. However, a complete survey can be accomplished with one panoramic exposure supplemented by upper and lower posterior bitewing intraoral films, thus accomplishing an acceptable dental survey in a minimum of time and with considerable reduction in the amount of ionizing radiation exposure to the patient.

This publication should serve as a valuable source of information concerning an often used but not fully understood dental radiographic technique.

Frequently, normal cranial structures are not recognized because their image is distorted owing to magnification by projection. This book will be helpful in recognizing some artifacts, such as those caused by failing to remove hair pins and small items of jewelry, that could be mistaken for foreign bodies in the region being radiographed.

I recommend that this text be made part of all dental radiographers' libraries as a reference and an aid in interpreting panoramic projections.

DONALD C. HUDSON, D.D.S.

Preface

Panoramic x-ray machines have been in use for about 20 years. In that time, little has been done to provide a concise treatise for the everyday practice of panoramic radiology. At the time of the introduction of this type of equipment, it was most commonly seen in dental schools and dental and radiology departments of hospitals and other health care institutions. Private practitioners were reluctant to invest in panoramic radiography for a variety of reasons.

Recently, however, a number of factors have contributed to a veritable boom in the sale of panoramic x-ray machines. During their education, dental students learn to appreciate the information that is available on panoramic films. The purchase of panoramic machines is much more cost effective and affordable today than it was in the earlier days. Many dental offices now use automatic processing for all of their dental films, so that the purchase of this equipment is not as much of a consideration relative to the purchase of the panoramic machine. Additionally, some panoramic machines can be operated from the same master control as that used with the intraoral unit. Perhaps more importantly, it is a generally accepted fact that one panoramic film delivers to the patient a dose of radiation which is equivalent to about one set of four bite wing intraoral films.

These important factors, along with others, including the greater ease and less time necessary to produce a single panoramic film as compared with the standard intraoral full mouth survey; the additional visualization of the areas of the body of the mandible beyond the periapical region, the ramus, the temporomandibular joint, the maxillary sinus, and the stylohyoid complex; and the dentist's professional responsibility to the patient to provide the best care possible, have undoubtedly led many dentists in general practice and various specialty areas to use panoramic radiology on a daily basis.

In our consideration of this subject, we have presented the material in a manner that we believe to be logical. We believe that understanding the principles of panoramic radiography is an essential step in acquiring technical and interpretative acumen. We have tried to trouble shoot some of the problems that some practitioners may have and have stressed the limitations of this type of radiographic examination in areas where this was appropriate. The emphasis of this book is on radiographic interpretation, presented in a logical manner, based on a sound understanding of the principles of panoramic radiography.

Our classification of disease is based on the radiographic pattern produced by the lesion in its mature phase and in its most common radiographic presentation. The other radiographic patterns that can be produced by a single disease entity in the early and intermediate phases of its development or unusual variations are covered in the same area as the classic lesion. We have done this to include all of the material relative to a single disease entity in one part of the book for greater ease of use. The exceptions to this rule are the special regional considerations when a disorder, such as an ameloblastoma, affects the maxillary sinus or the TMJ area. In this instance, we have repeated our coverage of a disease entity to illustrate any special considerations peculiar to these two anatomic locations. Additionally, we have covered other disorders peculiar to the maxillary sinus and TMJ area. In this instance we did not consider it practical to classify the abnormalities by radiographic appearance owing to the peculiar nature of these anatomic locations.

Our overall goal for this book is to provide the dental practitioner with a largely visual experience. We have made great efforts to try to provide excellent quality illustrations in which the various details of the abnormality can be visualized. We have given a brief overview of each condition, which usually includes its etiology and various other details such as the most common age, sex, and location and some comments on management. As a separate consideration for each condition we have described the radiographic features. We have concentrated on the classic, mature lesion in its most common presentation and have described and illustrated some variations where appropriate. Some disorders have not been included as we had no material to illustrate them; other extremely rare disorders were included because we did have the material. This book is meant to be a pictorial; therefore it is not verbose. Some detail is, however, provided in areas that have been either excluded or largely neglected by the standard reference texts, which are listed at the end of each chapter.

There are three ways to read this book: first, the dentist or student may read this book from cover to cover, leaving nothing out; second, the reader may concentrate only on the radiographic features described in this book; third, the reader can learn a great deal by simply looking at the illustrations and reading the legends. We sincerely hope that others will believe, as we do, that there is a need for a book like this and that this text will provide the information that the reader is seeking.

O. E. Langland
R. P. Langlais
C. R. Morris

Acknowledgments

The authors wish to express their appreciation to their many colleagues who generously and willingly gave permission to use illustrative material and diagrams from their published works. Also, we would like to acknowledge with gratitude those many individuals throughout the world who have contributed radiographs of their cases. Without their kind assistance this book would not have been completed. Additionally, we are especially grateful to our contributors, Steven Bricker, Michael Callihan, A. Peter Fortier, Birgit Junfin Glass, John Preece, William McDavid, Chris Nortjé, Gus Pappas, Carlos Portales, Frank Sammis, Jr., Doug Stoneman, Gunilla Tronje, and Ulf Welander. The contribution of their time, material, and expertise is the most important collective factor that made this book possible.

We wish to give special thanks to unnamed friends, advisors, students, and technicians who may recognize in this book the results of their help. Please acknowledge our indebtedness to you.

We are especially grateful to Ulf Welander, William McDavid, and Gunilla Tronje for the truly masterful job that they did in writing and illustrating Chapter 2, The Theory of Rotational Panoramic Radiography and to John Preece who wrote Chapter 3, The Biologic Effects of Panoramic Radiography.

We wish to acknowledge Ray Aldrete, Mary Etta Raborn, Alvin J. Julian, and Dennis Havel, photographers at UTHSCSA, Department of Education Resources, for their excellent work. Also, special recognition should be given Jack Faude of the Pennwalt Corp. for obtaining excellent quality Log E-tronic prints of a number of the radiographs included in the book.

The illustrations and diagrams were skillfully prepared by Nancy O. Reid, Charles D. Whitehead, and Tom Hudgins, medical illustrators of the UTHSCSA, Department of Education Resources. Their work speaks for itself. The cover illustration was drawn by Carolyn Wittlif of the same department, who masterfully portrayed the transformation of clinical anatomy to the panoramic image.

We are especially grateful for the tireless efforts, patience, sound advice, and cooperation given to us by the dental x-ray technologists of the Department of Dental Diagnostic Science, University of Texas Dental School at San Antonio. They are Leo Bedock, Felix Cordero, Joan Pluchinsky, and Emily Taylor.

We would like to thank our secretaries, Pat Brownlow, Rebecca Cox, Carol Rios, and Stella Schwab, who contributed unselfishly of their time, skillfully typing each chapter many times, and carefully collected illustrative material in the preparation of the manuscript.

We wish to express our sincere appreciation to our colleagues at the Department of Dental Diagnostic Science, The University of Texas Dental School at San Antonio, who gave us helpful suggestions, time, assistance, encouragement, and cases. They are Dr. Bill Baker, Dr. James Cottone, Dr. James Frazer, Dr. Jack Hartley, Dr. Richard Morse, and Dr. Vincent Segreto.

We are particularly grateful for the encouragement, guidance, and assistance given us by Carroll C. Cann and Robert W. Reinhardt of W. B. Saunders Company. Their understanding, support, and gentle urging were most helpful.

Lastly, we wish to recognize our wives, Ruth, Denyse, and Evelyn, whose encouragement, understanding support, and patience were deeply appreciated and to whom we dedicate this book.

Contents

Chapter 1
Introduction and History of Panoramic Radiography

ADVANTAGES AND DISADVANTAGES OF PANORAMIC RADIOGRAPHY

METHODS OF PANORAMIC RADIOGRAPHY
- Intraoral Source of Radiation
  - Koch and Sterzel, Co., Essen, Germany, 1954, Horst Beger, Dresden, Germany, 1943
  - Dr. Walter Ott, Switzerland, 1946
  - Dr. Sidney Blackman, England, 1960, Panograph
  - Three companies still manufacture units
    - Panoramix, Koch and Sterzel
    - Status-X, Siemens Corp.
    - Stat Oralix, Philips Medical Systems
- Rotational Panoramic Radiography
  - Dr. H. Numata, Japan, 1933
  - Dr. Y. V. Paatero, Finland
    - Parabolography, intraoral film, 1946
    - Parabolography, extraoral film, 1949
    - Pantomography, extraoral film, 1950
      - Tomography
        - Watson, 1938
      - Scanography
        - Posche, 1903
        - Albers-Schönberg, 1906
        - Gott and Rosenthal, 1912
        - Millwee, 1937
        - Heckmann, 1939
  - Dr. R. T. Nelsen and John Kumpula, 1950
    - University of Washington (Seattle)
    - Panography, intraoral film, 1950
      - Pilot apparatus
      - Automatic unit
  - Dr. Y. V. Paatero and John Kumpula, 1950–51
    - University of Washington (Seattle)
    - Pantomographic unit
      - Extraoral film method
      - Single axis or concentric rotational method
      - Double axis or eccentric rotational method
  - Dr. Y. V. Paatero, Helsinki, Finland, 1951–1954
    - Pantomographic prototype unit
    - Dr. Sidney Blackman, England
      - Rotograph, Watson & Sons, Ltd.
  - Dr. Y. V. Paatero, Helsinki, Finland, 1954–1960
    - Orthopantomography
    - Three rotational axes (two eccentric and one concentric)
    - First commercially available unit, 1961
  - Dr. Y. V. Paatero, 1961–1963
    - Moves to University of Turku, Finland, 1961
    - Death of Paatero, 1963
  - Col. Donald Hudson and John Kumpula, 1951–1956
    - National Bureau of Standards, Washington, D.C.
    - Double eccentric rotational axes method
    - Required two exposures
    - Hudson and Kumpula take out patent, 1956
  - Panorex (SSW/Pennwalt) Panoramic Unit
    - XRM/SSW patent on automatic chair shift mechanism for Hudson/Kumpula machine, 1957
    - Panorex first introduced to market, 1959
    - Panorex patent to interrupt radiation during chair shift, 1962
    - Panorex clinical evaluation studies, 1960–1967
  - Panelipse (General Electric) Unit
    - First introduced as GE-3000 in 1970
    - Continuously changing rotational axis
    - Follows semi-elliptical paths
  - Three arch forms to describe dental arches
    - Parabolic form
    - Elliptical form
    - Cantenary form
  - Panex-E (Morita) Unit
    - Introduced in 1970
    - Called "ellipsopantomography"
    - Marketed in U.S. as Panoral (Sybron/Ritter) unit
  - Dr. Ulf Welander, Sweden, 1971–1978
    - Contends rotational panoramic radiography is not a form of tomography
    - Basically, rotational panoramic radiography is a specific projection technique
  - Two new litter–borne panoramic units
    - Tomorex (SSW/Pennwalt)
    - Orthopantomograph OP6 (Palomex Oy)

The value of any diagnostic procedure depends on the amount and validity of the information that can be derived from it. The importance of the intraoral radiograph in dental diagnosis is well documented. However, the intraoral radiograph is somewhat limited in its overall coverage of the maxillomandibular structures. Of course, conventional extraoral radiographs can achieve better coverage, but these radiographs are frequently plagued by distorted images, lack of definition, and superimposition of anatomic structures.

Panoramic radiography has overcome many of these limitations of conventional extraoral radiography and displays the entire maxillomandibular region on a single film. Hence the term panoramic radiography is derived from panorama, "an unobstructed view of a region in every direction." It is a radiographic technique that has become an essential diagnostic procedure in many modern dental offices. Panoramic radiography does not replace the conventional dental film, but, when used as a supplemental diagnostic technique, it produces a comprehensive radiographic survey never before realized by the dentist.

There are several reasons for panoramic radiography's popularity including increased overall coverage of the dental arches and associated structures, the relatively undistorted anatomic images produced, reduced radiation dosage to the patient, and the simplicity of operation.

HISTORICAL DEVELOPMENT

Panoramic radiographs are made using two basically different methods: (1) the use of an intraoral source of radiation, and (2) the use of an extraoral source of radiation (rotational panoramic radiography).

INTRAORAL SOURCE OF RADIATION (PANORAMIC RADIOGRAPHY)

The intraoral type of panoramic radiography, as the name implies, employs an intraoral source of radiation. The radiation is directed from inside the mouth through the jaws and exposes a film molded to the outside of the face of the patient. No-screen or slow-speed screen films are used. The x-ray source, patient, and film are stationary during the exposure. Separate exposures are made of the mandible and maxilla.

This method depends greatly on the use of a small x-ray tube that can be introduced into the patient's mouth. It must have a very small focal spot (.10 to .15 mm width), utilizing a tube current of 0.5 to 1.0 mA and a kilovoltage ranging between 40 and 80 kVp (Fig. 1–1).

Van Aken reports that the Koch and Sterzel Company of Germany published a report in 1954 stating that a patent was issued to their firm in 1943 (during World War II) for the manufacture of a machine designed "to make radiographs with an x-ray tube which can be inserted into cavities of the human body." This patent mentions the name of Horst Beger of Dresden, Germany, as the inventor of this machine (Fig. 1–2).

Without prior knowledge of this 1943 patent, Dr. Walter Ott, a Swiss dentist, began developing an intraoral x-ray tube in 1946 that could be introduced into the patient's mouth. Ott's method was later modified by Dr. Sidney Blackman of England (1960a; 1961) and marketed by Watson & Sons, Ltd. as the Panograph. At present, only three companies still manufacture the intraoral anode type of panoramic x-ray unit. They are Koch and Sterzel Co. of Essen, Germany (Panoramix); Siemens Corp., Erlangen, Germany (Status-X); and Philips Medical Systems, Inc., Holland (Stat Oralix) (Fig. 1–3).

EXTRAORAL SOURCE OF RADIATION (ROTATIONAL PANORAMIC RADIOGRAPHY)

The rotational panoramic radiography method is by far the most popular method of panoramic radiography. Dr. H. Numata of Japan (Fig. 1–4**A**) was the first to propose (1933) and experiment (1934) with this method of panoramic radiography. Numata placed a curved film in the mouth lingual to the teeth and used a slit or narrow x-ray beam that rotated around the patient's jaws to expose the film (Fig. 1–4**B** and **C**).

Twelve years later, in 1946, Dr. Yrjö Veli Paatero (Fig. 1–5) of the Institute of Dentistry,

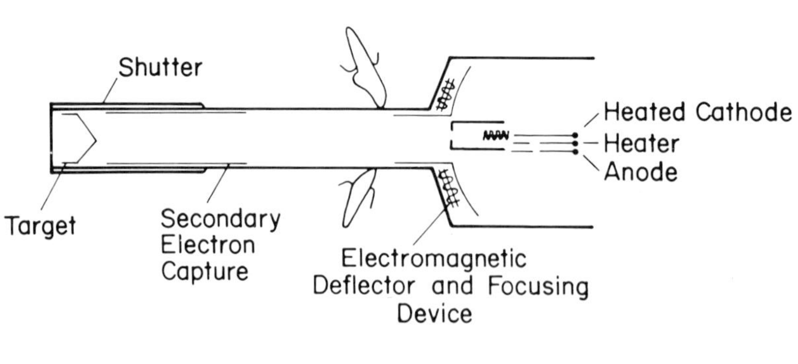

Figure 1–1. Intraoral x-ray source (panoramic technique) illustrated by a schematic drawing. The cone-shaped anode, a special extension of the x-ray tube, is placed within the patient's mouth. As the electrons strike the target of the anode, x rays are produced, which radiate in all directions.

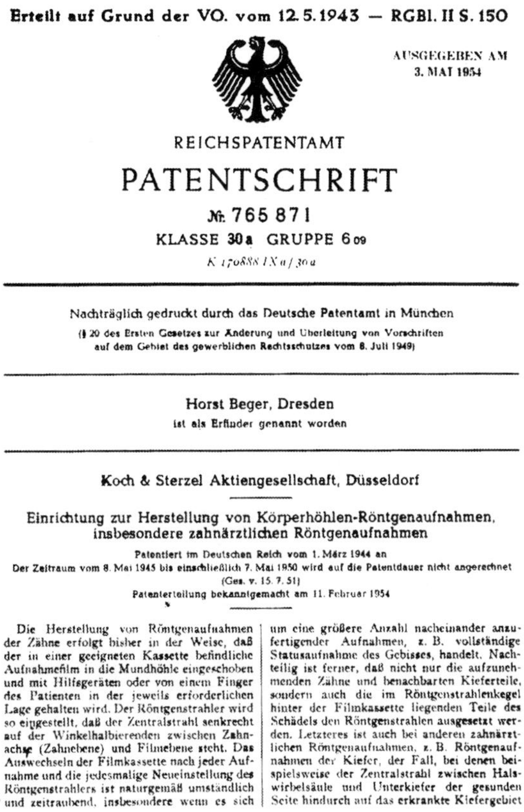

Erteilt auf Grund der VO. vom 12.5.1943 — RGBl. II S. 150

AUSGEGEBEN AM
3. MAI 1954

REICHSPATENTAMT

PATENTSCHRIFT

№ 765 871

KLASSE 30a GRUPPE 6 09

K 170888 IX a / 30 a

Nachträglich gedruckt durch das Deutsche Patentamt in München

(§ 20 des Ersten Gesetzes zur Änderung und Überleitung von Vorschriften auf dem Gebiet des gewerblichen Rechtsschutzes vom 8. Juli 1949)

Horst Beger, Dresden
ist als Erfinder genannt worden

Koch & Sterzel Aktiengesellschaft, Düsseldorf

Einrichtung zur Herstellung von Körperhöhlen-Röntgenaufnahmen, insbesondere zahnärztlichen Röntgenaufnahmen

Patentiert im Deutschen Reich vom 1. März 1944 an
Der Zeitraum vom 8. Mai 1945 bis einschließlich 7. Mai 1950 wird auf die Patentdauer nicht angerechnet
(Ges. v. 15. 7. 51)
Patenterteilung bekanntgemacht am 11. Februar 1954

Die Herstellung von Röntgenaufnahmen der Zähne erfolgt bisher in der Weise, daß der in einer geeigneten Kassette befindliche Aufnahmefilm in die Mundhöhle eingeschoben und mit Hilfsgeräten oder von einem Finger des Patienten in der jeweils erforderlichen Lage gehalten wird. Der Röntgenstrahler wird so eingestellt, daß der Zentralstrahl senkrecht auf der Winkelhalbierenden zwischen Zahnachse (Zahnebene) und Filmebene steht. Das Auswechseln der Filmkassette nach jeder Aufnahme und die jedesmalige Neueinstellung des Röntgenstrahlers ist naturgemäß umständlich und zeitraubend, insbesondere wenn es sich um eine größere Anzahl nacheinander anzufertigender Aufnahmen, z. B. vollständige Statusaufnahme des Gebisses, handelt. Nachteilig ist ferner, daß nicht nur die aufzunehmenden Zähne und benachbarten Kieferteile, sondern auch die im Röntgenstrahlenkegel hinter der Filmkassette liegenden Teile des Schädels den Röntgenstrahlen ausgesetzt werden. Letzteres ist auch bei anderen zahnärztlichen Röntgenaufnahmen, z. B. Röntgenaufnahmen der Kiefer, der Fall, bei denen beispielsweise der Zentralstrahl zwischen Halswirbelsäule und Unterkiefer der gesunden Seite hindurch auf das erkrankte Kiefergebiet

A

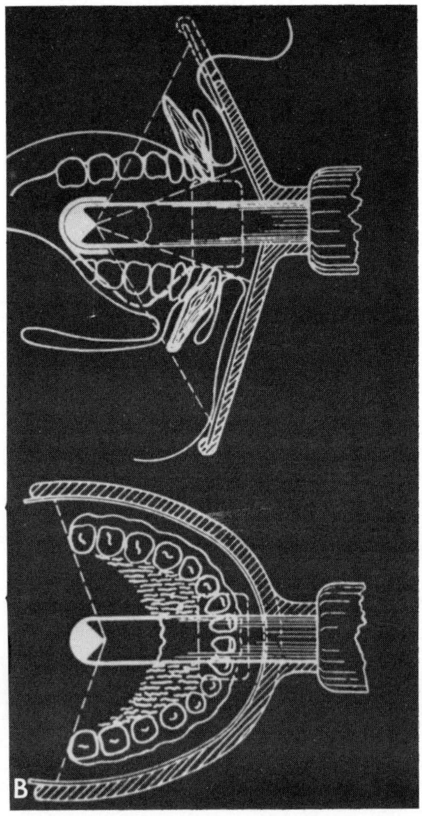

Figure 1–2. **A.** Intraoral x-ray source tube patent issued to Horst Beger in 1943. **B.** Original illustrations accompanying Beger patent. (Courtesy of Koch and Sterzel X-Ray Equipment Co., Essen, Germany.)

University of Helsinki, Finland, proposed (1946), experimented (1948), and demonstrated a slit beam method of panoramic radiography for the dental arches (1949a). This method was similar to the one proposed by Numata.

Paatero used a long curved film inserted lingual to the teeth in each jaw. Intensifying screens were required because, in 1946, the film speed was slow as compared with modern fast films. A separate radiograph was taken of each jaw. While the patient moved by means of a rotating chair, the exposure was made by a narrow beam of x rays emitted through a slit collimator. The x-ray source was stationary (Fig. 1–6). Paatero called this technique parabolography after parabolic, which was thought to be the normal arch form of the jaws by Angle (1907).

In 1949, Paatero observed that panoramic radiographs could be taken with the parabolographic technique by placing the film extraorally (1949b). In this method, the film cassette and patient revolved with the same velocity on a single vertical axis; the x-ray source remained stationary. This technique made it possible to radiograph the curved surfaces of the jaws by unfolding them onto one plane in a panoramic view (Fig. 1–7). Subsequently, in 1950, Paatero called this technique pantomography, a contraction of the words panoramic tomography, **panoramic** meaning "an unobstructed or complete view of a region in every direction," and **tomography** meaning "an x-ray technique for making radiographs of layers of tissue in depth, without the interference of tissue above and below that level" (Fig. 1–8).

Eleven years earlier, in 1938, Watson of England had read a paper on tomography emphasizing that the film need not be flat, that it could be curved or bent to any reasonable shape. This was contrary to the existing practice of tomography.

Paatero's pantomographic method was believed by many to be a combination of scanography and tomography applied to curved surfaces. Slit or scanographic radiographic methods are procedures that use a narrow, strictly limited beam of x rays. Motion is an

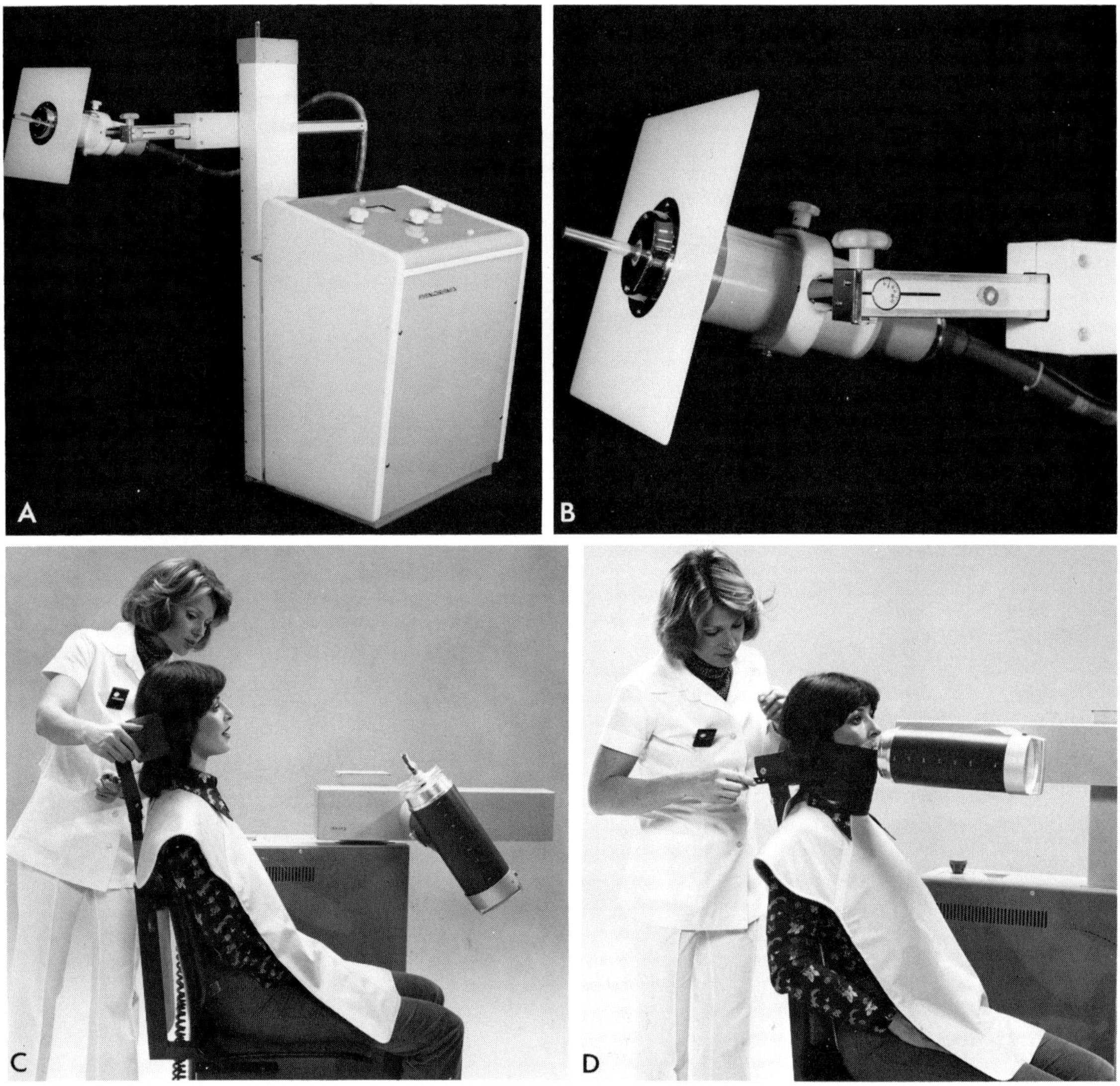

Figure 1–3. Intraoral anode-type panoramic units that are still being manufactured. **A** and **B.** Two views of the Panoramix (Koch and Sterzel, Germany). **C.** Status-X. Siemens Co., Erlangen, Germany. **D.** Status-X. Patient positioned to take mandibular projection. **E.** Maxillary and mandibular radiographs taken with Status-X. **F.** Stat Oralix. Philips Medical Systems, Inc., Holland. **G.** Stat Oralix. Close-ups; upper: radiograph being taken of left jaws; lower: disposable sanitary covering placed over anode. **H.** Stat Oralix, Completed radiographs of both sides of jaws (taken by two exposures).

Illustration continued on opposite page

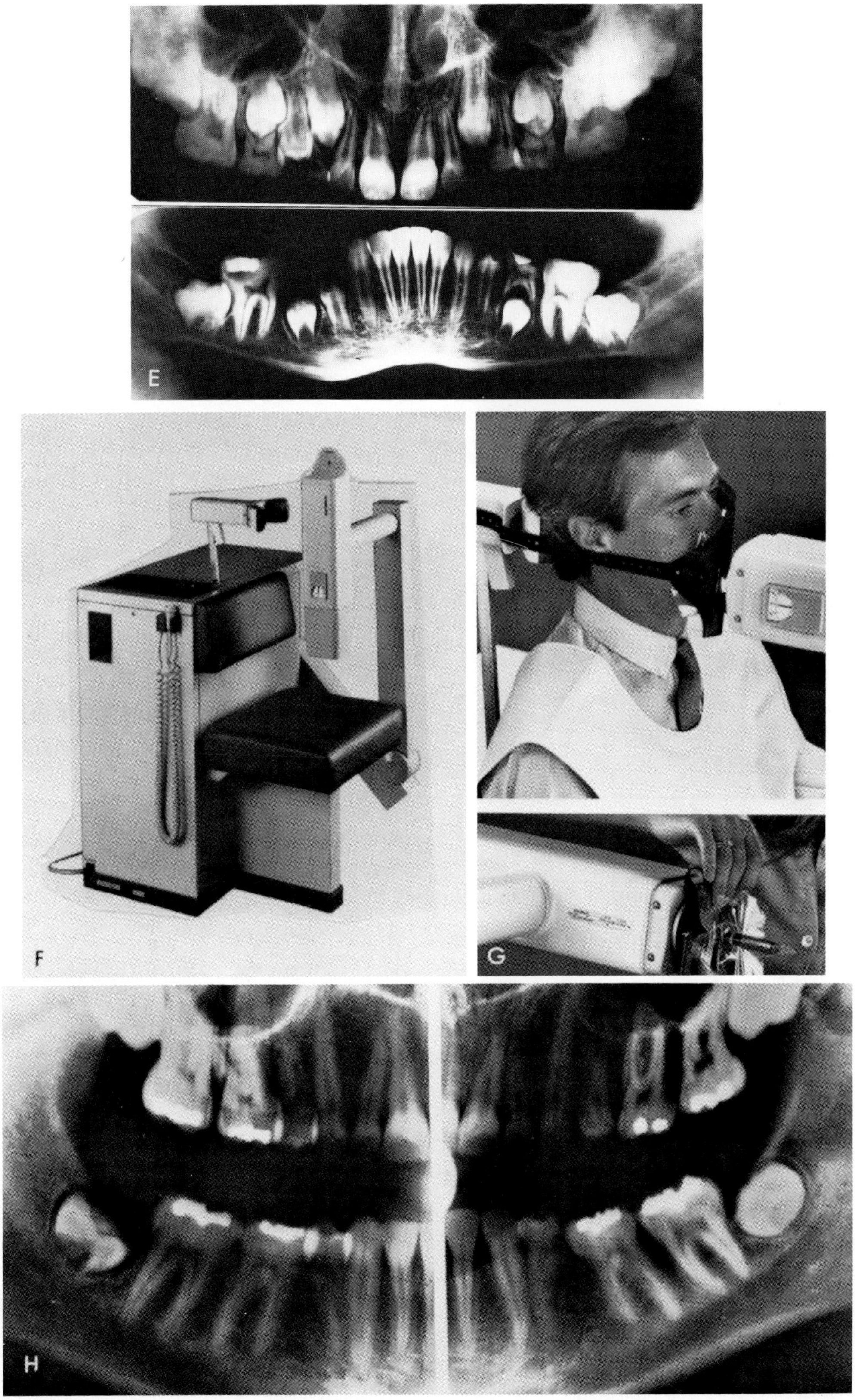

Figure 1–3. *Continued.*

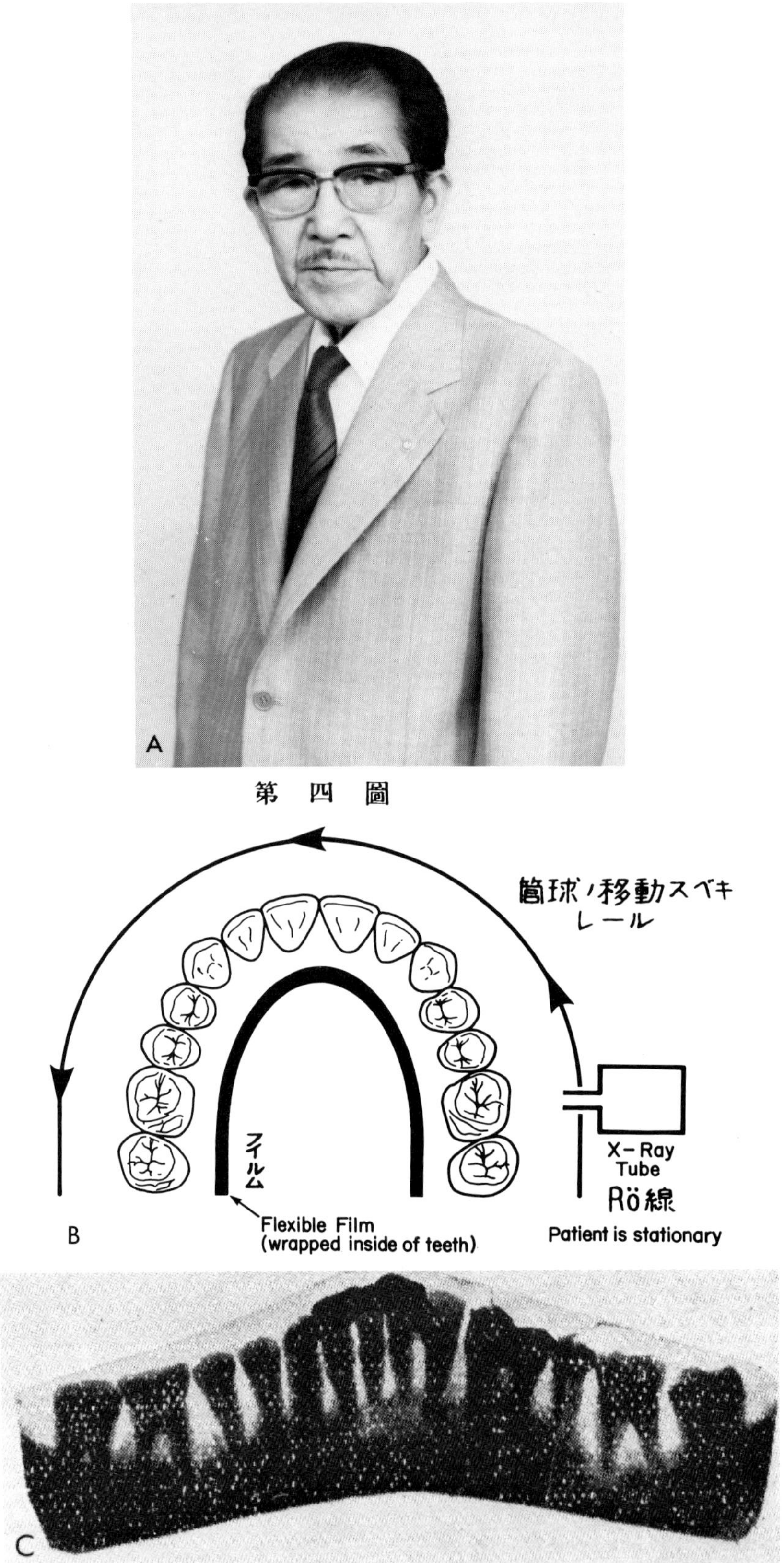

Figure 1–4. **A.** Dr. Hisatugu Numata. First to take panoramic radiograph of teeth in 1933. **B.** Diagram of panoramic technique used by Dr. Numata. A long curved film was placed lingually to the teeth, and the x-ray source rotated around the patient's head. **C.** Mandibular radiograph taken by Numata's method. (Figure 1–4 courtesy of Dr. Numata.)

essential part of slit radiography because without it only a narrow area would be exposed, and no actual radiograph would be produced. Slit radiography has been in existence for almost as long as conventional radiography. Some of the first slit methods used were described by Pasche, Albers-Schönberg, and Gott and Rosenthal.

Through the years, slit or narrow beam radiography (scanography) was used in the majority of cases to measure body organs and anatomic structures. However, it never really became a practical technique until fast films, fast screens, and more efficient x-ray machines were developed in the late 1930s. In 1937, Millwee published an article in which he described a method of slit radiography or scanography. He proposed to use this method to measure the heart (Fig. 1–9).

Two years later, in 1939, Heckmann, of Germany, wrote an article describing a slit beam technique for radiographing curved surfaces (Fig. 1–10). Interestingly, Heckmann discussed slit beam rotational radiography again in a chapter of a book published 28 years later. Heckmann's theory did not differ greatly from Paatero's pantomographic theory. Although Heckmann was first to record the theory of slit beam radiography of curved surfaces, Paatero must receive the credit for achieving the first practical application of the method.

Early in 1950, Dr. Robert J. Nelsen, Head of the Department of Dental Materials at The University of Washington, Seattle, assisted by John W. Kumpula, a predental student and machinist technician, developed a technique of panoramic radiography similar to Paatero's parabolographic intraoral film method. Nelsen called his method **panographic radiography.** In Nelsen and Kumpula's method, a narrow beam of radiation was directed onto a lead-backed, curved film placed in the mouth by means of a small film holder. Three radiographs were taken, one for each arch and a bitewing of the crowns of the teeth of both arches. Each radiograph was taken by coordinated motions between the x-ray tube and the chair. The posterior projections were made with the patient

Text continued on page 13

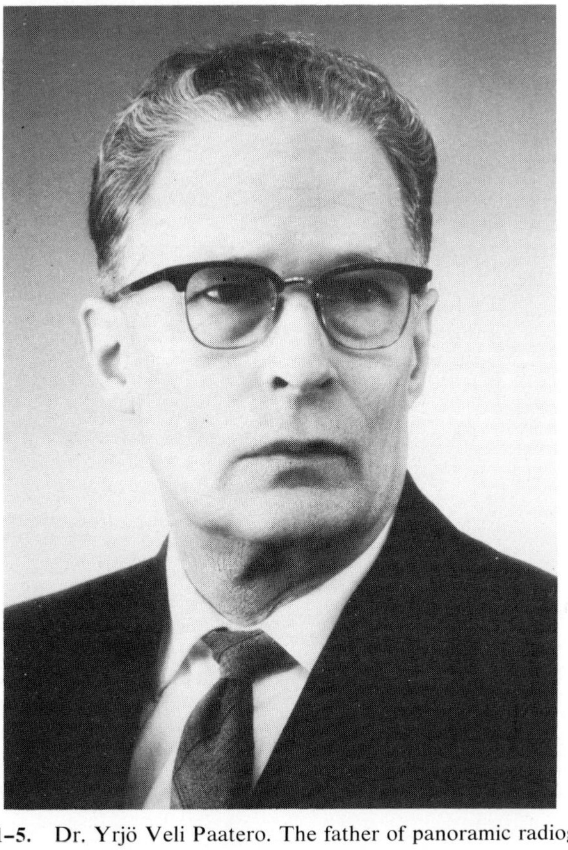

Figure 1–5. Dr. Yrjö Veli Paatero. The father of panoramic radiography.

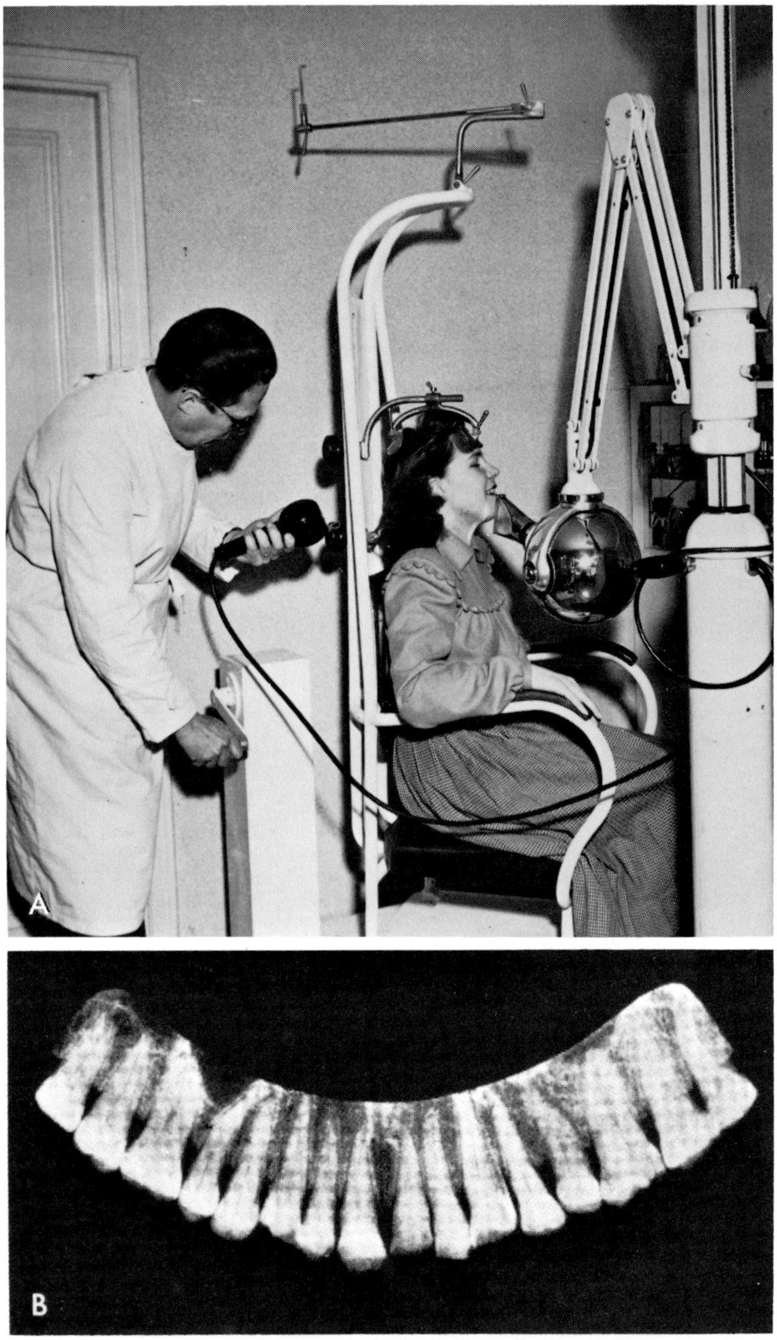

Figure 1–6. **A.** Rotating chair used in parabolography. Paatero rotated the chair while the x-ray source remained stationary. A long narrow film was placed intraorally. (Courtesy of Mrs. Paatero.) **B.** Parabologram of maxillary teeth. (From Tammisalo, E. H.: Prof. Yrjö V. Paatero—The pioneer of panoramic oral tomography. Dent.-Max.-Fac. Radiol. **4**:53, 1975.)

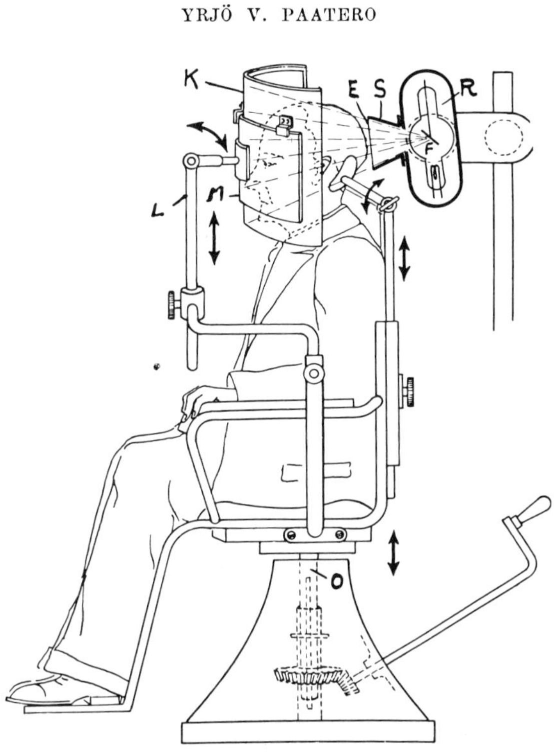

A

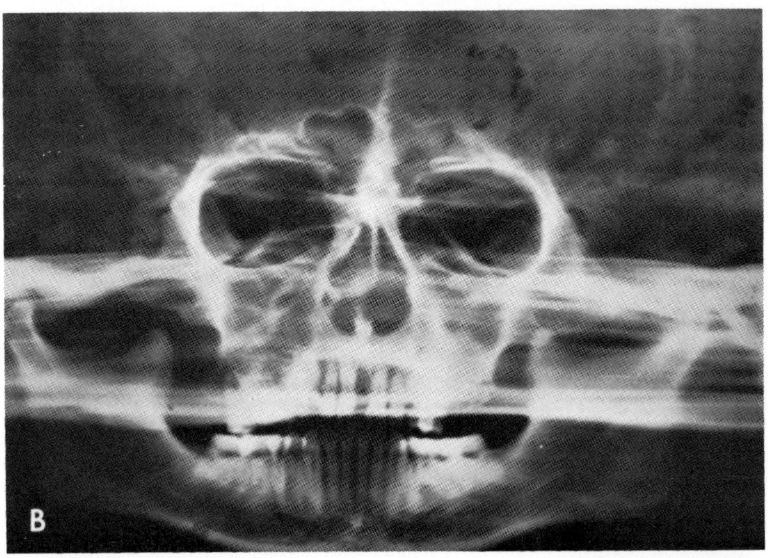

Figure 1–7. **A.** Schematic drawing of Paatero's parabolic apparatus, which made it possible to take panoramic radiographs by placing the film extraorally. X-ray tube (R) was stationary; the cassette holder (K) was semicylindrical and was attached to the chair. Chair and patient rotated 180° by hand or by electric motor. Paatero later called this method "pantomography." **B.** Semicranial radiograph taken by Paatero's extraoral parabolic method. (From Paatero, Y. V.: A new tomographical method for radiographing curved outer surfaces. Acta Radiol. **32**:177, 1949.)

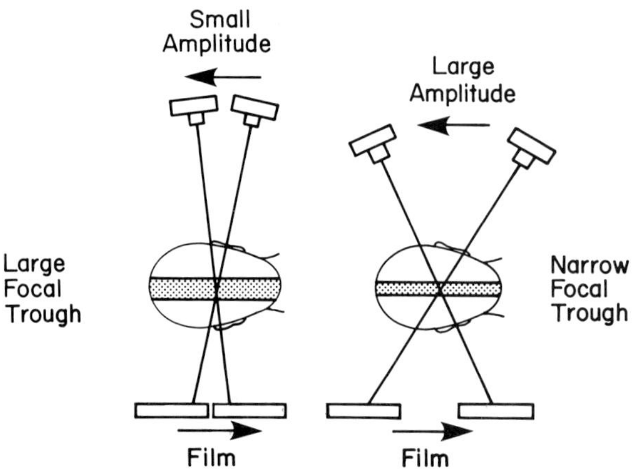

Figure 1–8. Tomography is a method of radiographically revealing a depth of tissue (focal trough) free from unwanted images of superimposed structures. This is accomplished by simultaneously moving the x-ray source and film in opposite directions at a constant speed during exposure. The amplitude (angle of movement) of the x-ray tube influences the width of the focal trough.

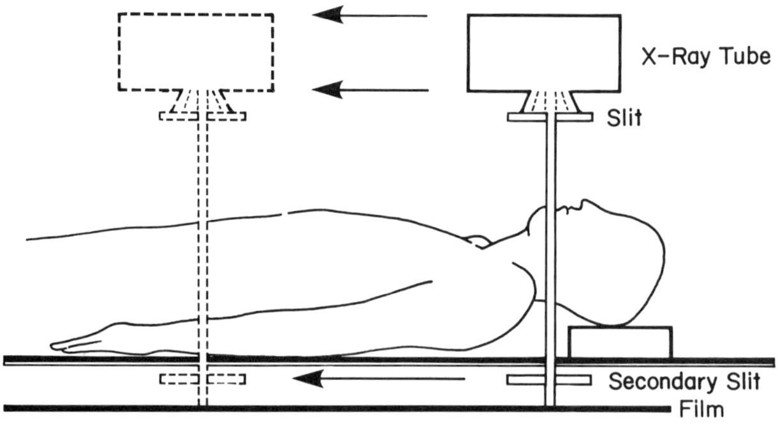

Figure 1–9. Scanography is a procedure by which a narrow x-ray beam scans a body part. Two slit collimators are usually used: one between the x-ray tube and the patient, and one between the patient and the film.

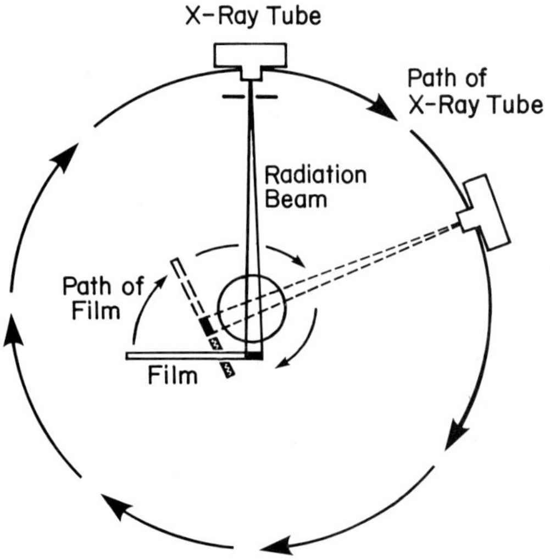

Figure 1–10. One of the seven tomographic methods proposed by Heckmann in 1939. The x-ray tube and film rotated simultaneously around the round object. The x-ray beam was limited by a slit collimator. This method was very similar to Paatero's pantomographic technique.

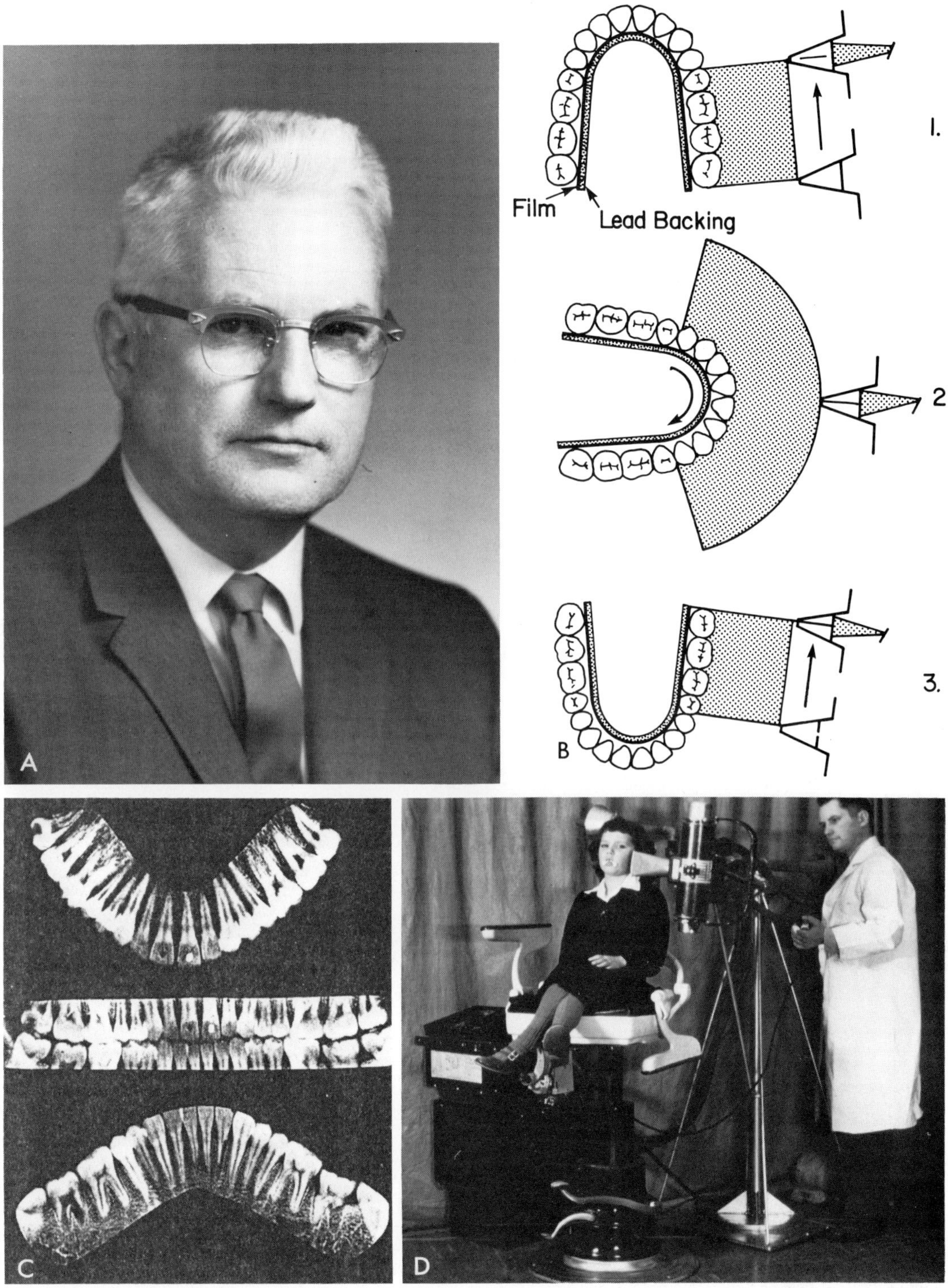

Figure 1–11. **A.** Robert J. Nelsen, first person to achieve practical application of panoramic radiography in the United States. **B.** Schematic drawing of Nelsen's panoramic technique. (1) Motion of x-ray tube in molar to premolar region. X-ray tube stops its horizontal motion and assumes correct vertical angulation for anterior region. (2) X-ray tube is stationary while patient rotates and anterior segment is exposed. Extent of rotation was adjusted to conform to size and shape of arch. (3) In third motion, the x-ray tube assumes the proper angulation for the posterior region and moves to expose the premolar to molar region while the patient is stationary. **C.** Complete radiographic survey and bitewing radiographs on three films taken by Nelsen's technique of a dry skull. (**B** and **C** from Nelsen, R. J., and Kumpula, J. W.: Panographic radiography. J. Dent. Res. **31**:158, April, 1952.) **D.** Dr. Robert Nelsen demonstrating his original panographic x-ray machine. Patient shown here is for demonstration purposes only. Nelsen used this machine for radiographing dry skulls only. (**A** and **D** courtesy of Dr. Robert J. Nelsen.)

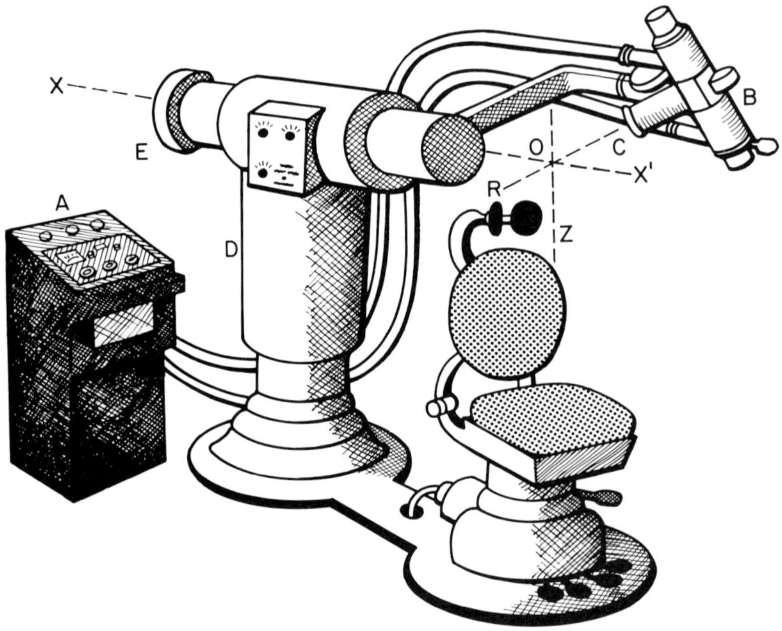

Figure 1–12. Drawing of Nelsen/Kumpula panographic x-ray machine with hydraulic mechanism to adjust the sequence of movement of the x-ray tube and/or the chair to the size or shape of the patient's jaw. (A) Control panel and transformer of x-ray machine; (B) x-ray tube; (C) lead-lined cone that passes narrow beam of radiation; (R) central beam of radiation, (Z) axis of chair rotation, which intersects axes X–X′ and R–C at O. (From Nelsen, R. J., and Kumpula, J. W.: Panographic Radiography. J. Dent. Res. **31**:158, April, 1952.)

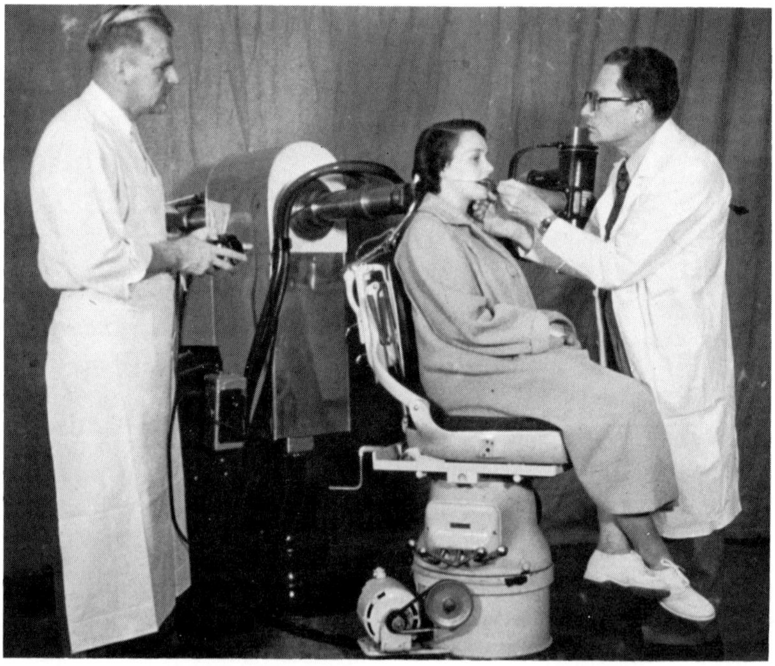

Figure 1–13. John W. Kumpula (left) and Y. V. Paatero (right) positioning patient prior to taking radiograph in intraoral automatic panographic unit designed at University of Washington in 1950. (Courtesy of Dr. Robert J. Nelsen, Mrs. Y. V. Paatero, and Mr. and Mrs. John W. Kumpula.)

stationary and the narrow x-ray beam moving, whereas the anterior projections were exposed with the patient rotating and the narrow x-ray beam stationary. Nelsen's pilot apparatus was primarily used to take radiographs of a skull (Fig. 1–11).

During this time (1950), Nelsen and Kumpula were also designing an automatic panographic unit with a hydraulic mechanism that would permit the operator to select any desired range or sequence of movements as determined by the size and shape of the patient's arch (Fig. 1–12). This was done manually in the experimental model.

It was through the efforts of Dr. Nelsen that Dr. Paatero was brought to the University of Washington in the summer of 1950 to work with Dr. Nelsen and Mr. Kumpula on the construction of the automatic panographic unit, which was completed in the fall of 1950 (Fig. 1–13). Within time, however, the panographic intraoral film method was abandoned. The main reason for this was possibly the limited space within the oral cavity to accommodate the size of film needed to reveal all the necessary dental structures of each arch. Also, separate exposures were required for each of the jaws, and scientists at that time were looking for a panoramic method that required only a single exposure.

While at the University of Washington from 1950 to 1951, Paatero constructed a prototype of the pantomograph for radiographing live subjects. He had been working on the pantomographic method in Finland before leaving for the United States (1949b). The basic principle of this method of rotational panoramic radiography was discussed in Paatero's patent application of 1950. His pantomographic method has been classified as a single axis or concentric rotational panoramic x-ray system. In this method, the patient and film rotate synchronously, whereas the narrow x-ray beam is stationary. The radiation must pass through two vertical slits: one between the tube and the patient and the other between the patient and the film (Figs. 1–14 and 1–15).

While experimenting with the single axis concentric rotational pantomographic system, Paatero found that by positioning the patient's mandible closer to the film and eccentrically in relation to the single axis of rotation, the x rays could be directed more perpendicular to the jaws and film. This placed the single center of rotation at approximately the left third molar region when radiographing the right side of the jaws and at the right third molar region when radiographing the left side (Fig. 1–16).

This produced a radiograph with better overall definition and less overlapping of teeth than the single axis concentric rotational type of pantomography, but it had a serious drawback

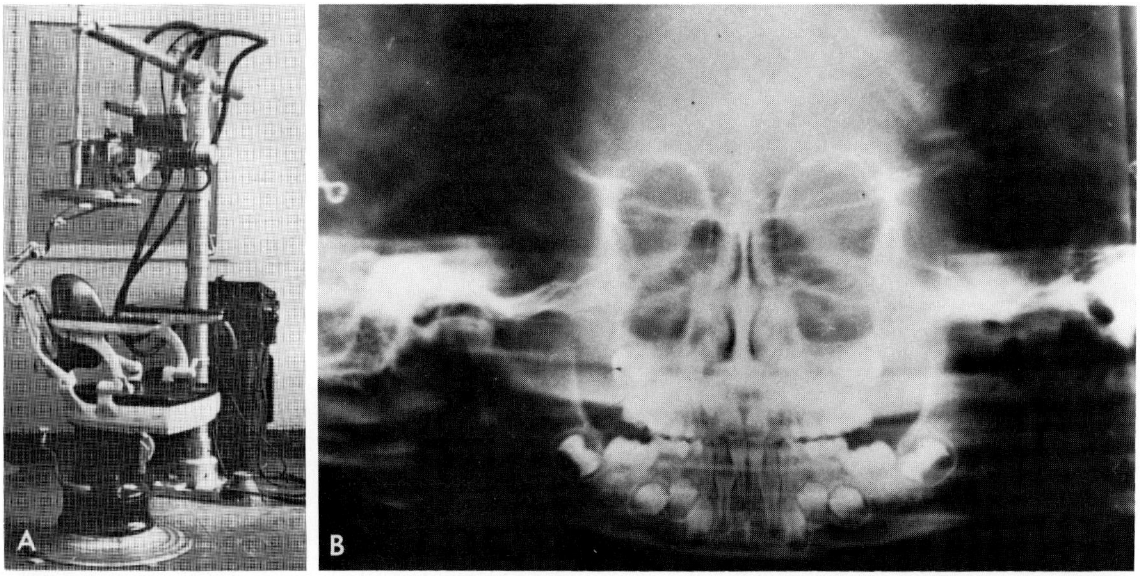

Figure 1–14. **A.** An early pantomograph set-up devised by Paatero in 1951 at the School of Dentistry, University of Washington (Seattle). **B.** Pantomography radiograph of the facial half of the skull of a seven-year-old child taken by Paatero's early pantomographic unit. (From Paatero, Y. V.: Pantomography and orthopantomography. Oral Surg. **14**:947, 1961.)

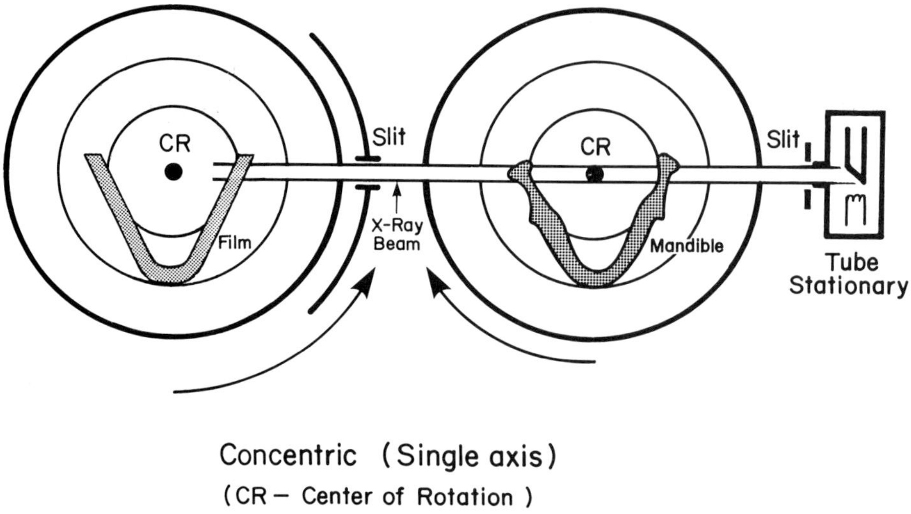

Figure 1–15. Pantomography (concentric–single axis method). A narrow x-ray beam was aimed through the axis of the object (mandible) and the film, which was bent on a film holder. The film and the object were rotated at the same angular speed.

in that separate exposures had to be made of each side of the jaws. This required repositioning the patient after each exposure. Paatero's eccentric rotational pantomographic technique was similar to the double eccentric rotational panoramic x-ray system developed by Hudson and Kumpula at the National Bureau of Standards in the 1950s, later known as the Panorex. However, in the Panorex system, the film and the tubehead are mobile and the patient is stationary during the exposure.

In 1951, Paatero returned to the Institute of Dentistry, University of Helsinki, where he built another prototype of the pantomograph (Fig. 1–17) and began to improve on the concentric rotational panoramic method (1952a, b, c; 1953). During this period, a Frenchman, Duhamel, did a mathematical analysis of Paatero's pantomographic method (1954, 1957).

In 1954, Dr. Sidney Blackman of England became interested in Dr. Paatero's pantomograph and visited him at Helsinki. Later, a slightly improved model of the pantomograph was manufactured in Helsinki and supplied to Dr. Blackman at The Royal Dental Hospital in London. Dr. Paatero was then invited to London where he collaborated with Dr. Blackman on further experimental work with the pantomograph (Blackman, 1955, 1960b). Soon after, Watson & Sons, Ltd., of England, in collabora-

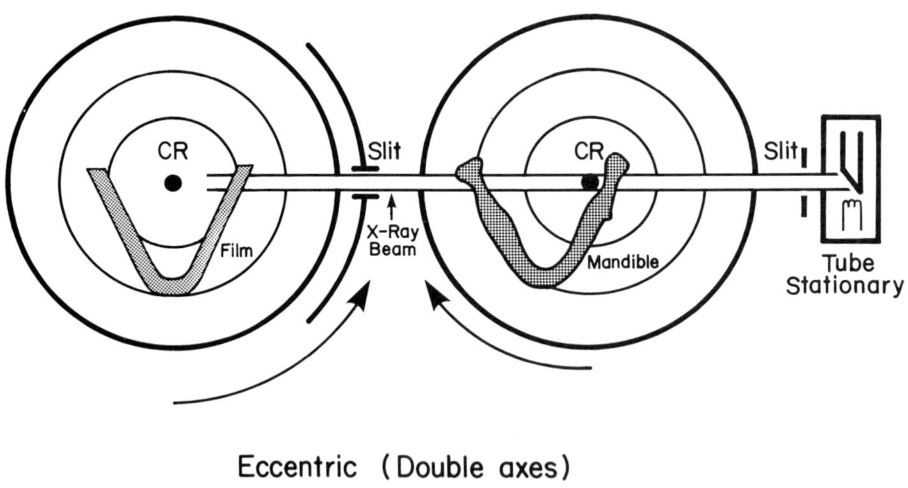

Figure 1–16. Paatero's eccentric (double axes) pantomography. In this method, the object (mandible) is positioned asymmetrically to the object's rotational axis. In doing this, the x-ray beam penetrates the jaws at almost a perpendicular angle (orthoradial projection).

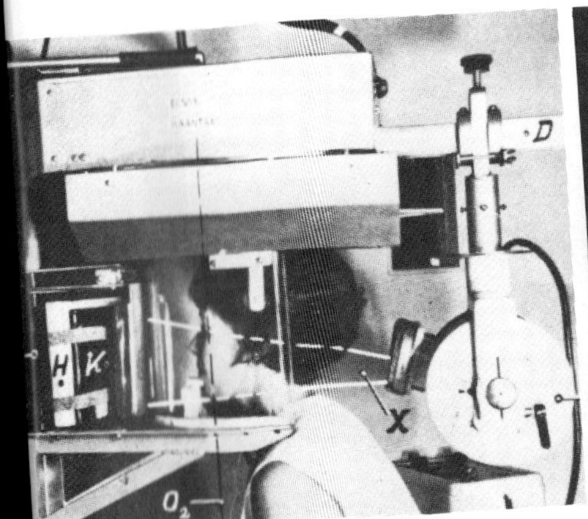

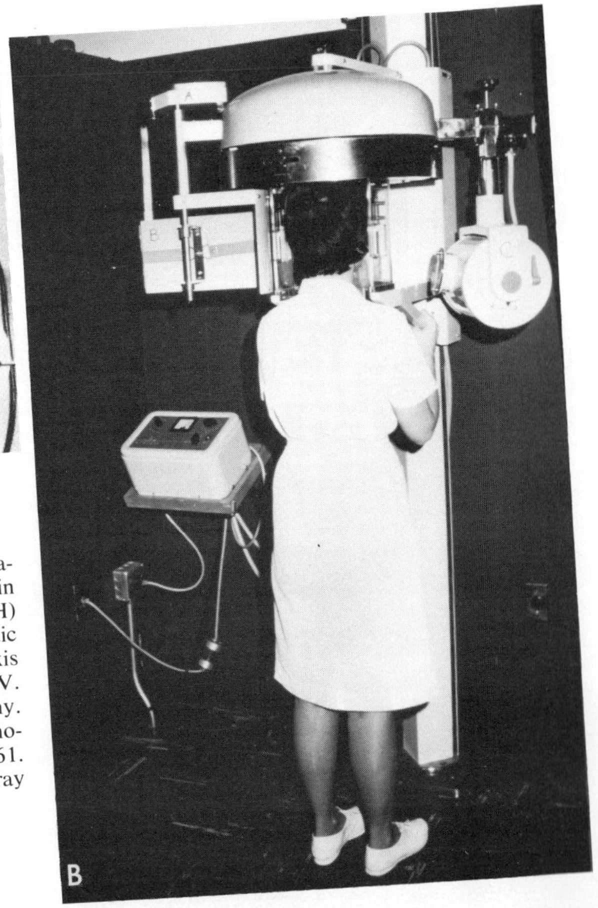

-21. **A.** The first Orthopantomograph capa-
king clinical radiographs was completed in
e unit is shown here. (R) X-ray tube; (H)
curved cassette holder; (K) flexible plastic
(X) narrow x-ray beam that turns about axis
om Tammisalo, E. H.: Professor Yrjö V.
The pioneer of panoramic oral tomography.
x.-Fac. Radiol. 4:53, 1975.) **B.** The Ortho-
raph became commercially available in 1961.
d flexible cassette is on the left and the x-ray
slit collimator is on the right.

e first commercially manufactured omograph became available in 1961 . At present, the Orthopantomograph ctured by Palomex Oy of Finland and by the Siemens Corp. of Erlangen, (Fig. 1–22). There are at least two opantomographic-type x-ray units on ese market today: Orthopantomo lda Electric Co.) and Panoramax entgen Mfg. Co.).

Dr. Paatero accepted an invitation to irst chair of Oral Radiology at the of Turku, Finland. Here he contin- search as intensely as he had during years. During this time the Univer- rku was building a new Institute of Expansive accommodations for re- d for the teaching of oral radiology included within the new building. li Paatero never saw the new Institute y building and its Department of Oral , which he had so anxiously awaited. d away suddenly on February 13, e age of 62. One of his last papers was in 1963 on a special orthopantomographic projection technique of the maxillary sinuses.

Erkki H. Tammisalo, Paatero's colleague and friend who (along with others) continued to research the orthopantomographic technique (1964a, b, c, 1967) after Dr. Paatero's death, said this of Dr. Paatero in an excellent biographical sketch, which he wrote in 1975:

> Yrjö V. Paatero's character was as exceptional as his career. A modest man, with a sense of humor, he held his fellow beings in high esteem. He possessed the perseverence of a pioneer and believed in his own work. More than anything else, he wanted to do his work in peace without fuss and expectations of fame — and above all, he had a resolute belief in the significance and future of dental radiology.

During the time Tammisalo was doing his research, the Japanese had begun their research endeavors into pantomographic and orthopantomographic techniques (Ando, 1964, 1970, 1971; Suzuki et al., 1965).

After Dr. Paatero moved back to Finland in 1951, John W. Kumpula, through the efforts of Dr. Robert Nelsen, took a position at the Na-

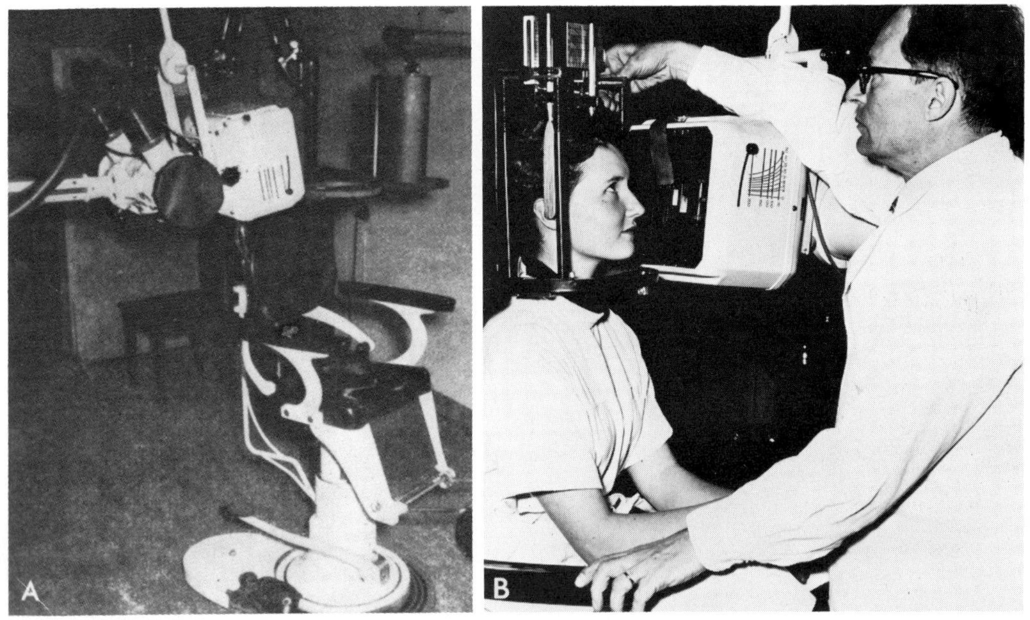

Figure 1–17. A. Pantomographic prototype unit built by Paatero after he arrived back in Finland. (From Tammisalo, E.: Professor Yrjö V. Paatero—The pioneer of panoramic oral tomography. Dent.-Max.-Fac. Radiol. **4**:53, 1975.) **B.** Dr. Paatero positioning patient in pantomographic prototype unit designed in Finland. (Courtesy of Mrs. Y. V. Paatero.)

tion with Dr. Blackman, manufactured and marketed a commercial model of the pantomograph, which they called the Rotograph (Fig. 1–18). One of the first Rotographs in the United States was received by Dean Seymour Yale of the University of Illinois Dental School in the early 1960s. At present, Watson & Sons, Ltd., has discontinued manufacturing the Rotograph.

In 1954, Paatero published a comprehensive article on pantomography (1954a). However, he was also working on a new idea. It was an orthoradial panoramic unit utilizing three rotational axes (two eccentric and one concentric). He was not satisfied with the old pantomographic radiograph because there was too much overlapping of teeth in the posterior regions. He found that by using two eccentric rotational axes on the sides of the jaws and a single concentric rotational axis in the anterior segment of the jaws, the resultant projection was more of an orthoradial projection (i.e., a projection in which the x rays penetrate the teeth perpendicularly), thereby eliminating the problem of overlapping.

As early as 1954, Paatero had worked out the theoretical basis and preliminary experiments for this new orthoradial panoramic unit with three rotational axes (1954b). In 1958, he built a miniature prototype of this apparatus (Fig. 1–19) and started experimenting with dry skulls (1958a, b, 1961). The results were so successful that he called the method **orthoradial jaw pantomography.**

It was Dr. Eiko Sairenji (1958, 1980) of Nihon University, Japan, who suggested the name orthopantomography to Dr. Paatero in 1958. Dr. Sairenji had been corresponding with Dr. Paatero since 1954, and he reasoned that since the prefix ortho meant correct or straight, it would be a good descriptive term for the new pantomographic technique. It was shortly thereafter that Paatero adopted the term orthopantomography for his technique.

In the orthopantomographic system, the patient sits or stands immobile while the x-ray tube rotates behind the neck and a curved film cassette moves around the face, rotating on its own axis. As a narrow beam of radiation is directed through the patient's neck onto the film cassette, it revolves on three successive rotational axes: one concentric rotational axis for the anterior portion of the jaws and two eccentric axes for each side of the jaws (Fig. 1–20).

Dr. Paatero completed the first orthopantomograph suitable for taking clinical radiographs in 1959, and it was subsequently proved to be clinically acceptable (1960). Timo Nieminen, an engineer, assisted Paatero in the design and construction of the first Orthopantomo-

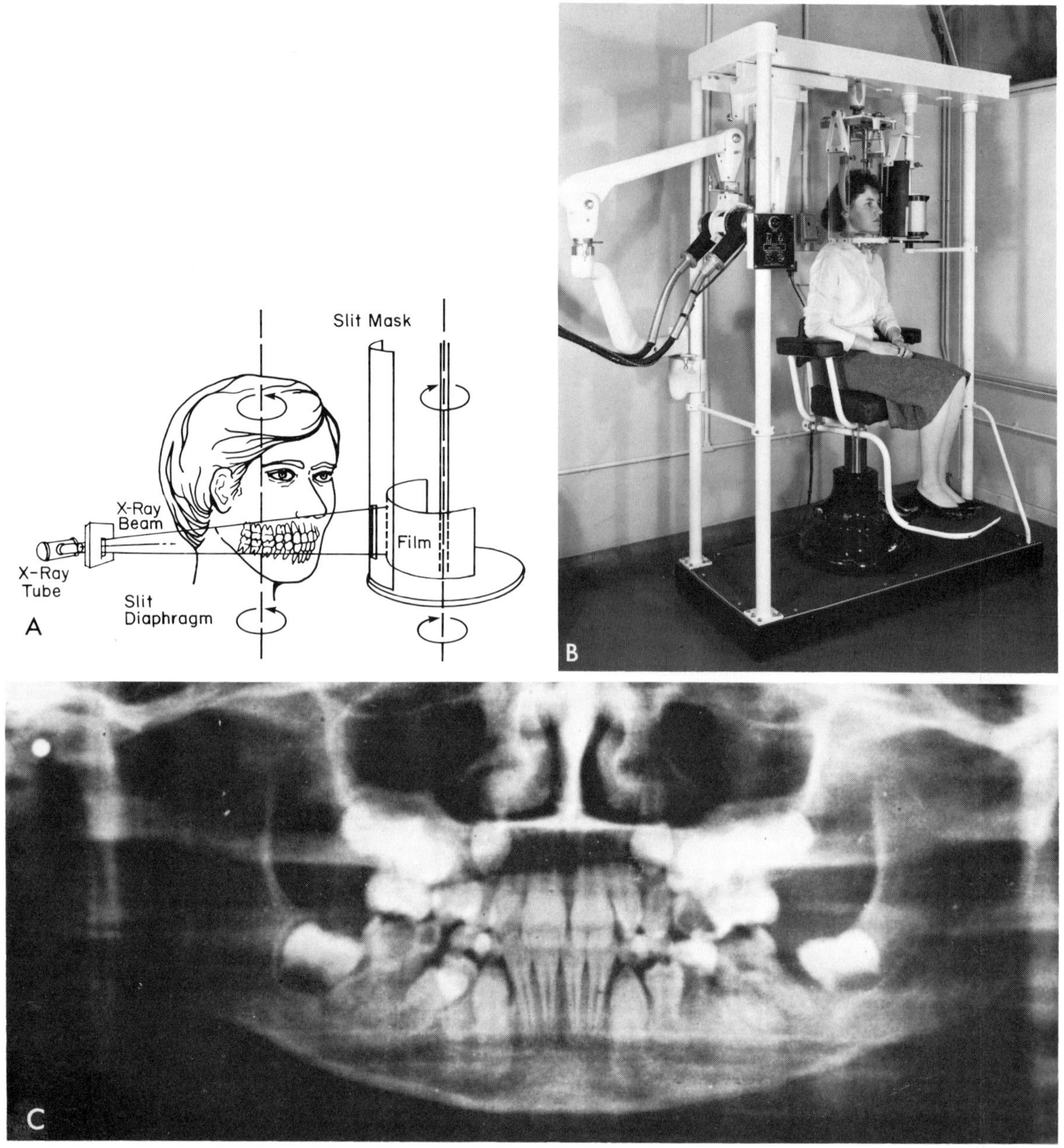

Figure 1–18. Rotograph. **A.** A rotary radiograph is made by rotating the patient and a curved film simultaneously on their own axes in opposite directions while a narrow beam of x rays from a stationary x-ray tube passes through the patient's jaws to the film. Only the regions remaining at a constant distance from the film are well defined. **B.** A cephalostat positions the head correctly. On the left is the x-ray tube with a slit collimator, and on the right, the rotating table carrying the film on a holder corresponding to the shape of the jaw. **C.** A complete mouth radiograph taken in a single exposure. (**A** through **C** courtesy of Watson & Sons, Ltd., Wembley, England.)

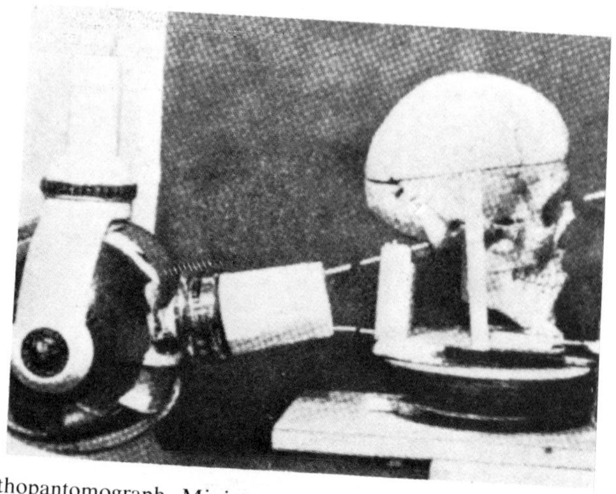

Figure 1–19. Orthopantomograph. Miniature prototype built by Y. V. Paate
Professor Yrjö V. Paatero – The pioneer of panoramic oral tomography. Dent.-M

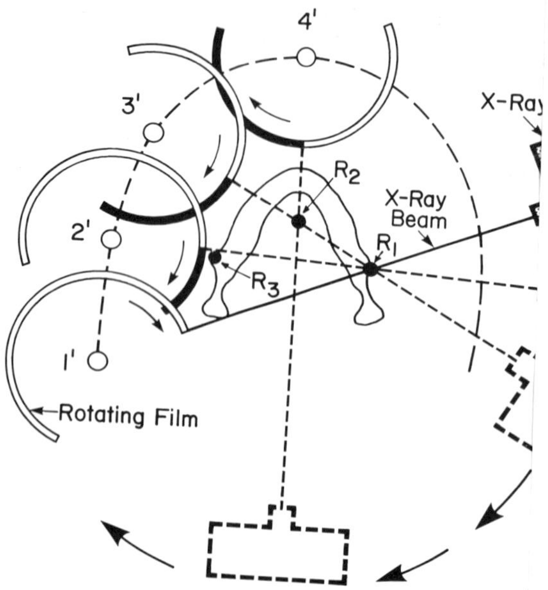

Figure 1–20. Orthopantomographic principle. Orthopantomography as designe
rotation: two eccentric rotational centers (R_1, R_3) and one concentric rotational cent
positions of x-ray tube and curved, rotating film in film holder. The procedure is repea

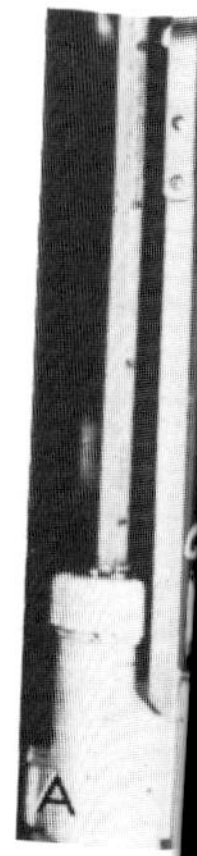

Figure
ble of t
1959. T
rotating
cassette;
(O_2). (Fr
Paatero–
Dent.-M
pantomo
The curv
tube wit

graph. T
Orthopant
(Fig. 1–21
is manufa
marketed
Germany
other orth
the Japa
N-70 (H
(Asahi R

In 1961
take the
Universit
ued his r
his earlie
sity of T
Dentistry
search a
were to b

Yrjö V
of Dentis
Radiolog
He pass
1963, at t
published

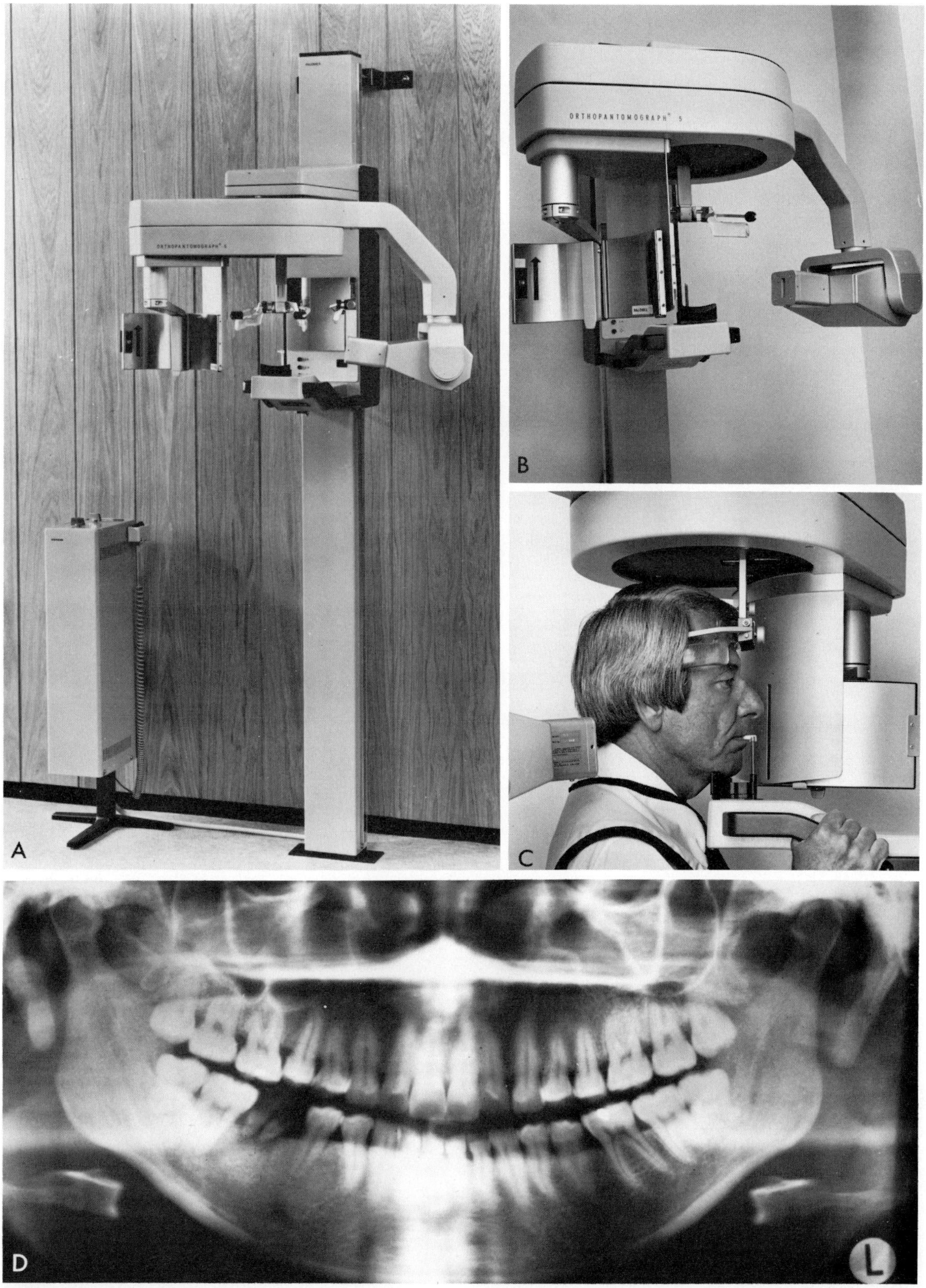

Figure 1–22. Orthopantomograph OP5. **A.** 1980 model. **B.** Close-up of **A.** Notice the curved metal cassette and slit collimator of x-ray tube. (**A** and **B** courtesy of Siemens Corp., Dental Division, Iselin, N.J.) **C.** This machine uses several patient positioning devices: bite fork, motor-driven head positioner device verified by a digital read-out, hinged mirror, light beams, and chin guide for special techniques. **D.** Radiograph taken with Orthopantomograph OP5.

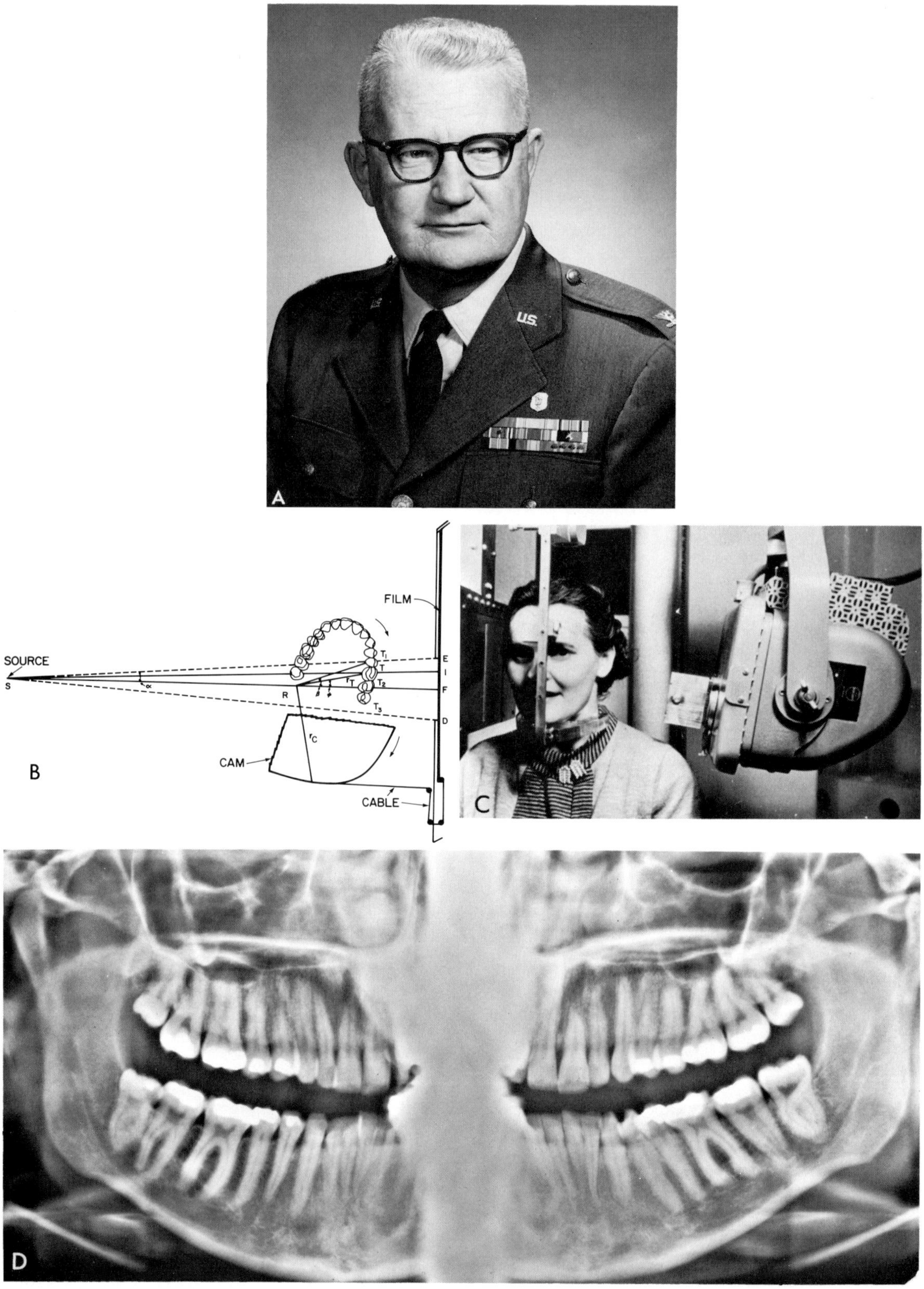

Figure 1–23. *See legend on opposite page.*

tional Bureau of Standards in Washington, D.C. Dr. Nelsen had become a research associate at the National Bureau of Standards a year earlier. It was during this time that the United States Air Force became interested in panoramic radiography. While Dr. Nelsen pursued other research projects at NBS, including the development of high-speed dental handpieces, Dr. Donald Hudson, an Air Force Colonel on temporary assignment to the National Bureau of Standards, and John Kumpula were assigned the project of designing and constructing a panoramic x-ray machine that could serve as a rapid method of recording the dental conditions of large numbers of people. Since Kumpula had worked previously with Drs. Paatero and Nelsen at the University of Washington, his knowledge of panoramic radiography was invaluable to the team headed by Dr. Hudson.

After experimenting with some of Paatero's earlier methods, Hudson's group decided to proceed with the double eccentric rotation axes system of panoramic radiography (Hudson, Kumpula, and Dickson, 1957). In this system, the tubehead and film cassette holder rotated in opposite directions around the patient's head, which remained stationary. There were two collimator slits: one between the tubehead and the patient and one between the patient and the film cassette. The film cassette was flat (instead of curved as in orthopantomography), and it moved in a translatory motion posterior to the collimator slit in the film cassette holder.

The two rotation axes were located at points just medial to the angle of the mandible on the side opposite the one being radiographed. The Hudson/Kumpula National Bureau of Standards panoramic machine required two exposures. After one side of the jaws was radiographed, the machine was stopped and the patient was manually repositioned on the chin rest, which was 1 3/4 in wider than the present design (Panorex). This repositioning oriented the patient's head to the opposite side of the arch. Then, the tubehead–film cassette assembly was manually swung about its own axis to the opposite side, where the machine again was started, and the second side of the jaws was exposed. The results convinced Hudson that the information recorded with this panoramic system was sufficient to be employed in mass screening surveys and that the machine could be especially useful in prosthodontics and surgery (Fig. 1–23). Since Hudson and Kumpula had arrived at a set of parameters for the function of their machine, they felt the mechanism should be analyzed mathematically. George Dickson, a physicist, performed this analysis, and the results were published in 1957. The prototype machine was field tested at Lackland Air Force Base in San Antonio, Texas.

In January of 1956, Hudson and Kumpula filed for a U.S. patent on their double eccentric rotational panoramic machine (Fig. 1–24). Immediately upon issuance, the patent would become public domain because the basic principles of panoramic radiography and the prototype machine were developed with government funds. Therefore, any person or company would have the right to the information contained in the patent.

In the fall of 1956, commercial x-ray manufacturers were invited to the National Bureau of Standards to see the Hudson/Kumpula panoramic x-ray machine. Henry Hollman, General Manager for the XRM Company of America, Great Neck, New York, was unable to attend the meeting but visited NBS two weeks later. He came back enthused about the concept of the panoramic x-ray machine and engaged the services of an outside consultant to do the paper design, which cost less than $1,000. The consultant's initial paper design incorporated

Figure 1–23. **A.** Colonel Donald C. Hudson, co-inventor with John W. Kumpula of double eccentric rotational panoramic unit, later marketed by XRM of America Company as the Panorex. (Courtesy of Donald C. Hudson.) **B.** Schematic drawing of Hudson/Kumpula double eccentric rotational panoramic unit later called the Panorex. Synchronization of image and film is obtained by moving a flat film by means of a cable passing around a cam, shaped to simulate the curve of the dental arch. (From Hudson, D. C., and Kumpula, J. W.: A panoramic x-ray dental machine. U. S. Armed Forces Med. J. **13**:46, 1957.) **C.** Prototype double eccentric rotational panoramic x-ray unit (Panorex). This panoramic machine required two exposures. After half of the jaw was radiographed, the unit was stopped and patient's head repositioned on the chin rest, which was 1 3/4 in wider than the present Panorex. (Courtesy of Donald C. Hudson and Mrs. John Kumpula.) **D.** Panoramic radiograph taken by Hudson/Kumpula's double eccentric rotational panoramic unit. The white band in the middle represents where unit was stopped and patient's head was repositioned on chin rest to opposite side of arch. Then, the tubehead and film cassette assembly was manually swung around on its own axis to opposite side, where machine was energized again to expose the other side of the jaws. (Courtesy of Dr. Donald C. Hudson.)

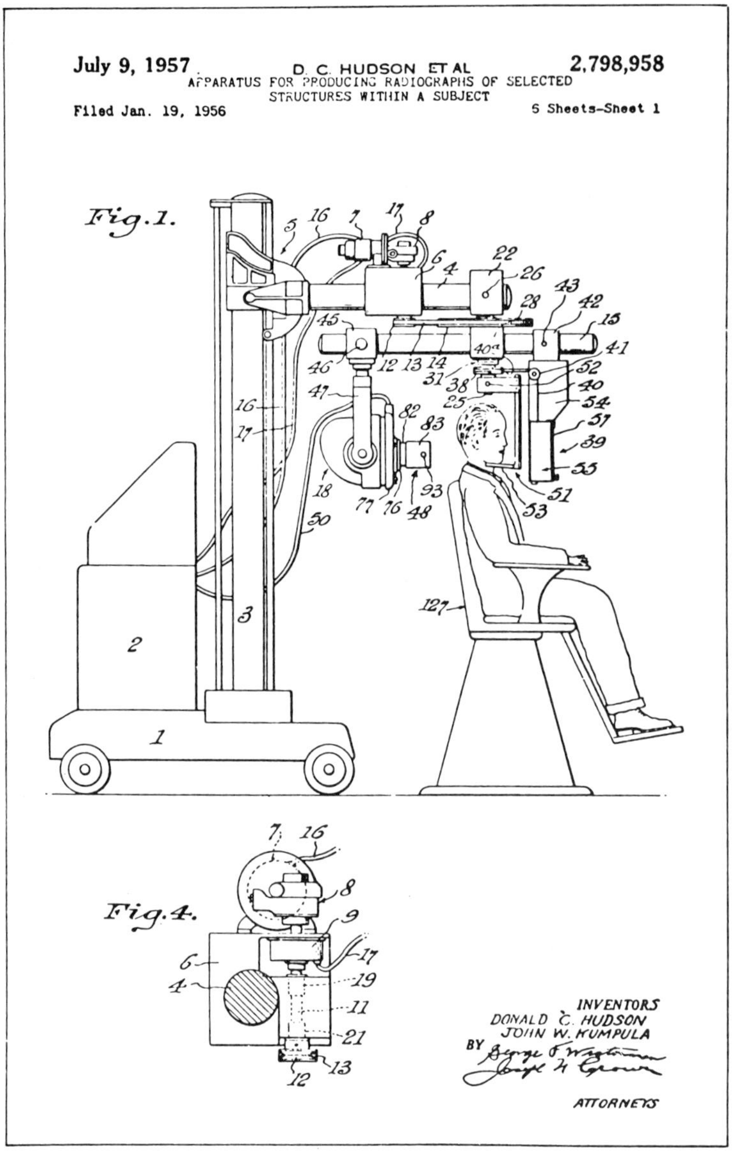

Figure 1–24. Reproduction of portion of a patent filed by D. C. Hudson and associates. January 19, 1956, for panoramic machine that later became known as Panorex x-ray machine.

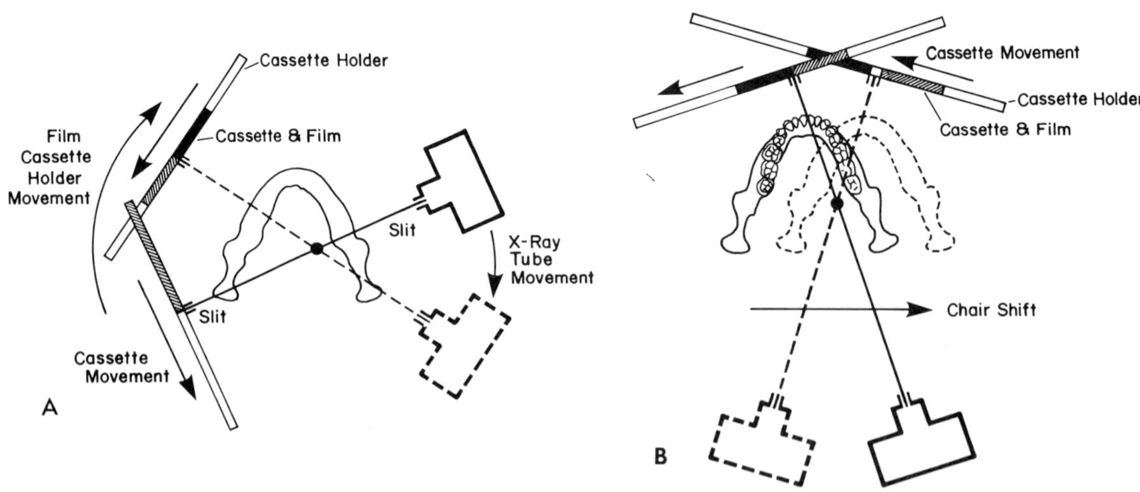

Figure 1–25. *See legend on opposite page.*

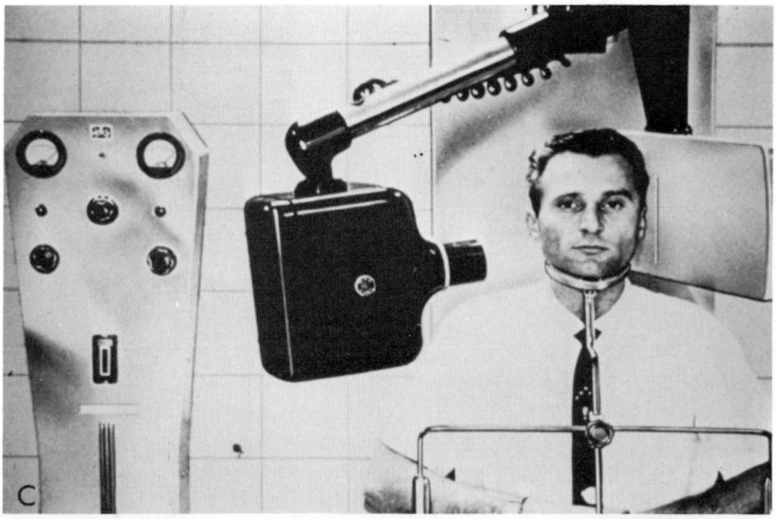

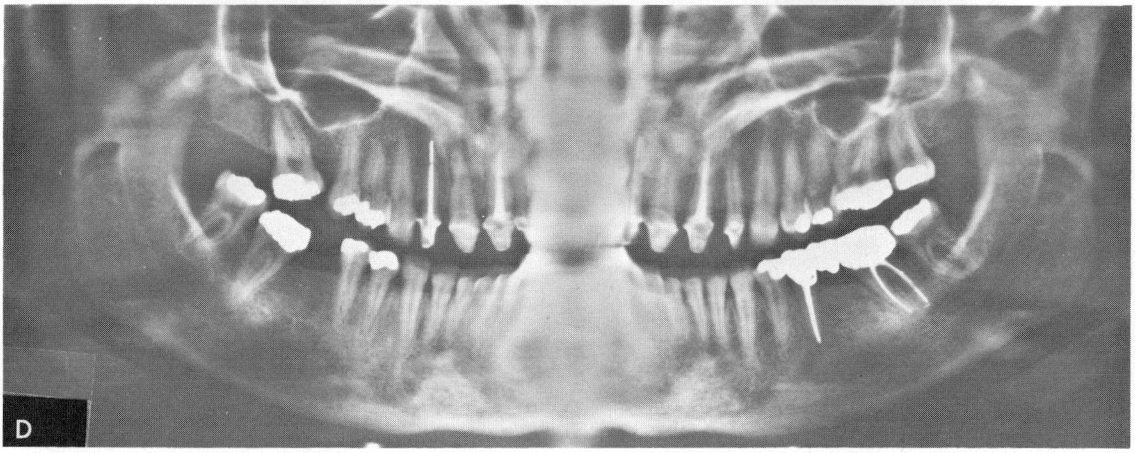

Figure 1–25. Panorex principle. **A.** Schematic drawing of half-cycle exposure. Patient is stationary; the x-ray source and the cassette holder rotate. The arrow indicates the movement of the film past the slit in the cassette holder. **B.** The center of the rotation changes midway in the cycle by the automatic lateral shift of the chair. (After Updegrave, W. J.: Panoramic dental radiography. Dent. Radiogr. Photogr. **36**:75, 1963.) **C.** Early Panorex, which was first introduced to the market in 1959. **D.** One of the first radiographs taken with the commercially available Panorex. During the first three years of production, the generation of x-radiation was continuous, including the time during the chair shift. This left a blurred area in the center. (**C** and **D** courtesy of Jack Faude, S. S. White, Dental Products Division, Pennwalt Co., Phila., PA.)

the novel idea of shifting the chair automatically so that the excursion scan could be continuous. This was the only patent held on the Panorex by XRM/S. S. White, but it was effective (Faude, 1980).

The first working prototype of the panoramic x-ray machine (later called the Panorex) was completed by XRM in mid-1958 and clinically tested at Fort Dix, New Jersey, with encouraging results. The original system was designed to record the dental structures on a 4- × 10-in film with the rotation cycle limited to 180°. The clinicians recommended, as an added value, that the rotation cycle be increased so that the temporomandibular joints could also be recorded. The machine was introduced on the market at the combined ADA/FDI Meeting in New York in October, 1959. The first installation was made in Newburg, New York, in December, 1959 (XRM, 1959). The new machine was called the Panorex (Fig. 1–25).

During the first three years of production, the

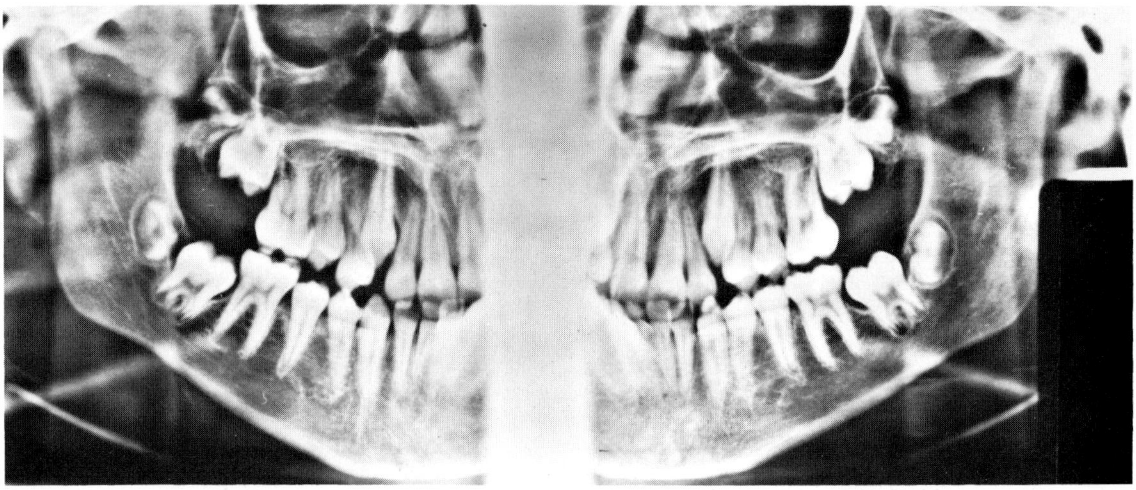

Figure 1–26. The clear, white band in the center of the Panorex radiograph became reality in 1962, when Jack Faude of S. S. White conceived the idea of interrupting x-ray generation during the chair shift.

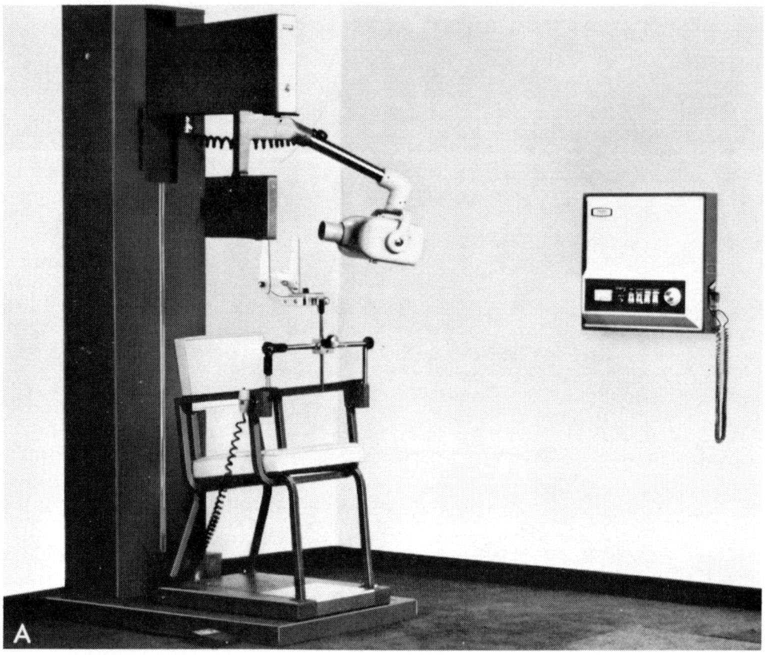

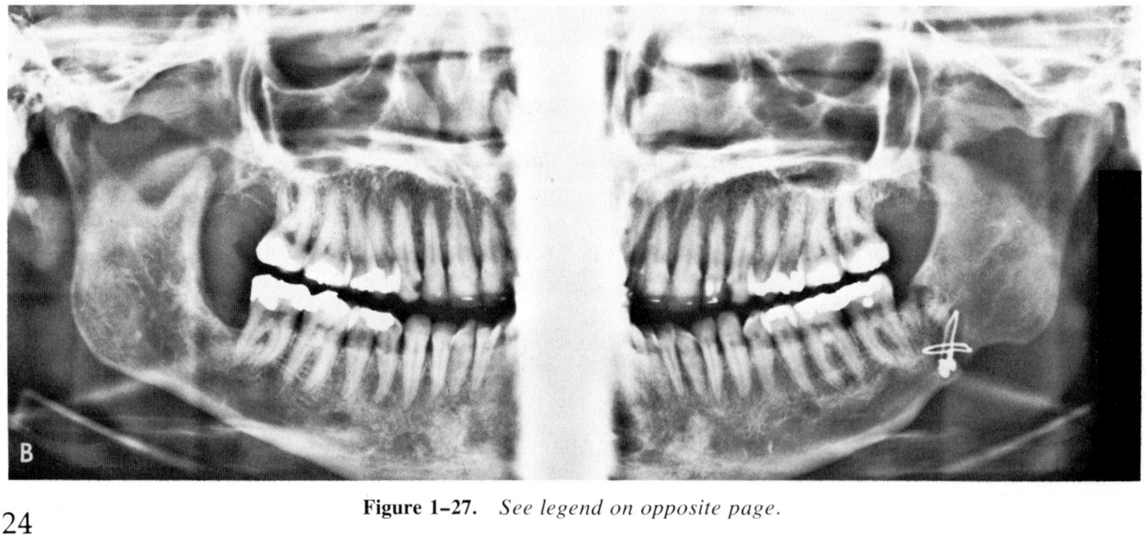

Figure 1–27. *See legend on opposite page.*

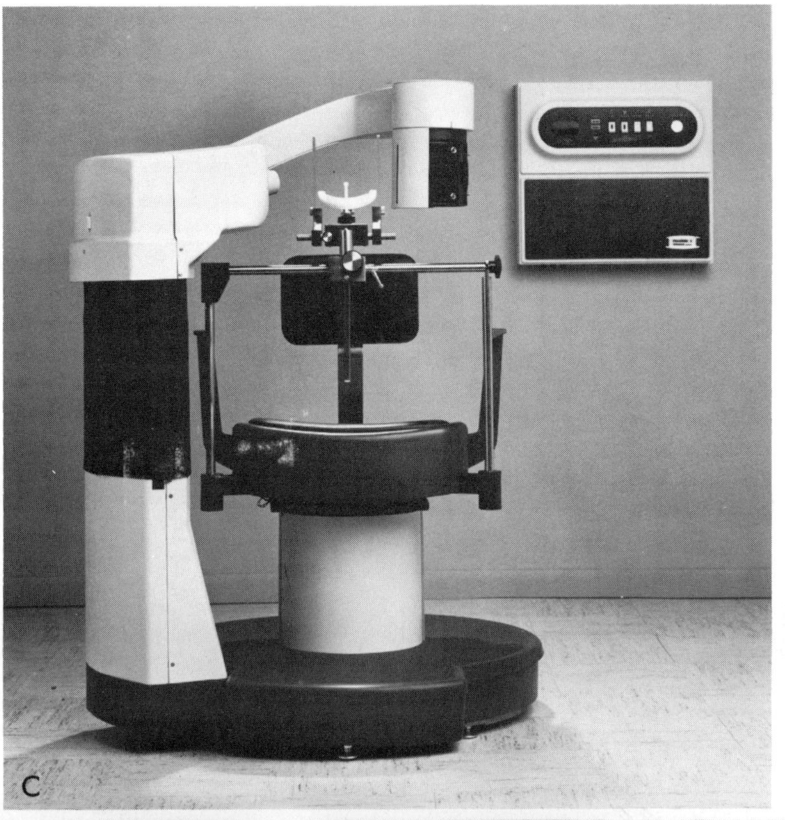

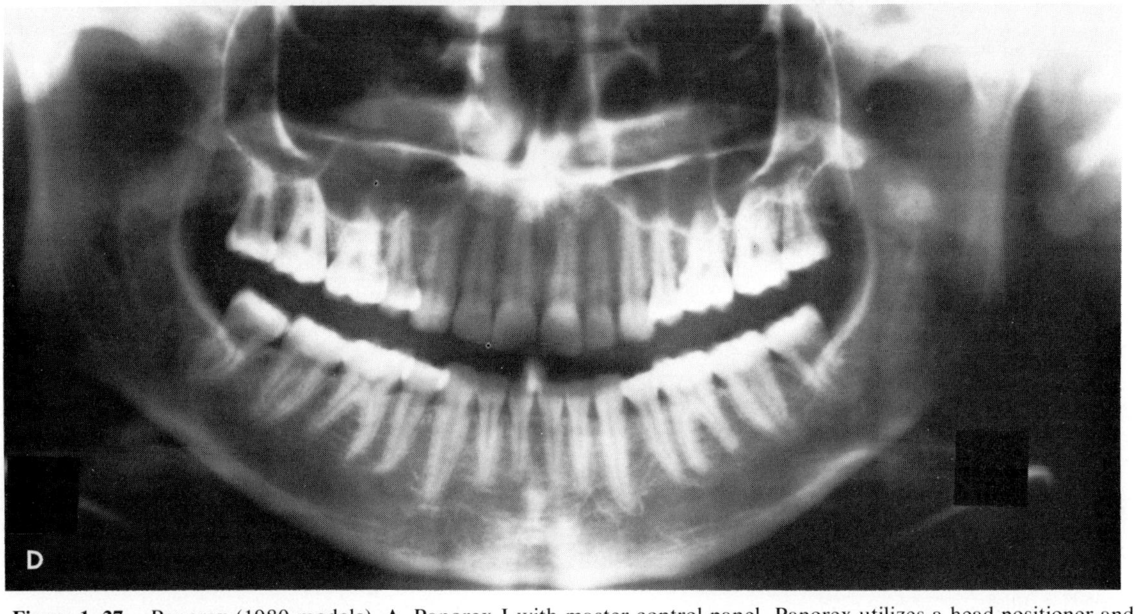

Figure 1–27. Panorex (1980 models). **A.** Panorex I with master control panel. Panorex utilizes a head positioner and chin rest to place patient's head in correct position. A flat metal cassette is used. **B.** Split-image panoramic radiograph taken by Panorex I. (Notice areas of healed fracture of mandible and composite restorations replacing incisal edges of maxillary anterior teeth.) **C.** New Panorex II model introduced in 1980. This unit can take both a split and a continuous radiographic image. (**A** and **C** courtesy of S. S. White, Dental Products Division, Pennwalt Corp., Phila., PA.) **D.** Continuous panoramic radiograph taken by Panorex II x-ray machine.

x rays were generated continuously, including during the chair shift. This left a blurred area in the center of the film. In early 1962, Jack Faude, an engineer with XRM/S. S. White, conceived the idea of interrupting the x-ray generation during the chair shift to reduce the patient's exposure time. Thus, the white or clear band in the center of the image was generated (Fig. 1–26). The Panorex is now marketed by the S. S. White Co. (Pennwalt Corp.), as XRM of America became a subsidiary of S. S. White (Fig. 1–27).

Although the prototype for the Panorex was originally developed by Air Force personnel in affiliation with the National Bureau of Standards, it was the United States Navy that first used it as a mass screening procedure for recruits. Kraske and Mazzarella (1960, 1961) reported that Navy personnel used the XRM Panorex on 905 patients at the United States Naval Training Center and United States Naval Hospital, Great Lakes, Illinois, from 1959 to 1960. They found that the machine produced moderately acceptable films of the maxillo-mandibular region with relative ease and rapidity, even in the hands of inexperienced operators.

One of the first studies of image distortion and radiation safety of the Panorex machine was done by Owen W. Kite and associates at the Massachusetts Institute of Technology in 1962. They determined that through the use of intraoral calibration direct measurements could be made on films with sufficient accuracy for clinical research and that the Panorex was radiologically safe for the patient and operator.

Louis Mitchell, of the Medical College of Virginia School of Dentistry, was one of the first to complete a clinical evaluation of the Panorex. In his study, several dentists compared 200 Panorex radiographs with intraoral full mouth surveys of the same patients. Although they concluded that the Panorex radiograph was of little value in revealing incipient caries and finer details of dental and osseous bone structures, it was particularly valuable for children, for adolescents when the clinical examination revealed no defects, for edentulous patients, and whenever extraoral projections were indicated.

During the early 1960s, various clinicians began to compare and evaluate the Orthopantomograph and the Panorex with two intraoral anode devices, the Panograph (Watson & Sons) and the Panoramix (Westinghouse). William Updegrave (1963, 1966), of Temple University, and T. M. Graber (1965), of Kennelworth, Illinois, wrote excellent articles evaluating panoramic radiography. A seminar-workshop on panoramic radiography was held in Chicago, Illinois, on February 26, 1966, under the auspices of the American Academy of Dental Radiology. Dr. Updegrave was chairman of this seminar-workshop. Some of the papers presented were by I. Brueggemann (St. Louis University) and Norris Knight (Marquette University), both of whom discussed the S. S. White Panorex X-Ray Machine; James E. Phillips (University of Pennsylvania) and Olaf Langland (University of Iowa), who evaluated the Siemens Orthopantomograph); and Sidney Blackman (Northwestern University) (1968) and C. A. Guzman (Eastman Dispensary), both of whom analyzed the Westinghouse Panoramix.

In June, 1967, the United States Air Force began routinely taking Panorex panoramic radiographs of all inductees. In 1969, Charles R. Morris and associates analyzed 5,556 Panorex radiographs taken of United States Air Force recruits at Lackland Air Force Base, Texas. From the results of this study they concluded that panoramic radiography was a simple and rapid method of recording the general dental health of a large population and that it provided information vital to treatment planning.

Throughout the years of investigation, three arch forms have continually been used to describe the dental arches, specifically, the elliptical, parabolic, and catenary forms. Black and Izard believed that the majority of normal arches were elliptical. Broomell, Angle, and Wheeler were all of the opinion that the normal arch form resembled a parabolic curve. Sicher believed that the normal arch form was elliptical in the maxillary arch and parabolic in the mandibular arch. He described the U-shaped

Figure 1–28. G. E. Panelipse. **A.** The axis of rotation (X) is constantly moving in an adjustable semielliptical path (dotted line) conforming to the patient's dental arch. This diagram shows three positions of x-ray tube and film cassette during their continuous movement around the stationary patient. The film cassette also moves simultaneously on its own axis during the exposure cycle. **B.** Radiograph taken with G. E. Panelipse. (Note low horizontal impaction.) **C.** 1980 model. A chair supports the patient in a sitting position facing the operator. The head positioner unit swings out to allow patient access and egress. It locks into place when brought into radiographic position. **D.** Control panel.

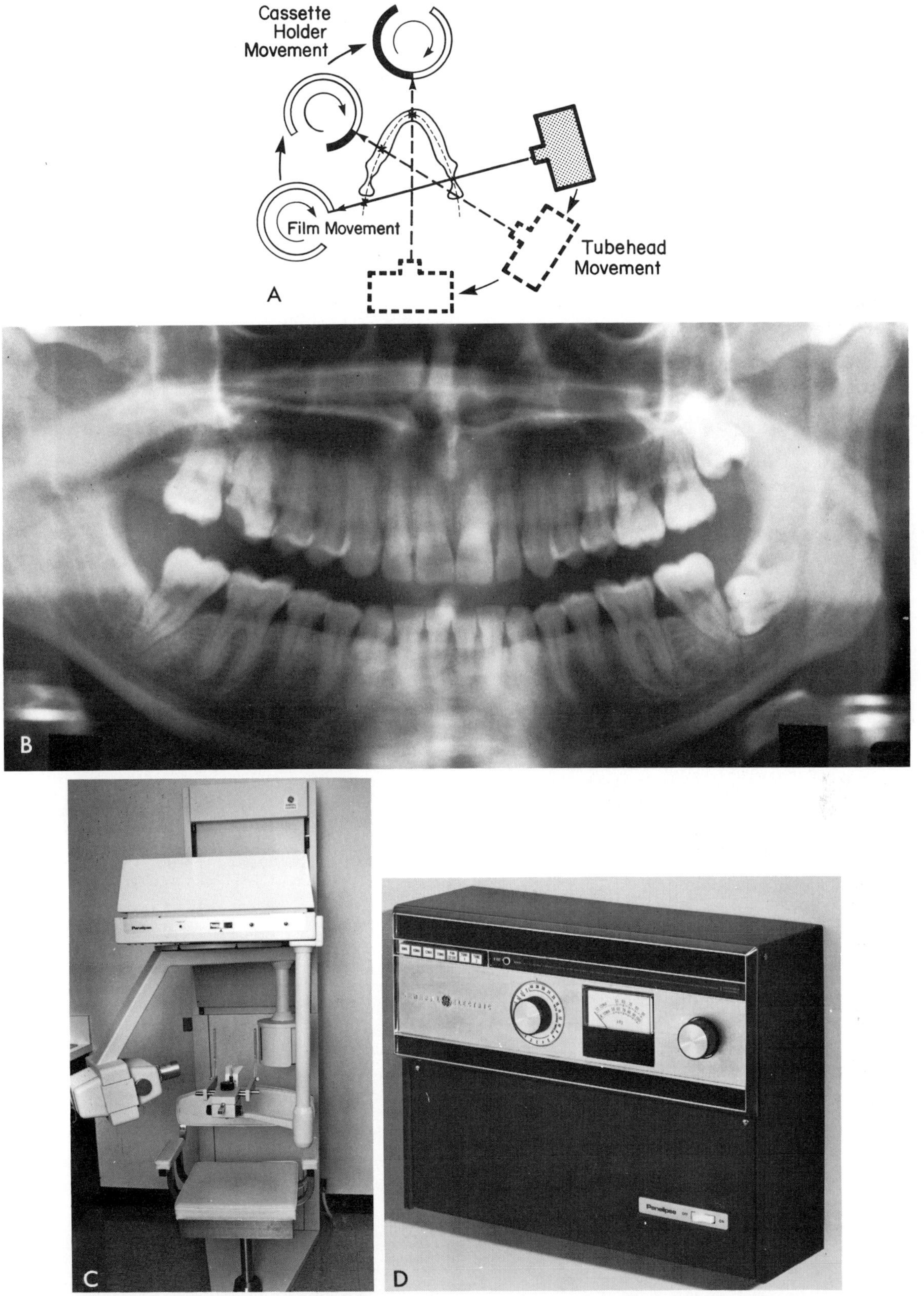

Figure 1–28. *See legend on opposite page.*

Illustration continued on following page

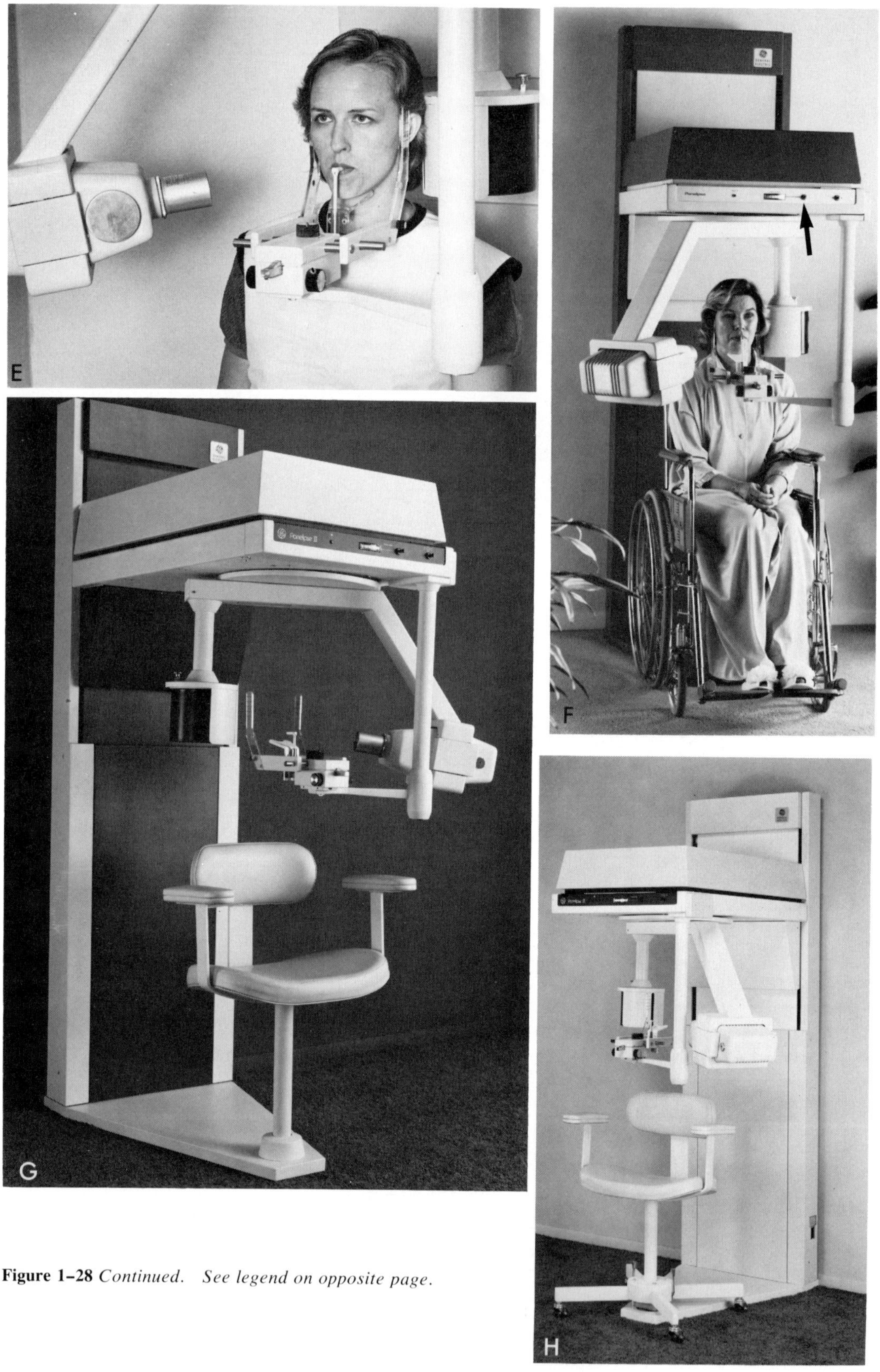

Figure 1–28 *Continued.* *See legend on opposite page.*

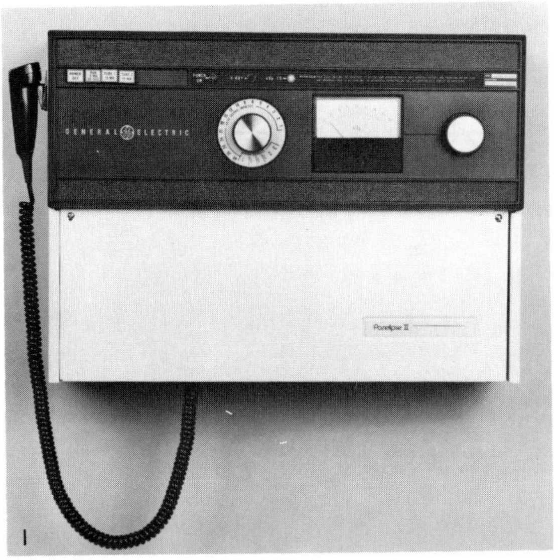

Figure 1–28 *Continued.* **E.** The head positioner is used to position the patient's dental arch in the sharply depicted image plane of the Panelipse. It also restrains the patient's head during the panoramic excursion and provides a method of measurement of the arch size. The chin rest assembly moves in or out when either knob on the side of the head positioner base is turned. A scale moves under the index line to obtain the proper index measurement or dental arch size for the patient. An electric motor, controlled by a knob on operator's control panel above patient, adjusts the rotational axis of the machine to correspond with the patient's dental arch size. A plastic bite guide or block is positioned between the teeth to separate them and to place them in edge-to-edge position. **F.** Special stand to accommodate wheel chair. **G.** Panelipse II. Stand shown with standard chair base. **H.** Stand with optional mobile chair base. **I.** Panelipse II master control panel. The mA setting has been reduced from 8 to 4 mA in the Panelipse II. (Figure 1–28 courtesy of G. E. Medical Systems Division, Milwaukee, WI.)

arch as having primitive characteristics. MacConaill and Scher and Scott described the normal arch forms as catenary curves. The catenary curve is formed when a perfectly inextensible cord of uniform density and cross section hangs freely from two fixed points.

In 1969, James Currier completed an interesting computerized geometric analysis of the human dental arch form of 25 Caucasian adults with "ideal" occlusions. He concluded that the ellipse conforms best to the outer curves of both maxillary and mandibular arches and that the parabola provides the best fit to the middle curves of both arches.

Paatero believed that the side portions of the jaws were flat, whereas the anterior portion was curved (1954a). His first orthopantomographic machine followed a parabolic curve; however, later models seem to follow a modified parabolic curve.

In 1970, the General Electric Company introduced a new panoramic x-ray unit called the GE-3000. The name was later changed to Panelipse. As in the Panorex technique, the patient is stationary and the narrow x-ray beam tubehead and film cassette rotate around the patient's head. The film cassette rotates on its own axis behind a narrow slit between the patient and the film cassette (Fig. 1–28).

The G. E. Panelipse employs a slit or narrow beam similar to that used in the Panorex and Orthopantomograph, but there is a fundamental difference in the movement of the rotational assembly. The Panelipse employs a continuously changing rotational axis that follows the arc of the mandible and maxilla in semielliptical paths. The G. E. engineers adopted an elliptical rotational movement because they believed that the Caucasian outer arch is elliptical rather than parabolic (Currier, 1969).

At about the same time that General Electric introduced the GE-3000 (1970), Morita Dental Manufacturing of Japan developed a panoramic machine called the Panex-E, which had some similarities to the G. E. Panelipse (Ando, 1971). The Panex-E uses a moving center of rotation, and the x-ray tube follows an elliptical path during exposure of the film (Fig. 1–29); this method is called ellipsopantomography. The Panex-E panoramic machine is presently marketed in the United States as the Sybron/Ritter Panoral machine (Fig. 1–30).

During the 1970s, Dr. Ulf Welander, a Swedish researcher, became interested in panoramic radiography. Previously, panoramic radiography had been described as a modified form of tomography. Paatero introduced his second method of panoramic radiography as a form of tomography and called it pantomography (1949b). The tomographic approach taken by Paatero was generally accepted by many authors including Hudson, Kumpula, and Dickson; Soila; Tammisalo (1964a, b, c); Ando (1971); Blackman (1955, 1964); Graber; Jung (1965); Manson-Hing; and Phillips.

In a series of research investigations, Welander and colleagues (1971, 1972, 1974, 1975, 1977, 1978a, b) concluded that rotational panoramic radiography should **not** be classified as a modified form of tomography unless tomography is defined in its most general terms as meaning "any layer-forming imaging system."

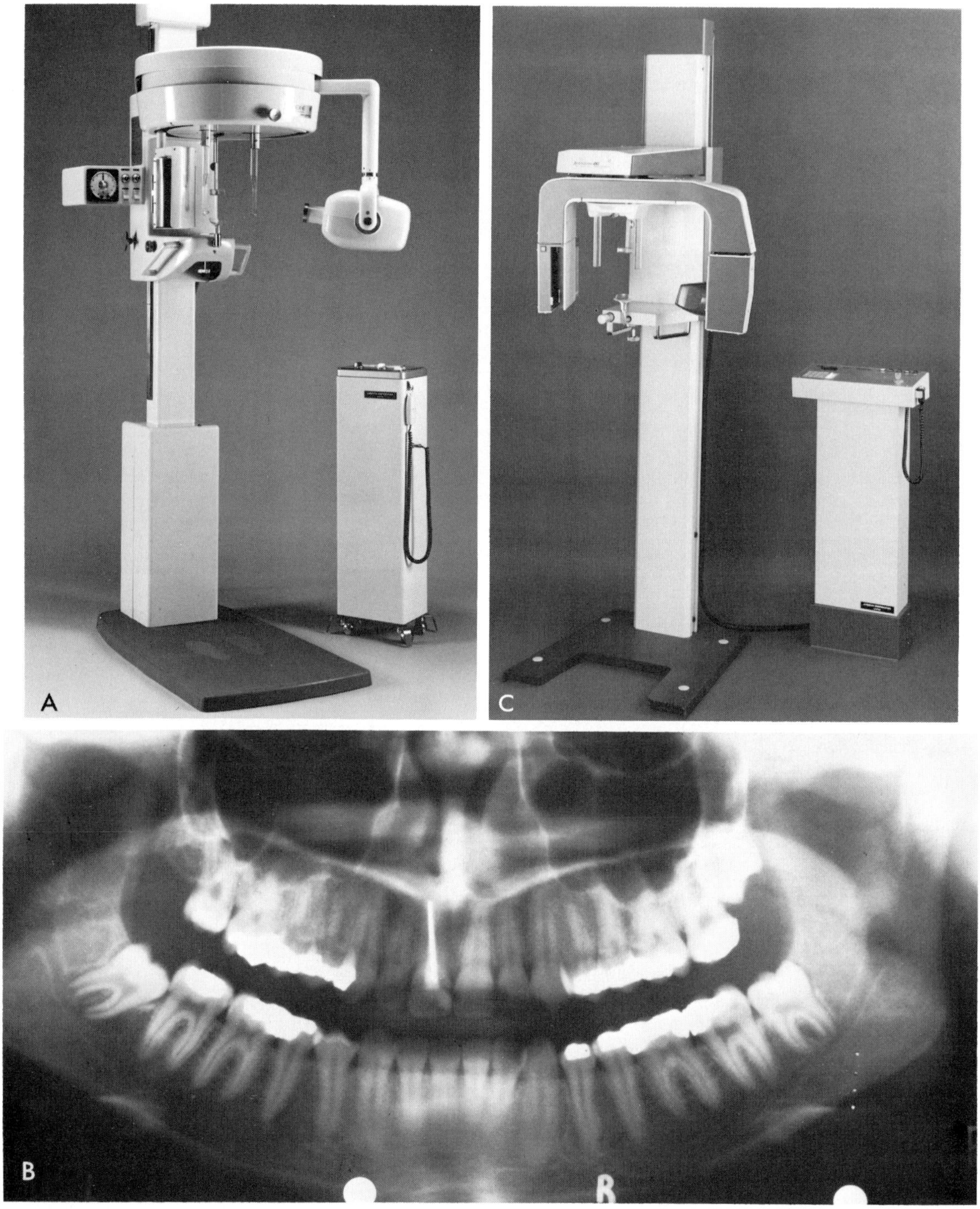

Figure 1–29. **A.** Panex E (1980 model). The first Panex came out in 1968 and was named "ellipso-pantomography" by Professor Eiko Sairenji, Department of Dentistry, Nihon University, Japan. The center of rotation of the x-ray beam of the Panex changes continuously, following an elliptical path during the exposure cycle. The patient stands facing the machine. The head is positioned by means of a head positioner, chin cup, and bite block. **B.** Radiograph taken by Panex E panoramic x-ray machine. **C.** Architron DC (Panex). Newest ellipso-pantomographic apparatus manufactured by Morita Corp. However, it is not in production as yet. It is provided with a D.C. x-ray generator and digital computer control. (**A** and **C** courtesy of J. Morita Corp., Kyoto, Japan.)

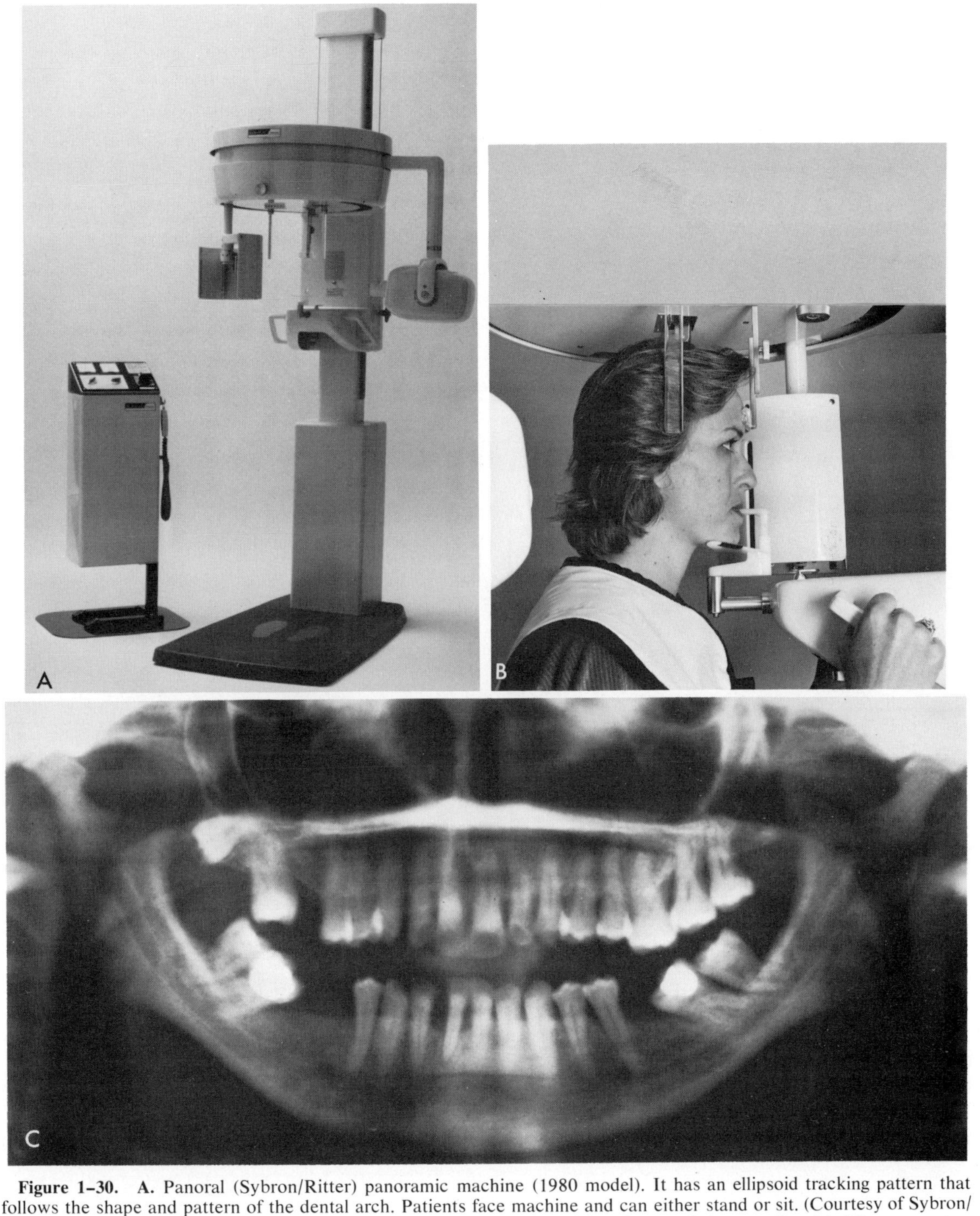

Figure 1–30. **A.** Panoral (Sybron/Ritter) panoramic machine (1980 model). It has an ellipsoid tracking pattern that follows the shape and pattern of the dental arch. Patients face machine and can either stand or sit. (Courtesy of Sybron/Ritter Corp., Dental Products Division, Romulus, MI.) **B.** Patient is positioned correctly by use of head-holding apparatus, chin rest, and bite block. The bite block is indented to assure that the anterior dentition of the patient is in the sharply depicted plane of the machine. **C.** Panoral radiograph.

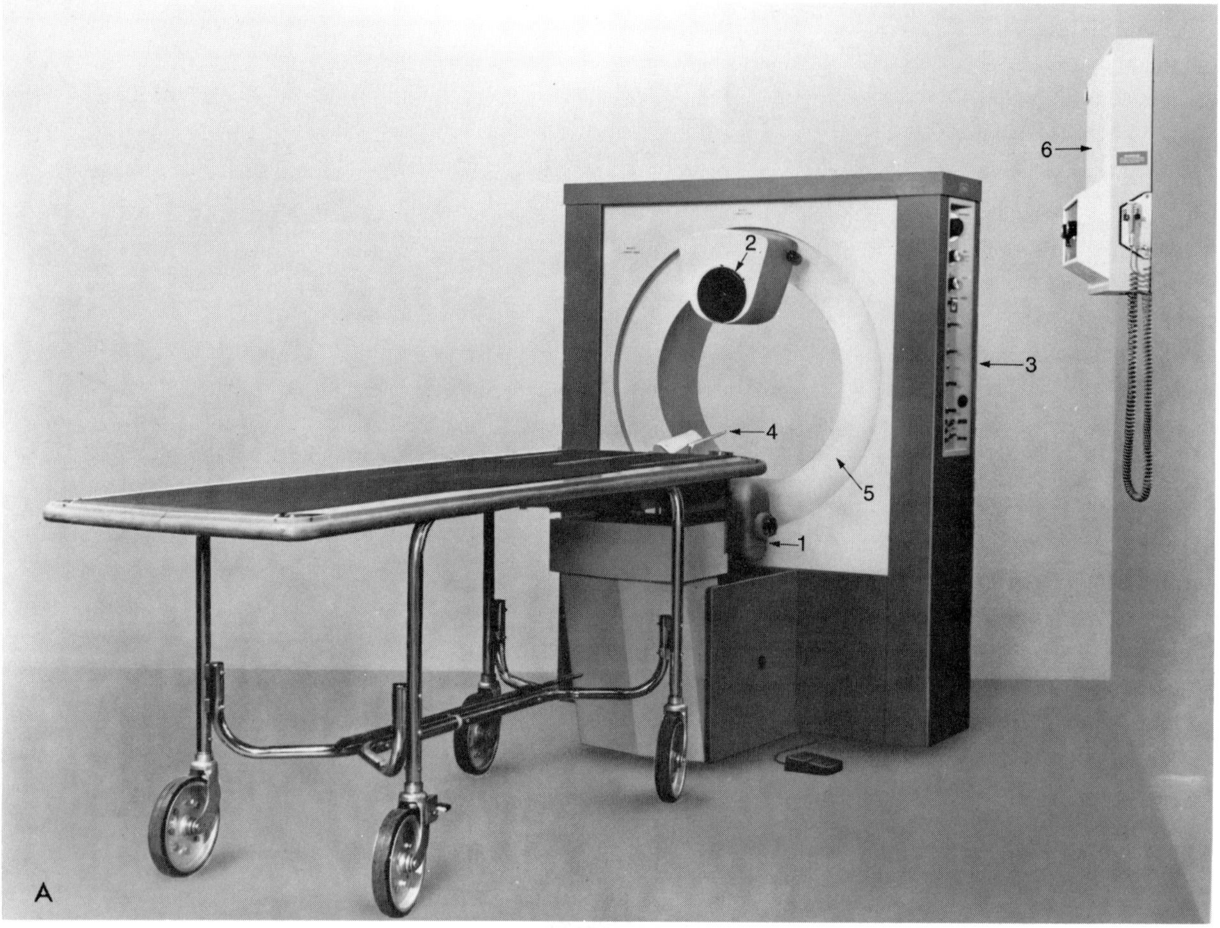

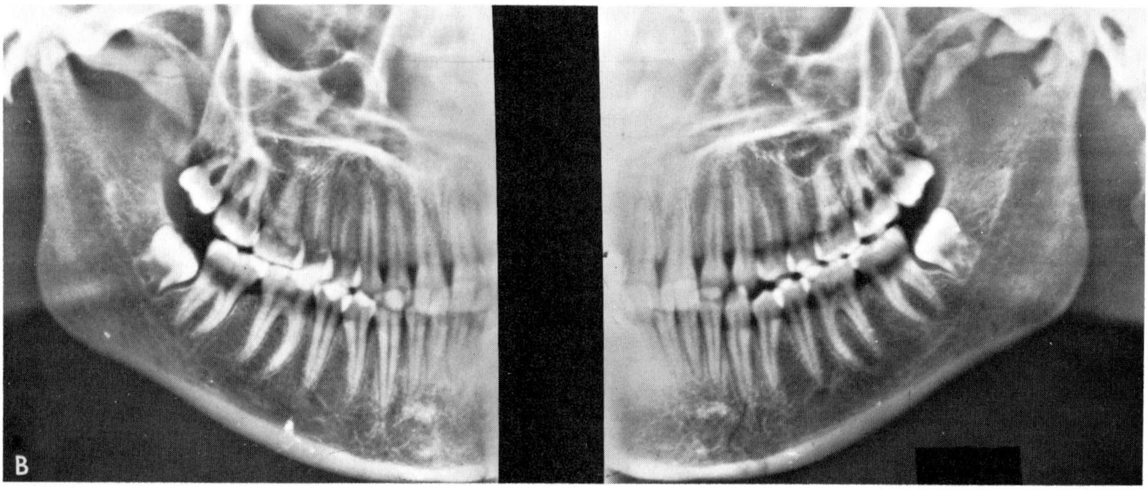

Figure 1–31. **A.** Tomorex panoramic machine. Designed to radiograph the injured, litter-borne patient. (1) Tomorex tubehead is specially designed to function at either 0 or 7° angulation. A built-in electronic control prevents the head rest from coming in contact with the tubehead. (2) Cassette assembly holds flexible film cassette. (3) Master control panel. (4) Head rest. (5) Rotating disc. (6) Remote control panel. (Courtesy S. S. White, Medical Products Division, Pennwalt Corp., Phila., PA.) **B.** Conventional split-image panoramic radiograph of jaws taken by the Tomorex. (Note overlapping of anterior teeth because cotton roll was not placed between incisal edges of anterior teeth.)

Illustration continued on opposite page

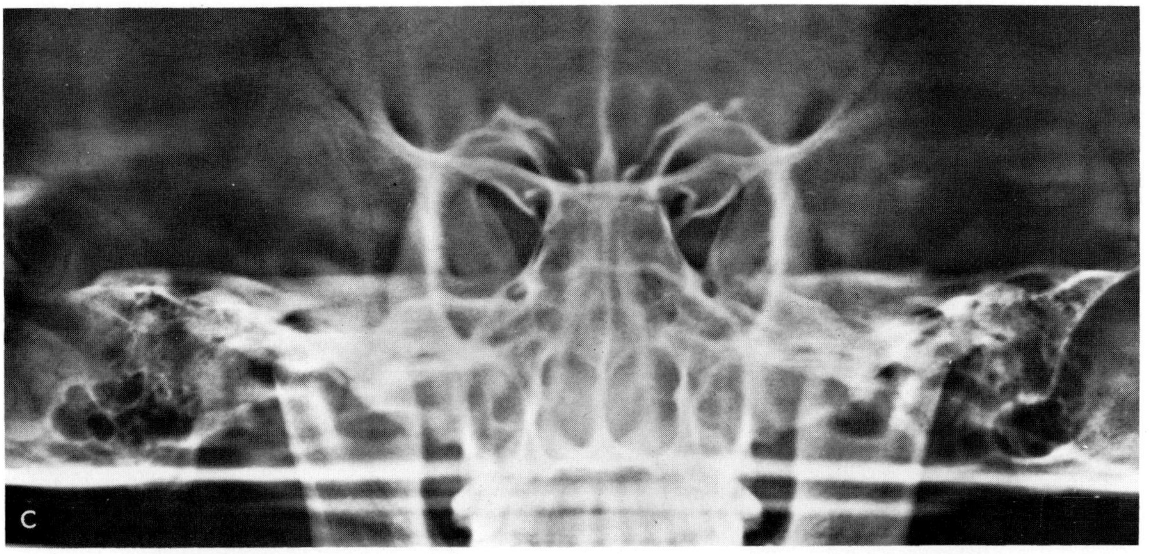

Figure 1–31 *Continued.* **C.** Mid-face postero-anterior (PA) projection taken by Tomorex.

Welander contended that the layer (sharply depicted plane) formed in rotational panoramic radiography has certain similarities to the tomographic layer, but the basic layer formation process is entirely different (1974, 1975). It was Welander's opinion, supported by a mathematical model (1974), which he and associates subsequently confirmed experimentally (1977, 1978a, b), that rotational panoramic radiography is basically a specific projection technique. See Chapter 2 for an explanation of Dr. Welander's theory.

During this same period (1970s), the form and thickness of the image layer of various rotational panoramic x-ray machines were analyzed experimentally. Among the researchers were Jung from Germany; Brown, Christen, and Jerman from the United States Air Force; Lund and Manson-Hing (1975a, b, c) from the University of Alabama; and Ogura and associates from Japan. Ogura and associates emphasized that an optimum panoramic imaging system could be obtained if the linear speed of the film could be optimally controlled and if the location of the desired layer could be determined for each patient.

Since 1974, many new panoramic x-ray machines have become available to the dentist. There are too many to list in this textbook. The Tomorex (Pennwalt) is rather unique in that it allows the operator to take a panoramic film of an injured or litter-borne patient (Fig. 1–31). This unit was designed by Charles R. Morris and Don Hudson. Dr. Morris, originally an oral surgeon, saw the need for such an x-ray device while working in emergency rooms at various hospitals. The patient is moved into position by means of a conveyor belt and radiographed while lying on a specially designed litter. The Tomorex operates in a manner similar to the Panorex, but the x-ray rotational center is changed half way through the exposure by the automatic movement of the tubehead–film cassette assembly instead of by shifting of the chair, as is done in the Panorex.

In 1980, Palomex Oy of Helsinki, Finland, introduced to the market a panoramic unit similar to the Tomorex, called the Orthopantomograph OP6 (Fig. 1–32).

Panoramic radiography has come a long way since the late 1940s when Dr. Paatero began experimenting with slit beam rotation methods to produce panoramic radiographs of the jaws. It has proved to be an excellent diagnostic aid for the medical and dental professions.

On September 23, 1980, Dr. Donald C. Hudson of San Antonio, Texas, died of cardiovascular disease. He was 69 years of age. Dr. Hudson was co-inventor of the Panorex and the Tomorex. Dr. Charles Morris, a friend of long standing, had this to say of Donald C. Hudson:

> Don Hudson was a very quiet, soft-spoken gentleman of the first order. He was always very proper and formal, maintaining a military bearing and a strong allegiance to the United States. He was also a

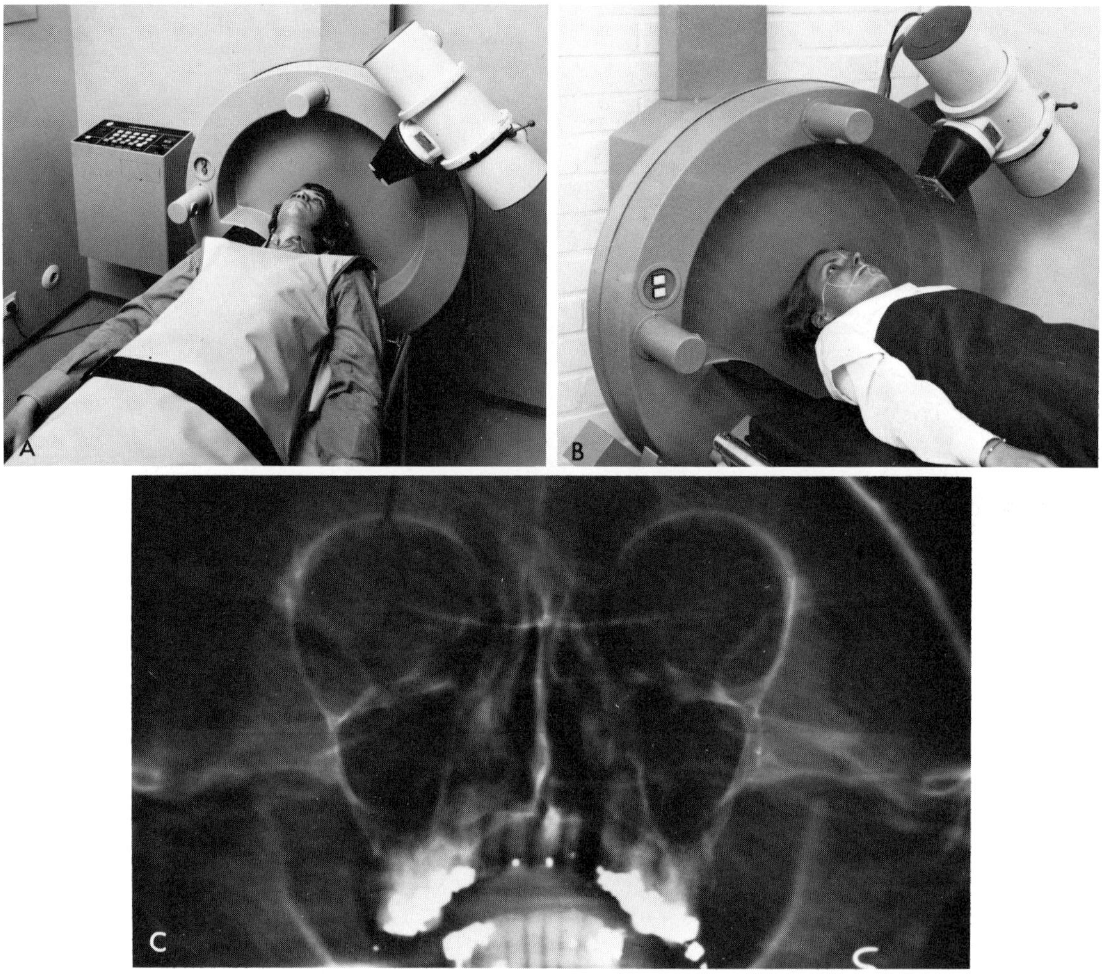

Figure 1–32. OP6 Orthopantomograph. **A.** A specially designed stretcher with head support minimizes handling of patient in prone position. Called "panoramic zonography" of head and neck, it employs a narrow-angle tomographic arc and strives to scan the whole of the object, undistorted and sharply defined. **B.** Permits uncomplicated patient positioning with the use of light beam lines, assuring reproducible and symmetrical images of pre- and postoperative radiographs. **C.** Waters view of mid-face. (Figure 1–32 courtesy of Palomex Instrument Co., Helsinki, Finland.)

very warm person, willing to share his knowledge and to help anyone requesting it. Don was a real scientist with sound reasoning power. Everyone who knew him loved and respected him. He will be missed and remembered for years to come.

REFERENCES

Albers-Schönberg, H. E.: Rontgentechnik. 6. Aufl. Bd. 1. Leipzig: Georg Thieme, 1941 (German).

Ando, S.: Present status of panoramic radiography. **J. Nihon Univ. Sch. Dent. 38**:173, 1964.

Ando, S.: Pantomography and orthopantomography. **Dent. Current** (Sin Shi-cho) **4**:179, 1970.

Ando, S.: **Orthopantomography.** Tokyo: Assoc. Oral Hygiene, 1971 (Japanese).

Angle, E. H.: **Treatment of Malocclusion of the Teeth,** 7th Edition. Philadelphia: S. S. White, 1907.

Black, G. V.: **Descriptive Anatomy of the Human Teeth,** 4th Edition. Philadelphia: S. S. White, 1902, pp. 130–135.

Blackman, S.: Panoramic tomography: Pantomography. **Dent. Pract. 5**:368, 1955.

Blackman, S.: Mass dental radiography. **Radiography 22**:21, 1956.

Blackman, S.: Pan-oral Radiography. **Dent. Pract. 10**:12, 270, 1960a.

Blackman, S.: Rotational tomography of the face. **Br. J. Radiol. 33**:408, 1960b.

Blackman, S.: Panagraphy. **Oral Surg. 14**:10, 1178, 1961.

Blackman, S.: Panoramic radiography: Rotational tomography. **Br. J. Oral Surg. 1**:209, 1964.

Blackman, S.: Anatomic structures as visualized on the panoramix. **Oral Surg. 26**:321, 1968.

Broomell, I. N.: **Anatomy and Histology of the Mouth and Teeth,** 2nd Edition. Philadelphia: P. Blakiston's Son, 1902, p. 91.

Brown, C. E., Christen, A. C., and Jerman, A. C.: Dimensions of the focal trough in panoramic radiography. **J.A.D.A. 84**:843, 1972.

Brueggemann, I. A.: Evaluation of the Panorex units. **Oral Surg. 24**:348, 1967.

Currier, J. H.: A computerized geometric analysis of human dental arch form. **Am. J. Orthod. 56**:164, 1969.

Duhamel, J.: A new form of photomography: The photopantomography of Y. V. Paatero. **Sci. Ind. Photogr. 25**:353, 1954 (French).

Duhamel, J.: Sur la correspondance entre espaces image et object dans les procedes de radiographie en coupe par faisceau diaphragme. **Sci. Ind. Photogr. 28**:225, 1957 (French).

Faude, J. H.: Personal communication. August 8, 1980.

Gott, T., and Rosenthal, J.: Uber un Verfahren zur Darstellung der Herzbewegung mettels. **Rontgenstrahlen. Munch. Med. Wochenschr. II**:2033, 1912 (German).

Graber, T. M.: Panoramic radiography in dentistry. **J. Canad. Dent. A. 31**:158, 1965.

Guzman, C. A.: Principles and function of the panoramix. **Oral Surg. 24**:196, 1967.

Heckmann, K.: Potentials of radiography and the development of new exposure technics. **Fortschr. Rontgenstrahlen. 60**:144, 1939 (German).

Heckmann, K.: Pseudofokale und bivisuelle Aufnahmetechnik, Kapitel VIII. *In* **Handbuch der medizinischen Radiologie,** Band III. von Vieten, R. (ed.), New York: Springer-Verlag, 1967 (German).

Hudson, D. C., Kumpula, J. W., and Dickson, G.: A panoramic x-ray dental machine. **U. S. Armed Forces Med. J. 13**:46, 1957.

Izard, G.: New method for determination of the normal arch by the function of the face. **Int. J. Orthod. 13**:582, 1927.

Izard, G.: Potentials of radiography and the development of new exposure technics. **Fortschr. Rontgenstrahlen, 60**:144, 1939 (German).

Jung, T.: Panoramic radiographic procedures in stomatology. **Rev. Belge Med. Dent. 20**:165, 1965 (French).

Jung, T.: Die Wiedergabe der Frontazhregion auf Panorama-Schlicht-Aufrahnen. **Dtsch. Zahnaerztl. Z. 27**:972, 1972 (German).

Kite, O. W., Swanson, L. T., Levin, S., and Bradbury, E.: Radiation and image distortion in the panorex x-ray unit. **Oral Surg. 15**:1201, 1962.

Knight, N.: Anatomic structures as visualized on the panorex radiograph. **Oral Surg. 26**:326, 1968.

Koch and Sterzel Co., Patentschrift No. 765871. Deutsche Patentamt. Munchen, 3 Mai (May) 1954.

Kraske, L. M., and Mazzarella, M. A.: Evaluation of panoramic x-ray procedures. **J. Dent. Res. 39**:693, 1960.

Kraske, L. M., and Mazzarella, M. A.: Evaluation of a panoramic dental x-ray machine. **Dent. Progr. 1**:171, 1961.

Langland, O. E.: The use of the orthopantomograph in a dental school. **Oral Surg. 24**:484, 1967.

Lund, T. M., and Manson-Hing, L. R.: A study of the focal troughs of three panoramic dental x-ray machines. Part I, The area of sharpness. **Oral Surg. 39**:318, 1975a.

Lund, T. M., and Manson-Hing, L. R.: A study of the focal troughs of three panoramic dental x-ray machines. Part II, Image dimensions. **Oral Surg. 39**:647, 1975b.

Lund, T. M., and Manson-Hing, L. R.: Relations between tooth positions and focal troughs of panoramic machines. **Oral Surg. 40**:285, 1975c.

MacConaill, M. A., and Scher, E. A.: The ideal form of the human dental arcade with some prosthetic application. **Dent. Rec. 69**:285, 1949.

Manson-Hing, L. R.: Advances in dental pantomography: The GE-3000. **Oral Surg. 31**:430, 1971.

Millwee, R. H.: Slit scanography. **Radiology 28**:483, 1937.

Mitchell, L. D.: Panoramic roentgenography: A clinical evaluation. **J.A.D.A. 66**:777, 1963.

Morris, C. R., Marano, P. D., Swimley, D. C., and Runco, J. G.: Abnormalities noted on panoramic radiographs. **Oral Surg. 28**:772, 1969.

Nelsen, R. J., and Kumpula, J. W.: Panographic radiography. **J. Dent. Res. 31**:158, 1952.

Numata, H.: Consideration of the parabolic radiography of dental arch. **J. Shimizu Studies 10**:13, 1933 (Japanese).

Numata, H.: A trial on the narrow beam radiography. **J. Shimizu Studies 12**:6, 1934 (Japanese).

Ogura, K., Kanno, T., Suzuki, Y., and Shimano, T.: Changes in image layer due to variable speed in pantomography. Paper read at the 4th International Congress of Dento-Maxillo-Facial Radiology, Malmo, Sweden, 1977.

Ott, W.: Panorama-Rontgentechnik. **Festschrift zur 50-Feier der Graubundner Zahnarzte-Gesellschaft.** Chur, 1961 (Swiss).

Paatero, Y. V.: A new radiographic method in dentistry. **Suom. Hammaslaak. Toimi. 87**:37, 1946 (Finnish).

Paatero, Y. V.: The use of a mobile source of light in radiography. **Acta Radiol. 29**:221, 1948.

Paatero, Y. V.: Parabolography — A new method for radiography of teeth and jaws. **Suom. Hammaslaak. Toimi. 96**:4, 1949a (Finnish).

Paatero, Y. V.: A new tomographic method for radiographing curved outer surfaces. **Acta Radiol. 32**:177, 1949b.

Paatero, Y. V.: Method of and apparatus for x-ray photographing curved surfaces, especially for medical purposes. U. S. Patent Number 2-684-446 (1954) (Application 1950).

Paatero, Y. V.: The use of line focus in pantomography. **Suom. Hammaslaak. Toimi. 48**:11, 1952a (Finnish).

Paatero, Y. V.: Thickness of layer produced on pantomogram in relation to location of the object, speed of rotation, and divergence of roentgen rays. **Suom. Hammaslaak. Toimi. 48**:113, 1952b (Finnish).

Paatero, Y. V.: Pantomographische Röntgenphotographie. **Fortschr. Kieferorthop. 13**:115, 1952c (German).

Paatero, Y. V.: Radiography of temporo-mandibular joint, a new method. **Ann. Chir. Gynaecol. Fenn. 42**:259, 1953 (Finnish).

Paatero, Y. V.: Pantomography in theory and use. **Acta Radiol. 41**:321, 1954a.

Paatero, Y. V.: Geometrical study on possibilities of making double-eccentric pantomograms with a single exposure. **Suom. Hammaslaak. Toimi. 50** (Supp II):36, 1954b.

Paatero, Y. V.: Orthoradial jaw pantomography. **Ann. Med. Int. Fenn.** (Supp. 28) **48**:222, 227, 1958a.

Paatero, Y. V.: Ortoradiaalenen leukapatnomografia. **Suom. Hammaslaak. Toimi. 54**:12, 1958b (Finnish).

Paatero, Y. V.: Clinical orthopantomograms. **Suom. Hammaslaak. Toimi. 56**:408, 1960 (Finnish).

Paatero, Y. V.: Pantomography and orthopantomography. **Oral Surg. 14**:947, 1961.

Paatero, Y. V., Neiminen, T., and Tammisalo, E.: Tomography of maxillary sinuses in transversal projection with an orthopantomograph. **Suom. Hammaslaak. Toimi. 59**:309, 1963.

Pasche, O.: Uber eine neue Blendew vorrichtung in der Rontgentechnik. **Fortschr. Rontgenstrahlen 6**:210, 1903 (German).

Phillips, J. E.: Principles and function of orthopantomograph. **Oral Surg. 24**:41, 1967.

Sairenji, E.: Panoramic radiography. **Dental Outlook** (Shikai Tembo) **15**:1140, 1958.

Sairenji, E.: Personal communication. March 29, 1980.

Scott, J. H.: The shape of dental arches. **J. Dent. Res. 36**:996, 1957.

Sicher, H.: **Oral Anatomy,** 2nd Edition. St. Louis: C. V. Mosby, 1952, pp. 262–263.

Soila, P.: General theory of narrow beam rotating tomography. **Acta Radiol. 55**:458, 1961.

Suzuki, M., Ando, S., et al.: Diagnostic effects of panoramic radiography in maxillo-facial region. **Dental Outlook** (Shikai Tembo) **26**:1119, 1965.

Tammisalo, E. H.: The dimensional reproduction of the image layer in orthopantomography. **Suom. Hammaslaak. Toimi. 60**:1, 1964a (Finnish).

Tammisalo, E. H.: Determination of the form of the image layer and calculation of its location within object in conventional and simultaneous orthopantomography. **Suom. Hammaslaak. Toimi. 60**:13, 1964b (Finnish).

Tammisalo, E. H., and Nieminen, T.: The thickness of an image layer in orthopantomography. **Suom. Hammaslaak. Toimi. 60**:119, 1964c (Finnish).

Tammisalo, E. H., and Karhuvaara, Y.: Radiation exposure in jaw orthopantomography. **Suom. Hammaslaak. Toimi. 60**:128, 1964d (Finnish).

Tammisalo, E. H., and Ainoma, J.: The orthopantomogram in quantitative assessment of marginal bone loss. **Suom. Hammaslaak. Toimi. 63**:132, 1967 (Finnish).

Updegrave, W. J.: Panoramic dental radiography. **Dent. Radiogr. Photogr.** (4) **36**:75, 1963.

Updegrave, W. J.: The role of panoramic radiography in diagnosis. **Oral Surg. 22**:49, 1966.

Van Aken, J.: Panoramic equipment. **J.A.D.A. 86**:1050, 1973.

Watson, W.: Differential radiography I. **Radiography 5**:81, 1939.

Watson, W.: Differential radiography II. **Radiography 6**:161, 1940.

Welander, U., and Nystrom, O.: Image-producing geometry and tomography in roentgenologic narrow beam methods, with special reference to "Pantomography." **Swed. Dent. J. 64**:641, 1971.

Welander, U., and Nystrom, O.: A new theory on the image-producing elements in pantomographic methods. **Dent. Max. Fac. Radiol. 1**:3, 1972.

Welander, U.: A mathematical model of narrow beam rotation methods. **Acta Radiol. Diag. 15**:305, 1974.

Welander, U.: Layer formation in narrow beam rotation radiography. **Acta Radiol. Diag. 16**:529, 1975.

Welander, U., and Wickman, G.: Blurring and layer thickness in narrow beam rotation radiography. **Acta Radiol. Diag. 18**:705, 1977.

Welander, U., and Wickman, G.: Image distortion in narrow beam rotation radiography: A mathematical analysis. **Acta Radiol. Diag. 19**:507, 1978a.

Welander, U., and Sjoblom, A.: Position, form and thickness of the image layer in narrow beam rotation radiography. **Acta Radiol. Diag. 19**:697, 1978b.

Wheeler, R. C.: **A Textbook of Dental Anatomy and Physiology,** 2nd Edition. Philadelphia: W. B. Saunders, 1952, pp. 196–215, 352–406.

XRM develops panoramic dental x-ray machine. **Dent. Ind. News 42**:75, 1959.

Chapter 2

Theory of Rotational Panoramic Radiography

Ulf Welander, William McDavid, and Gunilla Tronje

A basic knowledge of the physical principles underlying rotational panoramic radiography is necessary for the optimum use of the technique. Knowledge of the process of image formation in this type of equipment and of the resulting features, which are characteristic of the panoramic radiograph, is helpful both in formulating a proper technique for exposure and in intelligently evaluating the information contained in the resulting radiographs.

WORKING PRINCIPLE

The panoramic radiograph is unique in that the foci of the projection in the vertical and horizontal dimensions are not the same; in the horizontal dimension it is the rotation center of the beam that constitutes the functional focus, whereas in the vertical dimension it is the x-ray source. It is important to bear this in mind when studying image characteristics such as the distortion effects that arise in panoramic radiographs.

PRINCIPLE OF PROJECTION IN THE PLANE OF ROTATION

All dentists are, through the use of their conventional radiographic equipment, familiar with the so-called **central projection** (Fig. 2–1). If an x-ray source is placed intraorally and a perfectly circular segment of the jaws is exposed on a curved film bent around this segment, the resulting projection is still a true central projection (Fig. 2–2**A**). Exactly the same projection of the object will be created in the horizontal dimension if the stationary intraoral x-ray source is replaced by a rotating beam of negligible width (Fig. 2–3) with its rotation center at that point where the ray source was previously (Fig. 2–2**B**). In fact, the rotation center of the beam will form the effective focus,

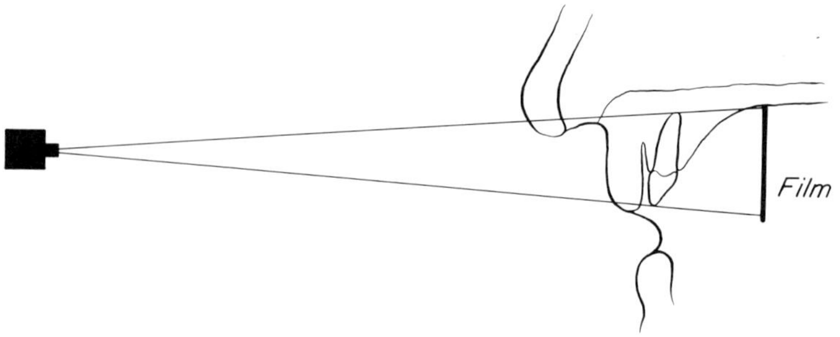

Figure 2–1. The conventional projection of an intraoral radiograph is a central projection. In a central projection the divergent rays have a common origin at a focal spot. The film is perpendicular to the central ray.

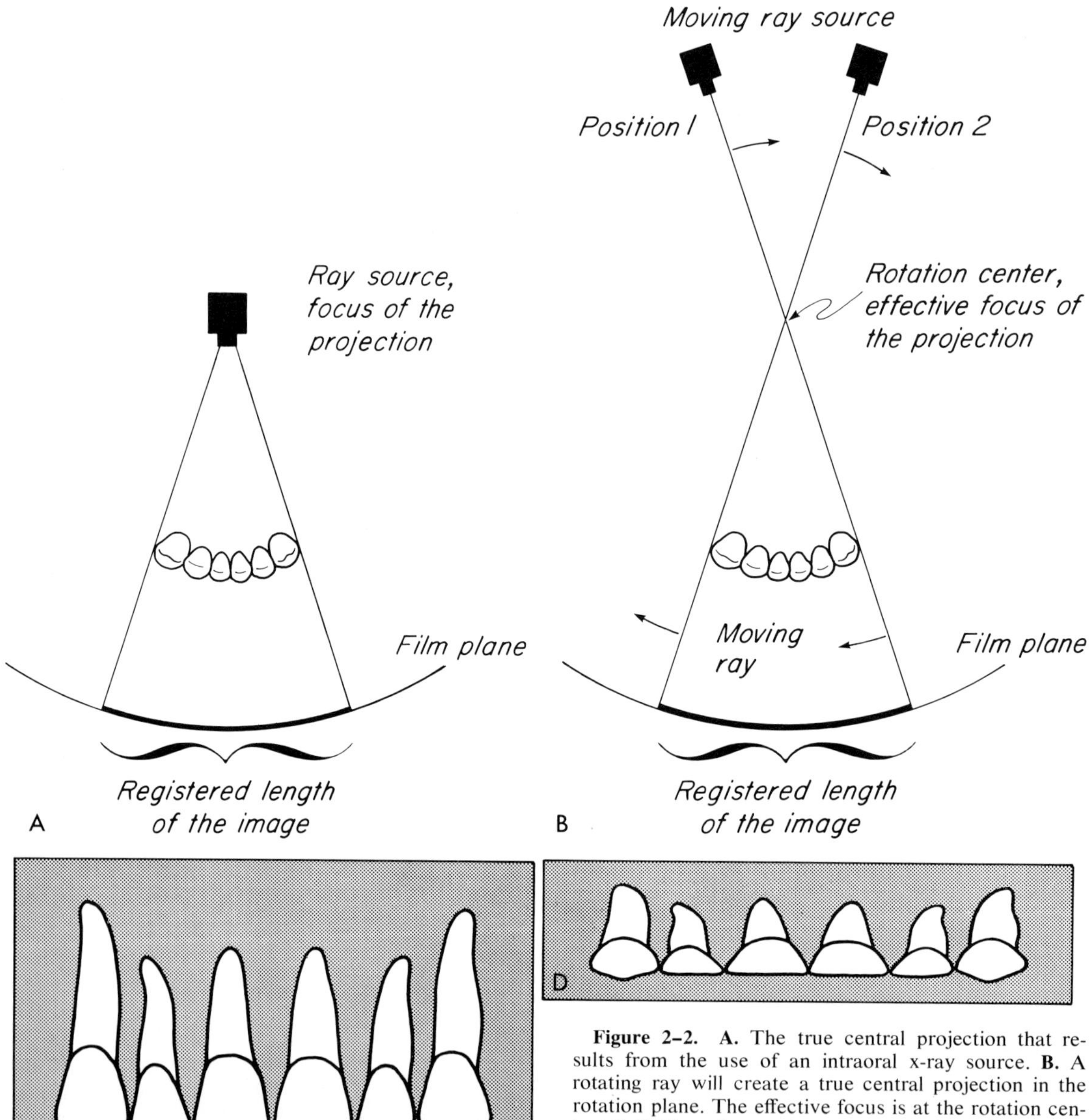

Figure 2–2. **A.** The true central projection that results from the use of an intraoral x-ray source. **B.** A rotating ray will create a true central projection in the rotation plane. The effective focus is at the rotation center. **C.** With an intraoral x-ray source, the ratio between the focus-to-film and focus-to-object distances is such that the magnification will be uniformly marked in all planes. **D.** Compare the magnification when a rotating beam projects the object onto a stationary film. It will be equal in the rotation plane but different in the vertical plane.

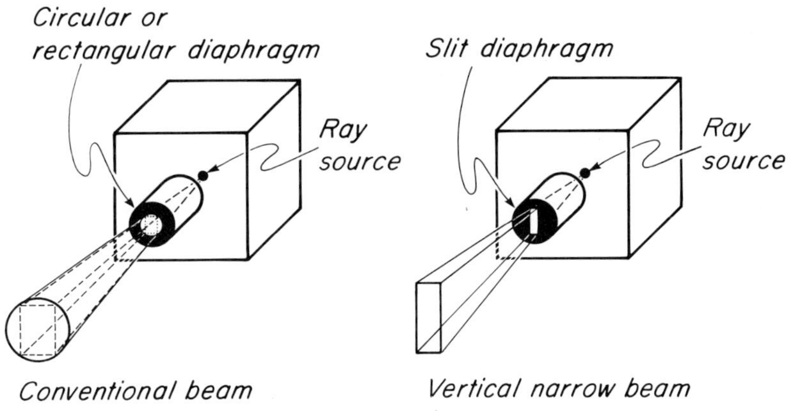

Figure 2–3. A narrow vertical beam is used in rotational panoramic radiography.

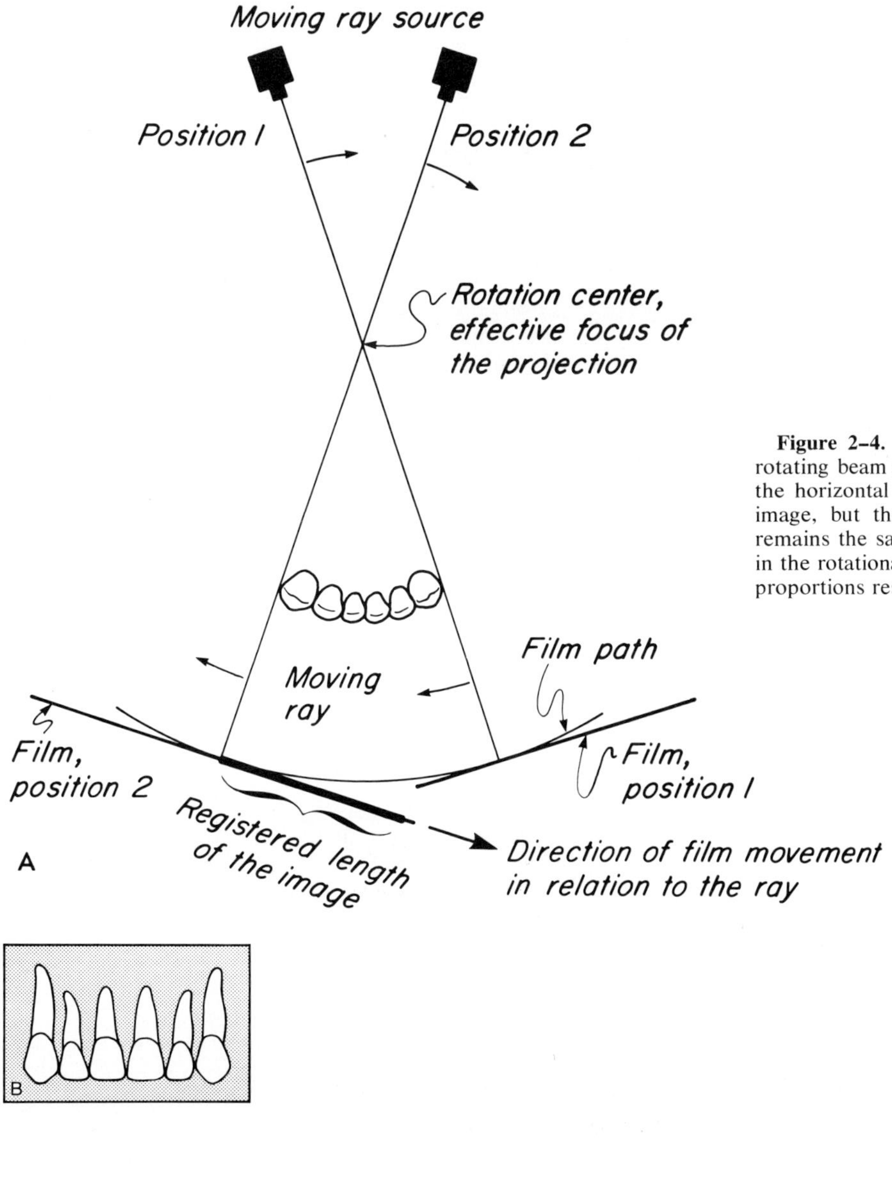

Figure 2–4. A. The combination of a rotating beam and a moving film changes the horizontal dimension of the recorded image, but the projection of the object remains the same. **B.** The resulting image in the rotational panoramic system has its proportions restored.

i.e., the effective center of the projection. In this case the object will be successively projected on the film as it is scanned by the rotating beam. The final image will be identical to the image exposed with the conventional central projection in the horizontal plane (Fig. 2–2**C** and **D**) but different in the vertical plane.

In the preceding examples, the film was assumed to be stationary. It is obvious that in such a geometrical projection as illustrated in Figure 2–2**A** and **B**, the relation between the focus-to-object distance and the focus-to-film distance is such that the magnification in the horizontal dimension will be marked (see Fig. 2–2**C** and **D**). It is important to remember that in this dimension the effective focus of the projection is the rotation center of the moving beam.

In rotational panoramic radiography the film is not stationary but moving. This does not affect the central projection of the object (Fig. 2–4**A**), but it does affect the length of the image recorded on the film. If the film moves in the same direction as the beam but at a slower speed, which is the case when a panoramic radiograph is exposed, the registered image will be foreshortened in the direction of the movement (Fig. 2–4**B**). Thus, the moving film changes the horizontal magnification of the image but not the projection of the object.

PROJECTION IN THE VERTICAL PLANE

In rotational panoramic radiography, the ray source constitutes the focus of the projection in the vertical plane. Thus, in the vertical dimension the panoramic image is the result of a conventional radiographic projection (Fig. 2–5).

PRINCIPLE OF LAYER FORMATION

When the previously described central projection technique utilizing a rotating beam is applied in practice, the beam must be of a certain width (see Fig. 2–3). When a beam of a finite width scans an object, the image is successively exposed on a stationary film as described previously (see Fig. 2–2**B**). However, there is also a successive build-up of unsharpness, since any point in the object will be successively projected onto the film by each ray in the beam. These rays do not project the point at the same spot along the film path (Fig. 2–6**A**). Thus, the projection of an object point moves at the film plane as the beam passes the point. The object point movement is in the same direction as the beam movement but at a lower speed. The fact that the projection of an object point moves along the film path in the same direction as the beam opens the possibility of eliminating some of the unsharpness created by the rotating beam. If the film moves at a speed that follows the moving projection of a certain object point, this point will always be projected on the same spot on the film (Fig. 2–6**B**) and will not appear unsharp in the resulting image. In rotational panoramic radiography the film is attached to the rotating system and moves in the same direction as the beam. The film is given

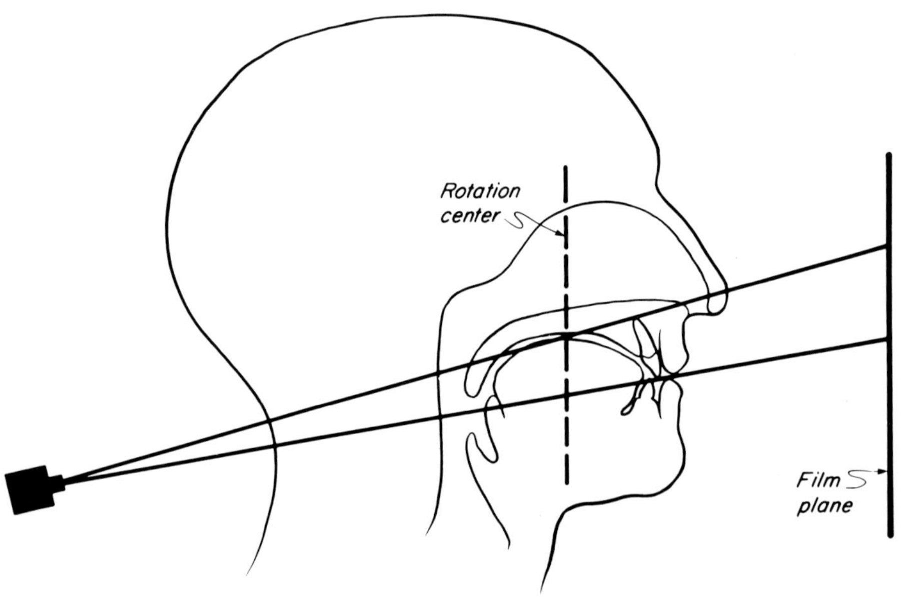

Figure 2–5. The projection in the vertical plane in rotational panoramic radiography.

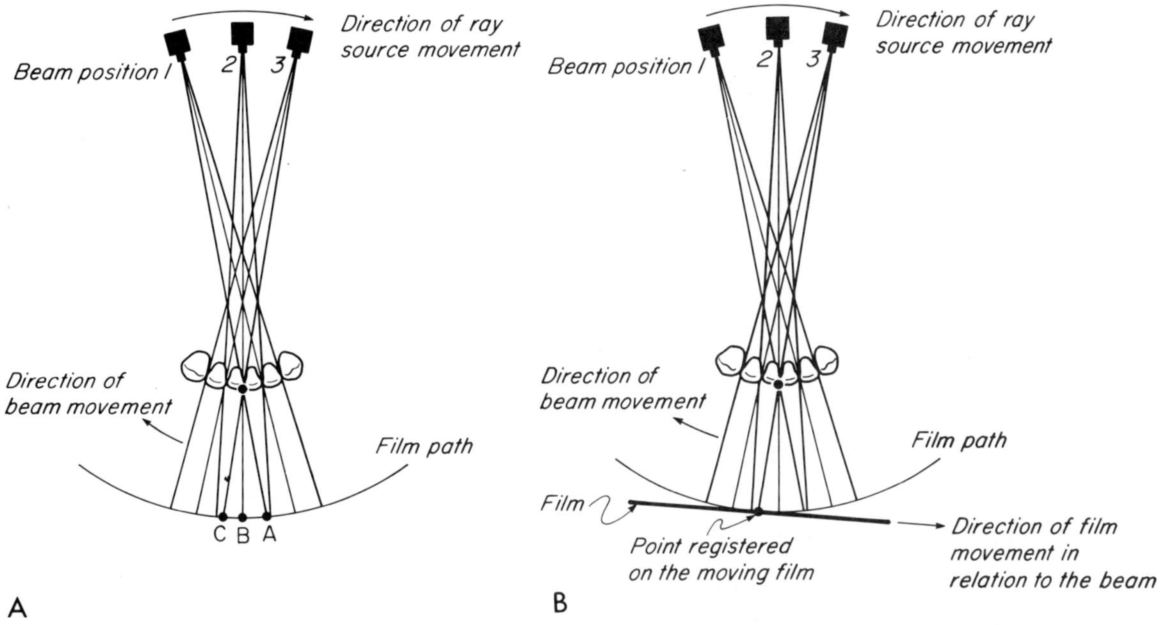

Figure 2–6. **A.** Successive rays do not project a given object point in the sharply depicted plane at the same spot along the film path. As the beam moves through positions 1, 2, and 3, the projection of a point moves through positions A, B, and C along the film path. **B.** If the film moves at the same speed at which the projection of the object point moves along the film path, the object point will be recorded as a single point on the film.

the correct speed by opposing this movement with a contrary movement relative to the beam.

The projection of object points outside the sharply depicted plane, either toward the rotation center of the beam or toward the film, will have a different projected speed at the film plane than the film itself (Fig. 2–7). As a result, the projection of these points will move in relation to the film, and they will be portrayed as lines on the film. Since the difference between the speed of the film and the speed of the projection of the points in the object will increase with the distance from the sharply depicted object plane, the unsharpness increases in both directions from this plane. At some distance the unsharpness will reach a level at which an object point is no longer perceptible in the image. In this way a zone in

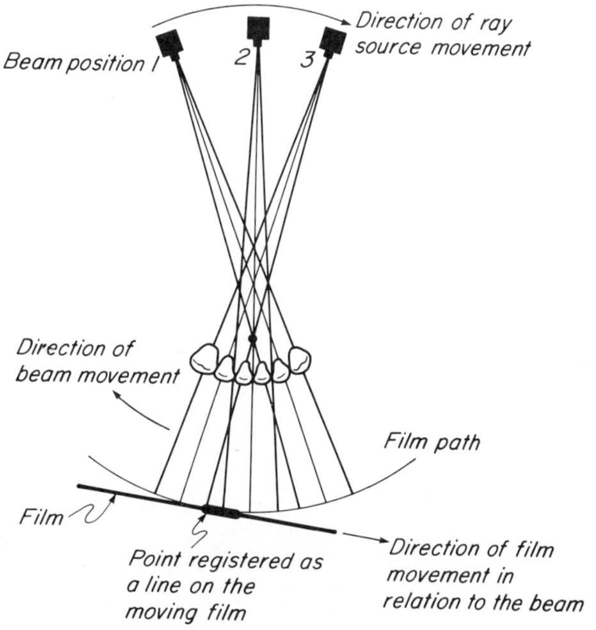

Figure 2–7. Since the film is programmed to follow object points located in the sharply depicted plane (see Fig. 2–6**A**), the speed of the projection of the points on the film does not match. Therefore, such object points will be depicted as lines, although smaller than the distance between A and C along the film path.

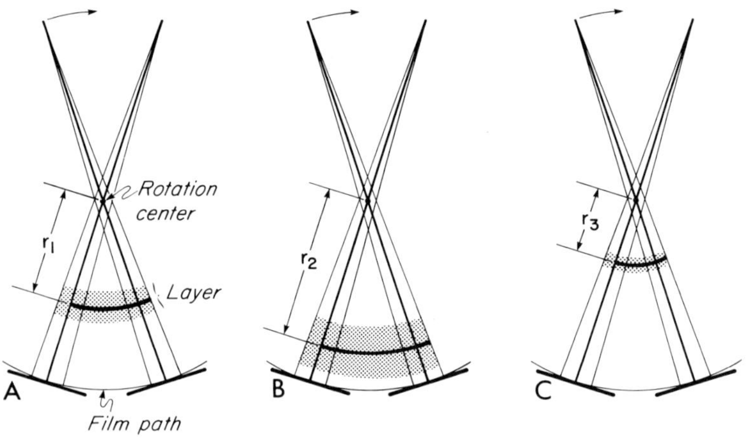

Figure 2–8. **A.** The position of the layer is dependent on the film speed, which is constant in this illustration. **B.** A relative increase in film speed places the layer away from the rotation center. **C.** A relative decrease in the film speed places the layer closer to the rotation center. Note the change in layer thickness between **A, B,** and **C.**

the object may be defined that contains those object points that are depicted with sufficient resolution so that they may be distinguished; this zone is referred to as the image layer.

A constant film speed in relation to the beam places the center of the image layer at a defined distance from the rotation center of the beam (Fig. 2–8**A**). If the speed of the film is increased the position of the layer will be shifted away from the rotation center (Fig. 2–8**B**), and if the speed of the film is decreased the position of the layer will be shifted toward the rotation center (Fig. 2–8**C**). Should the speed of the film not be constant during the exposure but increasing or decreasing, a continuous shift of the position of the layer will take place. Acceleration shifts the position of the layer successively away from the rotation center of the beam (Fig. 2–9**A**). Deceleration shifts the position of the layer successively toward the rotation center (Fig. 2–9**B**).

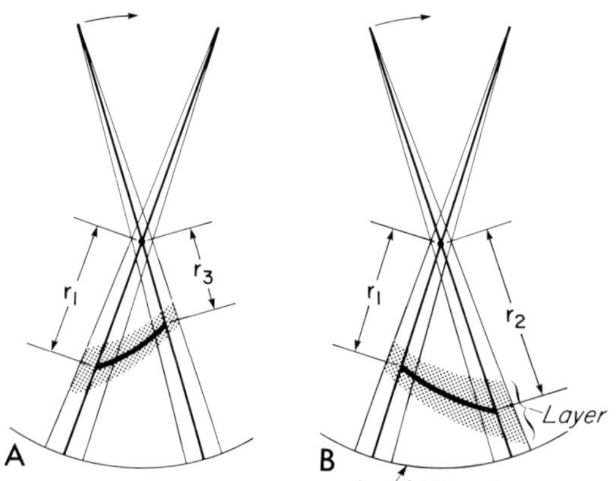

Figure 2–9. **A.** An acceleration of the film speed shifts the layer away from the rotation center. **B.** A deceleration shifts the layer closer to the rotation center. Note the simultaneous successive change in layer thickness.

The distance from the rotation center of the beam to the center of the image layer may be called the effective projection radius (see Figs. 2–8 and 2–9). The thickness of the layer is dependent on the length of this radius; the longer the radius, the thicker the layer. Thus, an altered film speed in relation to the beam not only changes the position of the layer but, indirectly, also the thickness of the layer.

The layer thickness is dependent on several parameters other than the effective projection radius. Among these, the width of the beam is of primary importance, the layer thickness being inversely proportional to the width of the beam. Thus, the layer thickness is doubled if the beam width is reduced by one half. As the beam width approaches zero the layer thickness approaches infinity. Theoretically, the projection technique utilized in rotational panoramic radiography would still work if only a single ray were used, but in this case there would be no layer formation. The image would be sharp at all object depths. It is, therefore, apparent the the formation of a layer, reminiscent of tomography, is a secondary effect in rotational panoramic radiography. Following this line of reasoning, the popular concept of rotational panoramic radiography as a modified form of tomography is questionable. The layer formation is a side effect resulting from the use of a beam of finite width to get an amount of radiation sufficient to expose the film.

PRACTICAL APPLICATION OF THE WORKING PRINCIPLE

BASIC PROJECTION SYSTEMS

So far, the fundamental principles of rotational panoramic radiography have been described assuming that the object is perfectly circular

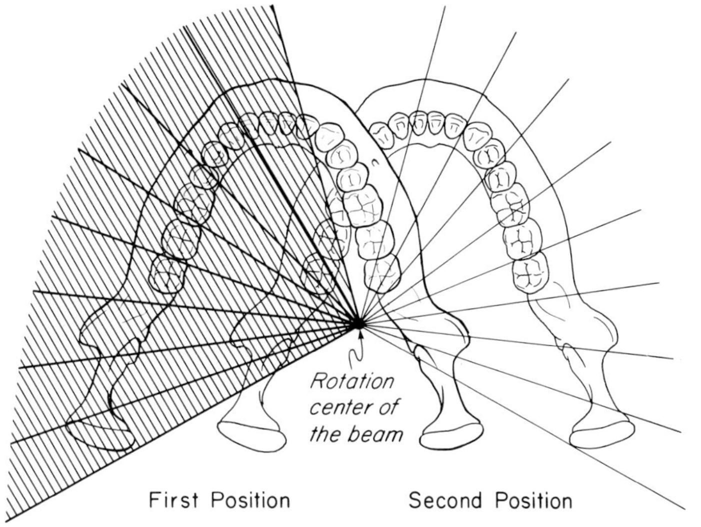

Figure 2–10. The projection of a so-called split image takes place in two sequences. Only one stationary rotation center of the beam is used. By moving the patient, two effective foci, one on each side, are created. (Examples: Panorex II, S. S. White, Dental Products Division, Pennwalt Corp., Phila., PA.)

and that the beam has one stationary rotation center. Since the jaws are not circular, a variety of different movement patterns for the beam have been developed by manufacturers. All of these patterns have one objective in common, namely, to adapt the previously described working principle to create a satisfactory projection of the average jaw. To understand how this is done it is necessary to remember two basic facts mentioned previously: (1) the rotation center of the beam is the functional focus of the projection, and (2) the speed of the film in relation to the beam defines the position of the layer. These two parameters are independent of each other.

The simplest projection technique applied in practice utilizes one stationary rotation center of the beam placed at one side of the jaws projecting the other side of the jaws onto the film (Fig. 2–10). One side of the jaws is exposed at a time and the position of the rotation center, i.e., the functional focus of the projection, is shifted symmetrically between the exposures by moving the patient. This projection technique creates the so-called **split image.**

In systems creating **continuous images,** several different movement patterns of the beam are utilized to achieve the desired projection of the jaws. The objective is to project each part of the jaws as close to perpendicular as possible. Two basically different techniques can be distinguished: (1) the utilization of several combined stationary rotation centers of the beam, and (2) the utilization of a continuously moving rotation center. In practice, many panoramic units have different hybrid movements, i.e., combinations of stationary and moving rotation centers.

STATIONARY ROTATION CENTERS

To produce a continuous image, a combination of three stationary rotation centers may be used (Fig. 2–11). During the exposure the beam first rotates around a laterally positioned rotation center, which serves as the functional focus while the major part of the opposite side is exposed. When the scanning beam approaches the anterior region the rotation center of the beam momentarily shifts to a midline position posterior to the dental arch. The anterior region is exposed with this second rotation center as the functional focus. During the continuous exposure the rotation center is once more shifted so that the movement pattern and,

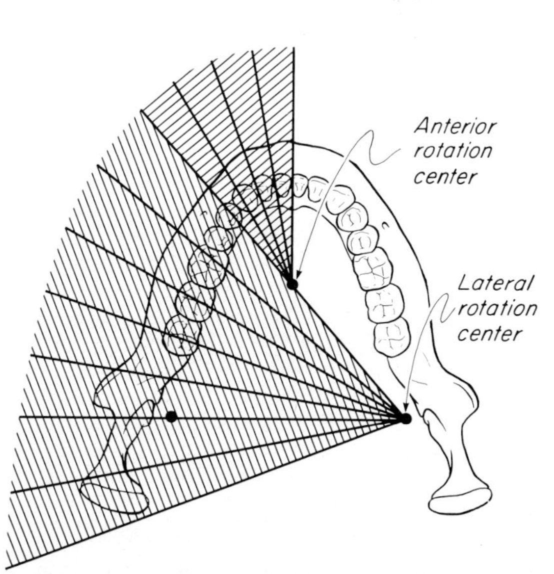

Figure 2–11. The projection of a continuous image utilizing three fixed rotation centers. (Example: Siemens Orthopantomograph, Model OP1.)

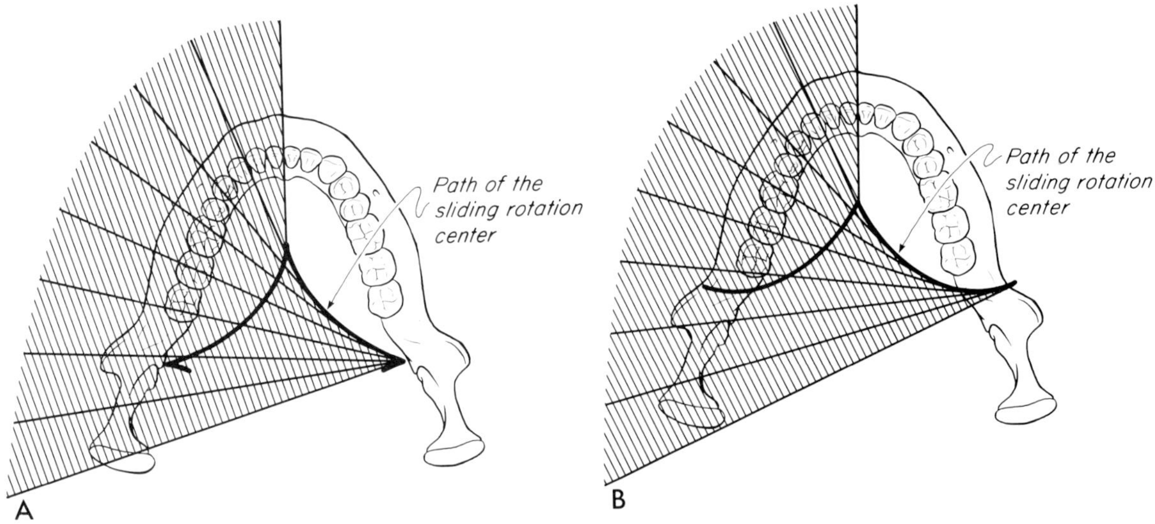

Figure 2–12. The projection of a continuous image utilizing a continuously sliding beam transmission. **A.** Examples: Panelipse; Morita Panex E; and the Sybron/Ritter Panoral. **B.** Example: Siemens Orthopantomograph, Model OP5.

therefore, the projection of the jaws are symmetric on both sides.

CONTINUOUSLY MOVING ROTATION CENTER

It is not necessary for the rotation center of the beam to be stationary at any instant during the exposure. The beam may be given a sliding movement throughout the total excursion (Fig. 2–12) so that the effective projection center, the functional focus, is continuously shifted along a defined path. The central ray of the beam is always tangential to this path at some point. The form of the path defines the direction of the beam and hence the projection of each successive part of the jaws.

COMBINED STATIONARY AND MOVING ROTATION CENTERS

Different combinations of the principal movement patterns described previously have been applied in practice (Fig. 2–13).

FORM AND THICKNESS OF THE IMAGE LAYER

The position and form of the image layer are independent of the movement patterns of the beam discussed previously. These movement patterns serve only to define the projection of the object, i.e., the jaws. Starting from any one of the possible beam movement patterns, the

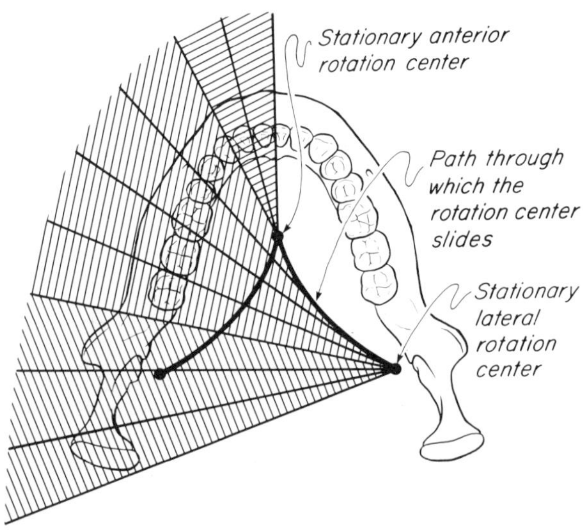

Figure 2–13. The projection of a continuous image utilizing a combination of stationary and moving rotation centers. (Examples: Siemens Orthopantomograph, Models OP2 and OP3; Phillips OrthOralix.)

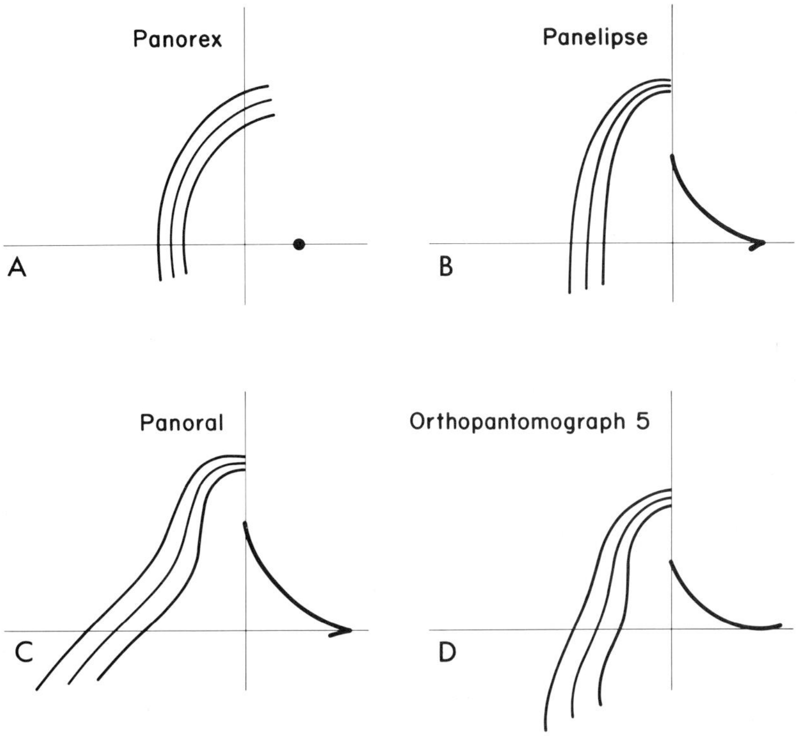

Figure 2–14. Examples of image layers. **A.** S. S. White Panorex 1. **B.** G. E. Panelipse. **C.** Sybron/Ritter Panoral. **D.** Siemens Orthopantomograph, Model OP5.

image layer may, in principle, be given any desired form and position by applying the proper film speed at each moment during the exposure. The faster the film moves in relation to the beam, the farther away from the rotation center is the center of the image layer.

By adjusting the film speed to place the layer at will, several basic layer forms have been built into commercial devices used in practice. These forms are all different approximations of the average form of the jaws (Fig. 2–14).

It has been pointed out previously that the layer thickness is highly dependent on the length of the effective projection radius. It follows that the layer thickness will vary in different regions in the panoramic radiograph. In the split image the projection radius varies only to a limited extent throughout the excursion, but it is slightly longer in the anterior region than in the lateral regions. Therefore, the split image has a layer thickness that is approximately the same all over the image, only slightly wider in the anterior region (see Fig. 2–14**A**). In the continuous image the projection radius is always short in the anterior region, and, consequently, the layer is more narrow in this region than in the lateral regions (Fig. 2–14**B**, **C**, and **D**).

BASIC IMAGE CHARACTERISTICS

The ideal panoramic radiograph should portray the primary object, the jaws, and all its different details without significant unsharpness or distortion. Since this ideal does not exist in practice, it is important to know within what limits the real panoramic radiograph is reliable when the diagnostic information is evaluated.

Most panoramic units have only one predesigned beam movement and one fixed form of the layer, adapted to an estimated average jaw. There are a few exceptions to this rule; the size, but not the form, of the image layer may, for instance, be changed in the General Electric Panelipse. However, in rotational panoramic radiography in general, the patient must be positioned as accurately as possible in a fixed system. The normal variations in the form and size of the individual jaw inevitably mean that some patients will not fit into the predesigned form of the image layer of a certain unit. Some parts of the jaws may be positioned outside the image layer, being displaced either toward the film or toward the rotation center of the beam. This will be visible in the radiograph both by unsharpness and by certain distortion effects that are typical of rotational panoramic radiography. Exactly the same effects will appear in the image when a patient is malpositioned in the unit, however close to the average the patient may be.

It will be shown that a correctly exposed panoramic radiograph, within certain limits, gives a reliable image of the object morphology. Knowledge of the appearance of ghost images, the characteristic distortion phenomena, and of the expected effects of unsharpness is, however, necessary if the form of an object or an object detail is assessed during the interpretation of the radiograph or if any measurements are carried out.

GHOST IMAGES

All objects or object details scanned by the beam in rotational panoramic radiography will be projected onto the film. This is also true regarding all structures positioned on the side of the jaws opposite the side within the layer, which is of primary interest. Objects with a high attenuation may, in certain instances, be observed in two positions in the panoramic radiograph. Only one of these images is intended, and the other is usually referred to as a **ghost image.** The projection of ghost images is explained schematically in Figure 2–15.

The ghost image is recognized by an unsharpness, which, in the horizontal dimension, is marked. Moreover, the ghost image is always projected at a higher position in the radiograph than its real counterpart. This results from the beam being directed from below. One important feature of ghost images is that they are always reversed, left and right being shifted. The explanation for this is that the ghost images are projected onto the film from a position on that side of the rotation center of the beam in which the direction of the beam movement is opposite that of the movement by which the beam is scanning the object layer of interest.

IMAGE DISTORTION

With a knowledge of the characteristic distortion effects of rotational panoramic radiography, it is possible to utilize the image to decide in what way and in what direction a patient has been malpositioned in the unit or in what way an individual differs from the average jaw used in the design of the unit. This information may be used to correct the positioning of the patient when retaking the radiograph or to correct distortion effects when evaluating the diagnostic information in the radiograph.

All the different distortion effects in panoramic radiographs are based on the fact that the vertical dimensions in the image are dependent on a projection that has the ray source as the focus, whereas the horizontal dimensions are dependent on a projection that has the rotation center of the beam as the functional focus. The horizontal dimensions are further affected by the speed of the film in relation to the beam.

In the vertical dimension the magnification factor varies relatively little with the object

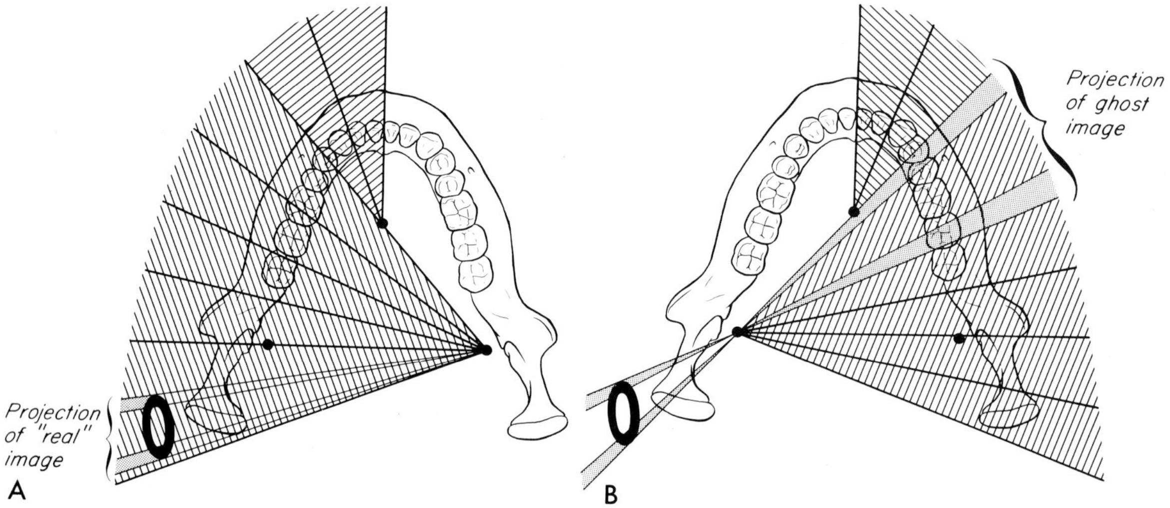

Figure 2–15. **A.** The real projection of an earring. **B.** The reversed ghost image is projected when the opposite side is scanned by the beam.

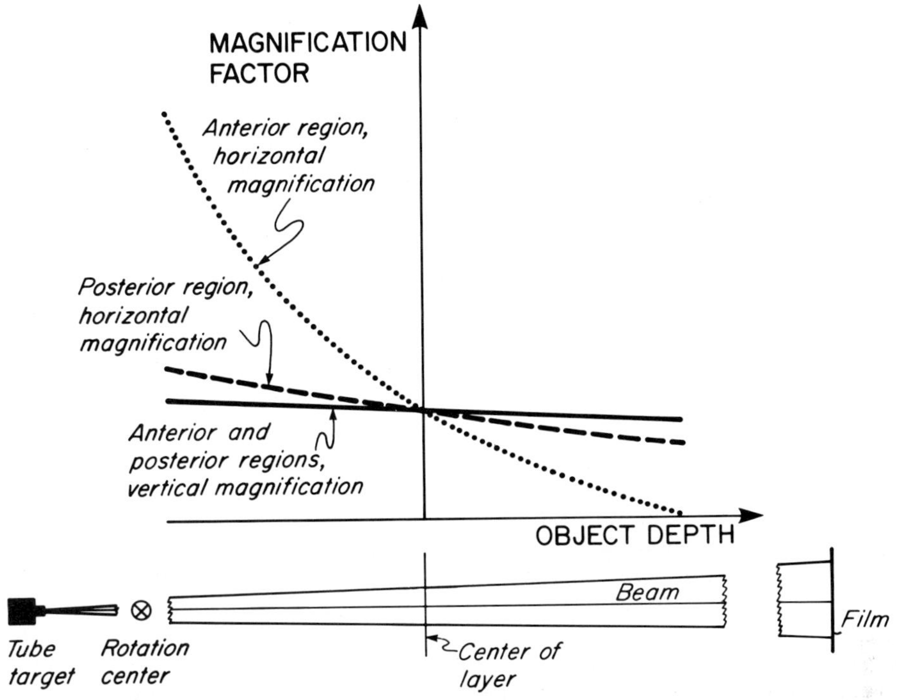

Figure 2–16. Variation in horizontal and vertical magnification factors with object depth.

depth. The magnification factor in the horizontal dimension increases markedly with the distance from the center of the layer toward the rotation center of the beam. Moving toward the film the magnification factor decreases, but this decrease is less marked than the increase on the opposite side. The variation with the distance from the center of the layer is more marked in regions where the effective projection radius is short than where it is long. Thus, the magnification outside the layer varies more in the anterior region of a continuous image than in the lateral regions. The vertical and horizontal magnification factors are identical at the center of the image layer (Fig. 2–16).

GENERAL PRINCIPLE OF DISTORTION

Since the magnification factors in the vertical and horizontal dimensions are the same at the center of the layer, there is no distortion in the image of this layer. A square and a circle placed at the center of the layer are portrayed as a square and a circle, respectively, in the image. Outside the center of the layer distortion effects appear that are characteristic of rotational panoramic radiography. These effects are easily explained and understood if a series of square planes in the object are considered (Fig. 2–17**A**). The central square will be projected with correct proportions in the image, whereas

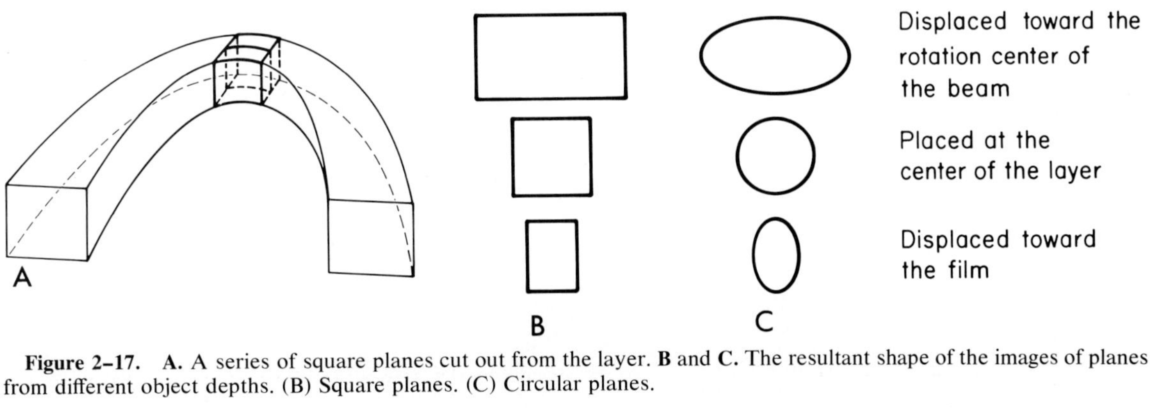

Figure 2–17. **A.** A series of square planes cut out from the layer. **B** and **C.** The resultant shape of the images of planes from different object depths. (B) Square planes. (C) Circular planes.

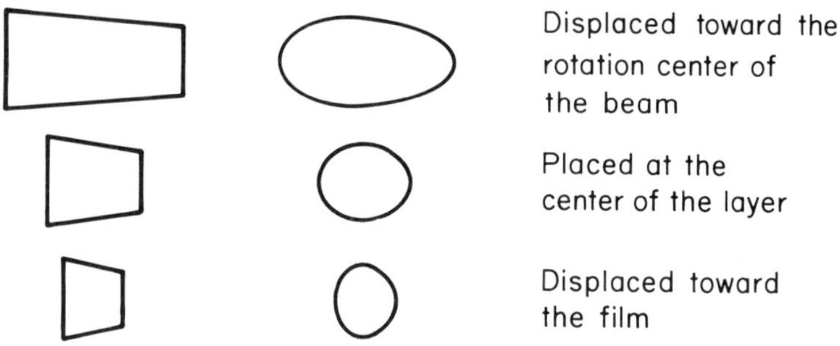

Figure 2–18. Image distortion resulting from a varying magnification within the radiograph and/or a varying effective projection radius.

squares positioned outside the layer will be magnified or diminished and distorted at the same time. Squares positioned toward the rotation center of the beam will be magnified more in the horizontal than in the vertical dimension. Therefore, they will be portrayed in the image with a rectangular form, the long axis being horizontal (Fig. 2–17**B**). Squares positioned toward the film will be diminished more in the horizontal than in the vertical dimension. These squares will also appear rectangular in the image, but their long axis will be vertical (see Fig. 2–17**B**). Circular cross sections at different object depths in a sphere will be distorted in analogous ways, but outside the center of the layer they will appear as ellipses (Fig. 2–17**C**).

This distortion principle holds true only in a circular movement system with a stationary rotation center. In the real radiograph, the overall magnification of the image may affect the basic distortion phenomena described previously. In several commercially available units the focus-to-object distance, i.e., the distance from the ray source to the center on the image layer, varies, whereas the focus-to-film distance is always constant. A varied focus-to-object distance results in a variation in overall magnification in different regions of the image. This will usually cause minor distortion effects but the principal result is illustrated in Figure 2–18. In the case of the square cross sections, all planes will be nonsymmetrical in the image, one end having a greater magnification than the other. In the case of the circular cross sections, ovoid forms will be created.

In all units the effective projection radius varies throughout the excursion. On circular cross sections of the object this will, principally, have the same effect as a variation in the focus-to-object distance (see Fig. 2–18). However, as long as the focus-to-object distance is constant the height dimension in the image remains the same. This means that a varied projection radius during the exposure changes the horizontal dimensions slightly, whereas the vertical dimensions remain the same. With respect to square cross sections, this means that rectangular forms are still to be expected.

So far, the principal distortions in the images of differently positioned object planes have been demonstrated separately for each plane. In the radiograph these planes, of course, overlap, and, since the angle of the beam is directed slightly from below, the overlapping planes will be somewhat displaced in relation to each other. The displacement is greater in the upper jaw than in the lower jaw because of a greater angulation of the rays intercepting the object (Fig. 2–19).

Distortion effects encountered for the whole object follow the same pattern: all planes will be magnified and distorted if the whole object is displaced toward the rotation center of the beam, and they will be diminished and distorted when displaced toward the film (Fig. 2–20).

The distortion effects in panoramic radiographs may be divided into some specific groups having different significance in the interpretation of the image. All of them have their explanation in the previously mentioned principal geometric effects.

In the following discussion, the main distortion effects will be outlined and some general considerations on the reliability of the panoramic radiograph with respect to certain measurements and to the evaluation of object morphology will be given. It is not possible to present universally applicable limits within which the

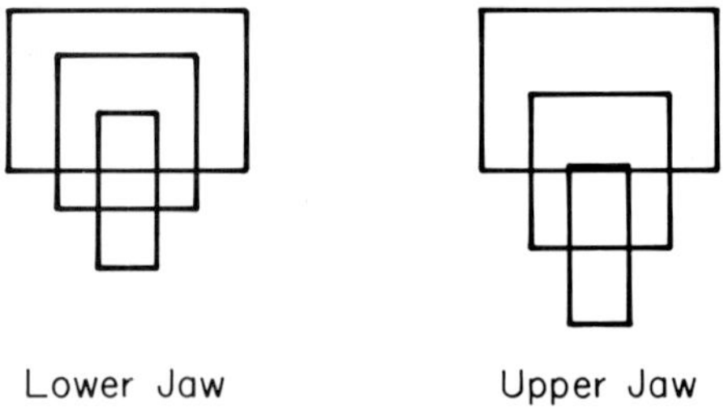

Figure 2–19. Schematic representation of the image of superimposed planes from different object depths.

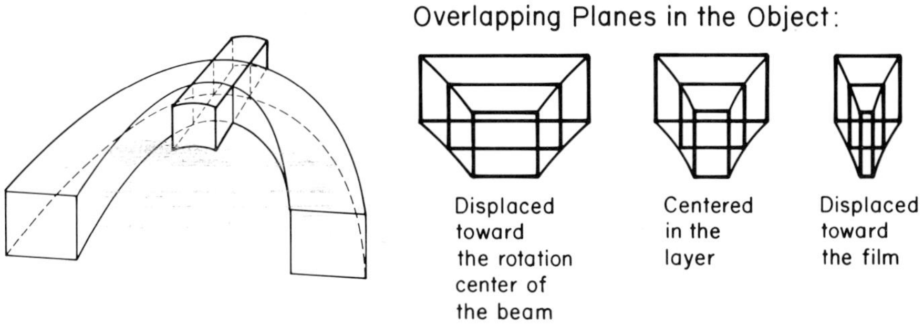

Figure 2–20. Schematic representation of the images of a cuboid object when positioned at different object depths.

panoramic radiograph is reliable, since these limits will vary with different units and, in most instances, with different regions in the same radiograph. They will also be highly dependent on the patient's position in the unit during the exposure and on how close the individual jaw conforms to the shape of the image layer in a specific unit. **Therefore, the statements that follow regarding the reliability of the panoramic radiograph refer only to the perfectly exposed image in which there is no marked distortion or unsharpness.**

LINEAR DISTORTION

The horizontal dimensions in a panoramic radiograph are very unreliable. It has been shown previously that the magnification factor in this dimension is a nonlinear function of the object depth (see Fig. 2–16), which varies in different regions of the image. As a result, two identical object details positioned at equal distances from the center of the layer but in different regions will have different horizontal dimensions in the image. The horizontal dimensions in the continuous panoramic radiographs are especially unreliable in the anterior region. The conclusion must be that, in general, the horizontal dimensions should not be relied upon, and horizontal distances should not be measured in panoramic radiographs.

The situation is somewhat different in the case of the vertical dimension. The magnification factor in this dimension varies with the object depth, but the variation is moderate (see Fig. 2–16). In units that have a constant or nearly constant distance between the ray source and the center of the layer throughout the excursion, the vertical magnification factor at a certain object depth is the same throughout the image. In units where this distance varies from region to region, the magnification at a certain depth in the object also varies with the regions. In this case, this variation is usually not very marked. It may therefore be concluded that vertical measurements can be performed in panoramic radiographs as long as only those distances are measured that, from anatomic considerations, are known to be near vertical. If such measurements are divided by the overall magnification factor in the unit, a distance such as that between the maxillary sinus and the alveolar crest may be estimated. An estimate of this kind may only be used for practical clinical purposes, and an error in the vicinity of ±10 per cent must be accepted.

Only a few distances of interest in clinical work are either vertical or horizontal. Most of them will be oblique in the object. In such instances the distortion to be expected may be demonstrated by studying the image of a line in the object (Fig. 2–21). Depending on the position of this line in relation to the center of the layer, on the region where it is located, on the inclination of the line, and so on, the degree of distortion will vary within relatively wide limits, but in all cases the line will appear curved in the image. It follows that distances between obliquely positioned object details or the length of inclined objects or object details cannot be relied upon in panoramic radiographs.

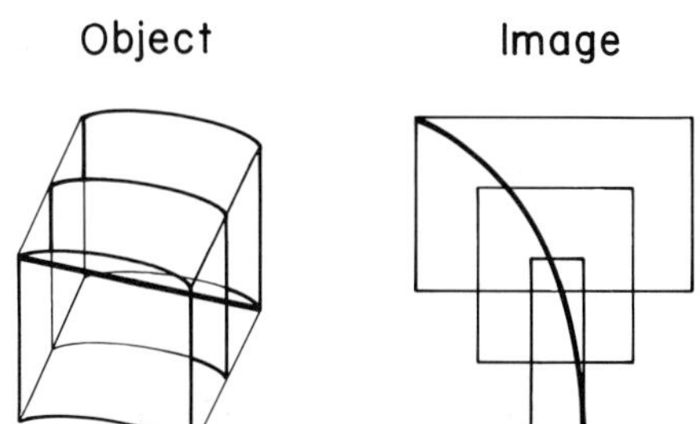

Figure 2–21. A straight line that passes through several object depths will appear as a curved line in the image.

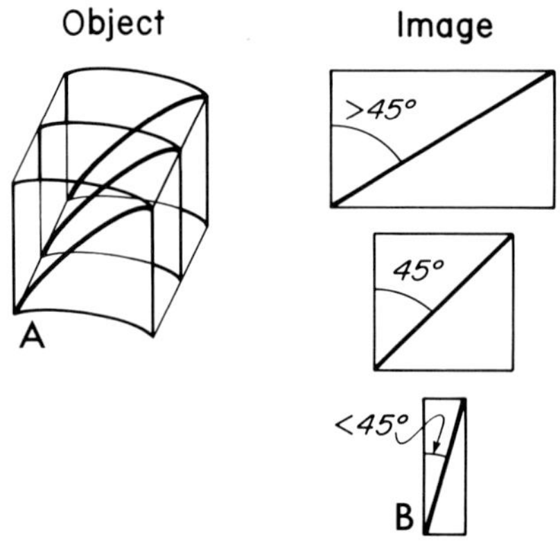

Figure 2–22. **A.** Images of diagonal lines from different object depths. **B.** As they would appear in a panoramic radiograph.

ANGLE DISTORTION

The angle in the image between inclined objects, such as teeth, will be dependent on the combined effects of the vertical and horizontal dimensions in the panoramic radiograph. When discussing the linear distortion, it was concluded that measurements in the horizontal dimension should never be performed or relied upon. In spite of this, angular measurements may be performed in panoramic radiographs.

Consider once again the series of square planes cut out from the object (Fig. 2–22). If the diagonal line is added to all the planes, a series of inclined model objects are created that have an inclination of 45° to the vertical plane. The images of the planes from different object depths, as they would appear in a panoramic radiograph, are illustrated in Figure 2–22**B** with the diagonal line added. In planes positioned toward the rotation center of the beam, the angle to the vertical plane in the image increases with the distance from the center of the layer. The opposite is true for object planes positioned toward the film. In this case, the angle to the vertical plane decreases with the distance from the center of the layer. Thus, an inclined object will be portrayed in the image with an angle that does not truly reflect the angle in the object. This is defined as angle distortion.

The angle distortion is much more marked in the anterior region of a continuous panoramic radiograph than in the lateral regions. In the lateral regions of a continuous image or in a full split image, the angle distortion is, in fact, small. If an error of, for instance, ±5° is tolerated — and such an error may be considered insignificant for most practical clinical purposes — angular measurements may be performed in the radiographs, and the obtained values are reliable. In the anterior region this is more critical. However, the previous statement still holds true if measurements are only performed in correctly exposed panoramic radiographs. If distortion effects or unsharpness is evident in the image, an angular measurement cannot be relied upon. Moreover, angular measurements may only be performed between nearby objects or object details that are portrayed in the same region of the radiograph.

Angular distortion is greatest for inclinations of 45° in the mesiodistal direction, decreasing continuously as the angle of inclination decreases or increases. For object details inclined 0 or 90° to the vertical plane, there is no angle distortion, only linear distortion.

One very important feature has not yet been discussed, namely, the effect of adding an inclination in the third dimension, i.e., the buccolingual direction. It may seem surprising, but buccolingual inclinations affect the angle distortion only to a limited extent. Only very marked buccolingual inclinations will deteriorate angular measurements. The explanation of this fact is simple. If a diagonal line is added to the previously illustrated cut-out planes in the object, a model object is created that is inclined 45° in all three planes in the object space (see Fig. 2–21). The image of this diagonal line will be curved, but its average angle to the vertical plane is still near 45°. Magnification on one side of the center of the layer is balanced by diminution on the other side.

Summing up, the angle distortion in panoramic radiographs is usually not greater than what can be accepted for measurements in clinical practice, but it must be repeatedly emphasized that these measurements are only reliable if performed in accurately exposed panoramic radiographs. It must also be remembered that the panoramic radiograph, like any other radiograph, is a two-dimensional image. An angular measurement gives the angle in one plane only. To evaluate the position and inclination of an object, such as an impacted tooth, at least one more projection is necessary.

FORM DISTORTION

The term form distortion refers to the way the object morphology is represented in the panoramic radiograph. Within this overall category, a distinction has to be made between the distor-

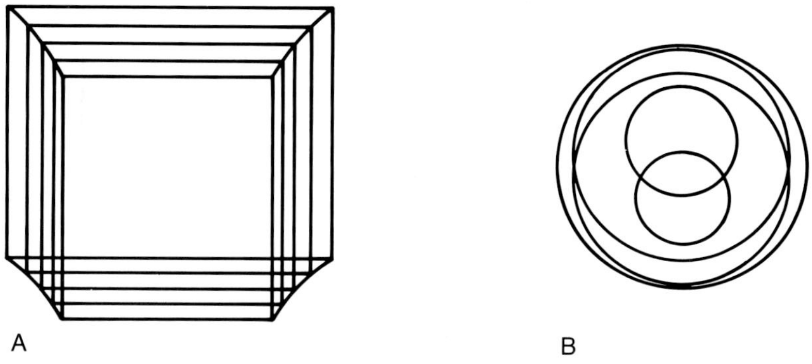

Figure 2–23. The image distortion is dependent on the form of the object; the rounder the form the less the distortion.

tion of the outer contour of different objects and the distortion and displacement of the inner structures of the objects.

The degree of distortion of the outer contour of an object in rotational panoramic radiography will depend on the form of the object itself. The more rounded the object, the more accurate is its representation in the image. This phenomenon is illustrated in Figure 2–23. Figure 2–23**A** illustrates once again the displacement and distortion of successive squares cut out from the image layer. The complete outer contour is now marked. The complete form is quite different from the sum of the squares that it represents. In Figure 2–23**B** an analogous series of cross sections cut out from a spherical volume in the layer are demonstrated. In this case the distorted planes fall mainly within the contour of the central cut. The sphere, centered in the layer, will appear basically circular in the two-dimensional image. Although the sphere, strictly speaking, is slightly distorted, this is hardly perceptible to the eye.

Since most objects within the jaws are more or less rounded, the sphere seems to be a good model to illustrate form distortion. The distortion effects to be expected when a spherical object is placed at different distances from the center of the layer are essentially the same as those for the circular object (Fig. 2–24). The spherical object will be portrayed as a distorted form resembling an ellipse. The ellipsoid image will have its long axis horizontally when the spherical object is displaced toward the rotation center of the beam. When the spherical object is displaced toward the film, the image will have its long axis vertically. There are relatively wide tolerance limits against form distortion, much wider in the lateral regions of a continuous image than in the anterior region. The tolerance limits regarding form distortion are, however, far less than those for angle distortion.

As in the case of circular objects, compressed or asymmetrically elongated forms can be expected when spherical objects are positioned in regions in which the effective projection radius varies during the exposure, i.e., during the time in which the beam scans the spherical object (see Fig. 2–18).

The inner structures of an object will suffer from both distortion and displacement when portrayed in the panoramic radiograph. A model object, symbolizing a trabecular pattern, may be created by once again cutting out planes from the layer and adding a random distribution of small squares to each plane (Fig. 2–25**A**). The sum of the series of planes results in a pattern such as that illustrated in Figure 2–25**B**. In Figure 2–25**C**, **D**, and **E**, the distorted pattern is demonstrated as it may appear in a panoramic radiograph. The three different patterns repre-

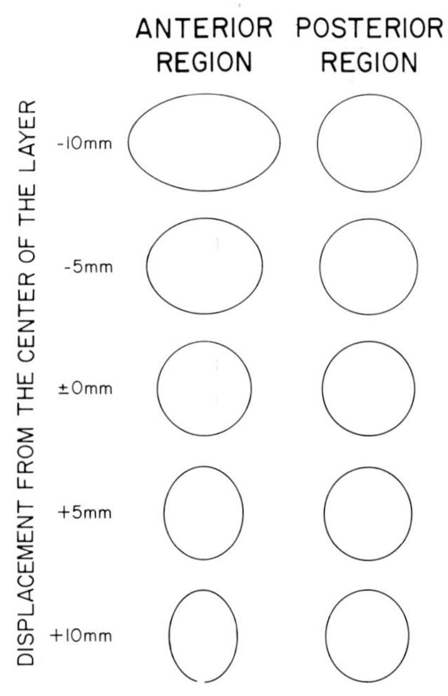

Figure 2–24. The distortion of a spherical object when positioned at different object depths in different regions of the jaws.

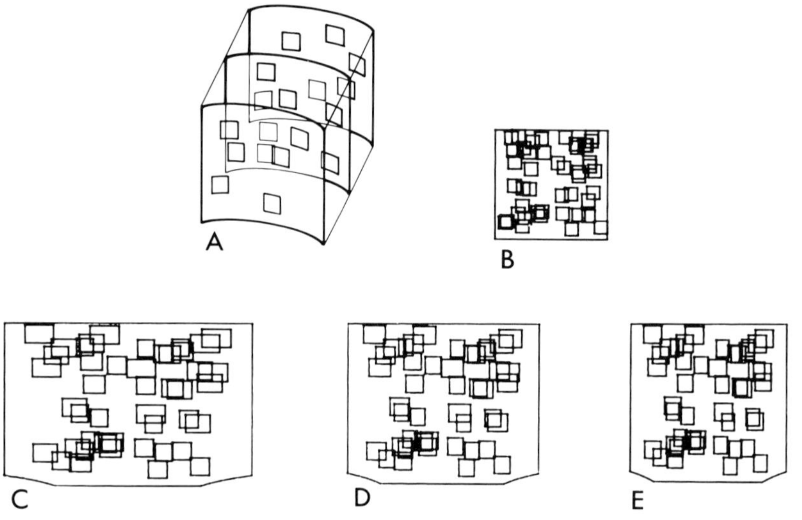

Figure 2–25. Distortion effects in a model of a trabecular pattern.

sent the images of the model object when it is placed at the center of the layer (**D**), toward the film (**E**), and toward the rotation center of the beam (**C**). Although the pattern is affected by the distortion effects inherent in rotational panoramic radiography, it is evident that the overall pattern can still be recognized.

The distortion effects in panoramic radiographs are dependent on a long series of parameters such as the distance between the ray source and the film, the distance between the ray source and the center of the layer, the effective projection radius, the speed of the film in relation to the beam, and the angle of the beam to the horizontal plane. There are many different panoramic units available on the market, and in all such units these parameters are different. Furthermore, the different distortion effects are, as has been shown, dependent on a particular object's position in relation to the layer and within the jaws. Because of the many variables involved in an analysis of the image distortion, the previous statements on the distortion and reliability of the panoramic radiograph are very generalized. An analysis of the distortion effects in rotational panoramic radiography indicates that when the panoramic technique is used at its optimum it gives, in many respects, an accurate and reliable representation of the object morphology.

UNSHARPNESS

In rotational panoramic radiography, a distinction should be made between the absolute unsharpness and the relative unsharpness in the image. The absolute unsharpness may be defined as the total projected length in the image of a point in the object. The absolute unsharpness increases continuously from the center of the sharply depicted object plane, i.e., the center of the layer (Fig. 2–26). This increase with distance from the center of the layer is more marked toward the rotation center of the beam than toward the film.

The relative unsharpness is found by dividing the absolute unsharpness of the image in the horizontal dimension by the magnification factor. The relative unsharpness is a linear function of the distance from the center of the layer, and it is symmetric on both sides of the layer (see Fig. 2–26).

Since the absolute and the relative unsharpness increase continuously outside the center of the layer, there are no distinct borders of the layer. The thickness of the layer may be defined in many ways. One common definition assumes that an unsharpness of, for instance, 0.3 or 0.5 mm may be considered tolerable. Since the magnification factor is different in different units, the relative unsharpness should be used when defining the layer thickness (Fig. 2–27). In this way, the effect of the magnification is eliminated, and the resulting values of the layer thickness are comparable from unit to unit.

In regions in which the effective projection radius is short, the unsharpness increases more markedly with increased distance from the center of the layer than when the projection radius is long (Fig. 2–28). This is the reason for the layer thickness being much less in the anterior than in the lateral regions in continuous panoramic radiographs.

Unsharpness in a panoramic radiograph is an indication that the patient has been malpositioned in the unit during the exposure or that the individual patient does not fit into the predesigned layer of the unit. The degree of unsharp-

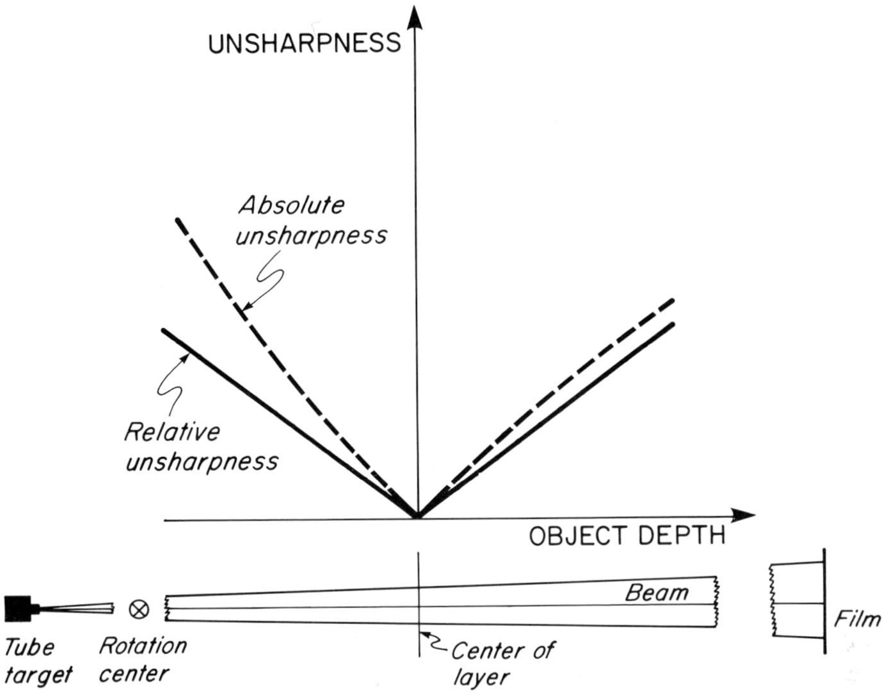

Figure 2–26. Diagrammatic representation of absolute and relative unsharpness as functions of object depth.

ness gives an indication of the magnitude of the discrepancy between the center of the layer and the patient's position.

Preferably, the layer thickness in rotational panoramic radiography should be great enough so that the whole depth of the jaws, which in themselves constitute a layer, can be sharply depicted in the image. This condition is never realized in practice. The layer is so narrow, especially in the anterior region of continuous

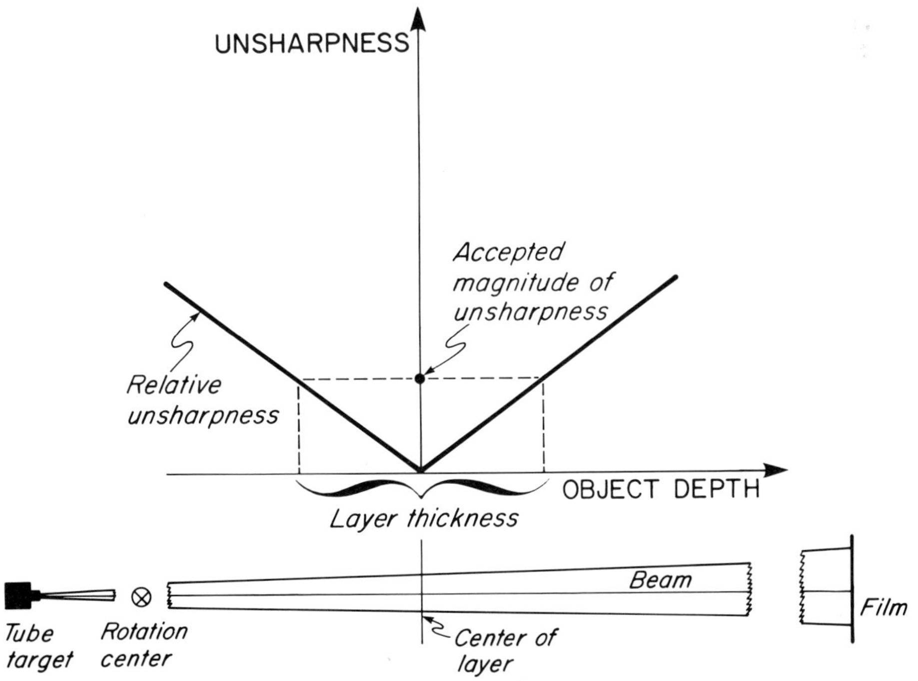

Figure 2–27. The layer thickness is defined by the accepted magnitude of unsharpness.

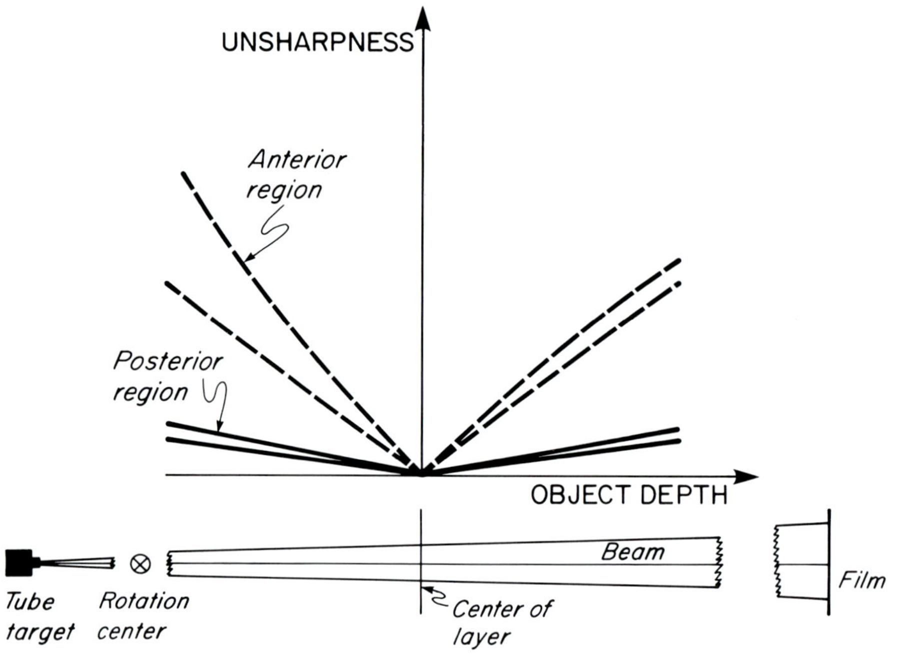

Figure 2–28. The absolute and relative unsharpness as functions of the object depth in different regions of the jaws.

images, that the position of the patient is critical. Unsharpness in this region, which decreases the diagnostic accuracy, is a frequent experience in clinical work with rotational panoramic radiography. Thus, although the unsharpness may be disturbing it is usually not great enough to conceal large object details. However, it may happen that a malpositioned tooth may be difficult or impossible to detect in the image if it is positioned toward the rotation center of the beam and at a great distance from the center of the layer. Unsharpness alone does not cause this effect in the image. The extreme magnification of objects displaced toward the rotation center is also a contributing factor.

CLINICAL NOTE

The unsharpness and the distortion effects are important criteria when evaluating panoramic radiographs. The fact that the teeth in a certain region appear too broad as compared with their length indicates, together with unsharpness, that this region has been malpositioned toward the rotation center of the beam during the exposure. A narrowing of the teeth, on the other hand, together with the accompanying unsharpness indicates that the region in question has been malpositioned toward the film during the exposure. This information is easily used to correct the patient's position when a retake shall be made.

Generally, if there is no significant unsharpness and distortion in a region of a panoramic radiograph or in the whole radiograph, this indicates that the image is essentially reliable when evaluating the morphology of normal or pathologically changed structures. Those measurements that may be relied upon (for instance, angular measurements) may be performed in such a panoramic radiograph.

Chapter 3

Biologic Effects of Panoramic Radiography

John W. Preece

RADIATION MEASUREMENT

UNITS OF MEASUREMENT

Dental x rays are a form of electromagnetic radiation; they are considered small invisible bundles or packets of pure energy called photons that travel through space in a wavelike fashion. Photons lose their energy by having it absorbed during collisions with the orbital electrons of any substance they come in contact with. When the energy of the absorbed x-ray photon exceeds the binding energy of the orbital electron, the electron will be propelled out of its orbit and can interact in a variety of ways with the nucleus and electrons of other atoms of absorbing material. The ability of x rays to remove electrons from substances is called ionization, and it is this process that permits the detection and quantitative measurement of radiation. In addition, ionization is the initiating event for all biologic damage.

The terms used to measure x-radiation are based on the photon's ability to deposit its energy in air, tissue, or other tissue-equivalent substances. Today, the most easily recognizable terms used to measure x-radiation are the roentgen, rad, and rem; however, the period between 1980 and 1985 will mark a changeover from these older units of radiation measurement to the new international system of units: the coulomb/kilogram (C/kg) (for the roentgen), gray (Gy) (for the rad), and sievert (Sv) (for the rem). Each of these units will be discussed briefly and their interrelationships described.

ROENTGEN (COULOMB/KILOGRAM)

The special unit of exposure is the roentgen (R). It is based on the ability of x radiation to ionize air molecules. The roentgen is defined and used only when measuring x- or gamma radiation and is the amount of radiation producing roughly 1.6×10^{12} ion pairs per gram of air. By performing the appropriate computations and conversions, an exposure of 1 roentgen can be demonstrated to be equivalent to a charge of 2.58×10^{-4}C/kg; this is the new exposure unit in the international system.

RAD (GRAY)

The rad is the special unit of absorbed dose and is used to describe the energy absorbed

TABLE 3–1. UNITS OF RADIATION EQUIVALENCE

Old Terminology					New Terminology			
*roentgen** *(R)*	*milliroentgens (mR)*	*rad/rem*	*millirad(s)†* *(mrad)*	*coulombs/kg (C/kg)*	*gray (Gy)*	*sievert (Sv)*	*Sv or Gy*	*Sv or Gy*
Exposure		*Absorbed Dose/Dose Equivalence*						
100	100,000	100	100,000	258×10^{-2}	1	1	1	
10	10,000	10	10,000	25.8×10^{-3}	0.1	0.1	10^{-1}	1 deci-Sv or Gy dSv or dGy
1	1,000	1	1,000	2.58×10^{-4}	0.01	0.01	10^{-2}	1 centi-cSv or cGy
0.1	100	0.1	100	2.58×10^{-5}	0.001	0.001	10^{-3}	1 milli-mSv or mGy
0.01	10	0.01	10	2.58×10^{-6}	0.0001	0.0001	10^{-4}	.1 milli- or 0.01 micro-mSv or mGy
0.001	1	0.001	1	2.58×10^{-7}	0.00001	0.00001	10^{-5}	.01 milli- or 0.1 micro-mSv or mGy
0.0001	0.1	0.0001	0.1					

*Technically, 1R = 0.87 rads or 86 ergs or 0.0086 J/kg; therefore 1.14R = 1 rad = 100 ergs = 0.01 J/kg in air.
†For x-rays, millirads and millirem are equivalent.

Notes: Roentgen and coulombs/kg are units of radiation exposure. Rad and gray are units of absorbed dose. Rem and sievert are units of biologic dose.

from all types of ionizing radiations (alpha, beta, gamma, x, neutron) by one gram of tissue. The rad is, by definition, equivalent to the deposition of 100 ergs of energy per gram of tissue. One roentgen is equivalent to 86.9 ergs per gram of air. In the new international system, the gray (Gy) is the unit of absorbed dose, and it is expressed in joules/kilogram (J/kg). One gray is equal to 1 joule/kilogram; 1 rad is equal to 0.01 joule/kilogram. An absorbed dose of 1 gray is therefore equivalent to 100 rads or 114 roentgens.

REM (SIEVERT)

It can be demonstrated experimentally that an absorbed dose of one type of radiation will not produce the same biologic effect as the same dose of another type of x-radiation. The radiobiological equivalent (RBE) is used to permit comparison of the biologic effectiveness of one type of radiation with a standard or test radiation in producing the same biologic effect, e.g., erythema, cataract formation, carcinogenesis, and so on. When the RBE is multiplied by the absorbed dose in rads a new unit is produced, the rem. The rem is the unit of dose equivalence and quantitatively expresses the biologic damage produced in an exposed individual on a common scale. Thus, a dose of 300 rem would be expected to produce an equivalent amount of biologic damage regardless of the type of radiation used. The RBE for x rays is 1; therefore, an absorbed dose of 1 rad and 1 rem are equivalent. In the new international unit system, the sievert is the unit of dose equivalence (gray × RBE = sievert [Sv]); for x-radiation, the gray and sievert are equivalent. One sievert is equal to 100 rem.

The roentgen, rad, and rem are quantitatively relatively large units. However, it is desirable to use smaller, more convenient units of measurement to describe the amount of radiation to patients from dental radiography. These smaller units are the *milli*roentgen, the *milli*rad, and the *milli*rem; they are equivalent to one-thousandth (1/1000) of a roentgen, rad, and rem, respectively. Table 3–1 lists equivalent units in both the old and new radiation unit systems.

Since it is difficult to conceptualize a quantity of radiation because it is invisible and we cannot see the ionization and energy deposition within the tissue, it may be useful, therefore, to consider a unit of radiation as a glass jar containing 1000 grains of rice; the entire container would be equivalent to the radiation unit, for example, a roentgen. One grain of rice from this container would represent in relative terms the quantitative difference between one roentgen and one milliroentgen. Quantitatively, one gray or sievert would be equivalent to 100,000 grains of rice.

RADIATION MEASUREMENT AND DOSIMETRY

Various methods have been developed to quantitatively measure radiation dose to the patient; some of these procedures are rather simple, whereas others require sophisticated, highly complex computer programs. Each method has its own advantages and disadvantages, and virtually all measuring methods provide only an approximation of patient dose. For a variety of legitimate reasons, literature references to patient dose from rotational panoramic radiography seldom agree because small differences in dosimeter location significantly affect the recorded dose.

At present, the most frequently used method to measure patient dose is through the use of thermoluminescent dosimetry (TLD), using small chips or capsules. The primary clinical advantage of this type of measuring system is that the dosimeters are small, relatively energy independent, and accurate over a wide range of radiation doses and they can be positioned in a variety of intra- and extraoral locations using patients or phantoms. The dose to various anatomic sites by various authors using TLD is reported for four rotational panoramic units (Tables 3–2 to 3–4). These measurements will be used in the discussion of potential risks associated with this type of radiographic procedure.

Efforts have been made to estimate the total energy absorbed by the patient during rotational panoramic procedures. Van Aken estimated a total dose of approximately 110 gram rads (110 grams of tissue received an average dose of 1 rad), whereas Sakamaki and associates reported a total dose of 896 gram rads. Both estimates were derived using different models of the Orthopantomograph, and each investigator used different methods for determining the total dose imparted to the patient. Such wide variations in results dramatically emphasize the difficulties encountered in attempting to quantitatively assess patient dose distribution and make the estimation of potential biologic risk difficult at best.

TABLE 3–2. DOSE IN MILLIRADS/MILLIREM FOR THE PANOREX I*

Anatomic Site	Author, Date *Kuba and Beck 1968*	*Weissman 1972*	*Bushong 1973*	*Altonen, Heikkilä, and Mattila 1974*	*Manson-Hing and Greer 1977*	*Wall et al. 1978*
Lens	27	7	24	7	6	2
Pituitary	45	11	–	36	8	–
Thyroid	37	14	27	28	22	2
First molar	–	22	–	–	40	–
Upper lip (midline)	–	14	–	–	9	11
Skin, back of neck (midline)	–	–	203	–	33	6
Parotid	354	366	–	266	60	87
Mandibular symphysis	–	–	22	9	20	–
Cervical spine	55	–	–	26	–	–
Submandibular gland	220	45	–	–	800	–
Highest dose (any site)	614	485	278	682	2419	220

*S. S. White, Dental Division, Pennwalt Corp., Philadelphia, PA.

TABLE 3–3. DOSE IN MILLIRADS/MILLIREMS FOR THE ORTHOPANTOMOGRAPH*

Anatomic Site	Author, Date, Model *Casebow 1973 NS†*	*Altonen, Heikkilä, and Mattila 1974 NS*	*Antoku et al. 1976 OP-2*	*Manson-Hing and Greer 1977 NS*	*Myers et al. 1978 OP-2*	*Wall et al. 1979 OP-G*
Lens	–	9	6	7	2	2
Pituitary	–	36	27	33	–	–
Thyroid	–	51	269	12	61	10
First molar	–	–	34	34	–	–
Upper lip (midline)	–	–	9	5	2	11
Skin, back of neck (midline)	–	–	187	80	–	120
Parotid	–	383	539	191	–	–
Mandibular symphysis	–	21	23	9	–	–
Cervical spine	–	57	150	–	–	–
Submandibular gland	–	–	–	740	–	–
Highest dose (any site)	1100	965	539	846	115	220

*Siemens, Palomex Corp., Helsinki, Finland.
†NS = Not specified.

TABLE 3–4. DOSE IN MILLIRADS/MILLIREMS

Anatomic Site	Panelipse* Author, Date *Manson-Hing and Greer 1977*	*Wall et al. 1979*	Panex-E† Author, Date *Antoku et al. 1976*	*Wall et al. 1979*
Lens	7	8	12	1
Pituitary	16	–	28	–
Thyroid	7	2	38	1
First molar	179	–	5	–
Upper lip (midline)	5	13	2	10
Skin, back of neck (midline)	140	94	12	47
Parotid	27	56	78	45
Mandibular symphysis	12	–	5	–
Cervical spine	–	–	19	–
Submandibular gland	1131	–	–	–
Highest dose (any site)	1384	100	78	74

*General Electric Co., Milwaukee, WI.
†J. Morita Co., Kyoto, Japan.

BIOLOGIC EFFECTS OF IONIZING RADIATION

CRITICAL ORGAN CONCEPT

When discussing potential biologic effects of ionizing radiation, two types of body tissues are discussed: somatic and genetic. Somatic tissues are those tissues comprising the skin, musculoskeletal, gastrointestinal, hematopoietic, and nervous systems. Somatic tissues are important to the irradiated individual only and do not affect the genetic viability of future generations. For radiologic health purposes, various somatic tissues have been designated as "critical" organs because of their potential for significantly diminishing the quality of life of the irradiated individual. Critical organs or tissues include the skin, thyroid, eye, and hematopoietic system. Exposure of the skin and thyroid gland to ionizing radiation has been demonstrated to increase the risk of these tissues to undergo carcinomatous changes, the lens of the eye because of its potential for cataract formation and the hematopoietic system because of its potential for leukemia induction. Genetic tissues are also regarded as "critical" organs because of the ability of ionizing radiation to produce potentially harmful genetic changes transferable from one generation to another.

The harmful effects of x-radiation do not show up immediately because of a time lapse or latent period between the irradiation and the biologic manifestation of the radiation damage. The latent period may vary from five to seven years for some leukemias to as long as 20 years or more for some skin cancers.

RISK ESTIMATION

The harmful effects of low doses of x-radiation associated with rotational panoramic radiographic procedures cannot be proved scientifically as a directly observable discrete change in a specific individual. The observable deleterious effects, if any, would manifest themselves not as specific changes in specific individuals but as a statistically demonstrable increase in the frequency of normally occurring disease states among the general population. In other words, a squamous cell carcinoma in an unexposed individual will have the same characteristics as a squamous cell carcinoma in an exposed individual; the only difference is that, from a statistical perspective, irradiated populations tend to have more of this kind of cancer than nonirradiated populations. The higher the dose, the higher the cancer rate and the easier it is to demonstrate a correlation between irradiation (the cause) and disease (the effect). On the other hand, at very low doses of radiation it becomes increasingly difficult to demonstrate the cause-and-effect relationship between radiation and disease, with the results being highly dependent upon the statistical approach used. As a result, the literature concerning effects of low doses of radiation tends to be highly confusing and frequently contradictory.

$$\frac{\text{No. cases irradiated with cancer}}{\text{No. cases irradiated without cancer}} \times \frac{\text{No. cases nonirradiated without cancer}}{\text{No. cases nonirradiated with cancer}} = r$$

Figure 3–1. Equation for deriving relative risk of biologic damage from radiation.

Risk of biologic damage is frequently expressed in terms of absolute or relative risk. Absolute risk is the *excess* risk due to irradiation; it is expressed as the difference between the risk in the irradiated population and the risk in the nonirradiated population. It is usually expressed as the number of extra cancers per million persons per year per rad. For example, Gregg estimates the risk of a typical complete dental radiographic survey causing cancer to be three chances in one million. Danforth and Gibbs estimate the risk of one panoramic radiograph causing cancer of any type to be two to seven chances in one million. The estimated "normal" cancer death rate in the United States is 1,790 per million population.

Relative risk is the ratio of the risk in irradiated populations and nonirradiated populations (Fig. 3–1). When the relative risk (r) equals 1.0 or less, there is no statistical association between irradiation and cancer; when the relative risk is above 1.0, there is an association between irradiation and cancer. The stronger the association, the higher the r value. The relative risks of some known carcinogens are listed in Table 3–5. For example, a study by Bithell and

TABLE 3–5. RELATIVE RISK OF CARCINOGENESIS*

CARCINOGEN	RELATIVE RISK
Ionizing radiation	1.1–9.5
Nonionizing radiation	2.5
Nickel compounds	4.9–800
Wood dust	500
Mustard gas	37
Asbestos	1.5–100
Vinyl chloride	1.6–(?)

*From Schottenfeld and Hass: **CA** *29*(3):144, 1979.

Stewart demonstrated an overall relative risk of 1.47 for the induction of tumors in children whose mothers received prenatal pelvic irradiation. Thus, an irradiated fetus would have a 47 per cent higher risk of developing a tumor than a nonirradiated fetus of the same age. Most dental risk estimates state radiation risk in terms of absolute risk.

The risk of harmful sequelae from ionizing radiation is dependent on a wide variety of factors such as the volume and type of tissue irradiated; type, intensity, and rate of irradiation, and individual host factors modifying an individual's susceptibility to biologic damage and repair processes. In discussing any potential harmful effects of radiation, it should be emphasized that the rotational panoramic unit irradiates a relatively thin, narrow band of tissue as it traverses through the patient's head, with some areas receiving relatively low doses and others relatively high doses (see Tables 3–2 to 3–4). The repair of radiation damage to a localized area is well documented as is evidence that tissue damage is never completely repaired and some residual damage persists within the irradiated tissues. The significance of this residual damage is at present poorly understood and largely speculative. The mechanisms for cancer induction are not well understood.

PANORAMIC RADIOGRAPHY AND THE RISK TO CRITICAL ORGANS

Radiobiologically, there are few absolutes in regard to calculating and evaluating the potential risk to a patient from rotational panoramic radiography. Available literature on patient dose will be correlated with doses reported to be associated with adverse biologic effects to each critical organ. On this basis, the reader is asked to make his or her own assessment regarding the potential risk to the patient from panoramic radiography.

It would be inordinately tedious to discuss separately the many fine papers dealing with radiation dosimetry to specific critical organs from several different rotational panoramic units (see Tables 3–2 to 3–4). Because of the imprecise nature of radiation dosimetry and the importance of small distances in influencing the resultant dose, it is perhaps more appropriate to develop a concept of "ball park dosimetry" to answer the question, What would be the approximate or ball park dose to the general area of a critical organ without regard to the specific x-ray units or the slight variations in experimental method? A ball park dose would therefore be an average of many literature sources for one area. Purists may be repulsed by the idea of such imprecision, but they are free to explore the literature and synthesize "order" from a plethora of sometimes apparently contradictory results. For the remainder of the discussion, ball park doses to critical organs will be derived by averaging all doses in a particular line for the four panoramic units listed in Tables 3–2 to 3–4.

SKIN

Rotational panoramic radiography produces wide variations in skin exposure, varying from an average of 8 mrem in the anterior midline (mandibular symphysis/upper lip), to an intermediate 89 mrem in the posterior midline (back of neck and cervical spine), to an average high dose at any somatic site of 558 mrem. Reports indicate a progressively increasing risk of skin cancer at doses of 25 rem (25,000 mrem) and above. Increased cancer risk is difficult to detect statistically at doses below 25 rem. The risk of any potential harmful effects to the patient's face arising in terms of carcinoma induction would therefore be derived from the relatively small dose range of between 8 and 558 mrem.

EYE

Panoramic radiographic exposures to the lens and cornea of the eye are extremely small, approximately 8 mrem per radiograph. Available literature indicates that it requires more than 200 rem (200,000 mrem) to experimentally induce cataracts in the lens of the eye. The risk of panoramic procedures contributing significantly to the occurrence of this problem appears to be extremely remote.

THYROID GLAND

During panoramic radiography, the thyroid gland may lie within the narrow primary beam of radiation on some units for a short period of time. As a consequence, the average dose is 32 mrem; the incidence of thyroid cancer has been reported to increase with doses of a few rem. Danforth and Gibbs estimate the risk to be about one to four radiation-induced cancers per million panoramic radiographs. Thyroid cancer is rarely fatal.

TABLE 3–6. DOSE IN MILLIRADS/MILLIREM FOR BONE MARROW

Author	Date	Anatomic Site	*Panorex*	*Panelipse*	*Orthopantomograph*	*Panex-E*
White and Rose	1979	Mandible	14	32	24	–
		Cervical spine	13	24	53	–
Wall et al.	1979	Bone marrow	4	3	5	2

HEMATOPOIETIC TISSUES

Very few authors have attempted to report panoramic exposure to the bone marrow. The skull contains approximately 13 per cent of the available bone marrow in the body, with the mandible accounting for less than 1 per cent of the total marrow. The risk of leukemogenesis is directly associated with the amount of hematopoietic tissue irradiated and the dose. The bone marrow dose reported by two authors for three to four panoramic units are illustrated in Table 3–6. The average bone marrow dose is 17 mrem. Reports indicate an increased risk of leukemia induction following relatively low doses of whole body exposure in the vicinity of 5 rem (5,000 mrem). Danforth and Gibbs estimate .04 to .06 cases per million examinations.

GENETIC TISSUES

The reproductive tissues of a patient receive radiation from panoramic radiography only as a result of scattered radiation from the head and neck. This amounts to approximately 0.2 mrem per radiograph when the leaded apron is not used. When an appropriately designed leaded apron covers the chest and back, reproductive exposure is reduced to the 0.01-mrem range. There have been no reports of doses in this range producing an increase in harmful genetic effects. Danforth and Gibbs estimate the risk of a first-generation defect to be nine chances in one billion.

BACKGROUND RADIATION LEVELS

It is considered inappropriate by some individuals to compare the radiation dose to a patient from panoramic radiographic procedures with that of normal background or environmental sources of radiation. The main reason for this is that panoramic or dental radiographic procedures are given in an "acute," relatively high exposure rate compared with background radiation, which occurs in a "chronic," low exposure rate over a longer period of time. Acute radiation exposure at high dose rates is known to produce more severe radiobiologic effects than similar exposures of less intensity. Unfortunately, background radiation levels are the only ones comparable in terms of total dose to many of the panoramic sites, at least in terms of annual dose. In addition, there are some experimental data for background radiation in terms of potential adverse biologic effects, and therefore such data are useful for indirect comparison. Background radiation amounts to between 90 and 130 mrem annually or 0.3 mrem/day and is within the same order of magnitude for some of the doses previously discussed regarding critical organs.

MAXIMUM PERMISSIBLE DOSE CONCEPT

The maximum permissible dose (MPD) for radiation protection purposes is the amount of radiation that, in light of present knowledge, *will not* produce any serious harmful effects in the individual receiving it. The MPD is defined for two population groups: occupationally exposed and nonoccupationally exposed. In addition, these guidelines provide maximum recommended limits for exposure to the whole body and localized areas of the body.

The MPD for occupationally exposed persons is 5 rem/year and 0.5 rem/year for nonoccupationally exposed persons for exposures covering the whole body, gonads, blood-forming organs, and lens of the eye. Permissible occupational exposure to isolated areas of the body such as the hands and forearms, head, neck, and feet and ankles is a maximum annual dose of 75 rem; nonoccupationally exposed persons are permitted to receive 1/10 of the permissible occupational exposure, or 7.5 rem. The primary purpose in mentioning these guidelines is to suggest that since these limits were established at a level considered not to endanger the life and welfare of a person receiving the radiation, diagnostic radiographic exposures below these levels may likewise be considered to involve minimal risk to the individual. When calculating the MPD, background radiation and radiation from medical and dental diagnostic procedures are specifically excluded from consideration because background radiation is unavoidable and medical and dental radiographic procedures serve to benefit the patient.

Based on available information, it must be assumed that all radiation exposures, whether acute or chronic, are potentially harmful and that it is desirable to overestimate the potential hazard rather than underestimate the risk and regret the consequences. It is therefore prudent, in light of the cumulative effects of small amounts of irreparable tissue damage from repeated radiographic exposures, to minimize a patient's exposure to ionizing radiation whenever and wherever possible. Present data suggest that the negative consequences of rotational panoramic radiography are extremely small compared with the potential diagnostic benefits gained by the practitioner in regard to evaluating the patient's facial complex.

RADIATION PROTECTION AND PANORAMIC RADIOGRAPHY

PATIENT PROTECTION

Leaded aprons do not reduce somatic exposure to the patient's face; they serve only to prevent scattered radiation from reaching the reproductive tissues and thorax. Genetic exposure from panoramic radiography is very small, approximately 0.2 to 0.3 mrem without the apron and .01 mrem with the apron. For panoramic radiography, the apron should cover both the front of the patient's chest and the back and shoulders, since the tubehead exposes the film from the posterior. A significant factor in the use of the leaded apron is that it is a readily observable, tangible demonstration to the patient of the clinician's concern for minimizing the patient's exposure.

Thyroid shields are reported to reduce thyroid exposure by approximately 40 per cent and thus are desirable, providing their positioning does not interfere with the projection of the radiographic image.

Proper darkroom procedures are essential to minimizing patient exposure by assuring the maximum development of the radiographic image following film exposure using minimum amounts of radiation. Key factors are (1) appropriate safelighting and light-tightness of the darkroom to minimize film fog, (2) maintenance of optimal solution concentrations and developing temperatures for optimum processing, and (3) appropriate cleanliness to prevent spotting and staining of films.

Staff training in the proper use and operation of the panoramic unit is essential to avoid retakes due to incorrect patient positioning and inappropriate exposure factors, cassette loading, and so on.

OPERATOR PROTECTION

Scattered radiation from panoramic x-ray units is relatively small owing to the narrow beam of radiation and the shielding designed into cassettes and cassette carriers. Of primary importance in radiation protection of the operator is the operator's distance from the unit during the exposure cycle. Manson-Hing and Greer report an exposure of approximately 0.1 to 0.15 mrem per exposure cycle at 1 meter using the highest available kilovoltage for the three units they evaluated. By observing recommendations for dental periapical radiography and standing at least 2 meters from the unit, an operator would receive a dose of 0.025 mrem per cycle. A majority of panoramic radiographs are exposed using a kilovoltage lower than the available maximum, and scattered radiation would therefore be less than the reported level. Using the MPD guideline for occupationally exposed persons of 100 mrem/week, an operator could conceivably expose 4,000 panoramic radiographs per week if he stood 2 meters from the unit or 1000 films per week if he stood 1 meter from the unit during exposure.

Zelac determined the radiation protective barrier requirements appropriate for a Panorex unit by assuming workloads of 20,000 mAs/week to be equivalent to 100 panoramic radiographs per week. He recommended a barrier thickness equivalent to 0.8 mm lead for high-use situations used in mass screening. However, for most conventional users "no shielding beyond that afforded by existing walls or partitions will be required, even for the operator."

REFERENCES

Altonen, M., Heikkilä, M., and Mattila, K.: A comparative study of radiation doses received during examinations with the Pantomograph, Orthopantomograph, Panorex, Status-X and conventional roentgen apparatus. **Proc. Finn. Dent. Soc. 70**:67, 1974.

Antoku, S., et al.: Doses to critical organs from dental radiography. **Oral Surgery. 41**:251, 1976.

Bithell, J. F., and Stewart A. M.: Pre-natal irradiation and childhood malignancy: A review of British data from the Oxford Survey. **Br. J. Cancer 31**:271, 1975.

Casebow, M. P.: Patient doses from Orthopantomograph dental x-ray exposures. **Br. J. Radiol. 46**:230, 1973.

Danforth, R. A., and Gibbs, S. J.: Diagnostic dental radiation: What's the risk? **CDA J.** 28, 1980.

Dunster, H. J.: Dose equivalent unit. **Health Phys. 36**:536, 1979.

Gregg, E. C.: Radiation risks with diagnostic x-rays. **Radiology 123**:447, 1977.

Kuba, R., and Beck, J. O.: Radiation dosimetry in Panorex roentgenography. **Oral Surg. 25**:393, 1968.

Manson-Hing, L. R., and Greer, D. F.: Radiation exposure and distribution measurements for three panoramic machines. **Oral Surg. 44**:313, 1977.

Myers, D. R., et al.: Radiation exposure during panoramic radiography in children. **Oral Surg. 46**:588, 1978.

National Academy of Sciences B.E.I.R. Committee: The effects on populations of exposure to low levels of ionizing radiation. Washington, D.C., Nov. 1972.

National Council on Radiation Protection: Dental x-ray protection. NCRP Report No. 35, 1970.

National Safety Council: **Accident Facts.** Chicago, 1979.

Preece, J. W., and Morris, C. R.: Efficient and effective use of x-radiation in the dental office. Part I — Patient protection. **G. P. Texas Acad. Gen. Dent. Pub. 6**(1): April, 1980.

Preece, J. W., and Morris, C. R.: Efficient and effective use of x-radiation in the dental office. Part II — Assessing dental radiation risks. **G. P. Texas Acad. Gen. Dent. Pub. 6**(2): August, 1980.

Sakamaki, K., et al.: Measurement of integral absorbed dose by chemical dosimeter in panoramic tomography. **Bull. Tokyo Med. Dent. Univ. 25**:109, 1978.

Schleien, B., Phoom, D., Tucker, T., and Johnson, D. W.: The mean active bone marrow dose to the adult population of the United States from diagnostic radiology. USDHEW, FDA Pub. 77-8013. Washington, D.C., 1977.

Schottenfeld, D., and Hass, J. F.: Carcinogens in the work place. **CA 29**(3):144, 1979.

Sonnabend, Von E.: Zur Dosis bei Panorama — Rontgenaufnahmen Dtsch. **Zahnartzl Z. 27**:984, 1972.

Van Aken, J., and Van der Linden, L. W. J.: The integral absorbed dose in conventional and panoramic complete-mouth examinations. **Oral Surg. 22**:603, 1966.

Wall, B. F., et al.: Doses for patients from pantomographic and conventional dental radiography. **B. J. Radiol. 52**:727, 1979.

Weissman, D. D.: Comparative absorbed doses in periapical radiography II Panorex. **Oral Surg. 33**:661, 1972.

Whitcher, B. L., Gratt, B. M., and Sickles, E. A.: Leaded shields for thyroid dose reduction in intraoral dental radiography. **Oral Surg. 48**:567, 1979.

Whitcher, B. L., Gratt, B. M., and Sickles, E. A.: A leaded apron for use in panoramic dental radiography. **Oral Surg. 49**:467, 1980.

White, S. C., and Frey, N. W.: An estimation of somatic hazards to the United States population from dental radiography. **Oral Surg. 43**:152, 1977.

White, S. C., and Rose, T. C.: Absorbed bone marrow dose in certain dental radiographic techniques. **JADA 98**:553, 1979.

Wycleaff, H. O.: The international system of units. **Radiology 128**:833, 1978.

Zelac, R. E.: Panoramic dental x-ray installation, structural shielding, and operator protection requirements. **Health Phys. 25**:521, 1973.

Chapter 4

Panoramic Films, Screens, and Processing

FILM PROCESSING
INTENSIFYING SCREENS AND PANORAMIC FILMS
- Intensifying Screens
  - Luminescence
    - Fluorescence
    - Phosphorescence
  - Calcium tungstate ($CaWO_4$)
  - Safe-light filters
    - Kodak ML-2 (light orange)
    - Kodak 6BX (dark orange)
    - Kodak 6B (brown)
    - Kodak GS-1 (reddish brown)
  - Newer intensifying screens
    - Barium fluorochloride (DuPont Quanta II)
    - Barium strontium sulfate (Kodak X-Omatic regular screens)
    - Yttrium oxysulfide (U.S. Radium Rarex B)
    - Rare earths of gadolinium and lanthanum (Kodak Lanex screens)
  - Phosphor composition and speed factors of various intensifying screens
  - Type of panoramic cassettes
  - Care of intensifying screens
- Panoramic Film
  - Size of panoramic film
  - Speed of panoramic film
  - Composition of emulsion of panoramic film
  - Type of panoramic film and recommended processing
- Typical Screen/Film Combinations
- Identification on Film
  - Identification of right or left side
  - Patient information identification
    - Commercial leaded tape
    - Commercial imprinter
    - University of Texas at San Antonio Dental School imprinter

FILM PROCESSING
- Manual Processing
  - Film hangers
  - Sequence of steps in manual processing
    - Developing solution
      - Composition
      - Mode of action
      - Replenisher solution
        - Composition
        - Performs double function
        - Mode of action
    - Rinsing
    - Fixing solution
      - Composition
      - Mode of action
      - Replenishment
        - Composition
        - Mode of action
    - Washing
      - Object of washing
      - Cause of staining
  - Manual processing trouble chart
    - Fog
    - Stain
    - Marks or defects
- Automatic Processing
  - Advantages and disadvantages
  - Basic mechanism
  - Difference of processing solutions
  - Differences in processing temperatures
  - Replenishment system important
  - Routine schedule of maintenance
    - Weekly cleaning
    - Monthly cleaning
  - Preventative maintenance
    - Check transport sections daily
    - Lubricate moving parts monthly
    - Replenishment on regular basis
    - Check temperature of processing solutions regularly
    - Cover of processor kept slightly open when not in use
  - Film feeding recommendations
  - Automatic processing trouble chart
    - Light density films
    - Dark density films
    - Wet or tacky films
    - Film discoloration
      - Brown
      - Greenish-yellow
    - Fogged films
    - Streaking
    - Surface marks
    - Shiny films
    - Jams or failure of film to transport

FILM PROCESSING

There is a tendency to underestimate the importance of film processing. A high-quality radiograph can be rendered unsatisfactory by even the slightest disregard for the simplest of processing procedures. Processing produces, by physical and chemical means, a visible radiographic image of the invisible latent image present on the film. The latent image is the undetectable change in the silver halide crystals induced by the remnant radiation exiting from the patient. A high-quality radiographic image can be obtained by adhering to the basic principles of film processing. The following is a review of some of these basic principles.

INTENSIFYING SCREENS AND PANORAMIC FILMS

Panoramic film has a photosensitive emulsion and is used in cassettes with intensifying screens. Intensifying screens are used because they decrease the x-ray dosage to the patient and still produce a high-quality film. Direct exposure of the film in panoramic radiography would require large patient doses.

The intensifying screen absorbs x-ray energy that has penetrated the patient and converts this energy into light, which forms a latent image on the x-ray film. The intensifying screen works on the principle of luminescence, i.e., the emission of light from a substance that is energized by various kinds of stimuli (e.g., light, chemical reactions, and ionizing radiation). There are two types of luminescence — fluorescence and phosphorescence. Fluorescence as used in radiography is the ability of crystals of certain inorganic salts (phosphors) to emit light promptly (within 10^{-8} seconds) after absorption of an x-ray photon. Phosphorescence is a delayed emission of light (delay of 10^{-8} seconds or more) after absorption of an x-ray photon. This is known as afterglow and is not seen in intensifying screens but is seen in fluoroscopic screens.

The phosphor originally used in x-ray intensifying screens was crystalline calcium tungstate ($CaWO_4$). It is used in panoramic screens and is still the most widely used phosphor in intensifying screens. Calcium tungstate phosphors produce light in the blue region of the visible light spectrum, and panoramic film is sensitive to most of the light emitted by this screen. Panoramic film is not sensitive to red light, so darkroom safelights with dark orange (Kodak 6BX) and brown filters (Kodak 6B) are recommended. The Kodak 6BX safelight filter is a new, universal safelight filter that can be used in darkrooms in which both intraoral and extraoral dental films are handled. This filter permits higher levels of illumination than the Kodak 6B filter (brown) but lower levels than the Kodak Morlite (ML-2) filter (light orange). The visible light spectrum colors are arranged in order of their wavelengths from longest to shortest — red, orange, yellow, green, blue, and violet. Although the Kodak 6BX filter is primarily meant for darkrooms using automatic processors only, it may be used successfully in darkrooms with manual processors provided film handling under safelight conditions is limited to approximately 2½ minutes.

The Kodak Morlite (ML-2) filter cannot be used when panoramic or extraoral screen films are being processed because it transmits light that is within the color-sensitivity range of panoramic film x-ray emulsions.

Some of the newer films, such as Kodak Ortho G, a slow-speed film used with Kodak Lanex rare-earth screens in cephalometry, are green light-sensitive films and require a Kodak GS-1 filter (reddish brown). The Kodak GS-1 filter is shifted more toward the red side of the spectrum and thus removes the green light from illumination. Although the Kodak 6B filter is suitable for blue-sensitive panoramic film, it is not suitable for use with ortho films (green-sensitive).

Several factors determine the speed of the intensifying screen including the thickness of the phosphor layer, the size of the phosphor crystals, the presence or absence of light-absorbing dyes, and the conversion efficiency of the phosphor. However, there is usually a price to pay with screen speed. High-speed screens record less detail. Since 1973, newer phosphors have been developed for intensifying screens including barium fluorochloride, barium strontium sulfate, yttrium oxysulfide, and rare-earths gadolinium and lanthanum. Barium strontium sulfate phosphors (Kodak X-Omatic regular screens) have a greater conversion efficiency than calcium tungstate and, therefore, are twice as fast as conventional par speed screens. Conversion efficiency is dependent on the ability of the phosphor crystal to absorb x-ray photons and convert these photons to light. Some manufacturers use special activators to increase the conversion efficiency of calcium tungstate, such as DuPont Hi Plus

TABLE 4–1. PHOSPHOR COMPOSITION AND SPEED FACTORS OF VARIOUS SCREENS

Screen	Phosphor	Principal Light Emission	Relative Speed Factor	Kodak Filter Recommended
Detail (DuPont)	Calcium tungstate ($CaWO_4$)	Blue	1	6B or 6BX
Par (DuPont)	Calcium tungstate ($CaWO_4$)	Blue	4	6B or 6BX
Hi Plus (DuPont)	Calcium tungstate ($CaWO_4$)	Blue	8	6B or 6BX
X-Omatic Regular (Kodak)	Barium strontium sulfate	Ultraviolet	8	6B or 6BX
Lanex* Regular (Kodak)	Oxysulfide compounds of gadolinium and lanthanum (rare-earths)	Green	32	GS-1

*Not used in panoramic screens; other intensifying screens with similar speeds are DuPont's Quanta III, U.S. Radium's Rarex BG, and 3M's Alpha 8.

screens, which are twice as fast as conventional par speed screens (Table 4–1).

The panoramic cassette is the light-tight holder containing the screens (always in pairs) and the film. Some cassettes are rigid and some are flexible (Fig. 4–1).

Screens should be kept meticulously clean because dust and other foreign particles will absorb light and cast an area of lessened density on the film. They should be cleaned periodically with a commercial product containing an antistatic compound and a detergent. Apply gently with cotton or a lint-free cloth. Allow the screens to dry completely before closing cassettes. If screens are wet, the film emulsion will stick to the screens, which could cause permanent damage.

It is important not to damage the screens by impulsively grabbing the film out of the cassette with the fingernails. This will nick, scratch, or chip the screens. Also, care in removing the film from the box or the cassette will prevent static electricity marks.

There are various types of panoramic films available (Table 4–2). Usually, they are 5 × 12 or 6 × 12 in. Panoramic film speeds are rated slow, medium, and fast. An emulsion is said to be fast if a small exposure produces a radiograph of adequate density (blackening). The emulsion is a homogeneous combination of gelatin and silver halide crystals. The silver halide is light sensitive and consists of approximately 95 per cent silver bromide and 5 per cent silver iodide. The addition of AgI produces a higher sensitivity in the emulsion than if pure AgBr were used. The differences in speed and contrast of films are controlled by how the emulsion is mixed by the manufacturer. Each manufacturer's mixture is a closely guarded secret. Some of the panoramic films (e.g., Kodak X-Omat) are specially made for automatic processors so that their emulsions will not swell excessively during developing. If the emulsion becomes too soft, it will stick to the rollers of the automatic processor and jam the machine. All panoramic films are double-emulsion films, except for one single-coated film, which tends to have a wider latitude and more contrast than double-emulsion films. However, single-emulsion films have a coarser grain structure than double-emulsion films.

Screens and films are manufactured to go together. For best results, follow the recommendations of the panoramic x-ray machine manufacturer in selecting your screen-film combination (Table 4–3).

IDENTIFICATION

The patient's name and relevant information can be identified on the film in several ways. One method is to use commercial leaded tape, which is placed on the cassette with the desired information typed or written on the tape. When the film is exposed, the information will be photographically imprinted on the film (Fig. 4–2). Another method is to use a commercial imprinter, which records the pertinent information on the panoramic radiograph by means of a semitransparent card placed between the film and the imprinter light. Care must be taken not to imprint the information on an area of the film that will block out diagnostic information (Fig. 4–3).

It is equally important to identify the right and left sides of the patient on the radiograph. This can be done by placing "R" or "L" lead markers on the cassette or the cassette holder (Fig. 4–4).

Text continued on page 74

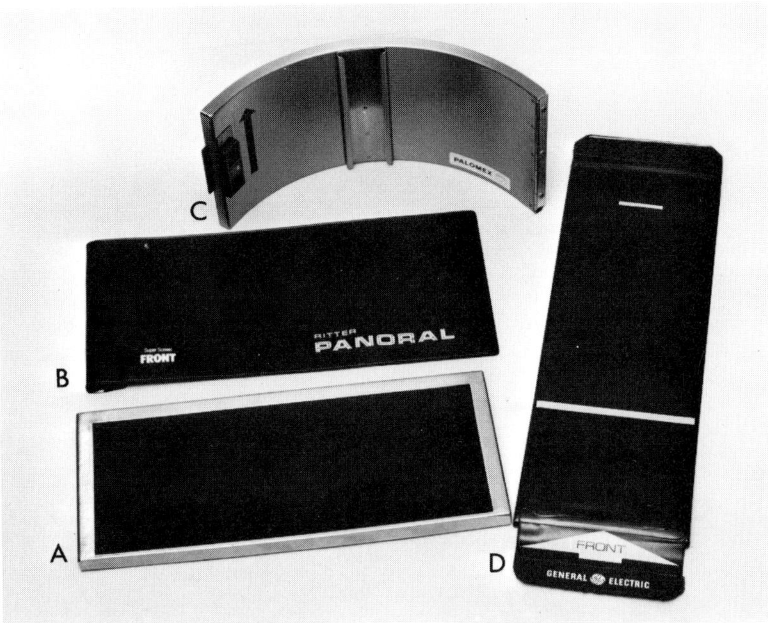

Figure 4–1. **A.** Flat metal cassette (S. S. White (Pennwalt), Panorex I). **B.** Flexible plastic cassette (Sybron/Ritter, Panoral). **C.** Curved metal cassette (Palomex, Orthopantomograph). **D.** Flexible plastic cassette (G. E., Panelipse).

TABLE 4–2. PANORAMIC FILM

Brand Name	Size (inches)	Speed and Color Sensitivity	Recommended Processing
Kodak Blue Brand DF-65, DF-66	5 × 12 6 × 12	Medium blue	Manual, longer-cycle automatic
Kodak X-Omat RP (XRP) DF-75, DF-76	5 × 12 6 × 12	Medium blue	All types of automatic
Kodak SB (single coated) DF-85, DF-86	5 × 1[illegible] 6 × 12	Medium blue	Manual, longer-cycle automatic
Kodak X-Omat G (XG) DFG/5	5 × 12	Slow blue	Manual or automatic
Kodak X-Omat R DF-95, DF-96	5 × 12 6 × 12	Fast blue (half exposure of Kodak medium speed)	All types of automatic
Kodak Ortho G and Kodak Ortho L	Not available in panoramic film	Both slow green (Ortho L has more latitude)	All types of automatic
DuPont Cronex 2DC	5 × 12 6 × 12	Medium blue (high contrast)	Manual, longer-cycle automatic
DuPont Cronex 4	5 × 12 6 × 12	Medium blue (high contrast)	Manual or automatic
DuPont Cronex 6	5 × 12 6 × 12	Medium blue (medium-scale contrast, wide exposure latitude)	Manual or automatic
DuPont Cronex 6 Plus	5 × 12 6 × 12	Medium blue (dual contrast and overexposure latitude)	Manual or automatic
DuPont Cronex 7	5 × 12 6 × 12	Slow blue	Manual or automatic
3M Trilite	5 × 12 6 × 12	Medium blue (high contrast)	RP automatic, manual

TABLE 4–3. TYPICAL SCREEN/FILM COMBINATIONS

System Speed*	Film Speed and Color Sensitivity†	Screens	Screen Phosphor	Color Emitted
1×	Medium blue	DuPont Cronex Par-Speed	$CaWO_4$	Blue
	Slow green	Kodak Lanex Fine	$Gd_2O_2S{:}Tb$	Green
	Slow blue	Kodak X-Omatic Regular	$BaSO_4{:}SrEu$	Ultraviolet
	Slow blue	DuPont Cronex Hi-plus	$CaWO_4$	Blue
2×	Medium blue	DuPont Cronex Hi-plus	$CaWO_4$	Blue
	Medium blue	Kodak X-Omatic Regular	$BaSO_4{:}SrEu$	Ultraviolet
	Medium blue	GE Blue Max 1	LaOBr:Tb	Blue
	Slow green	Kodak Lanex Medium	$Gd_2O_2S{:}Tb$	Green
4×	Medium blue	DuPont Cronex Quanta II	BaFCl:Eu	Blue
	Slow blue	DuPont Cronex Quanta III	LaOBr:Tm	Blue
	Medium blue	GE Blue Max 2	LaOBr:Tb	Blue
	Slow green	Kodak Lanex Regular	$Gd_2O_2S{:}Tb$	Green
	Slow green	3M Trimax 8	$Gd_2O_2S{:}Tb/Y_2O_2S{:}Tb$	Green

*System speed may be doubled by substituting medium blue film for slow blue film or medium green film for slow green film. Speeds are based on data supplied by manufacturer. Speeds may differ, depending on exposure conditions and processing.

†Typical films: **SLOW BLUE:** Kodak X-Omat G (XG), DuPont Cronex 7; **MEDIUM BLUE:** Kodak X-Omat RP(XRP), DuPont Cronex 4; **SLOW GREEN:** Kodak Ortho G (OG), 3M Trimax XD; **MEDIUM GREEN:** Kodak Ortho H(OH), 3M Trimax XM. (Films of similar sensitivity are manufactured by and are available from other companies.)

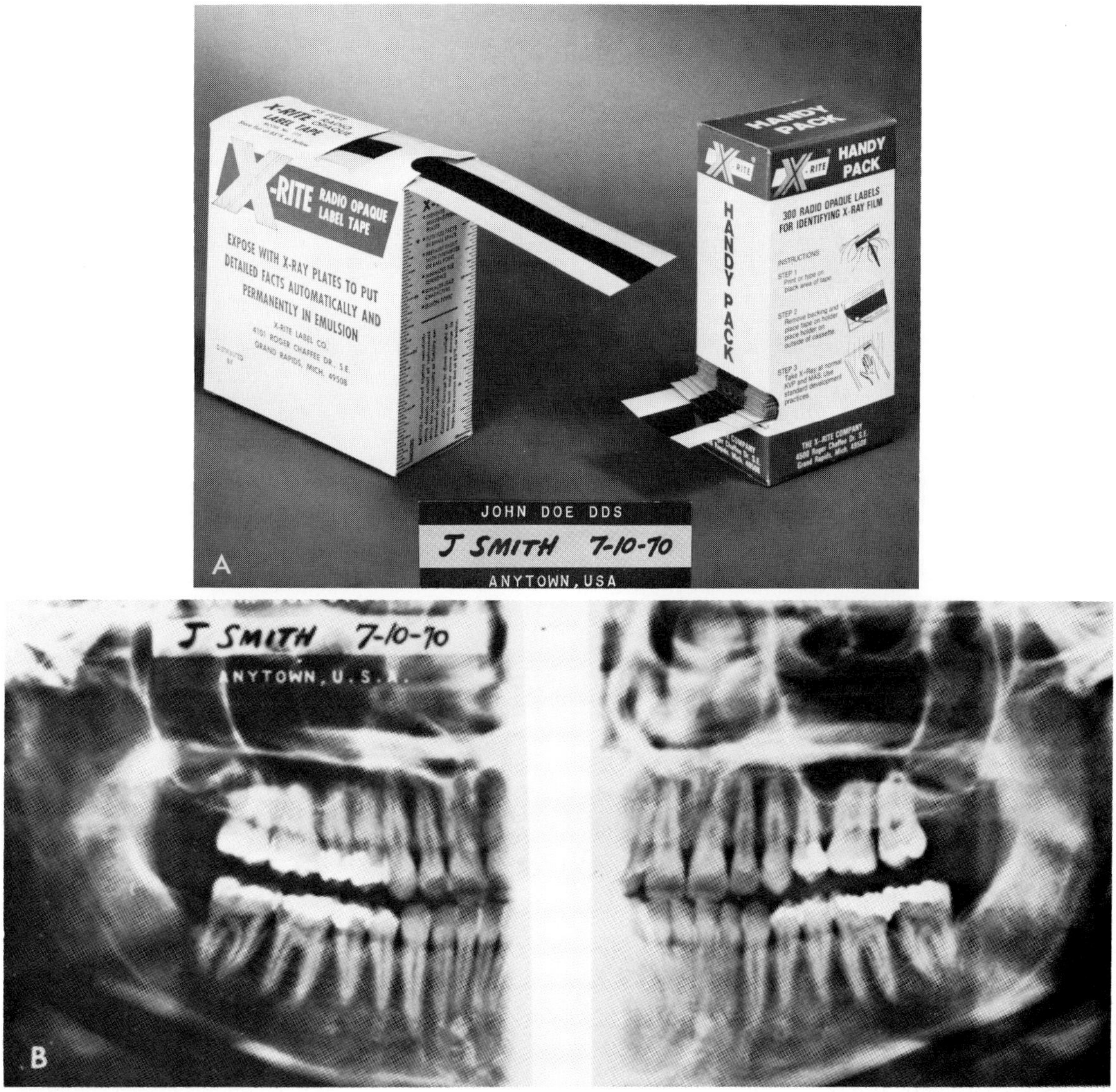

Figure 4–2. Use of leaded-type label to record patient's pertinent information on radiograph. **A.** Use of leaded-type labels to identify x-ray film. Provides positive legal identification at time of exposure. Print or type on black area of tape. Remove backing and place tape on a special holder. Place holder on cassette and take radiograph in normal manner. **B.** A Panorex radiograph taken with radiopaque identification label. (Figure 4–2 courtesy of X-Rite Label Co., Grand Rapids, MI.)

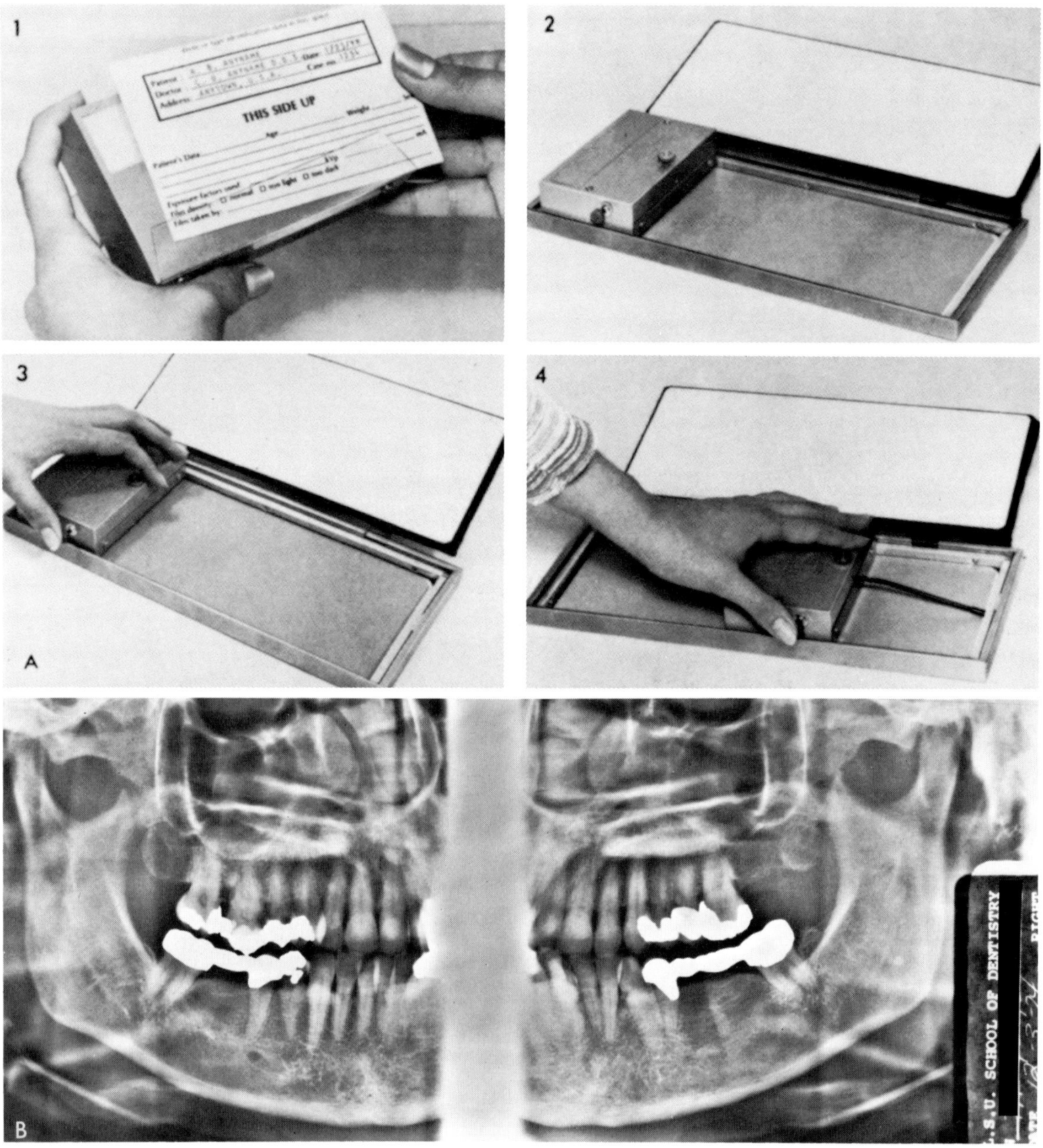

Figure 4–3. **A.** Panorex R.D.F. printer. *1*. Patient information typed on card, and card placed over illumination window. *2*. Illuminator placed on exposed film under safe-light conditions. *3*. Illuminator exposing film for imprinting side of radiograph. *4*. Imprinter exposing white band area in middle of Panorex radiograph. (Courtesy of S. S. White, Dental Products Division. Pennwalt Corp., Philadelphia, PA.) **B.** Card imprinter used on side of a Panorex radiograph. The area where patient information is to be imprinted must be blocked out with lead on outside of the cassette.

Illustration continued on opposite page

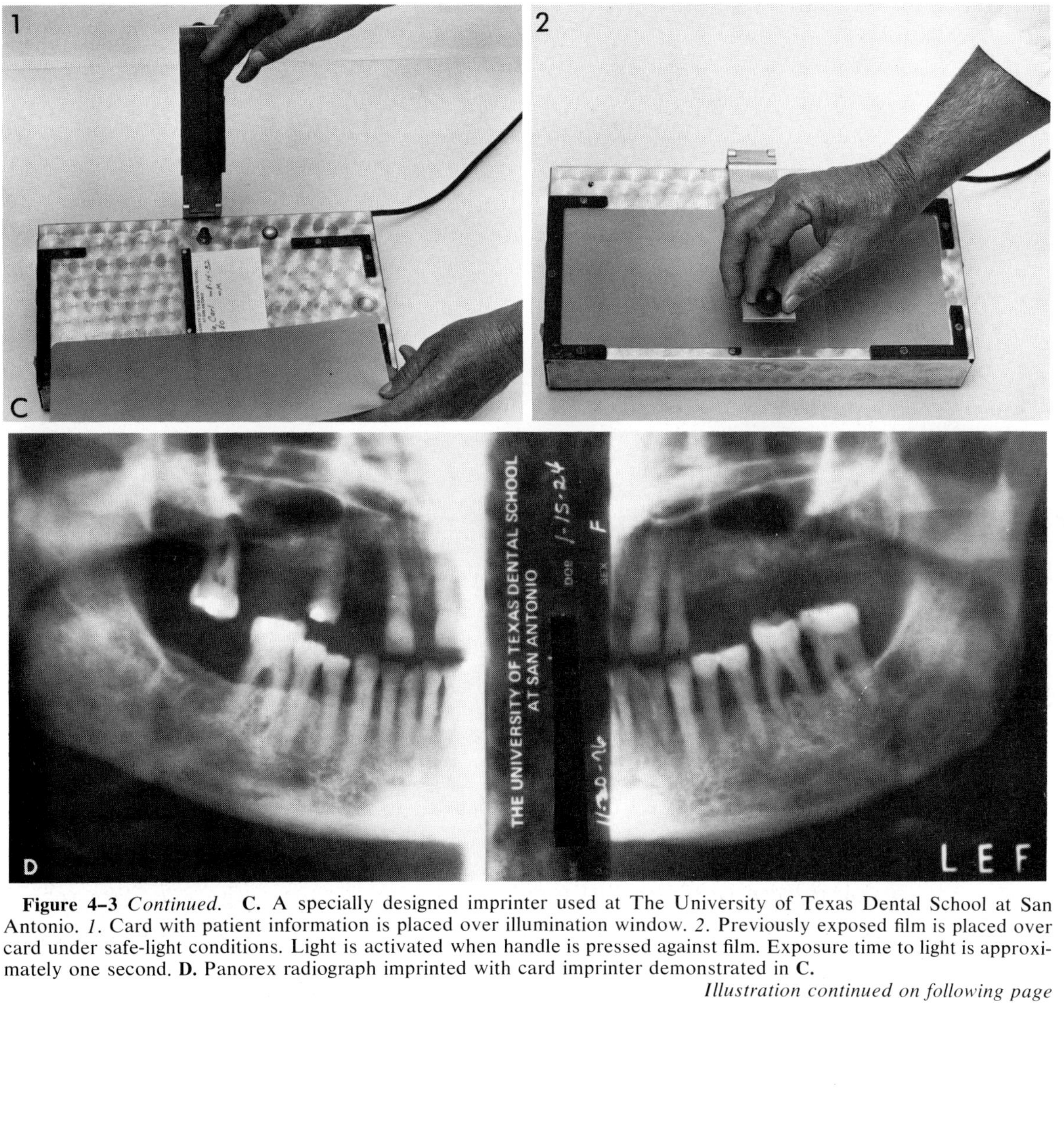

Figure 4–3 *Continued.* **C.** A specially designed imprinter used at The University of Texas Dental School at San Antonio. *1.* Card with patient information is placed over illumination window. *2.* Previously exposed film is placed over card under safe-light conditions. Light is activated when handle is pressed against film. Exposure time to light is approximately one second. **D.** Panorex radiograph imprinted with card imprinter demonstrated in **C.**

Illustration continued on following page

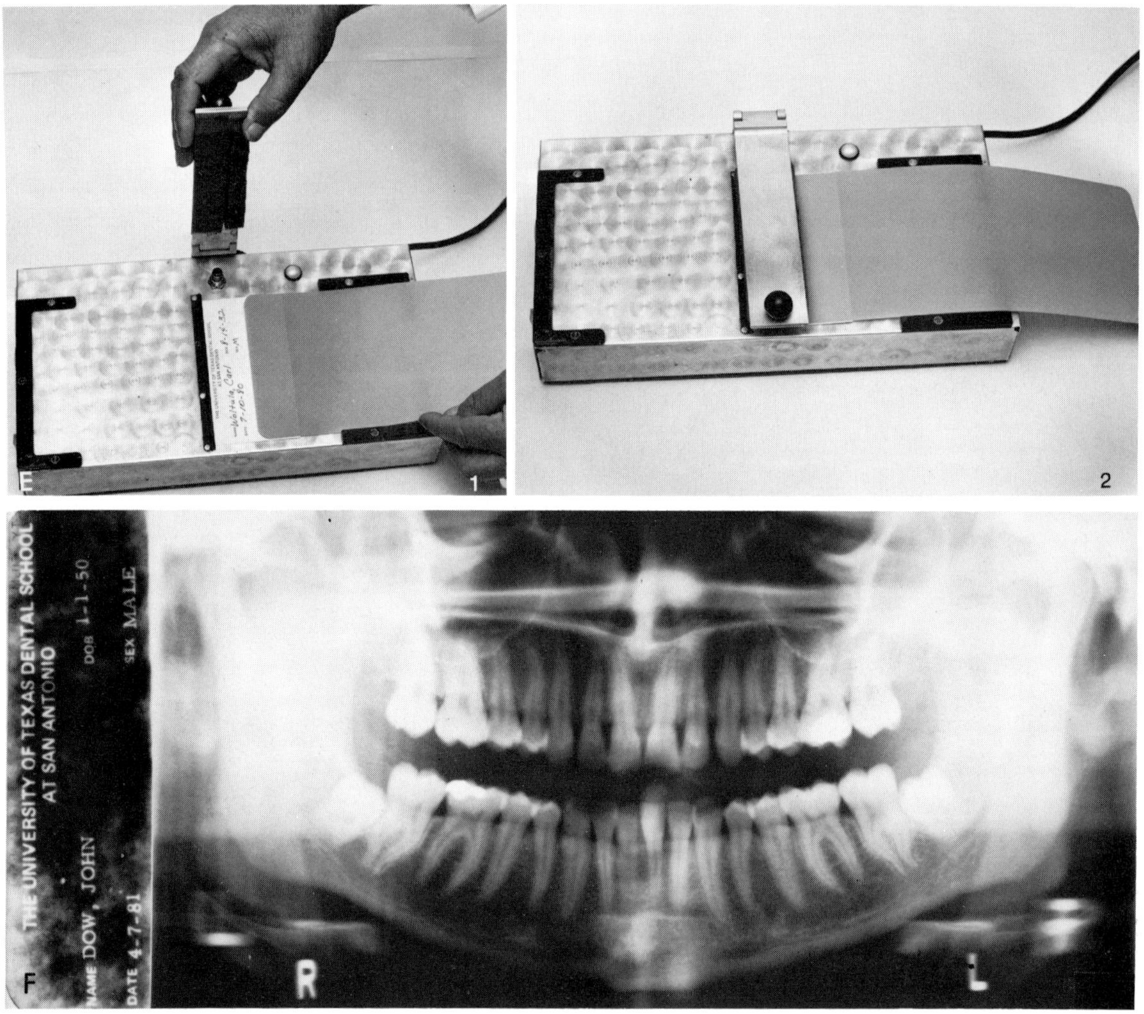

Figure 4–3 *Continued.* **E.** Procedure for imprinting patient information on side of panoramic radiograph. This is procedure to use with the continuous panoramic radiographs such as Panelipse, Orthopantomograph, Panoral, Panex-E, and Panorex II. **F.** Panelipse radiograph identified by University of Texas Dental School card imprinter.

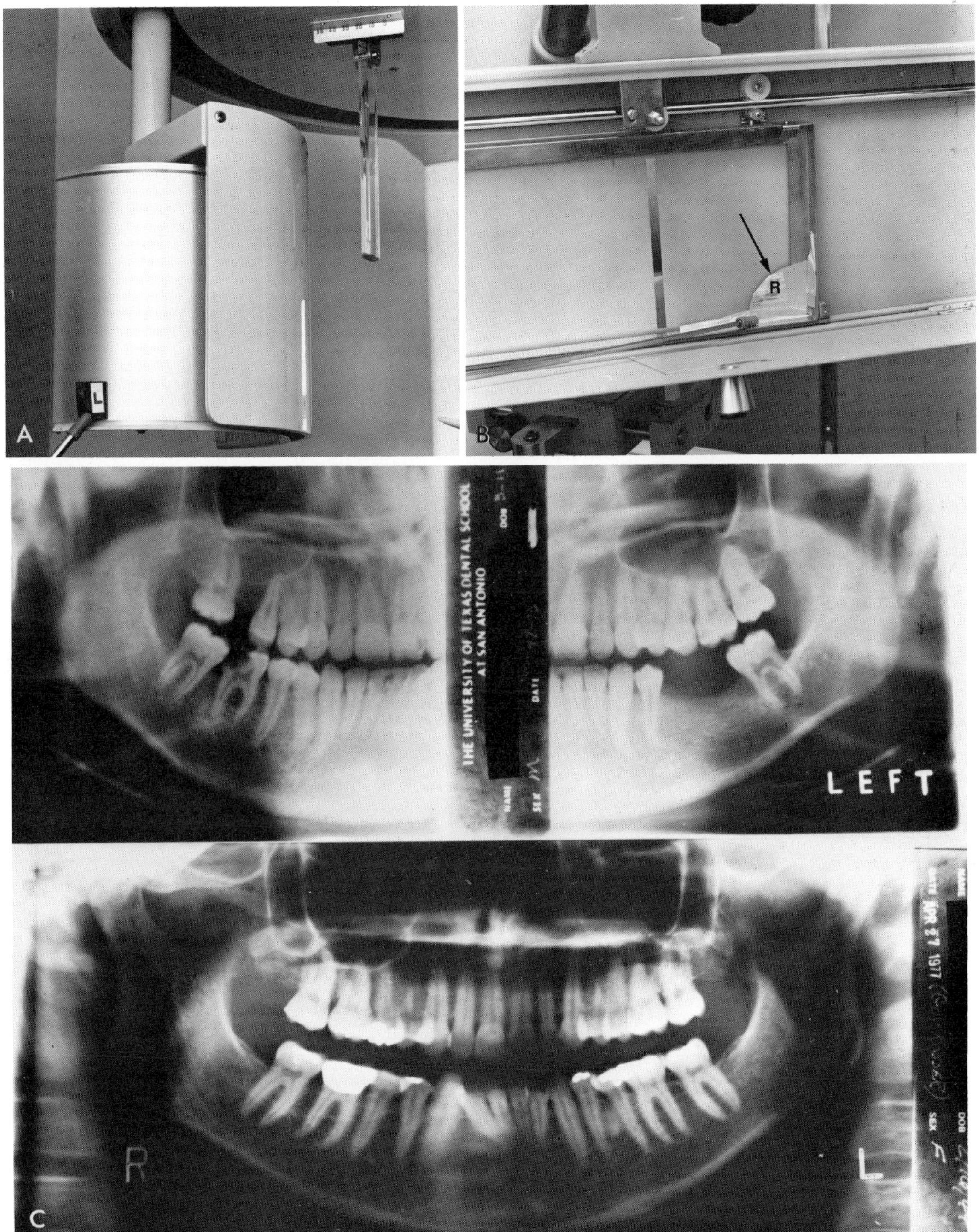

Figure 4–4. Identification of patient's right and left sides. **A.** Placement of letter "L" identifying the patient's left side on Panoral. **B.** Placement of letter "R" identifying patient's right side on Panorex. **C.** Upper radiograph taken by Panorex I machine. Patient's left side is identified by radiopaque letters "LEFT." Lower radiograph taken by Panoral. Letters "R" and "L" identify patient's left and right sides.

MANUAL FILM PROCESSING

Although manual film processing is gradually being replaced by automatic processing, there will always be a need for manual processors because automatic processors do break down. Therefore, it is judicious to have a manual processor to use when the automatic processor is inoperable. Also, some people prefer manual processors to automatic processors because the radiographs produced by manual processors, when done correctly, have a better quality.

In the manual processing of panoramic radiographs, the film is prepared for development by attaching it securely to a 6 × 12 or 5 × 12 in. film hanger. In doing so, the film should be handled only by the corners with dry hands. This must be done under safe light illumination.

It is important that the film hangers be kept clean. This can be done when the film is washed by passing water over the hangers. This will prevent subsequent staining and streaking of films by unclean hangers. Also, film hangers should not be placed too close to each other during the development, fixing, and drying procedures. If two films stick to each other, artifacts on the film will result.

Film processing refers to the entire procedure of (1) conversion of the latent image to a visible image, and (2) the preservation of the visible image. This primarily involves development, rinsing, fixing, washing, and drying. The sequence of steps in manual processing is outlined in Table 4–4.

DEVELOPMENT

The basic action of development is the reduction (addition of electrons) of the silver in the AgBr or AgI crystal into black metallic silver as follows:

$$Ag^+ \text{ (ion in x-ray–exposed AgBr crystal)} + \text{electron (from developing agents)} \rightarrow Ag \text{ (metallic)}$$

The silver in an AgBr or AgI crystal that is not exposed (i.e., does not contain the latent image) can be reduced by the developing agents but does so at a much slower rate. Therefore, time is a significant factor in the developing process.

Other important factors in the development process include the temperature and concentration of the developer. Manufacturers of radiographic film and developing chemicals have carefully established the optimum conditions of time, temperature, and concentration of chemicals for proper development. By following the manufacturer's directions, the development action will stop when the difference between the exposed (developed) crystals and the unexposed (undeveloped) crystals is the greatest.

The developer or reducing solution used in manual processing is a mixture of hydroquinone and metol (Elon). This mixture has a faster development rate than the sum of the development rate of each agent alone. As the developing agents reduce the silver ions to metallic silver, they become inactivated by the process of oxidation. Along with this chemical reaction is a liberation of hydrogen ions. The developer is alkaline because it serves as a buffer to control the hydrogen ions liberated during the development reaction. A combination of hydroquinone and phenidone (rather than metol) is used in automatic processing because the speed of this combination is of value in the rapid processing of film.

In addition to developing agents, the developer contains (1) an alkali to maintain the pH in a

TABLE 4–4. SEQUENCE OF STEPS IN MANUAL PROCESSING

STEP	PURPOSE	APPROX. TIME
Wetting	Alkaline developing solution softens and opens up gelatin so developing agents can act on silver halide crystals	15 sec
Development	Production of visible image from latent image; exposed silver halide crystals are reduced to metallic silver, forming radiographic image	5 min
Rinsing	Termination of development and removal of excess chemicals from emulsion	30 sec
Fixation	Removal of unexposed silver halide crystals from emulsion; hardening of gelatin	10 min
Washing	Removal of excess chemicals (if fixing agent [ammonium thiosulfate] is left in emulsion, it will eventually change deposited black silver to brown silver sulfide)	30 min
Drying	Removal of water and preparation of radiograph for viewing	30 min

range of 10 to 11.5; (2) a preservative (sodium sulfite) to decrease the rate of oxidation of developing agents, especially hydroquinone; and (3) restrainers (potassium bromide) to prevent the development of unexposed silver halide crystals, which cause fogging of the radiographic image.

DEVELOPER REPLENISHMENT

The developer is affected by rate of oxidation (by use and aeration), number of films processed, contaminants, and accumulation of byproducts of development reactions including oxygen, hydrogen ions (causing reduced alkalinity of solution), and bromine ions. All of these factors weaken, or exhaust, the developer. Unless measures are taken to compensate for this exhaustion, underdevelopment will result, adversely affecting the contrast of the films. Also, some of the developer is removed from the developing tank with each film, which lowers the level of the developer.

REPLENISHMENT SYSTEM

The principle of developer replenishment is to add a stronger developer to the original solution to compensate for its exhaustion and, subsequently, to permit a constant development time.

It should be emphasized that the replenisher solution is not merely original-strength developer. If the replenisher is to maintain the activity level of the developer, it must be free of bromide because this ion accumulates in the developer. It also must have higher concentrations of hydroquinone, metol, and alkali because these ingredients are disproportionately exhausted with continued use of the developer. The replenisher performs the double function of maintaining both the liquid level in the developing tank and the activity level of the developer. After adding the replenisher, the developer must be stirred thoroughly.

With the replenishment method, the films should be removed from the developer quickly, not allowing the excess solution to drain back into the tank. About ½ oz of replenisher will permit proper replenishment for development of one panoramic film. Replenisher solution should be added in relatively small quantities, stirring vigorously after each addition.

Replenishment should not be continued indefinitely. The developer should be discarded after three months because of the accumulation of gelatin, sludge, and impurities.

RINSING

After development, the film should be rinsed in clean, circulating water for 30 seconds. This will remove most of the adhering chemicals. Without thorough rinsing after development, the acidity of the fixer is rapidly reduced because the alkali of the developer will gradually neutralize the acid in the fixer. The fixer then will not act evenly on the emulsion, and the radiograph will be streaked and stained.

FIXATION

During fixation, the unexposed silver salts are dissolved out of the emulsion and the gelatin is hardened to prevent damage from future handling. A common fixer, which forms stable complexes with silver ions, is thiosulfate in the form of a sodium or ammonium salt. The fixer is called the clearing agent because it clears up the milky appearance of the film. It changes the unexposed and undeveloped silver halide crystals in the emulsion (milky appearance) to soluble silver salts, which are readily removed by washing the film in water. The fixer or clearing agent (hyposulfite or sodium thiosulfate — $Na_2S_2O_3$) is called hypo, a name given by photographers years ago.

A typical reaction of the hypo with a silver bromide crystal is as follows:

silver bromide + sodium thiosulfate (hypo) →
silver thiosulfate complex + sodium bromide

The time required for the fixer to dissolve the undeveloped silver halide on the film (clear up the original milky opacity) is called the clearing time. As the clearing action subsides, the hardening action begins, resulting in the shrinking and hardening of the gelatin emulsion containing the silver image, which was untouched by the clearing agent. Do not turn the white light on in the darkroom until the film is entirely clear (can see through clear areas) or it will become fogged (darker density) by the light exposing the unexposed silver halide crystals.

The hardener is usually a chromium or aluminum compound. The fixing solution also contains an acid, a stabilizer, and a buffer (to maintain the acid pH level).

Fixing time depends on the age and number

TABLE 4–5. MANUAL FILM PROCESSING TROUBLE CHART

Condition	Cause
1. **Low density and contrast**	a. **Underdevelopment** 1) time too short 2) temperature too low 3) combination of both 4) inaccurate thermometer b. **Exhausted developer** c. **Diluted developer** d. **Incorrectly mixed developer**
2. **Fog** (generalized darkening of film)	a. **Exposure to light leaks** in darkroom b. **Unsafe safelight** (too high bulb wattage, incorrect filter, crack in filter, too short safelight-to-workbench distance) c. **Exposure of films to white light** before films are cleared by fixer d. **Exposure of films to unwanted x-radiation** (store films safe distance from x-ray source or in lead-lined boxes) e. **Chemical fog:** 1) overdevelopment (time) 2) development at high temperatures 3) oxidized, exhausted developer (may stain emulsion brown) 4) repeated inspection of films during development 5) contaminated, corroded tanks
3. **Stain**	a. **Yellow or brown:** exhausted developer, oxidized developer; insufficient rinsing; exhausted fixer (hypo later reacts with silver to produce silver sulfide); prolonged fixing b. **Variegated (different colors in streaks or spots):** careless rinsing, causing fixer to act unevenly on emulsion; exhausted developer or fixer; contaminated developer or rinse water c. **Green:** insufficient washing d. **Grayish white scum:** incomplete rinsing (excess developer carried into fixer precipitates hardening agent, resulting in white sludge in solution and white scum on film; can be prevented by proper rinsing)
4. **Marks or defects**	a. **Crinkle marks:** curved black or white lines caused by film bending or rough handling of film b. **Static marks:** lightning or treelike marks on film caused by static electricity produced by friction between film and intensifying screen or when removing fresh film from box; usually occurs during periods of low humidity c. **Water marks:** caused by water droplets on film d. **Screen marks:** white spots on film caused by dust particles, small foreign objects, defects in screen e. **Streaking (uneven density):** 1) failure to rinse films prior to fixation* 2) failure to stir processing solutions thoroughly after replenishment 3) failure to agitate films in developer and fixer 4) unclean film hangers

*Streaking from improprer rinsing is due to the fact that one or two minutes may elapse before the alkali in the developer carried over by the film is neutralized by the acid in the fixer bath. During this time, development of the film will continue, causing streaks on the film.

of films processed. A freshly mixed fixer should clear a screen film in less than one or two minutes. It takes an equal amount of time to harden the film. Thus, the total fixing time is approximately twice the clearing time.

Fixing time can be kept at a minimum by replenishing the fixer (periodically adding fresh fixer after an equal volume of old fixer is removed). Replenishment also prolongs the life and maintains the activity level of the fixer.

The level of the fixing solution generally remains constant, since films and film hangers carry about the same amount of liquid into the fixer tank as they carry out of it when removed. Therefore, it is important to remove an equal amount of the exhausted solution before adding the replenisher.

When the original clearing time has increased by a factor of three, the fixer is exhausted and should be replaced.

Fixing, like developing, must be properly timed. Too short a fixing time can result in inadequate hardening, slower drying, and the possible loss of permanence of the image. Prolonged fixing may cause the hypo to be bound to the emulsion so that it cannot be removed in washing, thereby causing an eventual brown discoloration on the radiograph. Also, if the film is left in the fixing solution, for instance, for an hour or more, it will cause bleaching of the image, resulting in a loss in density.

WASHING

The object of washing is to remove residual processing chemicals and silver salts from the radiograph. If these chemicals are not removed, the radiograph will discolor, impairing its value as a permanent record.

You have seen radiographs that have turned brown with age. This is a result of improper washing. The retained hypo in the emulsion reacts with the silver image to produce a brown silver sulfide in much the same way as silverware tarnishes when exposed to the hydrogen sulfide of cooking gas. The general reaction is:

hypo + silver = silver sulfide (brown) + sodium sulfide

The washing procedure requires clear water running at a rate of approximately 8 tank volumes per hour. Hangers should be well spaced and completely immersed in the tank so that chemicals can be removed from the tops of the hangers. The time required in the wash tank depends on water temperature, rate of flow, and type of fixer. Washing is usually complete in 20 to 30 minutes. Table 4–5 lists common problems in manual film processing.

AUTOMATIC FILM PROCESSING

Manual film processing is gradually being replaced by automatic processing. There are many reasons for this. First, automatic processors shorten the processing time from 50 to 60 minutes to 1½ to 5 minutes. Second, the automatic processing cycle produces constant end-results. Of course, this is dependent on proper maintenance of the equipment. Automatic processors require less floor space than manual processors and have daylight-loading capabilities. Also, film hangers and film dryers, used in manual processing, are not required in automatic processing. Still another decided advantage is that automatic processing eliminates wet reading of films, which drips solution all over the office. Furthermore, a dry film is more useful diagnostically than a wet film.

The basic mechanism of automatic processors is usually a series of rollers that transport the films through the various sections — developer, fixer, washer, and dryer (Fig. 4–5). These rollers are driven by a series of gears, chains, and pulleys; any change in their speed, size, or tension alters the rotating speed of the rollers, which in turn affects the processing time in each section. Spacing of the rollers must be carefully adjusted to prevent jamming and slipping of the film during transport.

In addition to assuring continued movement, the rollers have other functions. They provide a massaging action, which contributes to the uniform processing of the films in the developing and fixing sections. Also, there are special squeegee rollers that remove processing solutions from the film surfaces, which reduces the amount of solution carry-over from one tank to the next. This prolongs the life of the fixer and increases the effectiveness of the washing procedure. The squeegee rollers in the wash section remove most of the water from the film emulsion prior to transport of the film to the drying section, allowing the film to dry uniformly and rapidly. In the drying section, the film is quickly dried by jets of heated air before the film drops into the discharge receptacle.

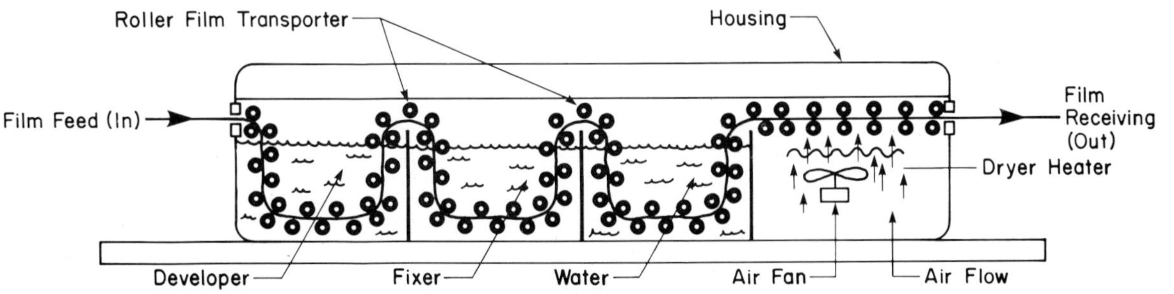

Figure 4–5. Diagram of automatic film processor. (From Kasle, M., and Langlais, R.: Basic Principles of Oral Radiology, Vol. 4, Exercises in Dental Radiology. Philadelphia: W. B. Saunders, 1981.)

Since the total processing time is reduced in automatic processing, the chemical concentration and temperature of the solutions must be increased. Phenidone is substituted for metol (Elon) as a developing agent because, when combined with hydroquinone, it provides the rapid chemical reaction necessary for automatic processing. In the 90-second automatic processors, the temperature is kept between 90 and 95°F in the developer, fixer, and wash sections and 135°F in the dryer section. The longer-cycle automatic units process at temperatures of approximately 83°F for a 4.5-minute cycle.

To prevent the emulsion from softening and sticking to the rollers, a special hardening chemical, glutaraldehyde, is added to the developer. Sulfate compounds are also added to the developer to minimize the swelling of the emulsion so that the films can be transported by the rollers uniformly.

With automatic processors, a rigid schedule of replenishment is necessary to maintain the proper concentrations of the solutions and to neutralize the unwanted by-products of each reaction. To maintain the alkalinity of the developer, the acidity of the fixer, and the chemical strength of both solutions, a replenisher must be added at a constant rate for each film processed.

If continued satisfactory results are expected, automatic processors must be cleaned routinely and preventative maintenance procedures followed. Experience has shown that the greatest cause of automatic processor breakdown is failure to keep the rollers clean. A schedule should be established for cleaning the rollers and replenishment and changing of solutions. A proposed schedule is listed below.

1. **Replenish solutions and check levels and temperature daily.** Temperature of developer should be 81 to 83°F for longer-cycle automatic processors (80°F for 5½-min cycle, and 83°F for 4-min cycle). It is best to drain water section each night. Always run a cleaning film through each morning before use.
2. **Weekly cleaning of roller racks with warm running water.** Soak and wash roller sections thoroughly for 10 to 15 minutes only. Remember to run at least two panoramic cleaning films through processor before use (exposed films will do).
3. **Change solutions every two to four weeks,** depending on rate of use of processor. Be sure to use rapid-processing developer and fixer solutions specially made for automatic processors. Do not use processing solutions or films designed for manual processing.
4. **Monthly cleaning**
   a. **Clean developer section with special developer cleaner.** (Failure to do so will cause foggy or streaked films.)
   b. **Clean fixer section with warm water only.** This will prevent crystals from forming on fixer rollers.
   c. **Clean wash section with household bleach/water solution.** This will prevent scum forming in the water and leaving spots and artifacts on films.
   d. **Rinse all racks thoroughly with water after removing from cleaning solutions.**
   e. **Visually check dryer; dust as needed.**

Preventative maintenance procedures are important, and a few of them are listed for your convenience.

1. **Check each day to see if transport sections are aligned properly.** The films will fall through to the bottom of the tanks if the transport sections are not aligned properly.
2. **Lubricate moving parts monthly.** Gears, sprockets, idlers, bearings, drive mechanisms, and ring points must be lubricated on a regular basis. Failure to do so will cause excessive wear of moving parts and will eventually slow down the speed of the rollers and, in turn, affect film quality. Do not allow any oil to get on rollers.
3. **Replenish the solutions on a regular basis according to the rate of films processed.** After four panoramic films, add approximately 6 ounces. Failure to do so will result in low levels of exhausted developer and fixer. This will cause smudgy, low-density films.
4. **Check the temperature of the processing solutions regularly.** Changes in temperature of the developer will cause changes in density of the processed film. (It only takes a change in temperature of a few degrees to affect the density. It is important to be sure that the thermostat on the processor is accurate.)
5. **Keep the cover open slightly when the processor is not in use.** After each day's operation, leave cover slightly open so the chemical fumes can escape. Failure to do so could lead to fogging (blackening) of films.

The following is a quick test to check your automatic processor. First, process an unexposed film. It should be clear, clean, and dry. If it is not, check (1) solutions (exhausted developer will create and increase film fog); (2) safe light; (3) darkroom light leaks; and (4) rollers (they may need to be cleaned). If the film is not dry, check dryer temperature and fixer. Second, process a film that has been exposed to light. It should be black and dry. If it is not, check solutions and dryer temperature.

Here are a few important recommendations for feeding the film into the processor.

1. **Feed the films slowly and carefully.** Enter the panoramic films into the processor in a straight line with the roller system. Failure to do so could cause a jam-up in processor.
2. **If film is bent,** insert the unbent side of the film into machine first.
3. **Do not feed damp or wet films** into machine, as it will contaminate rollers and cause streaking of subsequent films.
4. **Do not feed films too quickly** in succession. They may stick to each other and jam the machine.

Several brands of automatic processors are available (Fig. 4–6). Although they are competitive in performance and price, the decision on which brand to buy usually rests on the availability of competent repair service. Table 4–6 lists problems commonly encountered with automatic film processing.

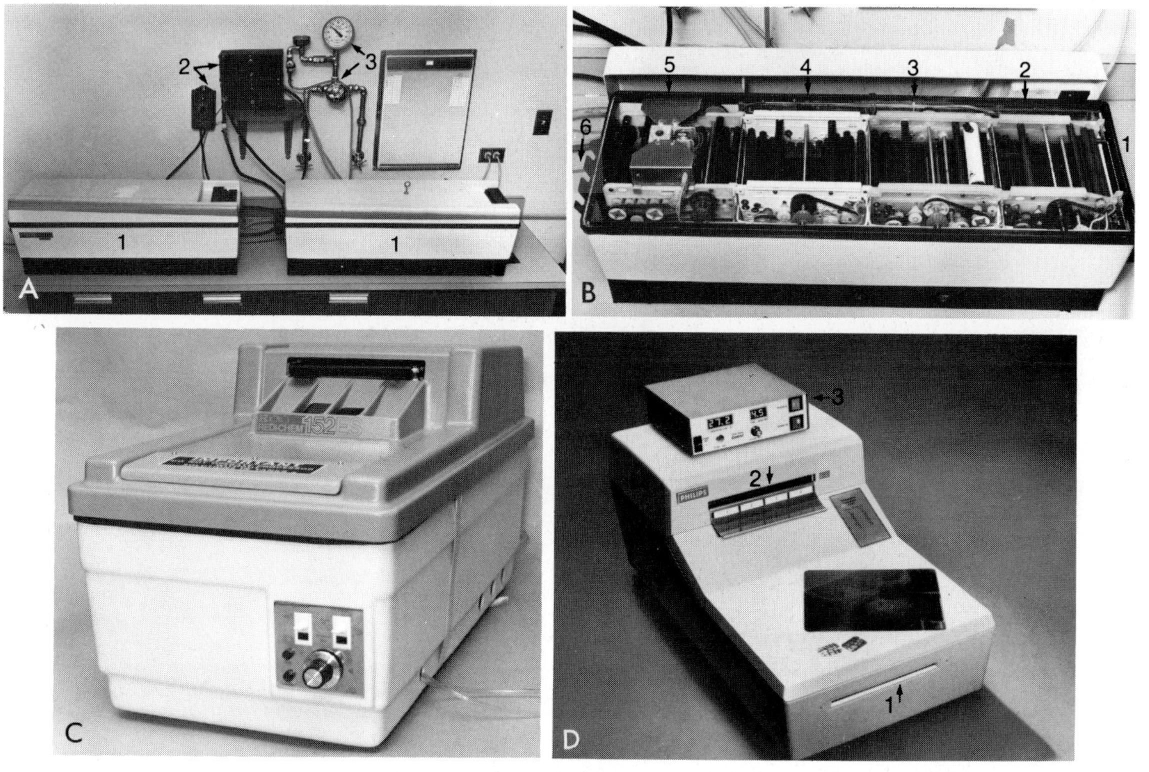

Figure 4–6. Commercially available dental automatic film processors. **A.** The Xonics (Xonics Medical Systems) automatic processor with replenishment systems. (1) Xonics automatic processor (P-6). Processing time is 4½ minutes dry to dry. Does not require hard plumbing, but utilizes flexible plastic tubing for wash drain and wash water supply. (2) Replenishment system uses a diaphragm-type pump. Replenisher solutions located in cabinets below processors. Activation of system is related to film usage. (3) Mixing valve plumbing system to control water temperature. **B.** Xonics processors are gear driven via a belt from main drive motor to drive shaft. The individual rack rollers are belt driven. A roller transport system is used to carry film. Daylight loaders are available for all size dental films. (1) Film inserted at this end. (2) Development rack. (3) Fixer rack. (4) Wash rack. (5) Dryer. (6) Film exit. **C.** Newer Xonics REDI-CHEM 152ES automatic processor (1981 model). **D.** Philips 810 automatic processor (Philips Dental Systems). May be installed with external plumbing into water and drain hook-ups or with an optional water recirculator, eliminating the need for external plumbing. Processing time and temperature can be varied from 50 seconds to 6 minutes (20 to 35° C [68 to 95° F]). An archival-quality film is provided in 4½ minutes at 28° C (83° F). (1) Film is inserted here. (2) Film exits here. (3) Time/temperature control system.

Illustration continued on following page

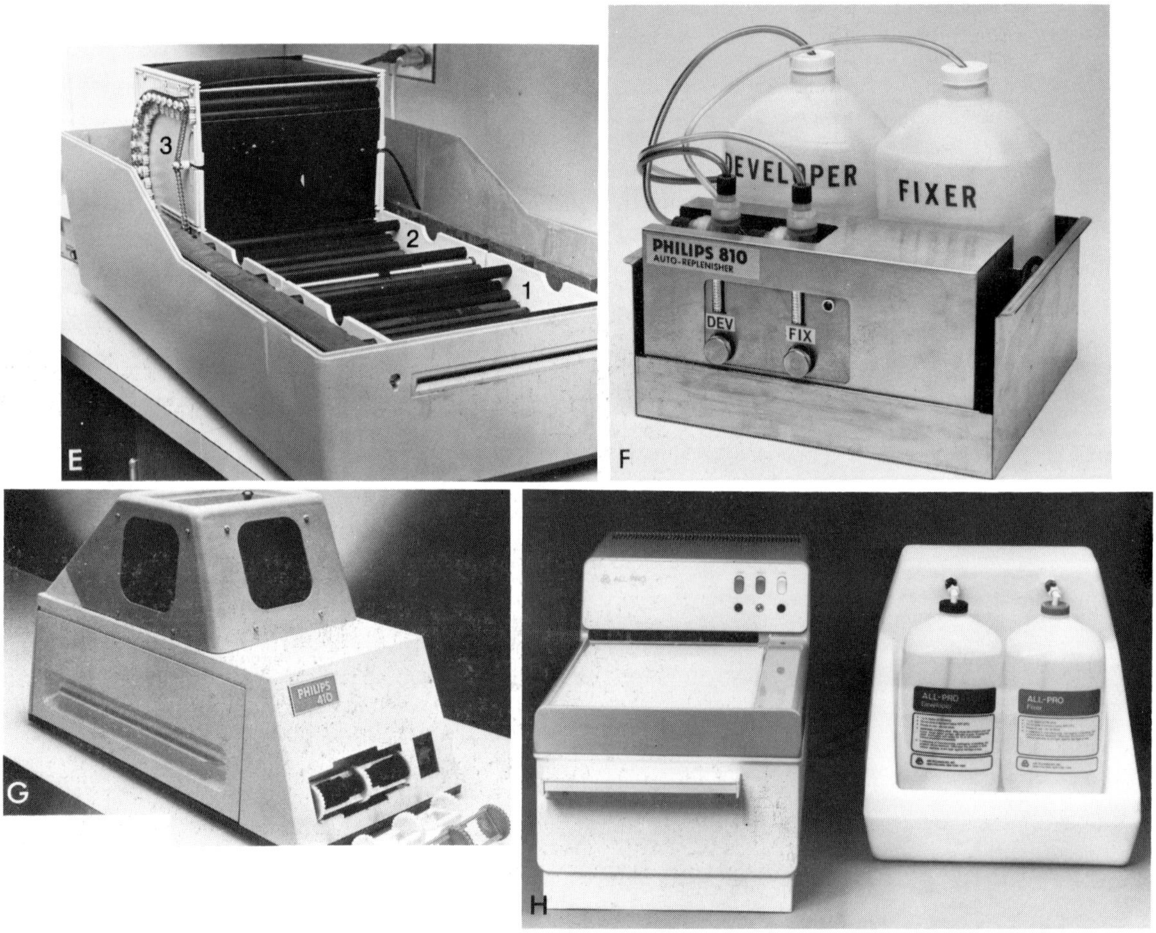

Figure 4–6 *Continued.* **E.** Philips 810 employs a bicycle and ladder–type drive system with stainless steel chains and gears. The film transport system uses plastic and rubberized rollers. Two daylight loaders are available, one for the larger panoramic and 8 × 10 films and one for intraoral films only. (1) Developer transport module. (2) Fixer transport module. (3) Washer/dryer mode, which employs a patented spray-wash feature, eliminating the conventional standing water bath. **F.** Philips 810 replenishment system employs dual metering controls for developer and fixer. The pump is automatically activated by a microswitch and provides replenisher in direct proportion to size of film processed. (*D* and *F* courtesy of Philips Dental Systems, Division of Philips Medical Systems, Inc., Stamford, CT.) **G.** New Philips 410 automatic processor for intraoral x-ray film only (1981 model). Provides wet reading in 3½ minutes and dry film in 6½ minutes. **H.** All-Pro (Air Techniques, Inc.) automatic processor requires water and waste hook-ups. Processing time preset at the factory from 5 minutes, dry to dry. This time can be changed to 3½ minutes by changing the pulleys on the main motor drive and the main drive shaft. An automatic replenisher is available, which can be installed alongside the All-Pro as shown here. It maintains the proper chemistry level and strength automatically.

Illustration continued on opposite page

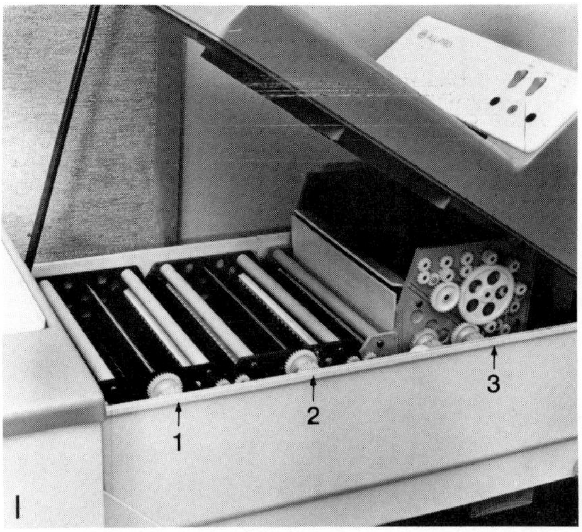

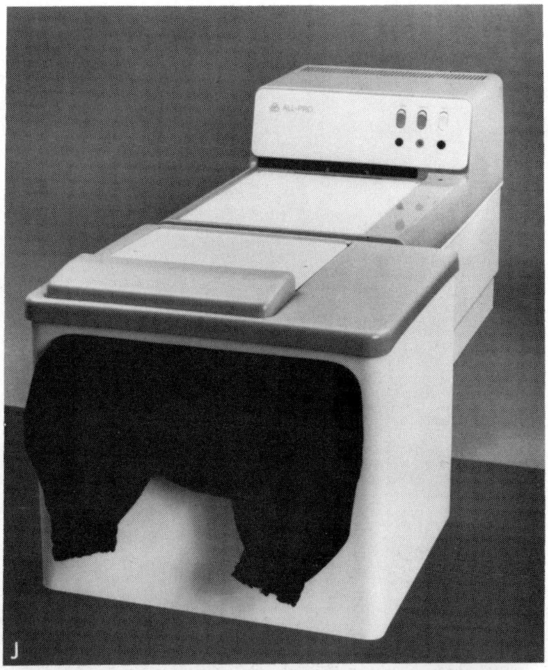

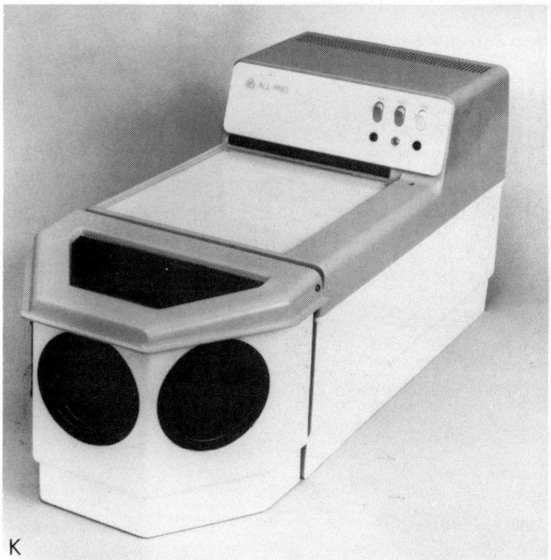

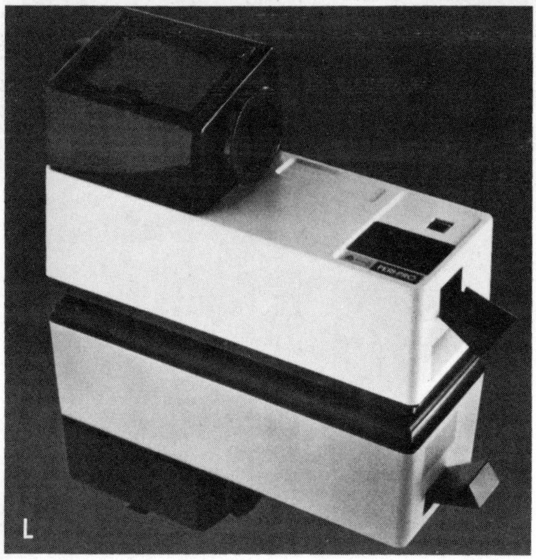

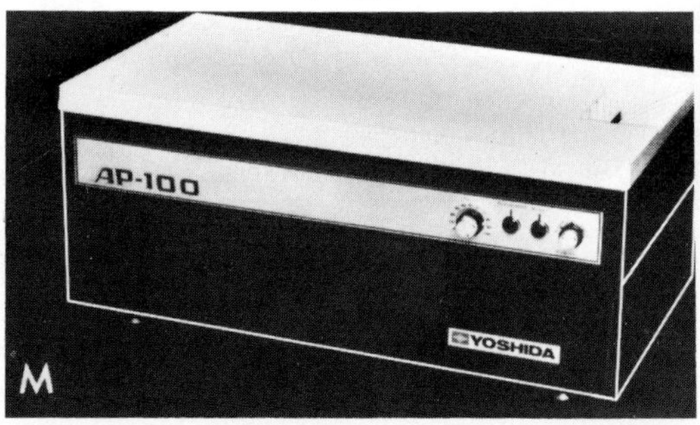

Figure 4–6 *Continued.* **I.** All-Pro employs a roller transport system, which is gear driven. There are three separate transports: (1) developer, (2) fixer, and (3) wash/dry transports. **J.** All-Pro daylight loader for all size dental films, including panoramic and cephalometric films. **K.** All-Pro daylight loader for intraoral film only. **L.** Peri-Pro (Air Techniques, Inc.) automatic processor used for intraoral film only (1981 model). Optional daylight loader is shown on top. (*H, J, K,* and *L* courtesy of Air Techniques, Inc., Hicksville, NY.) **M.** Yoshida/Kaycor AP100 automatic film processor (Yoshida Dental Mfg. Co. Ltd., Tokyo, Japan) handles intraoral, panoramic, and cephalometric films. Adjustable speed from 90 seconds to 5.75 minutes. Optional daylight loader and replenisher system available. (*M* courtesy of Kaycor International Ltd., Evanston, IL.)

TABLE 4–6. AUTOMATIC FILM PROCESSING TROUBLE CHART

Condition	Cause
1. **Low-density films**	a. Solution temperature too low b. Exhausted developer (underreplenishment) c. Improper agitation or massaging action of rollers d. Processing too fast
2. **High-density films**	a. Solutions overheated b. Light leaks in processor cover c. Too much replenisher
3. **Wet or tacky films**	a. Dryer and developer temperatures too low b. Dryer thermostatic control or heater inoperative c. Dryer air circulation inadequate (high humidity in dryer section) d. Wrong chemistry and/or film e. Processing too fast
4. **Film discoloration (brown)**	a. Contamination of fixer in developer
5. **Film discoloration (greenish yellow)**	a. Fixer solution exhausted (underreplenishment) b. Processing too fast c. Wrong type of film for processor
6. **Fogged films (unwanted density)**	a. Incorrect or defective safelight filter or bulb b. Light leaks in darkroom c. Developer temperature too high d. Improper storage of films
7. **Streaking (uneven density)**	a. Underreplenishment b. Rollers and crossovers encrusted with chemical deposits c. Dirty wash water d. Film not hardened properly by chemicals
8. **Surface marks**	a. Foreign materials or irregularities on surface of rollers b. Rough handling of film prior to processing
9. **Shiny films**	a. Excessive hardening b. Wash water not turned on
10. **Films chalky or dirty**	a. No wash water or dirty wash water b. Precipitate in fixer
11. **Jams or failure of film to transport**	a. Chemicals contaminated or diluted b. Chemical temperature too high c. Films excessively soft and not adequately hardened; when enough gelatin lubricates the rollers, films will jam up with one another d. Dirty rollers e. Racks not seated properly f. Dirty wash water g. Incorrect dryer temperature h. Hesitation in drive assembly, causing film to pause in transit i. Film not tracking through processor in straight course (improper feeding of films)

REFERENCES

Bloom, W. L., Hollenbach, and Morgan, J. A.: **Medical Radiographic Technic,** 3rd Edition. Springfield, Ill.: Charles C Thomas, 1969.

Bushong, S. C.: **Radiologic Science for Technologists.** St. Louis: C. V. Mosby, 1975.

Christensen, E. E., Curry, T. S., and Dowdey, J. E.: **An Introduction to the Physics of Diagnostic Radiography.** Philadelphia: Lea & Febiger, 1978, pp. 110–151.

Darkroom Techniques for Better Radiographs Processed Manually or Automatically, E. I. DuPont DeNemours & Co., Inc.

Fuchs, A. W.: **Principles of Radiographic Exposure and Processing,** 2nd Edition. Springfield, Ill.: Charles C Thomas, 1979.

Kasle, M. J., and Langlais, R. P.: **Exercises in Dental Radiology,** Vol. 4, Basic Principles of Oral Radiography. Philadelphia: W. B. Saunders, 1980.

Langland, O. E., and Sippy, F. H.: **Textbook of Dental Radiography,** Revised 3rd Printing. Springfield, Ill.: Charles C Thomas, 1981, pp. 170–200, 227–229.

Lawrence, D. J.: Kodak X-Omatic and Lanex screens and Kodak films for medical radiography. **Med. Radiogr. Photogr.** 53(1):2, 1977.

Manson-Hing, L. R.: **Panoramic Dental Radiography.** Springfield, Ill.: Charles C Thomas, 1976, pp. 157–164.

Manual Processing of Extraoral Kodak Dental X-Ray Films. Eastman Kodak Co., 1977.

Selman, J.: **The Fundamentals of X-Ray and Radium Physics,** 6th Edition. Springfield, Ill.: Charles C Thomas, 1978.

Skucas, J., and Gorski, J.: Application of modern intensifying screens in diagnostic radiology. **Med. Radiogr. Photogr.** 56(2):25, 1980.

The Fundamentals of Radiography. Rochester, N.Y.: Health Sciences Markets Division, Eastman Kodak, 1980, pp. 93–106.

Thunthy, K. H., Fortier, A. P., and Knapp, W. B.: Automatic film processing in the dental office. **Quintessence Int.** (9):75, 1977.

Wuehrmann, A. H., and Manson-Hing, L. R.: **Dental Radiology.** St. Louis: C. V. Mosby, 1977, pp. 30–33, 183–201.

Chapter 5

Common Errors Made in Panoramic Radiography

To produce panoramic radiographs with consistent image quality, common errors must be kept to a minimum. What are some of these common errors? Faults in technique, i.e., errors related to preparing the patient for the film exposure; errors in film exposure and processing; and errors in handling the film.

ERRORS IN PREPARING THE PATIENT FOR FILM EXPOSURE

It is imperative that the patient be positioned correctly in the panoramic machine. This is related to the size and shape of the focal trough, or the sharply depicted layer. Objects lying outside this layer will appear blurred on the radiographic image. Blurring of the object is an example of motion unsharpness caused by a moving tubehead.

In theory, only objects lying within the sharply depicted layer will attain maximum sharpness; however, in practice, structures near the layer will have acceptable diagnostic sharpness, as they will exhibit only a slight increase in motion unsharpness. The structures become less sharp as the distance is increased from the sharply depicted layer. For each panoramic machine there is a thickness of tissue volume considered to have maximal sharpness, called the sharply depicted layer or the focal trough.

The widths of the focal troughs of various panoramic machines are illustrated in Figure 5–1. As can be noted from the diagrams, the

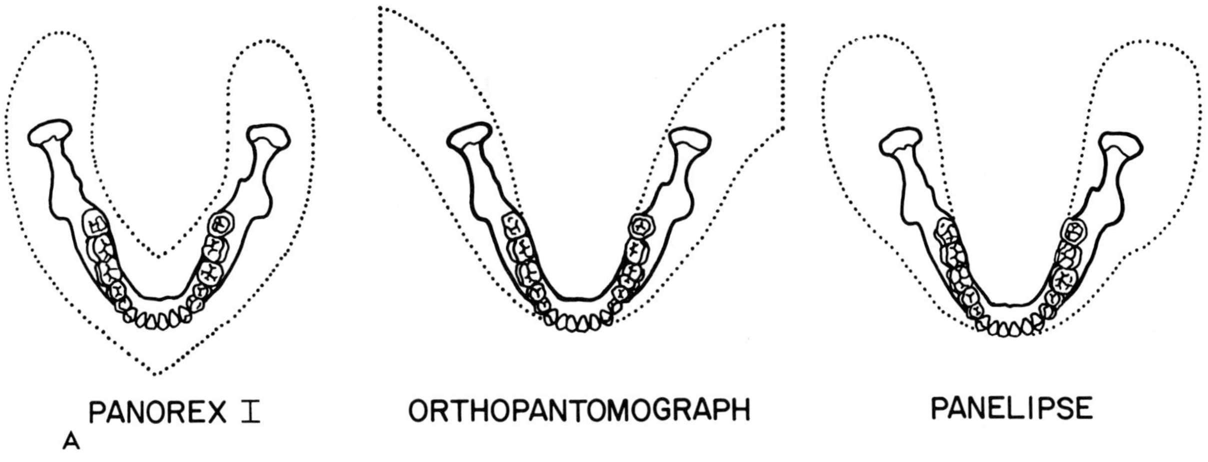

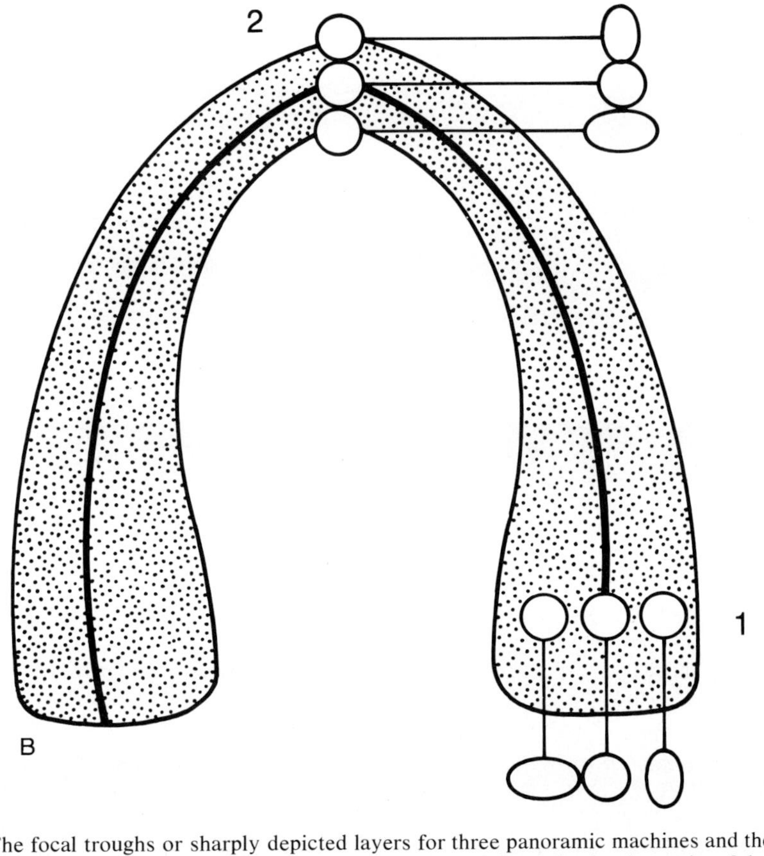

Figure 5–1. **A.** The focal troughs or sharply depicted layers for three panoramic machines and their relationship to an average mandible. (From Lund, T. M., and Manson-Hing, L. R.: A study of the focal troughs of three panoramic dental x-ray machines. Part I: The area of sharpness. Oral Surg. **39**:325, 1975.) **B.** Image magnification in Panelipse x-ray unit. Black line represents plane in focus or sharply depicted plane. The shaded area is the approximate field of focus, called the focal trough. To illustrate horizontal magnification, three steel balls have been placed equidistant to the sharply depicted plane in the posterior area (1) and anterior area (2). The outline drawings of the steel balls represent the approximate radiographic image that would be created. If the object (anatomy) is located more inside the sharply depicted plane (further from the film), it will be overmagnified horizontally and will be less distinct. If the object is more outside the sharply depicted plane (closer to the film), it becomes narrower in width and less distinct. Notice that horizontal magnification is more sensitive to the position of the steel ball than is vertical magnification. (Courtesy of G. E. Dental Systems, Milwaukee, WI.)

Panorex I has a wider focal trough or sharply depicted layer in the anterior region than the Orthopantomograph and the Panelipse. This wider, more sharply depicted layer in the anterior region in the Panorex I provides for a greater margin of error in the anterior positioning of the patient. In the Orthopantomograph and Panelipse, the positioning of the patient in the anterior region is more critical because of the thinness of the focal trough. Therefore, the use of a bite block is required to position the patient correctly in the Panelipse and the Ortho-

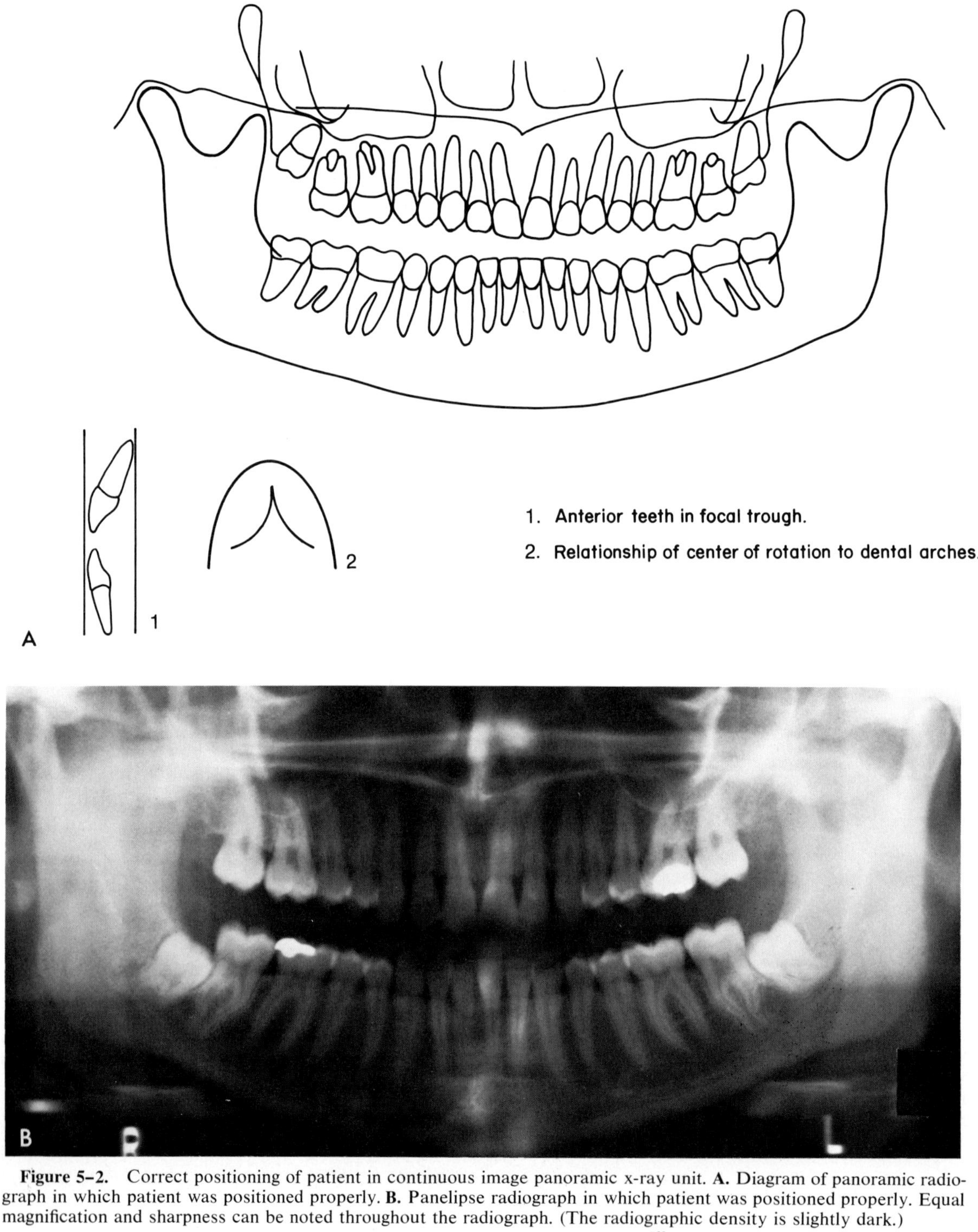

Figure 5–2. Correct positioning of patient in continuous image panoramic x-ray unit. **A.** Diagram of panoramic radiograph in which patient was positioned properly. **B.** Panelipse radiograph in which patient was positioned properly. Equal magnification and sharpness can be noted throughout the radiograph. (The radiographic density is slightly dark.)

Illustration continued on opposite page

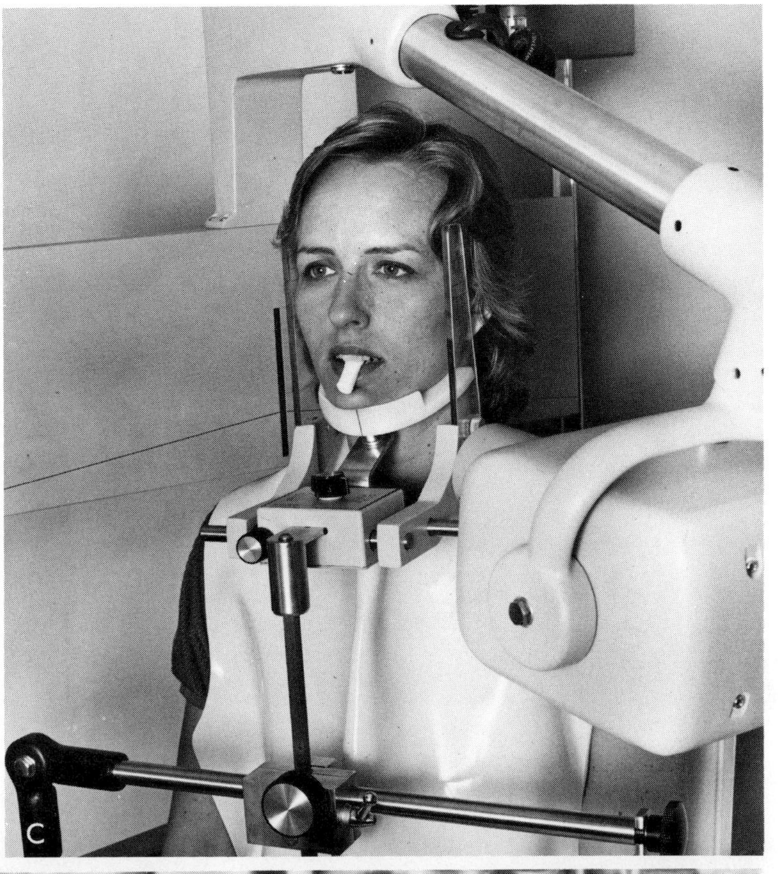

Figure 5–2 *Continued.* **C.** Correct positioning of patient's head in Panorex I x-ray unit. The patient's head should be tilted downward so that the tragus-ala line is 5° down and forward. The midsagittal plane of the patient's head is aligned with the vertical center line of the chin support. A cotton roll is placed between the teeth to prevent overlapping of crowns. **D.** Panorex I radiograph taken with patient's head positioned correctly. Equal magnification and sharpness can be observed throughout the radiograph.

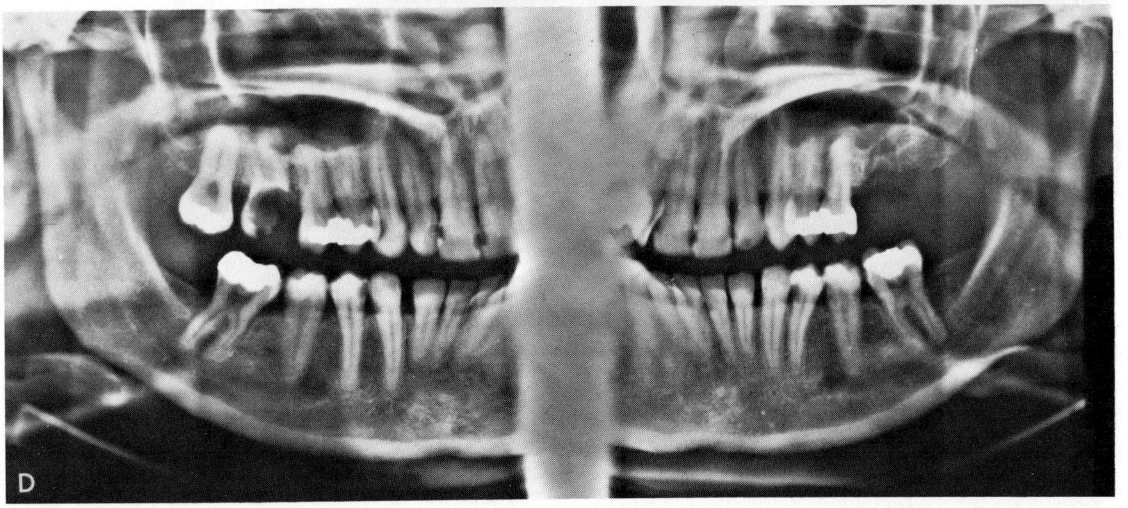

pantomograph. All panoramic units use some sort of head-positioning device and a chin rest to stabilize the patient's head during the relatively long exposure cycle.

CORRECT POSITIONING OF PATIENT

1. **Have patient remove jacket or bulky sweater.** This allows more room between bottom of cassette holder and patient's shoulder.

2. If unit requires patient to sit, be sure patient's buttocks are against backrest of chair.

3. **Have patient sit or stand erect with back straight.** A cushion may be placed between patient's back and chair in units requiring patient to sit during exposure.

4. **The patient's head should be tilted downward so that the tragus-ala line is 5° down and forward.** This will, in most cases, position the

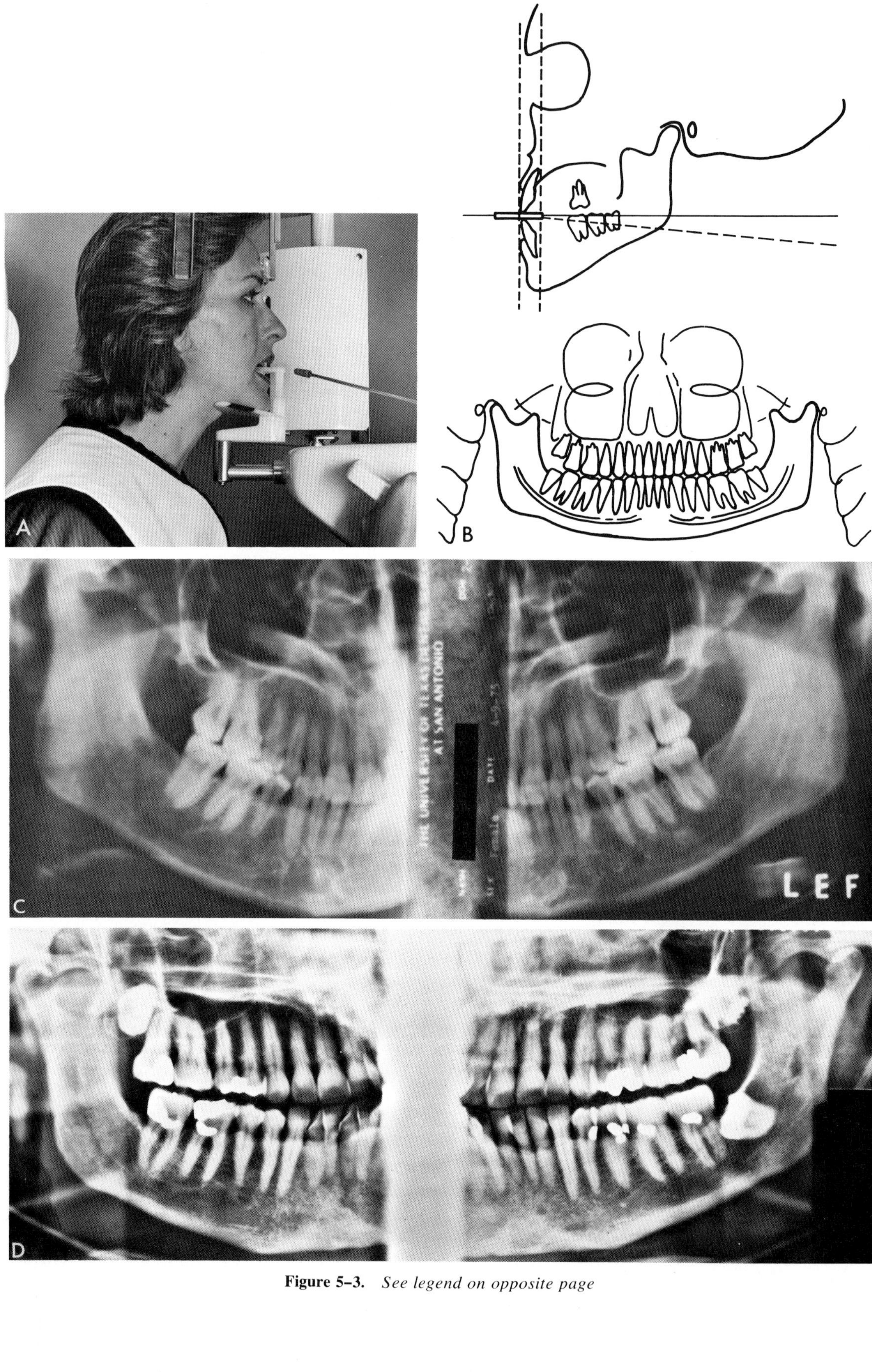

Figure 5–3. *See legend on opposite page*

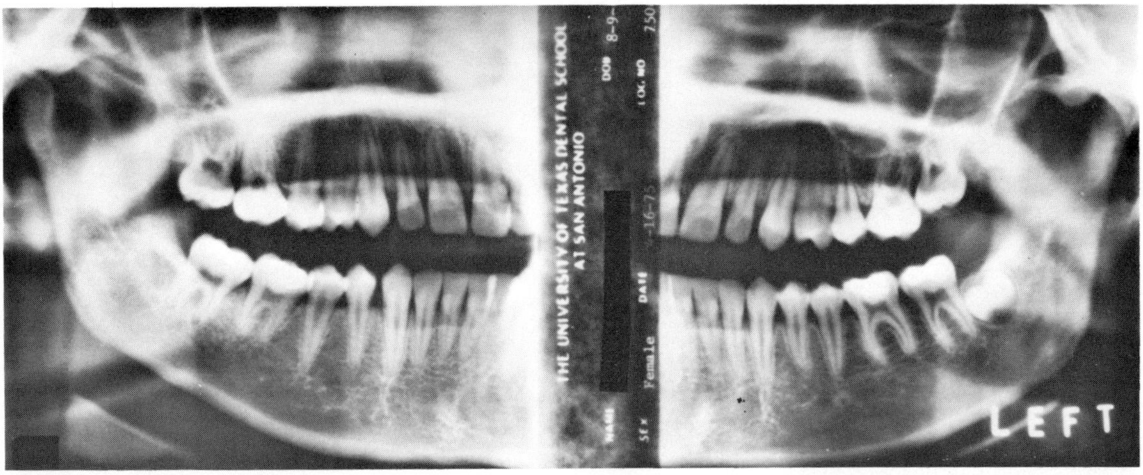

Figure 5–4. Tongue not placed on roof of mouth, resulting in dark shadow above the tongue representing the air space between the tongue and the palate.

occlusal plane slightly downward toward the floor. If the patient has a low palatal vault, increase the occlusal plane angulation slightly; if the patient has a high palatal vault, decrease the occlusal plane angulation slightly. Center the lower border of the mandible on the chin rest equidistant from each side.

5. **Align the midsagittal plane of the patient's head** with the vertical center line of chin rest.

6. **Explain to the patient how the machine works** and that the cassette holder will not strike him, although it may gently rub his ear and head at the limits of the excursion.

Figure 5–2 illustrates panoramic radiographs taken with the patient's head positioned properly.

PREPARING THE PATIENT

1. **Insert a cotton roll or bite block between incisal edges of the maxillary and mandibular teeth.** This will prevent the teeth from overlapping vertically, which would obscure caries and defects of the crowns of the teeth. Figure 5–3 illustrates the use of a cotton roll or bite block. Besides correcting for vertical overlapping of the crowns of the teeth, a bite block or cotton roll aids in placing the teeth in the focal trough and prevents undue shape distortion.

2. **Have the patient close his lips and place his tongue against the roof of the mouth.** If this is not done during exposure, a dark shadow above the tongue will result, which will obscure the apices of the maxillary teeth (Fig. 5–4).

3. **The patient should remove glasses and metallic items** from the head and neck. These items will appear as radiopacities on the radiograph and will obscure diagnostic information. The following items should be removed:

a. Napkin chains, necklaces, and neck chains (Fig. 5–5).
b. Nose jewelry and earrings (Fig. 5–6).
c. Eyeglasses (Fig. 5–7).
d. Other objects that may be projected onto the radiograph, such as metallic paste on make-up sequins, chewing gum, hearing aids, hairpins, and turtleneck sweaters with metal fasteners or zippers.

4. **Dentures (full and partial)** should also be removed from the oral cavity (Fig. 5–8).

5. **The lead aprons** currently used may produce artifacts on the panoramic radiograph

Figure 5–3. Use of cotton roll or bite block to prevent overlapping and distortion. **A.** Patient positioned correctly in Panoral x-ray machine using bite block to keep incisal edges apart and placing anterior teeth in focal trough. **B.** Diagrams illustrating use of anterior bite block to prevent overlapping and distortion by placing anterior teeth in focal trough. **C.** Panorex radiograph taken without placing cotton roll between the anterior teeth, resulting in severe overlapping of incisal edges. **D.** Panorex radiograph taken with cotton between anterior teeth. Overlapping has been corrected.

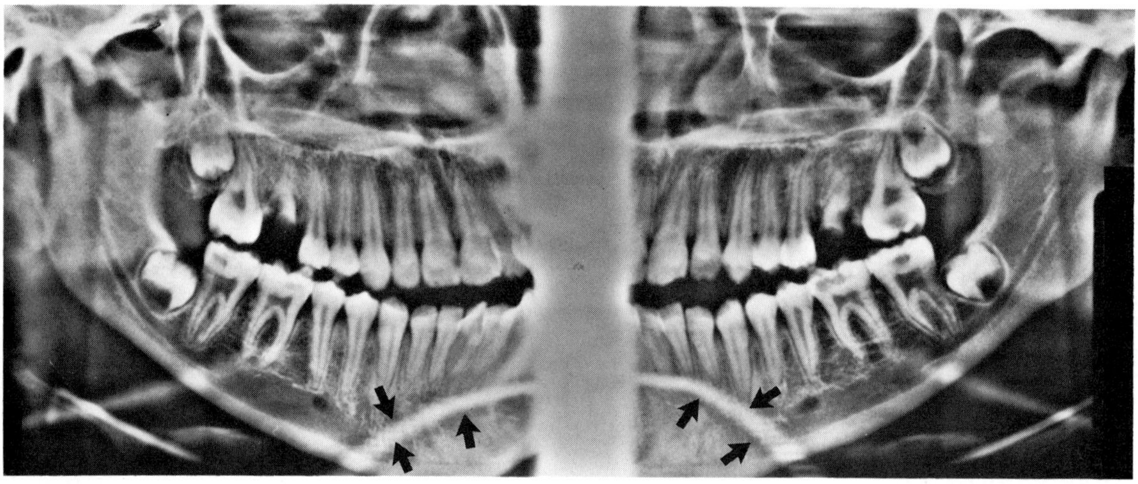

Figure 5–5. Necklace artifacts. Panorex radiograph in which necklace was not removed from patient (see arrows). This shows necklace on posterior portion of neck.

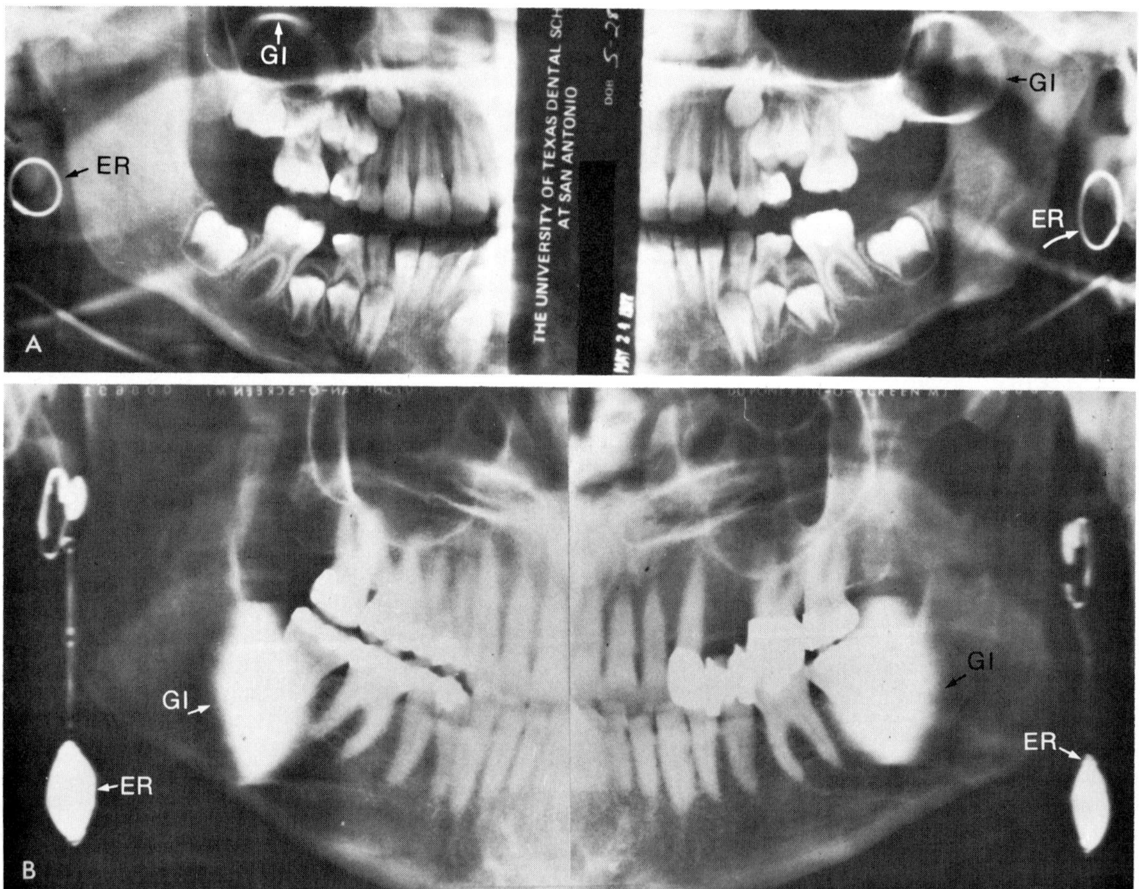

Figure 5–6. Ear jewelry artifacts. **A.** Small round earring (ER) not removed. GI = ghost image of earring. **B.** Long earrings not removed.

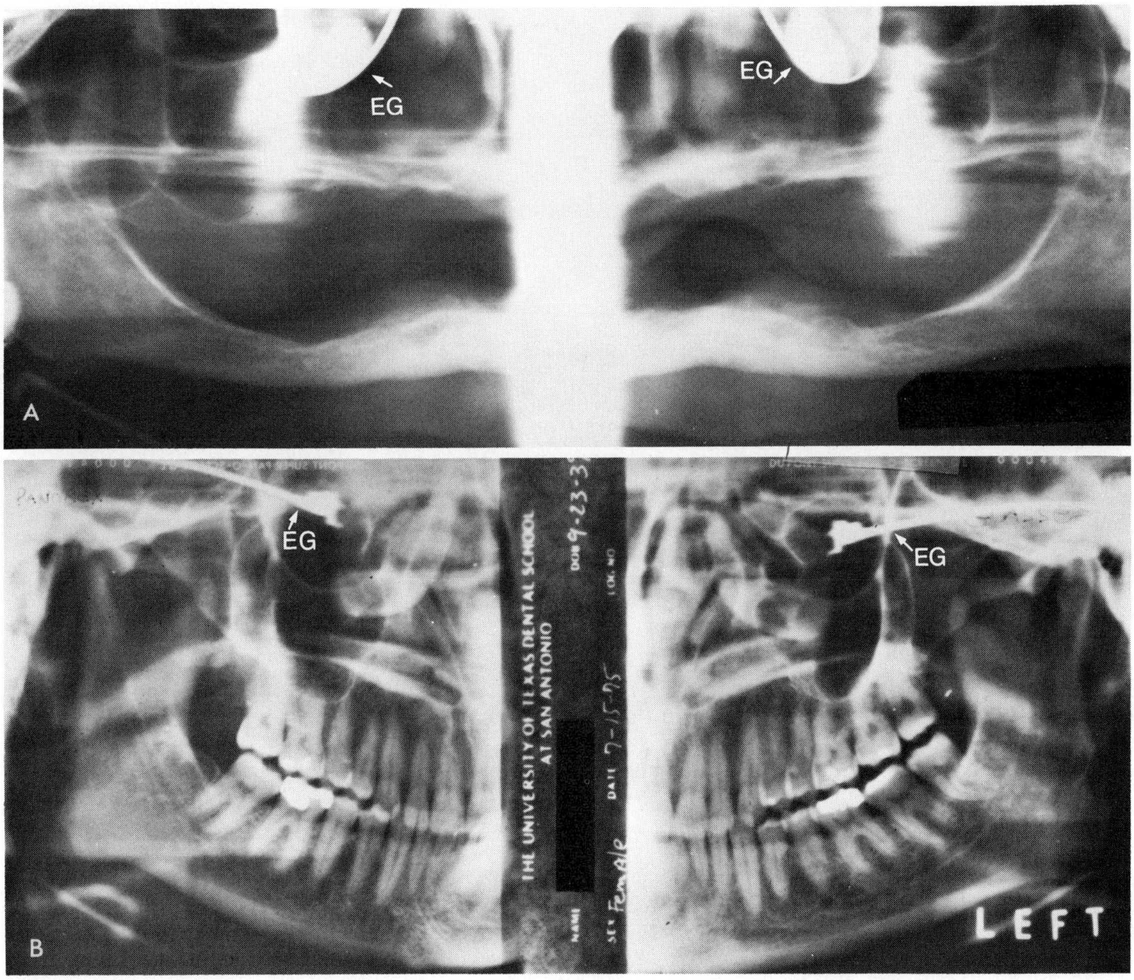

Figure 5–7. Eyeglasses artifact. **A.** Eyeglasses (EG) not removed from edentulous patient with severely resorbed ridges. **B.** Eyeglasses not removed. Teeth are overlapped because cotton roll was not placed between incisors.

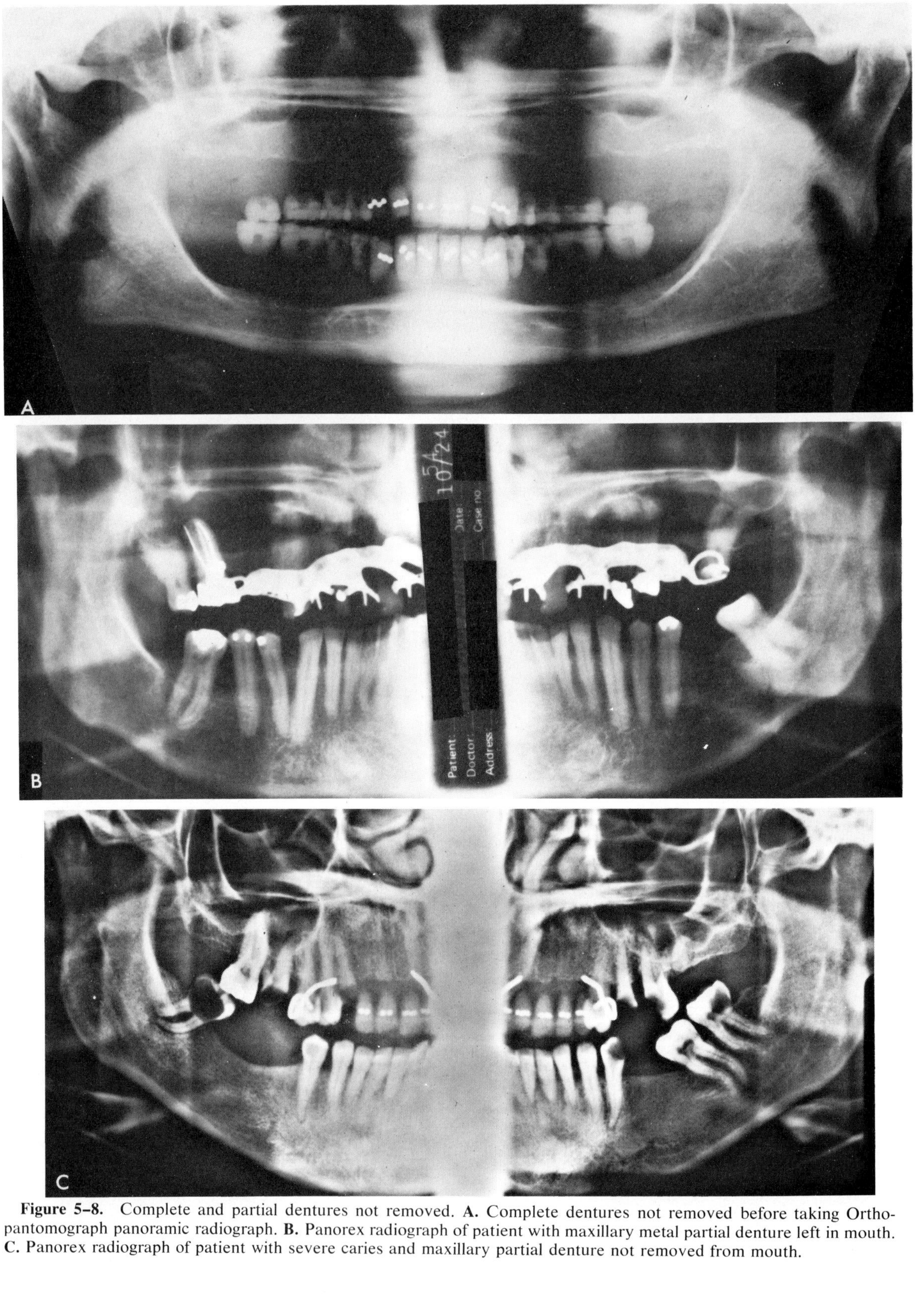

Figure 5–8. Complete and partial dentures not removed. **A.** Complete dentures not removed before taking Orthopantomograph panoramic radiograph. **B.** Panorex radiograph of patient with maxillary metal partial denture left in mouth. **C.** Panorex radiograph of patient with severe caries and maxillary partial denture not removed from mouth.

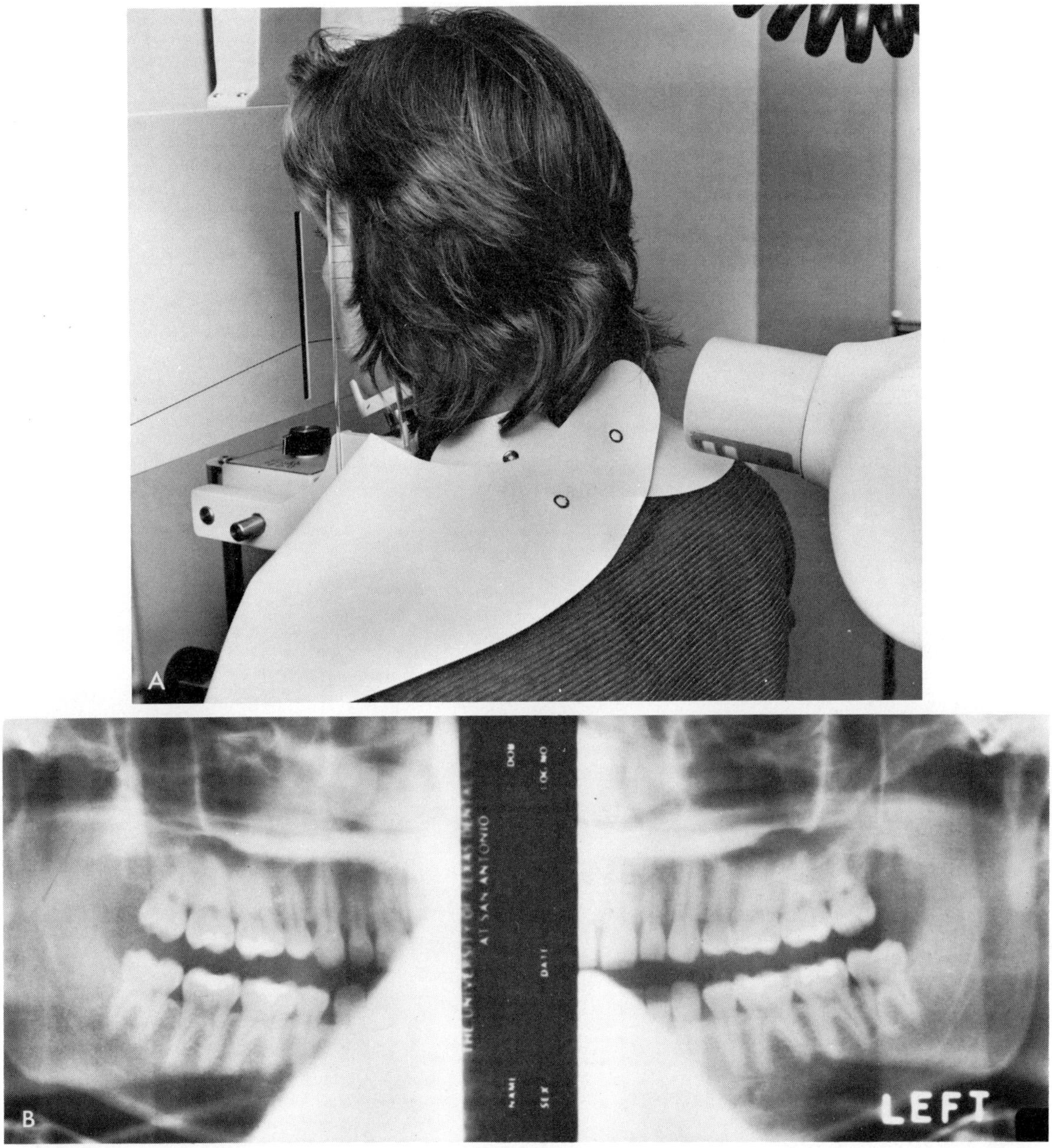

Figure 5–9. Apron placed too high on patient's neck, resulting in a radiopacity on radiograph. **A.** Patient positioned in Panorex x-ray machine with lead apron too high on back of neck. Actually, this is not the proper lead apron to use for panoramic radiography. The lead apron should cover both front and back of patient for panoramic radiographic projections. **B.** Panorex radiograph taken with lead apron too high on patient's neck, resulting in a radiopacity in lower middle portion of film.

when placed above the clavicles of the patient (Fig. 5–9). However, Witcher and associates have reported of an experimental leaded apron they designed that resulted in a 40 per cent reduction in thyroid exposure, without producing film artifacts. Usually, though, a cervical shield is not recommended for use in panoramic radiography because it produces a radiopaque area in the mandibular portion of the radiograph. See Figure 5–10 for a lead apron recommended for panoramic radiography.

ESTABLISHING EXPOSURE FACTORS

1. **Depending on the type of panoramic unit used and the film-screen combination,** select the

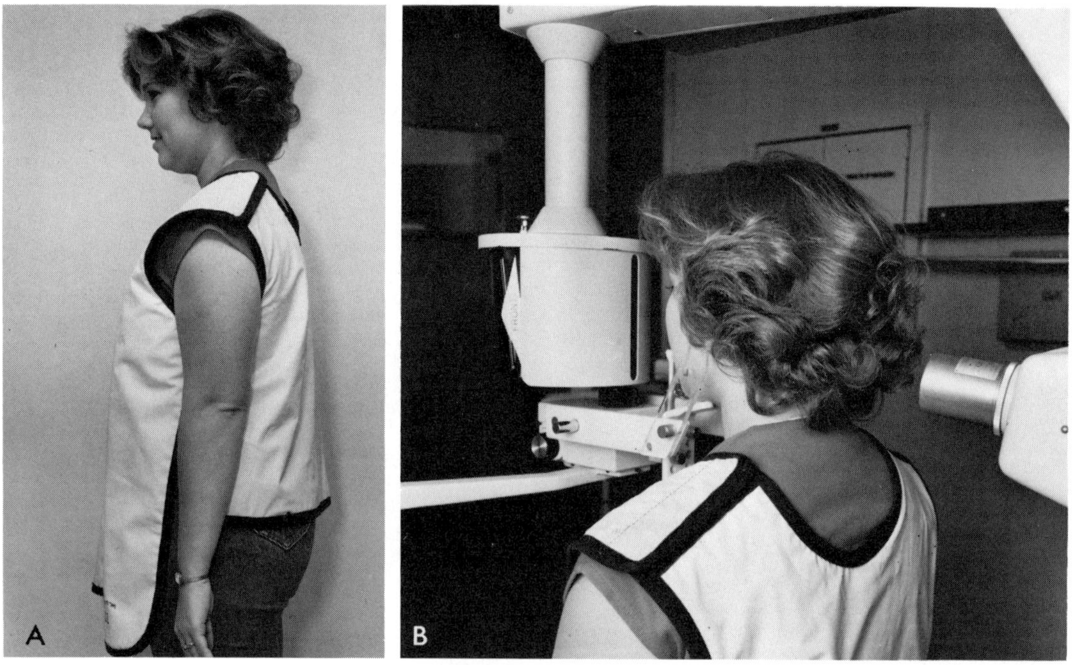

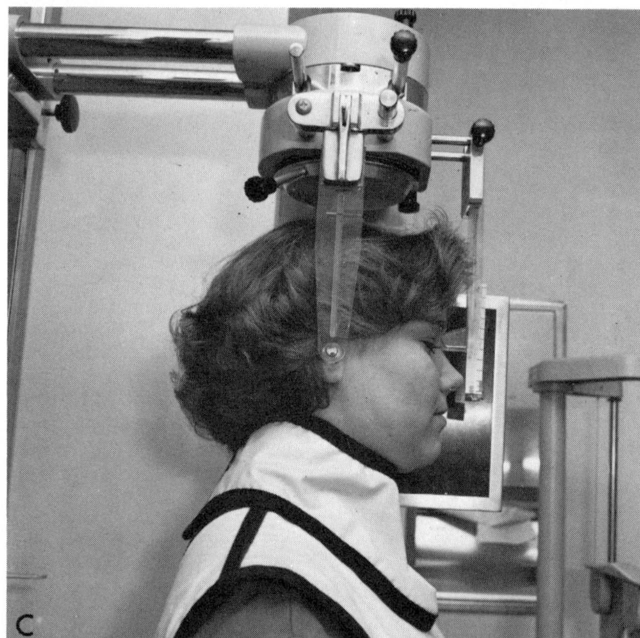

Figure 5–10. **A.** The panoramic lead apron should cover both the front and the back of the patient because both sides are exposed in panoramic x-ray projections. This apron is specifically designed for the panoramic "sit-down" machines (i.e., Panorex and Panelipse). **B.** Patient positioned in Panelipse machine with panoramic lead apron in place. A leaded cervical collar cannot be worn, as it will cause an unwanted radiopaque area in the mandibular arch. **C.** A leaded cervical collar can be used without interfering with the skull anatomy when taking a cephalometric radiograph. Of course, the cervical collar cannot be used if the clinician needs to see the cervical vertebral column on the radiograph.

proper kVp and/or mA recommended by the manufacturer (this varies with size of patient). The exposure time is fixed in panoramic radiography. It is approximately the time needed to complete one excursion of the film-tubehead assembly.

2. **The exposure factors (kVp and/or mA)** should be adjusted accordingly when taking a panoramic radiograph under the following circumstances:

a. If patient has darker skin pigmentation, use the higher kVp and/or mA setting.
b. If patient has heavy soft tissue and/or bone structure about the face and neck, use the next higher kVp and/or mA setting.
c. If patient is small and has narrow facial bone structure, use the next lower kVp and/or mA setting.
d. If patient is edentulous, use the next lower kVp and/or mA setting.

ERRORS IN POSITIONING THE CASSETTE

1. **Alternating vertical dark and light bands** on the radiograph result from improper movement of either the cassette in back of the slit in the cassette holder or the tubehead–cassette holder assembly around the patient's head. A common error is the patient's shoulders touching the cassette holder during its movement in the exposure cycle (Fig. 5–11). If the patient has a short neck and well-developed shoulders, then have him stretch his neck upward as much as possible. Elevate the chin, if possible, until the tragus-ala line is horizontal to the floor. If necessary, position the cassette holder 1/2 in

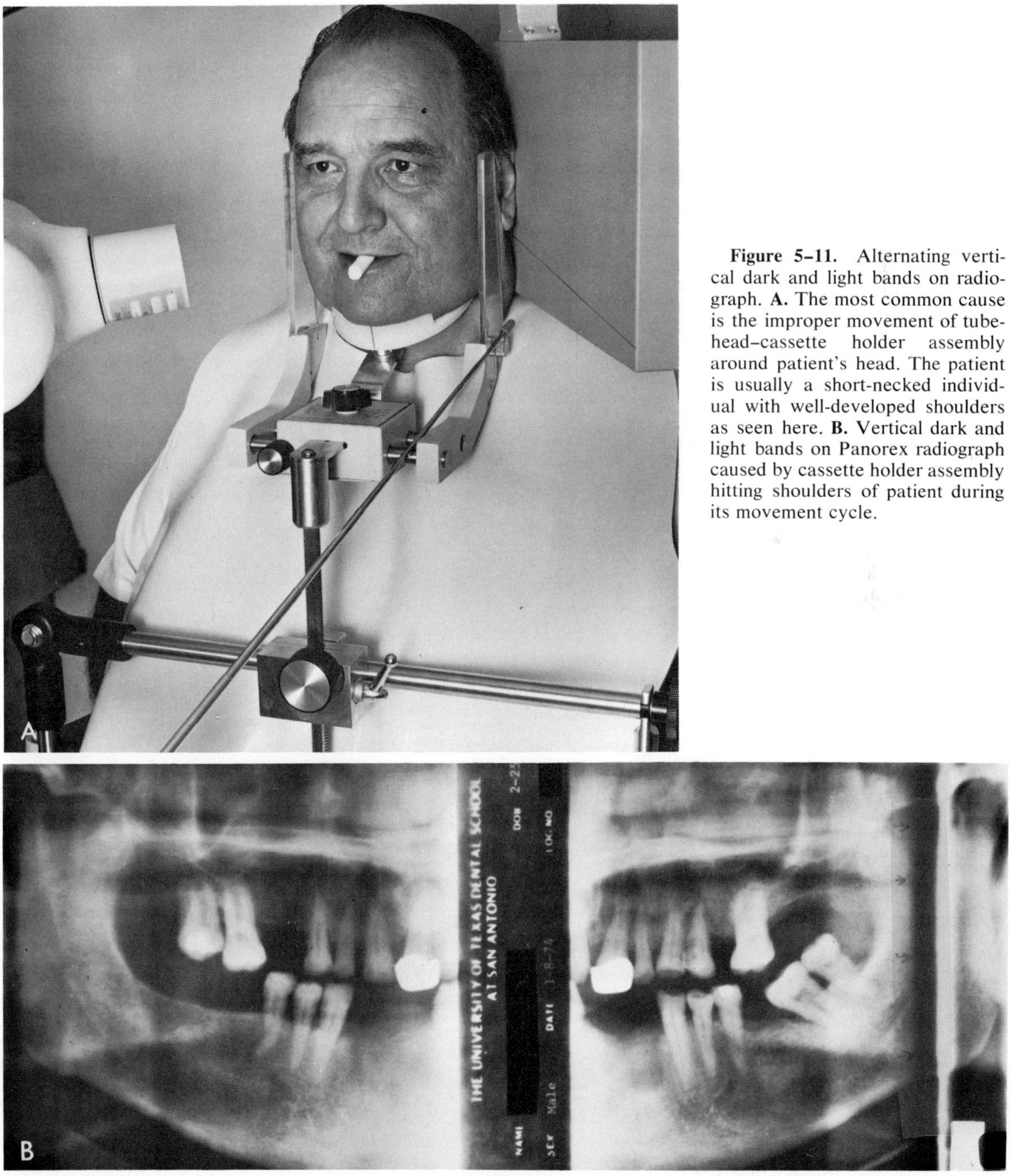

Figure 5–11. Alternating vertical dark and light bands on radiograph. **A.** The most common cause is the improper movement of tubehead–cassette holder assembly around patient's head. The patient is usually a short-necked individual with well-developed shoulders as seen here. **B.** Vertical dark and light bands on Panorex radiograph caused by cassette holder assembly hitting shoulders of patient during its movement cycle.

higher than usual, especially when using the Panorex. Be careful not to position the cassette too high, as it will cut off the lower border of the mandible (Fig. 5–12).

2. When the **cassette is placed too far below** the mandible, diagnostic information in the maxilla will be cut off (Fig. 5–13).

3. If **two exposures are taken on a single film,** the resulting radiograph will have a higher density and superimposition of anatomic structures. The radiograph in almost all cases is undiagnostic (Fig. 5–14). To prevent double exposures, exposed and unexposed films should be kept separate at all times. When a film has been exposed, it should be immediately developed or the cassette placed in a container or pass box marked "EXPOSED"; otherwise, the likelihood of double exposure is increased.

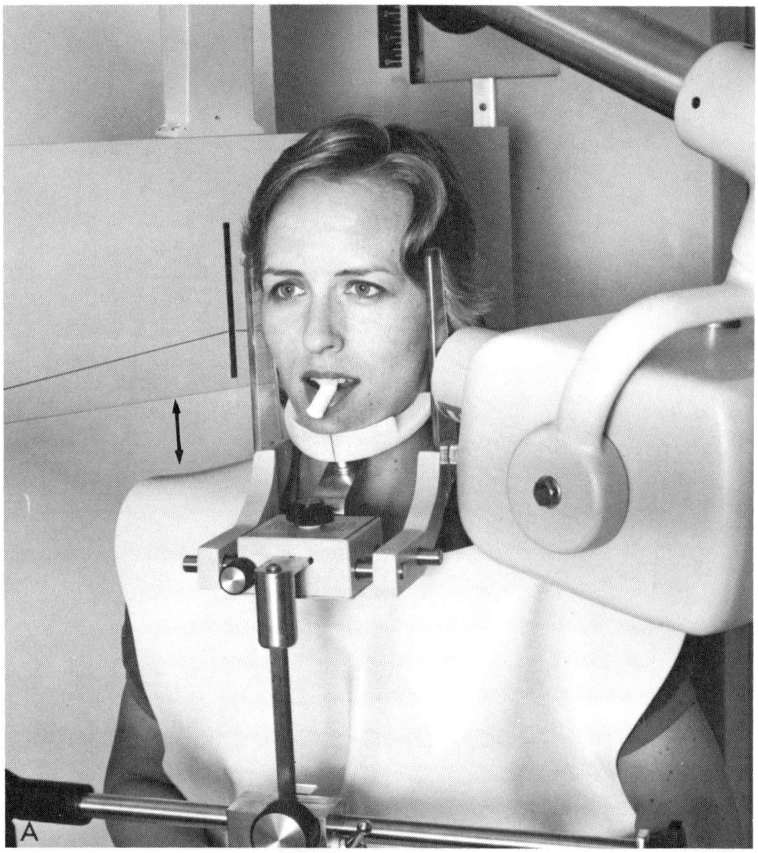

Figure 5–12. **A.** Panorex cassette holder assembly is placed too high for this patient. **B.** Panorex radiograph taken with cassette holder assembly placed too high. The lower border of the mandible is missing.

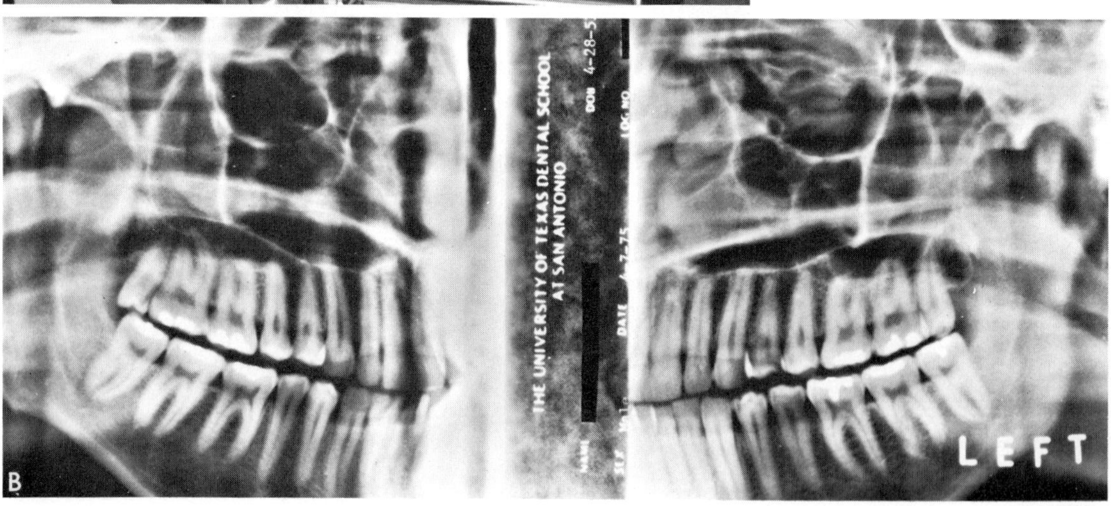

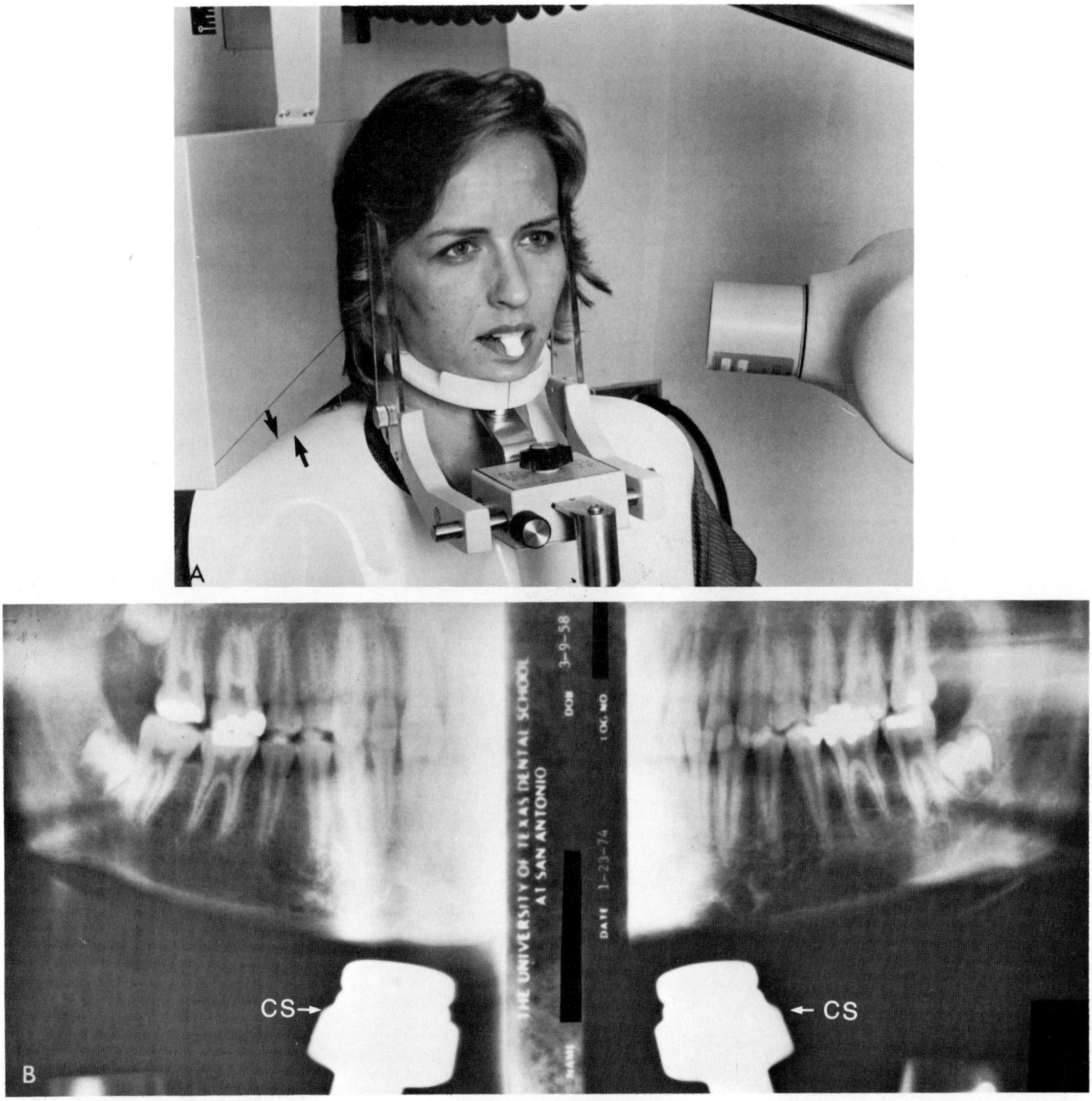

Figure 5–13. **A.** Patient positioned in Panorex with cassette holder assembly positioned too low. **B.** Panorex radiograph with cassette assembly placed too low, resulting in loss of maxillary sinuses and temporomandibular joints. Also, no cotton roll was placed between the teeth, resulting in vertical overlapping. CS = metal chin rest supports.

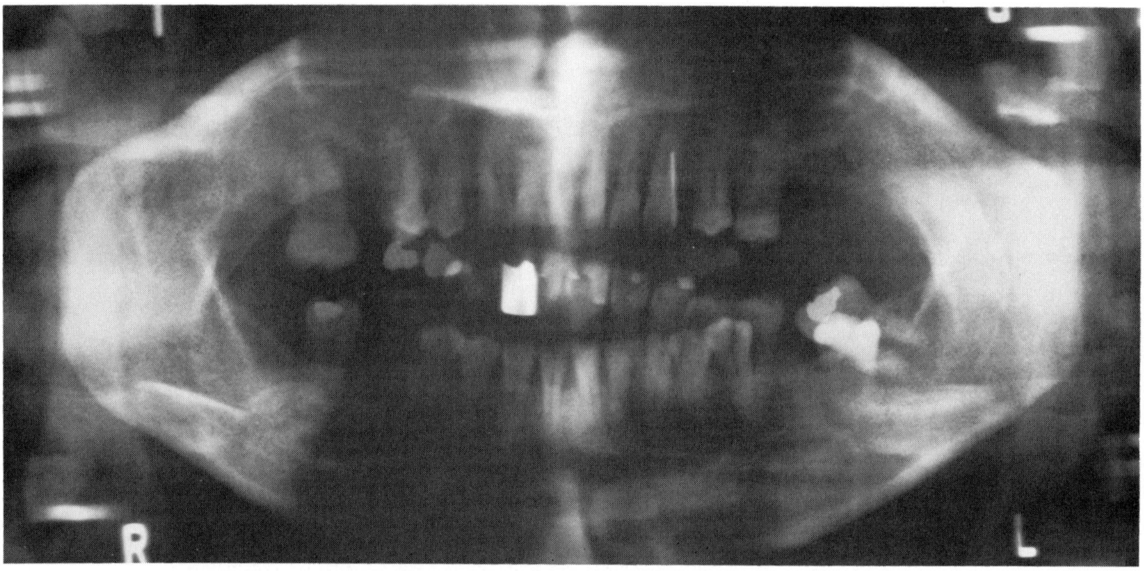

Figure 5–14. Double exposure. Two Panelipse radiographs taken on a single film.

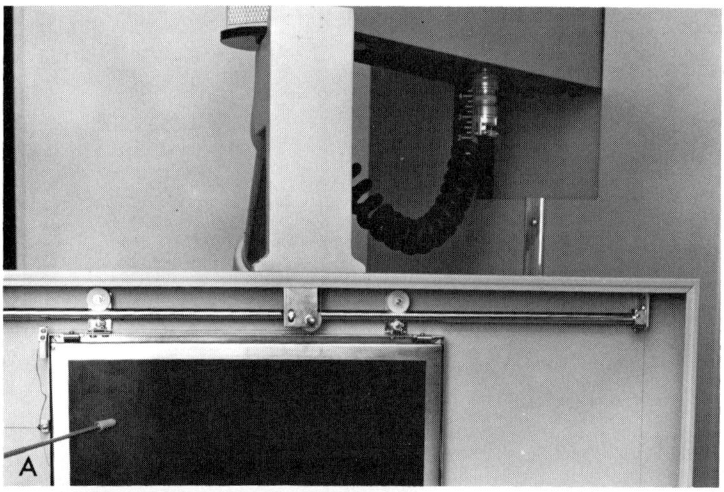

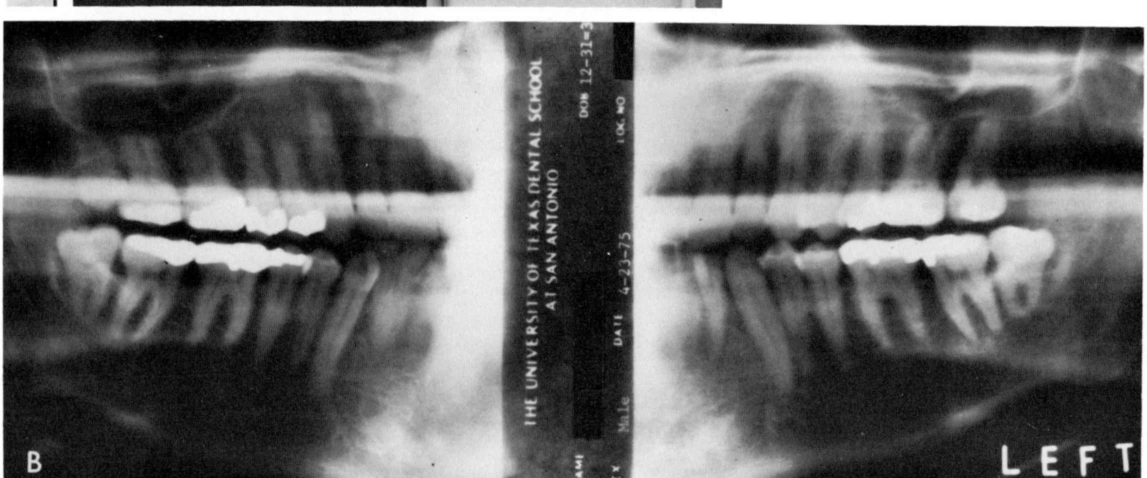

Figure 5–15. A. Panorex cassette placed backwards in cassette holder. **B.** Broad radiopaque horizontal line through middle of Panorex radiograph indicates that cassette was placed backward in cassette holder.

4. **When the cassette is placed backwards,** especially in the Panorex, the x rays must penetrate the metal latch, which will present a radiopaque broad horizontal line through the middle of the radiograph (Fig. 5–15).

ERRORS IN POSITIONING THE PATIENT

1. **Anterior Teeth Positioning Error.** Blurring of the anterior teeth will occur if they are positioned outside the focal trough. The apices of the anterior teeth are located normally more posteriorly to their incisal edges. Therefore, to place the anterior teeth in the anterior focal trough, the occlusal plane must be tilted downward in the anterior region and the teeth placed in an end-to-end position. Many panoramic units have narrow anterior focal troughs, and accurate anterior positioning is very important in these units. Figure 5–16 illustrates unsharpness caused by improper positioning of the anterior teeth outside the focal trough, too far forward or too far backward.

2. **Midsagittal Plane Positioning Error.** If the symphysis of the mandible is not aligned with the midline of the chin rest or if the midsagittal plane is off center, the image of the structures farthest from the film will be magnified, whereas, on the opposite side, the image of the structures closest to the film will be decreased in size. Figure 5–17 shows the distortion caused by not positioning the patient symmetrically in the chin rest. If the head-positioning device in the Panelipse machine is not locked in place, the patient's head can be asymmetrically aligned in the machine, resulting in a poor-quality radiograph (Fig. 5–18). If the patient's head is too large and cannot be centered on the chin rest of the Panorex, rotate the cassette holder assembly 5 to 10° (with radiation off), position the head in the usual position, switch on the exposure, and complete the exposure cycle.

3. **Spinal Column Positioning Error.** Incorrect vertebral column positioning will result in an unexposed area in the middle inferior portion of the film or sometimes in the ramus/condylar area. If the spine is not kept erect, the radiation will be excessively absorbed by the spinal column, resulting in the low-density area near the lower center of the film (Fig. 5–19). One of

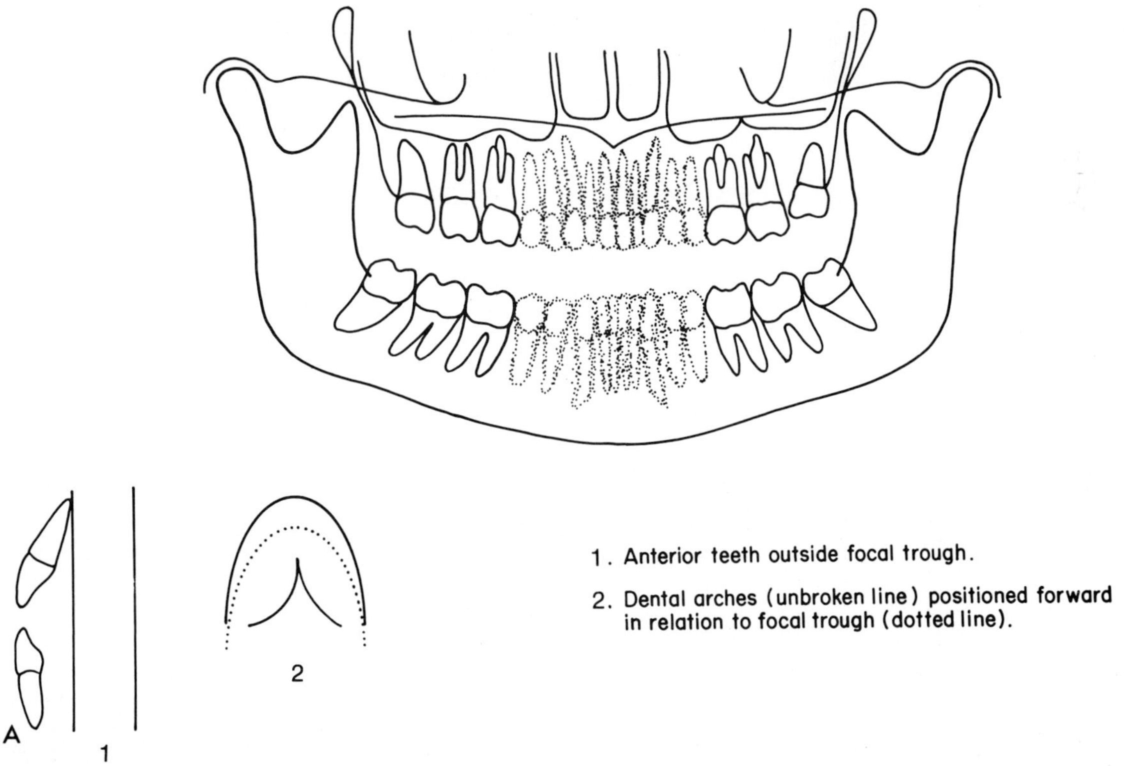

Figure 5–16. Anterior teeth positioning error. **A.** Diagram of continuous image panoramic radiograph with anterior teeth positioned too far forward outside the focal trough.

Illustration continued on following page

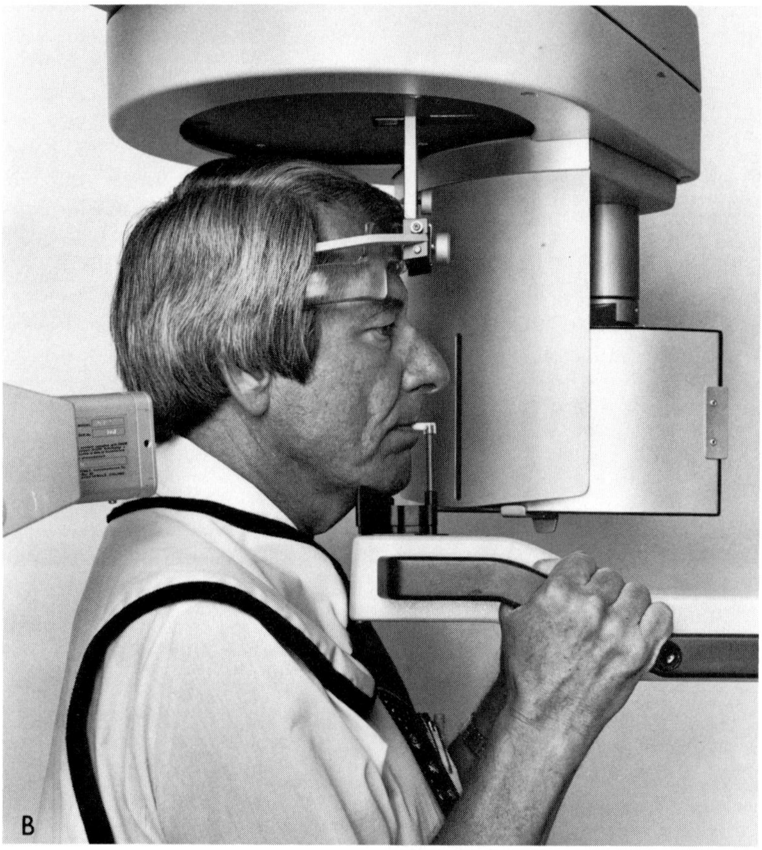

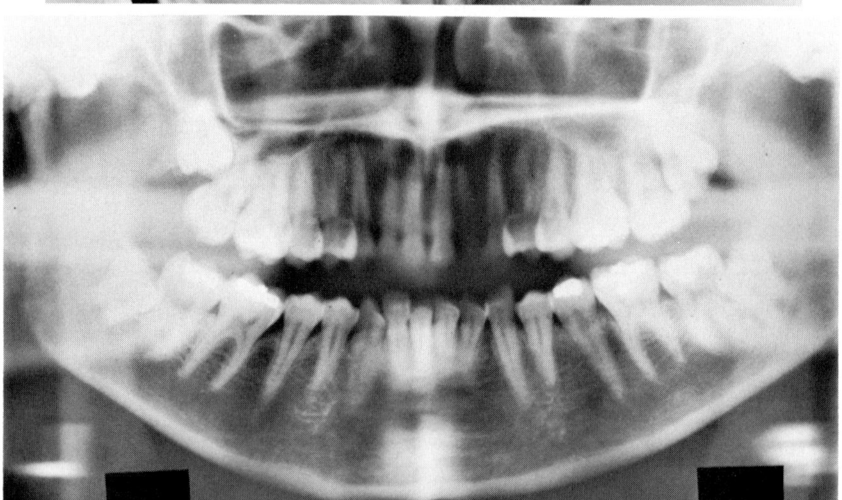

Figure 5–16 *Continued.* **B.** Patient placed too far forward in Orthopantomograph. This will cause narrowing and blurring of anterior teeth images. **C.** Patient placed too far forward outside the focal trough, resulting in blurring and narrowing of maxillary anterior teeth.

Illustration continued on opposite page

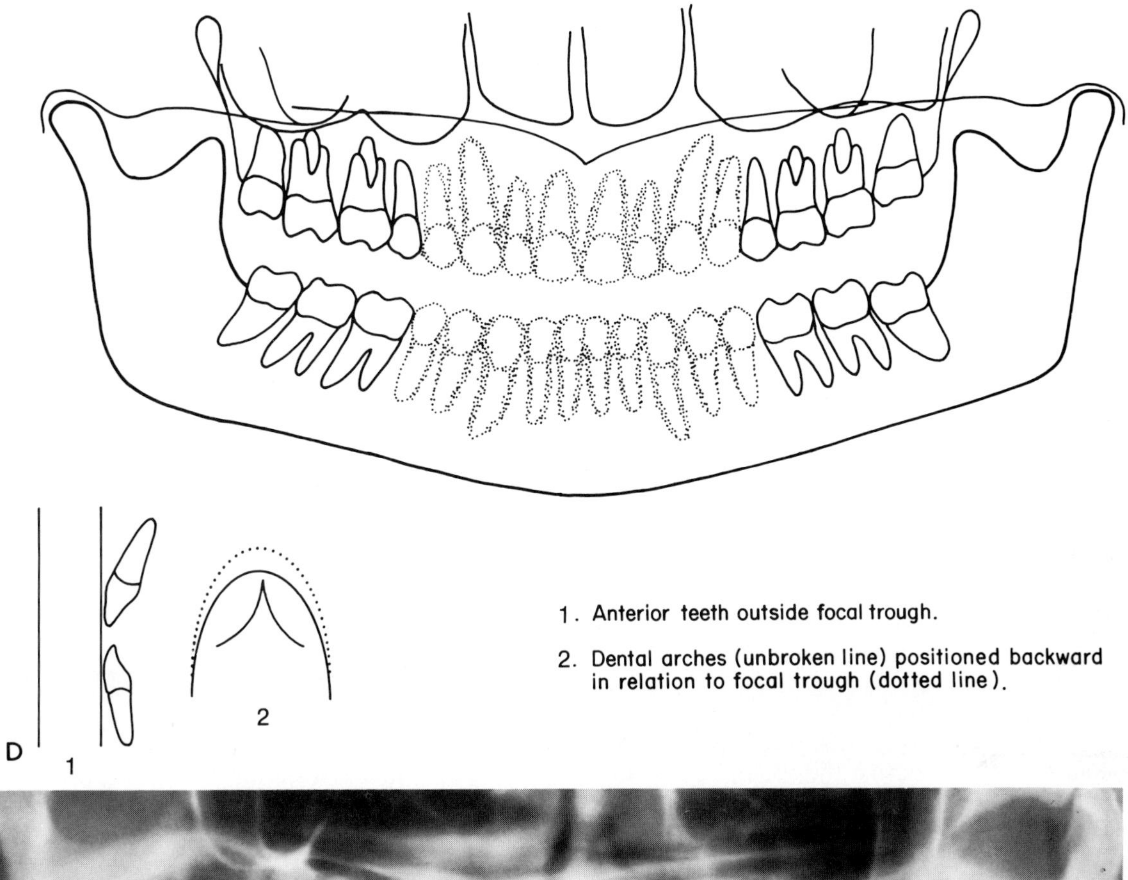

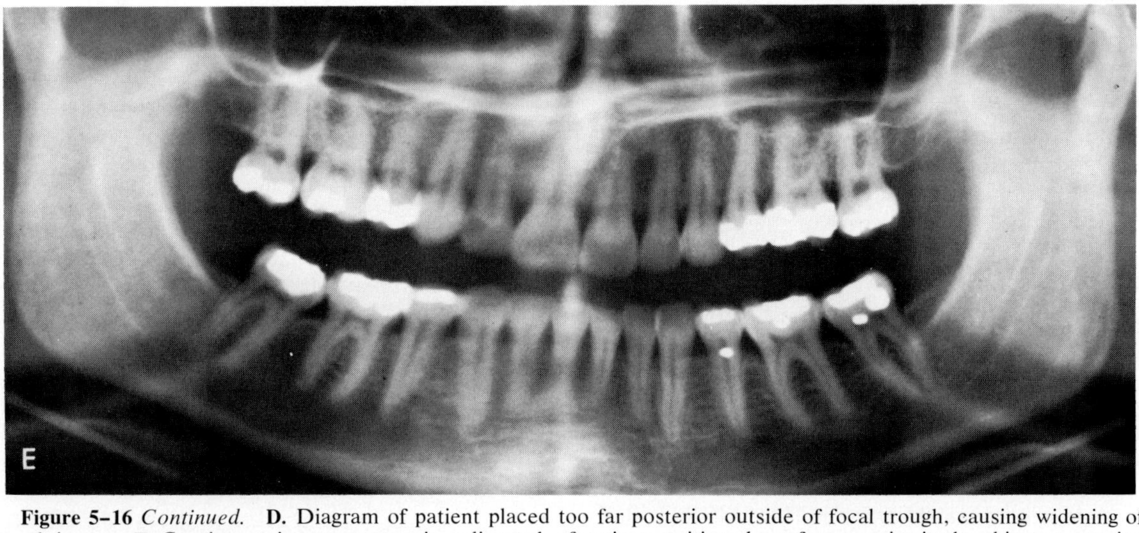

Figure 5–16 *Continued.* **D.** Diagram of patient placed too far posterior outside of focal trough, causing widening of tooth images. **E.** Continuous image panoramic radiograph of patient positioned too far posterior in the chin rest, causing widening of teeth images.

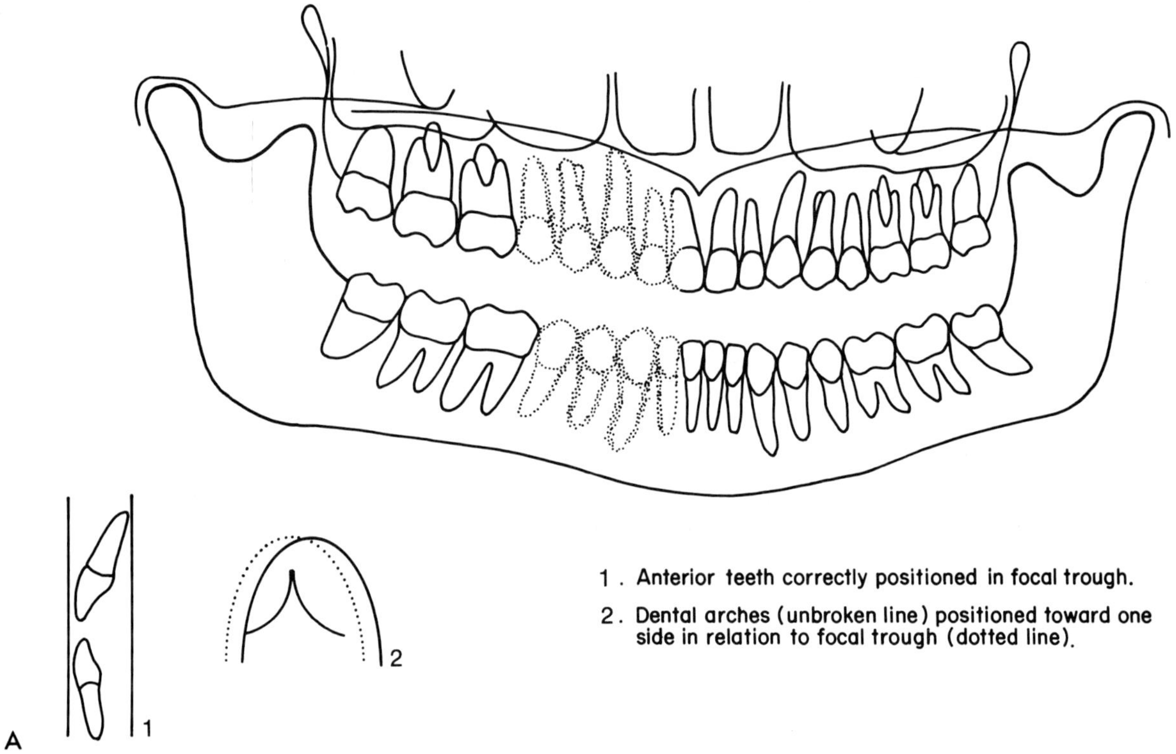

Figure 5–17. **A.** Diagram of radiograph of patient positioned toward one side and outside of focal trough toward the film cassette causing distortion of tooth images.

Illustration continued on opposite page

the authors believes that the radiopaque area in the anterior portion of the radiograph produced by slumping of the patient's neck and shoulders is caused by the phenomenon of "ghosting" (see Fig. 5–5). Gratt and coworkers demonstrated that the use of an inclined footrest for nonshifting, front-seating dental panoramic x-ray units (such as the GE Panelipse) improves the sitting posture of the patient (back arched and neck extended), which, in turn, reduces the spine-radiopacity artifact (Fig. 5–20).

4. **Occlusal Plane Positioning Error: Upward Overangulation.** If the occlusal plane is positioned parallel to the floor rather than slightly down and forward, it will produce the following faults or conditions:

a. Superimposition of the hard palate on the maxillary anterior tooth apices.
b. A loss of density in the middle of the radiograph, usually characterized by an hourglass shape.
c. The loss of either one or both temporomandibular joints.
d. When the chin is tipped upward, the back of the patient's head is usually positioned posteriorly. This will cause magnification of the maxillary anterior teeth. Figure 5–21 illustrates incorrect positioning of the patient's chin (too high). This error may also cause interference of the back of the patient's head with the cassette holder, thereby preventing the operator from positioning the patient's head symmetrically in the chin rest.

5. **Occlusal Plane Positioning Error: Downward Overangulation.** This overangulation (tragus-ala line greater than 5° downward and forward) results in a severe curvature in the occlusal plane and a consequent lack of definition of the incisors on the radiographic image. Figure 5–22 illustrates this error.

6. **Distortion Due to Patient Movement.** The patient will occasionally move during the exposure of a panoramic radiograph. This can give rise to a series of artifacts or distortion effects that are usually localized to only one region of the radiograph, namely, the region the rotating beam was scanning when the patient moved. The following are the primary image artifacts or distortion phenomena caused by patient movement (Samfors and Welander):

a. Should the patient move slowly in the same

Text continued on page 115

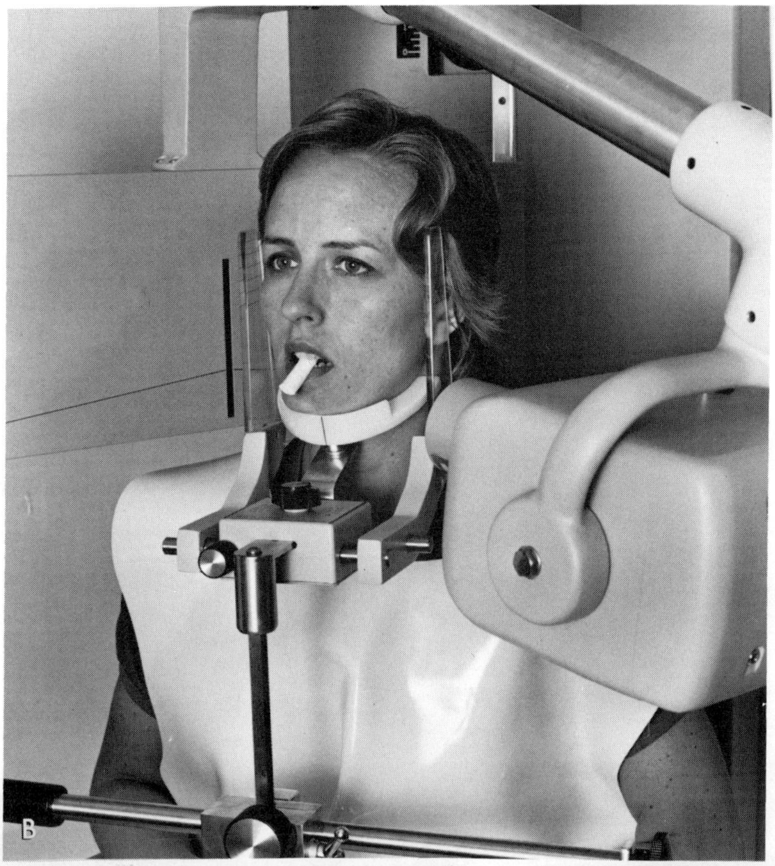

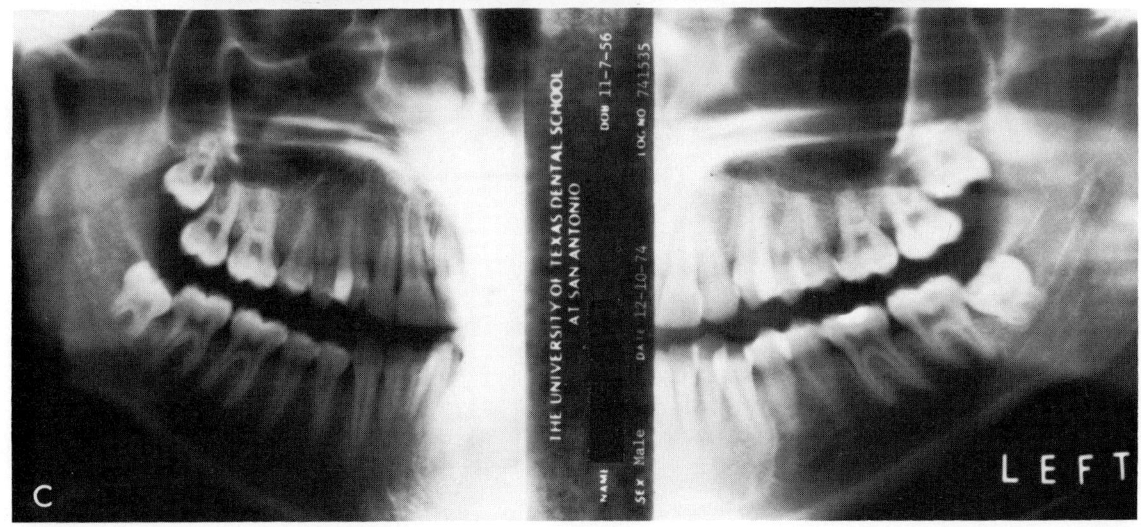

Figure 5–17 *Continued.* **B.** Patient positioned asymmetrically in Panorex chin rest too far toward (film cassette on patient's right side). **C.** Panorex radiograph taken with patient positioned asymmetrically in chin rest. Images of structures farthest from the film will be magnified, whereas images of structures closest to the film will be decreased in size.

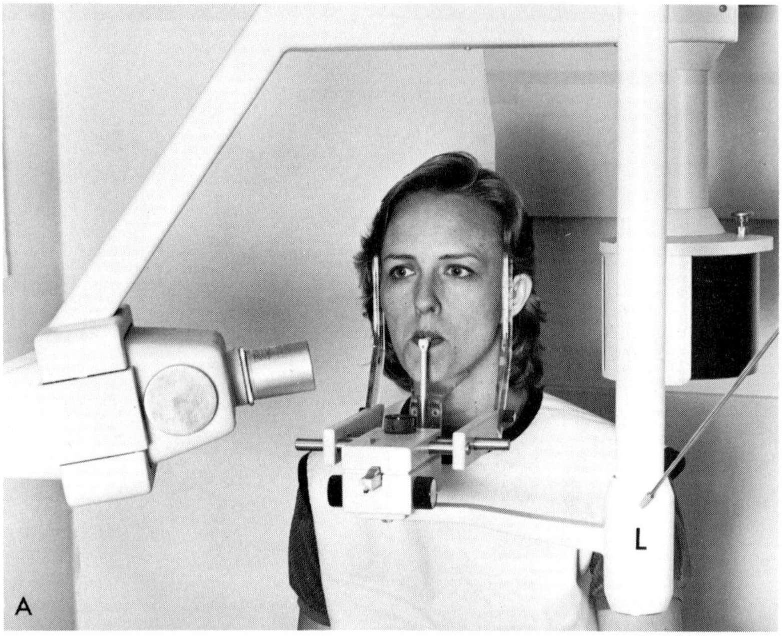

Figure 5–18. **A.** Patient misaligned to focal trough because Panelipse head positioner is not locked in place. L = head positioner locking mechanism. **B.** Panelipse radiograph taken with patient positioned asymmetrically in x-ray unit because head positioner was not locked in place.

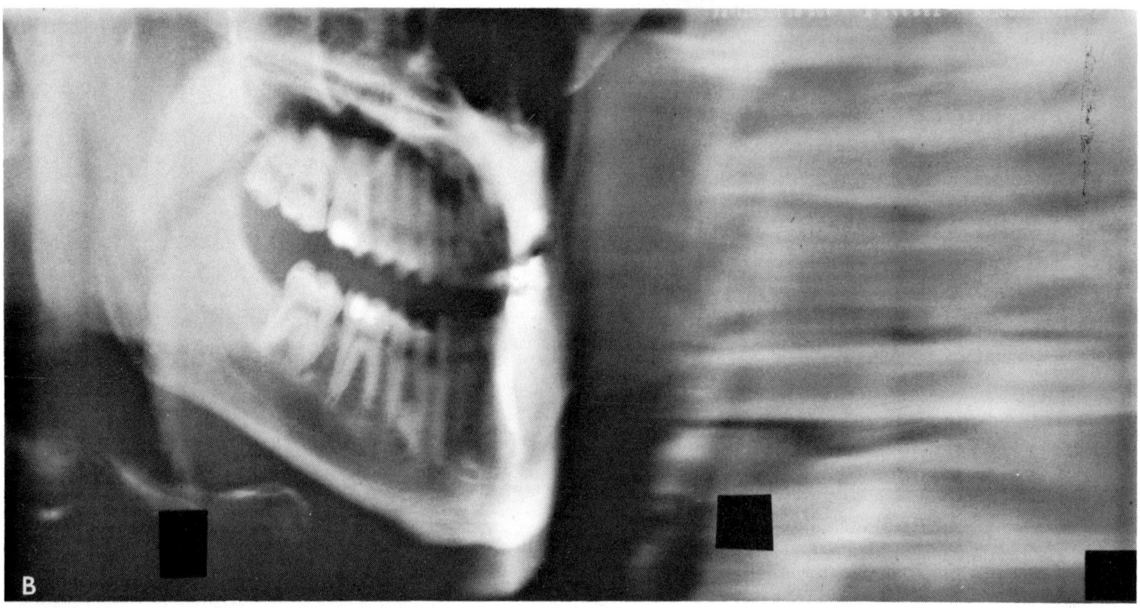

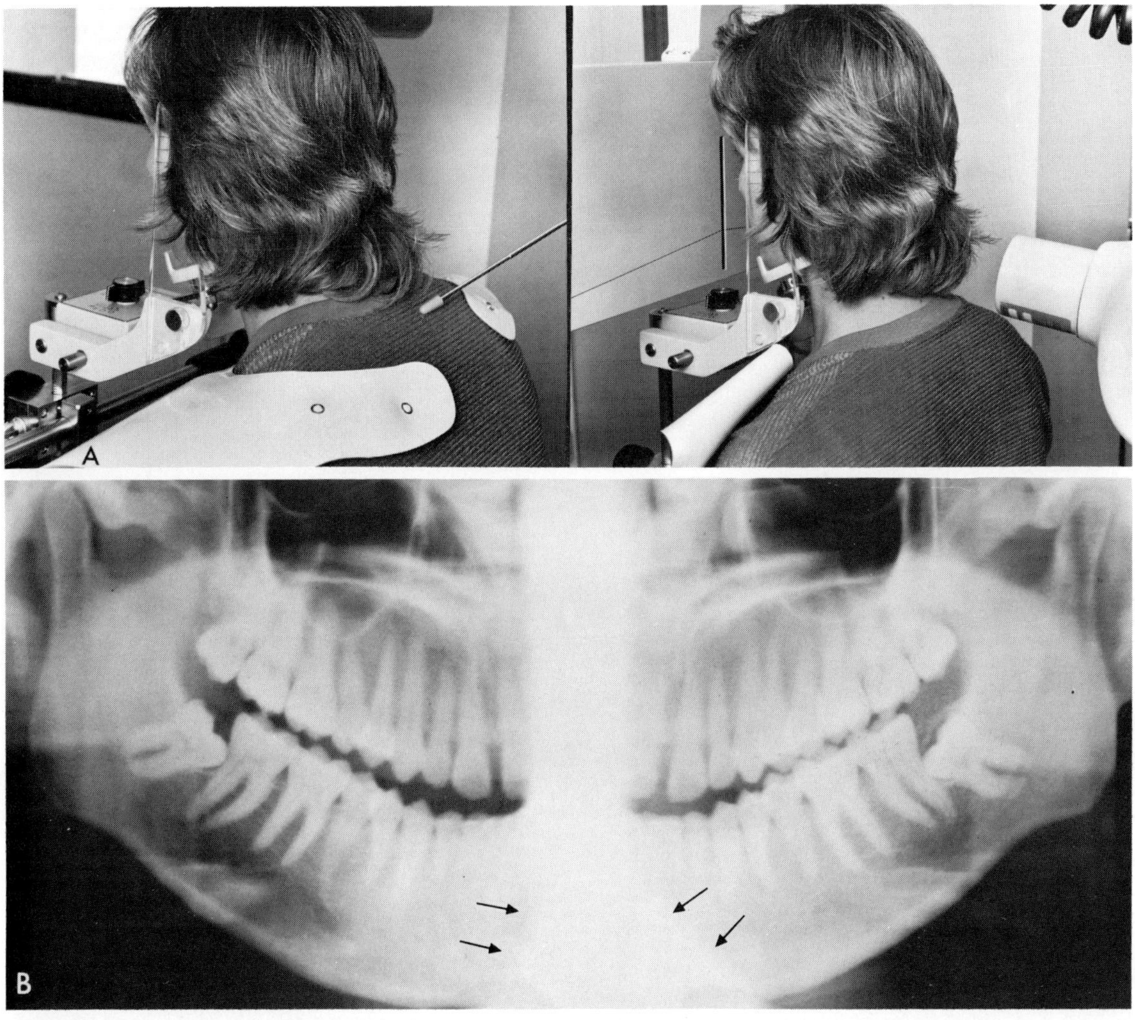

Figure 5–19. **A.** Left, patient positioned in Panorex with spinal column not erect. Right, patient positioned correctly with spinal column erect (apron has been removed to show correct positioning). **B.** Panorex radiograph of patient with spinal column not erect, causing radiopaque area in lower center of radiograph.

Illustration continued on following page

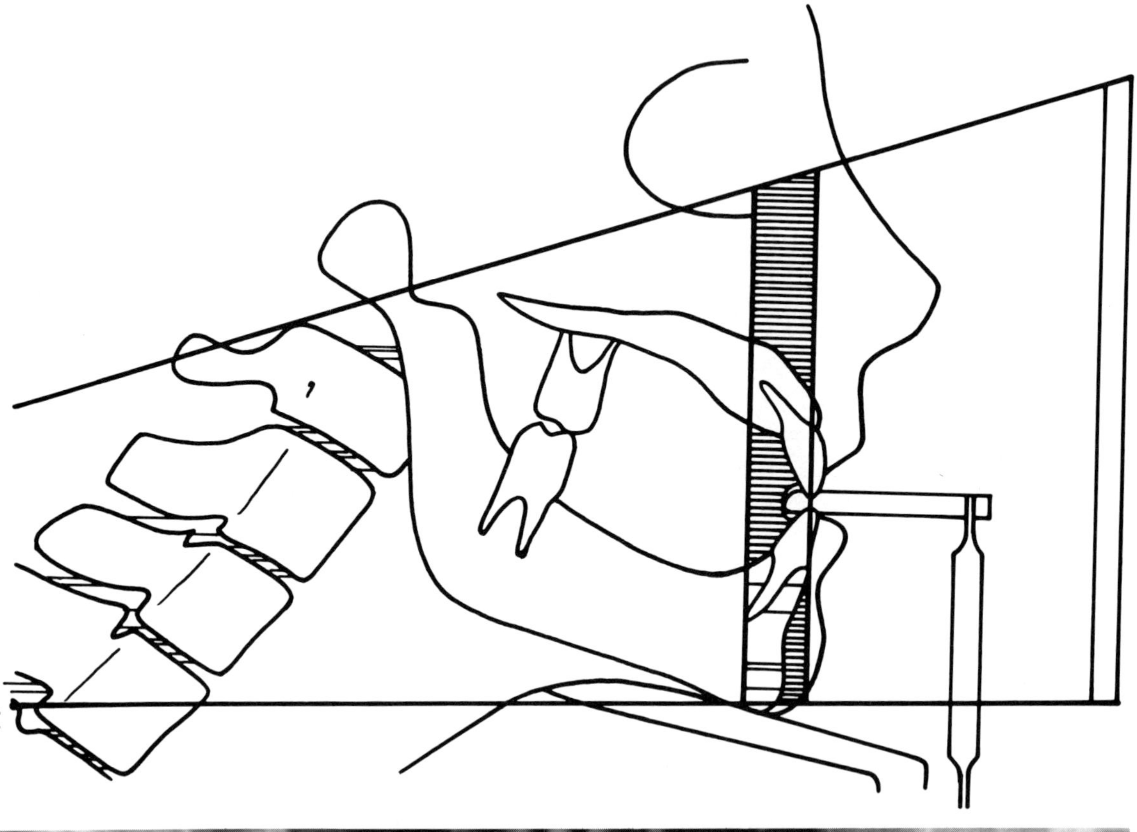

C

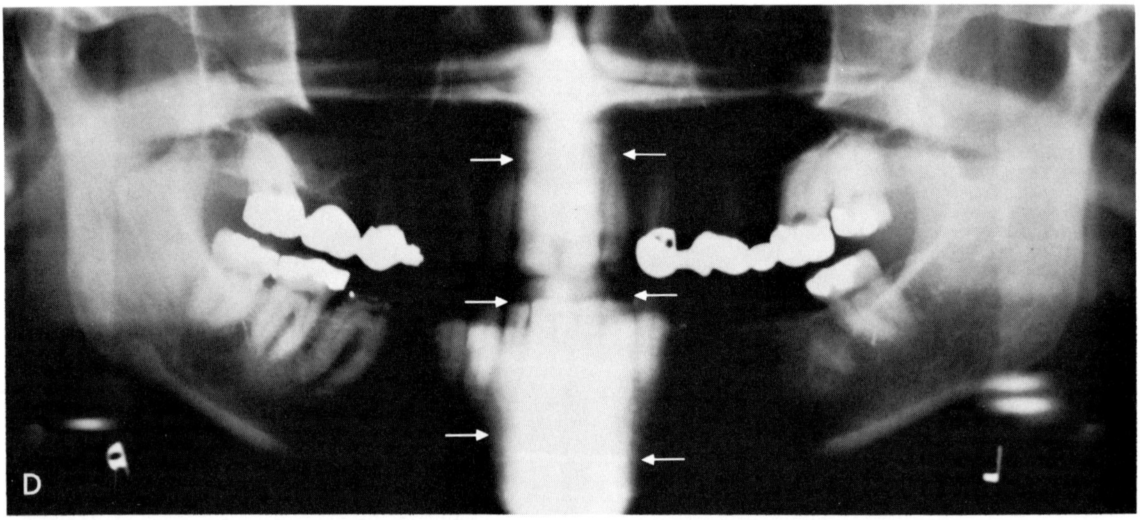

Figure 5–19 *Continued.* **C.** Diagram of a patient positioned in the Panelipse panoramic unit. The patient's occlusal plane is properly positioned (tilted slightly downward), but the neck is in a slumped position rather than the proper straight position. (Courtesy of G. E. Dental Systems, Milwaukee, WI.) **D.** Panelipse radiograph with an obscuring spinal column radiopacity in the center of the radiograph. This is caused by the patient's neck being placed in a slumped position, which projects the cervical spine image over the maxillary and mandibular anterior regions. (Courtesy of Felix Cordero, San Antonio, TX.)

Illustration continued on opposite page

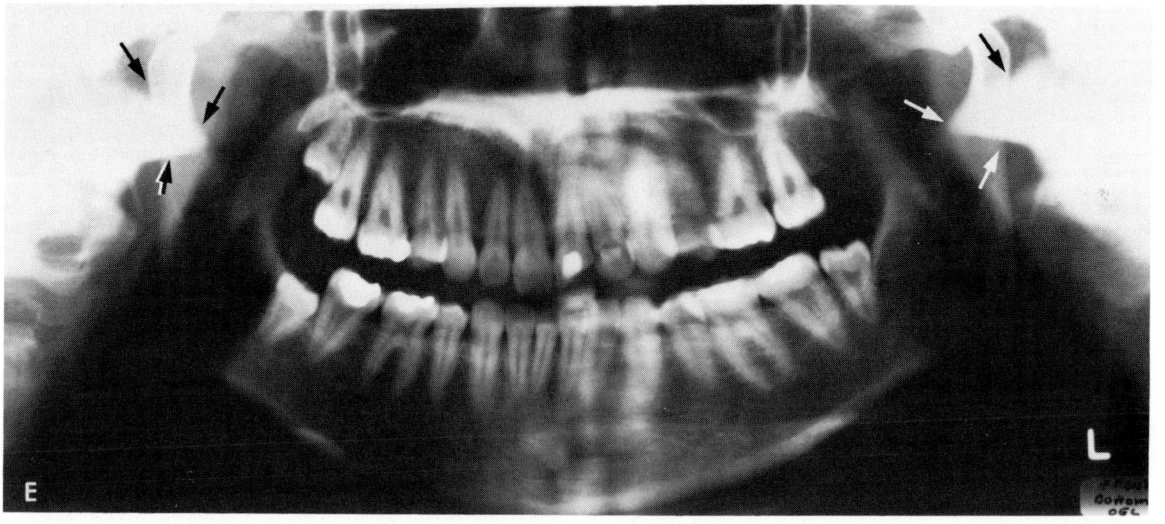

Figure 5–19 *Continued.* **E.** Notice the superimposition of a portion of the spinal column over the neck of the condylar process of the mandible caused by improper positioning of the spinal column.

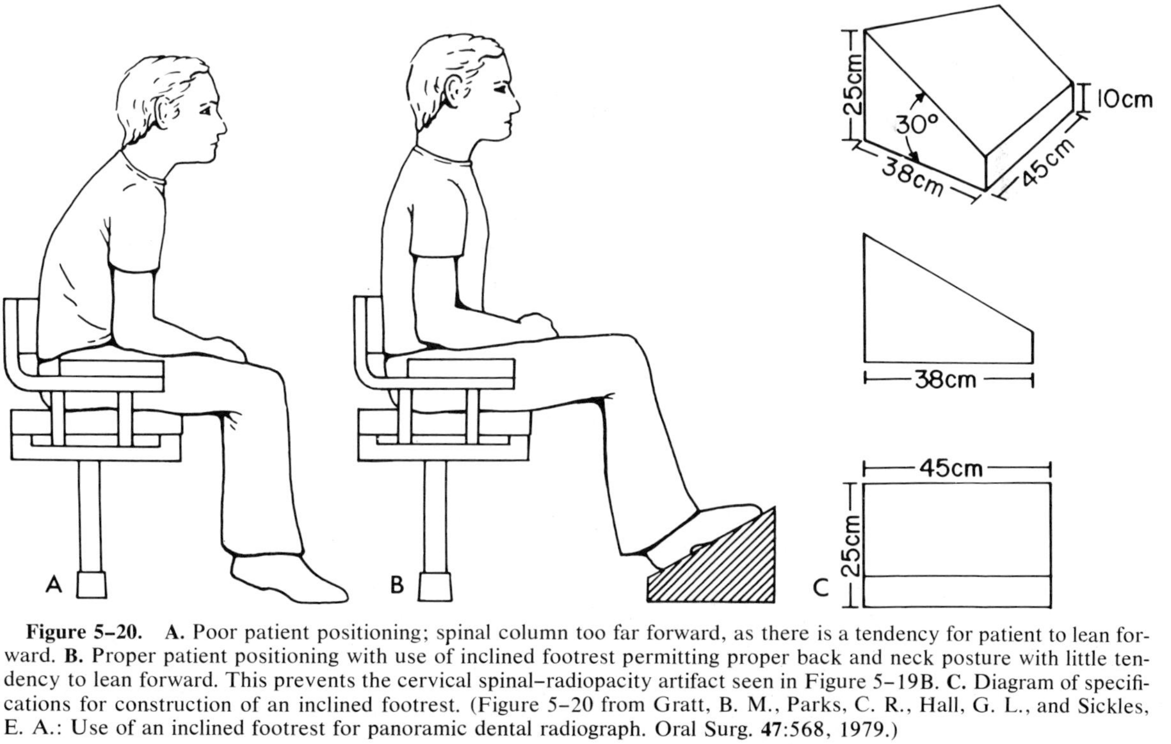

Figure 5–20. **A.** Poor patient positioning; spinal column too far forward, as there is a tendency for patient to lean forward. **B.** Proper patient positioning with use of inclined footrest permitting proper back and neck posture with little tendency to lean forward. This prevents the cervical spinal–radiopacity artifact seen in Figure 5–19B. **C.** Diagram of specifications for construction of an inclined footrest. (Figure 5–20 from Gratt, B. M., Parks, C. R., Hall, G. L., and Sickles, E. A.: Use of an inclined footrest for panoramic dental radiograph. Oral Surg. **47**:568, 1979.)

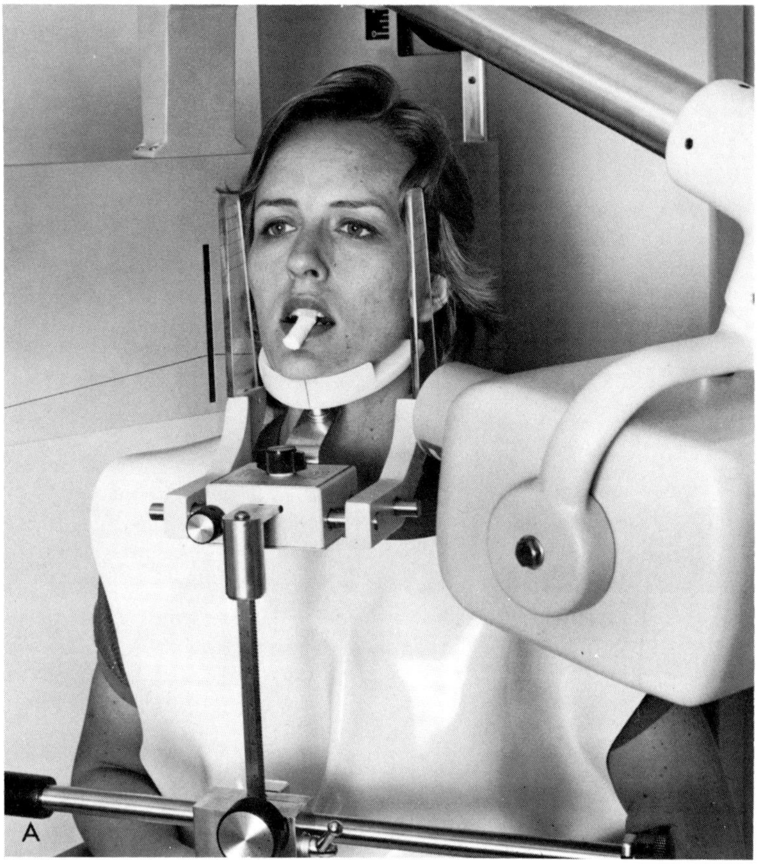

Figure 5–21. **A.** In panoramic radiography, it is recommended that the patient's head be positioned with the tragus-ala line 5° below the horizontal plane. Patient is positioned in Panorex unit with occlusal plane at a positive degree of angulation above the horizontal plane. **B.** Diagram showing that when chin is placed too high and the maxillary arch anterior teeth are positioned outside the focal trough away from the film cassette, magnification will result.

Illustration continued on opposite page

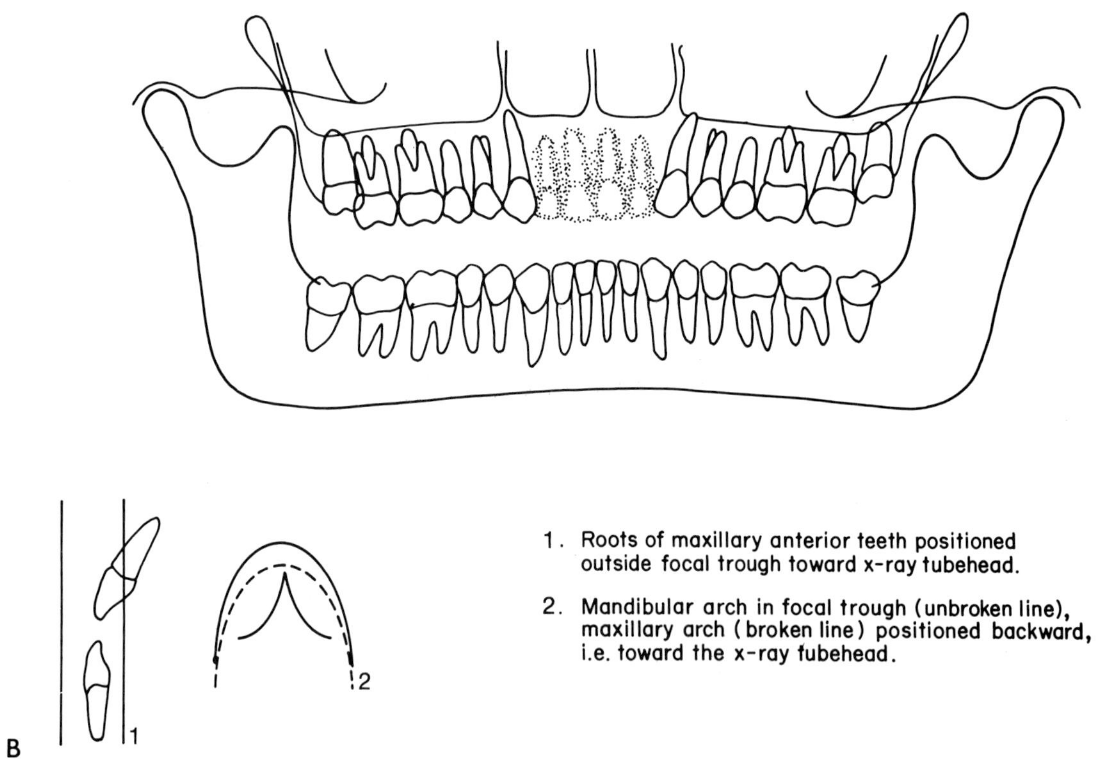

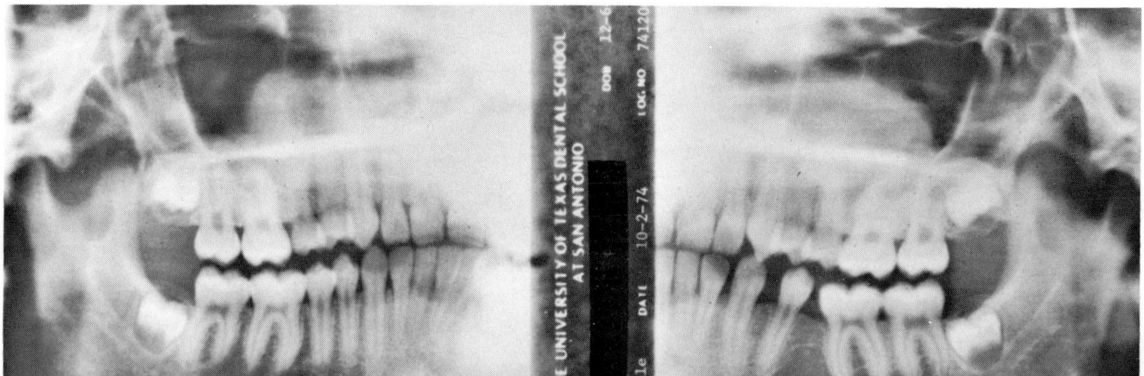

Figure 5–21 *Continued.* **C.** Panorex radiograph taken with patient's head positioned with chin too high, resulting in the hard palate superimposed over the maxillary anterior tooth apices. **D.** Panoral radiograph taken with chin positioned too high, resulting in magnification of maxillary anterior teeth and loss of both temporomandibular joints.

Illustration continued on following page

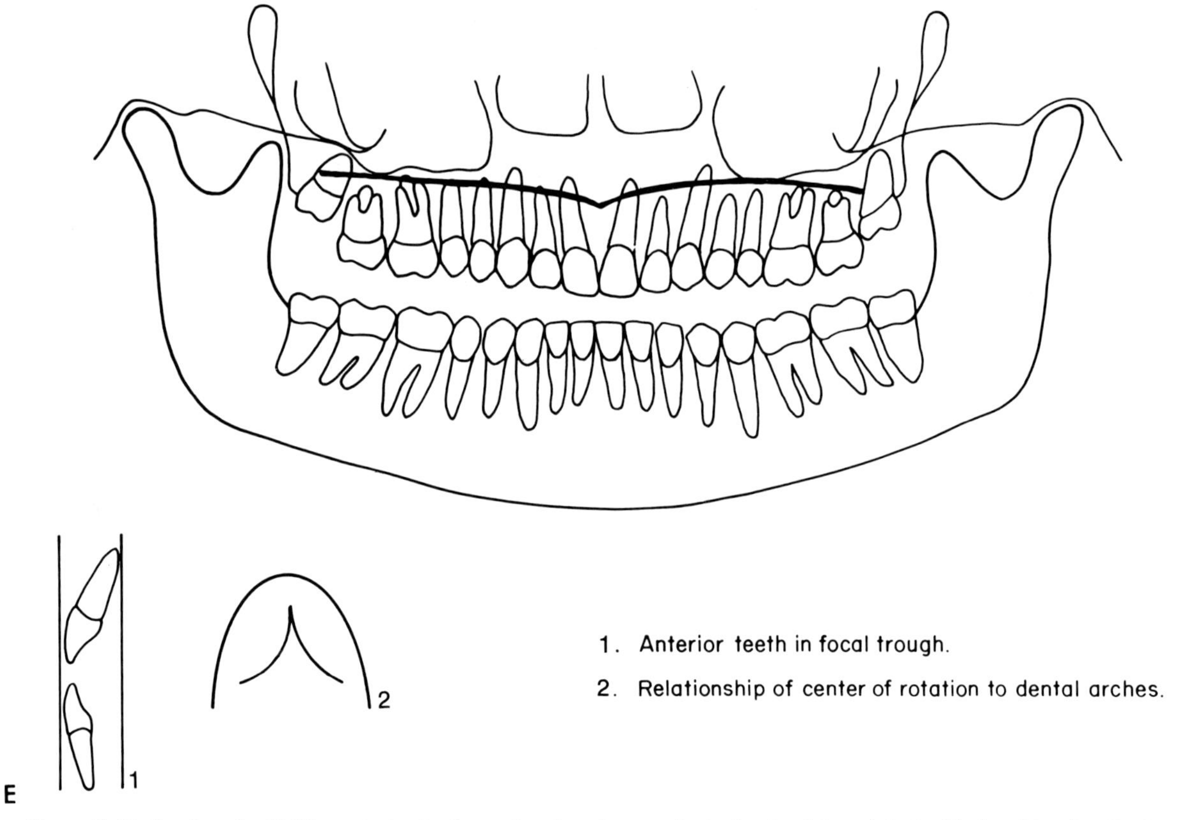

Figure 5–21 *Continued.* **E.** The anterior teeth can be placed correctly in the focal trough but with the chin of patient positioned too high, as shown in this diagram. The maxillary anterior teeth will not be distorted, but the maxillary palate will be superimposed over the roots of the maxillary teeth.

Illustration continued on opposite page

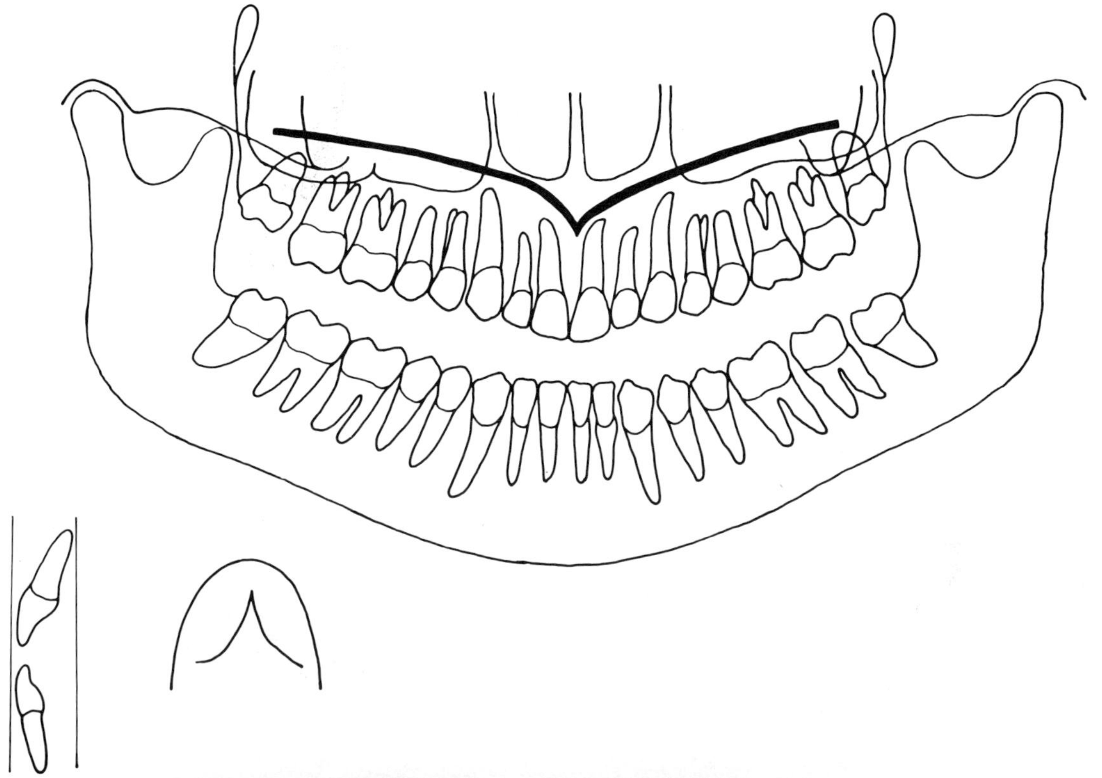

F

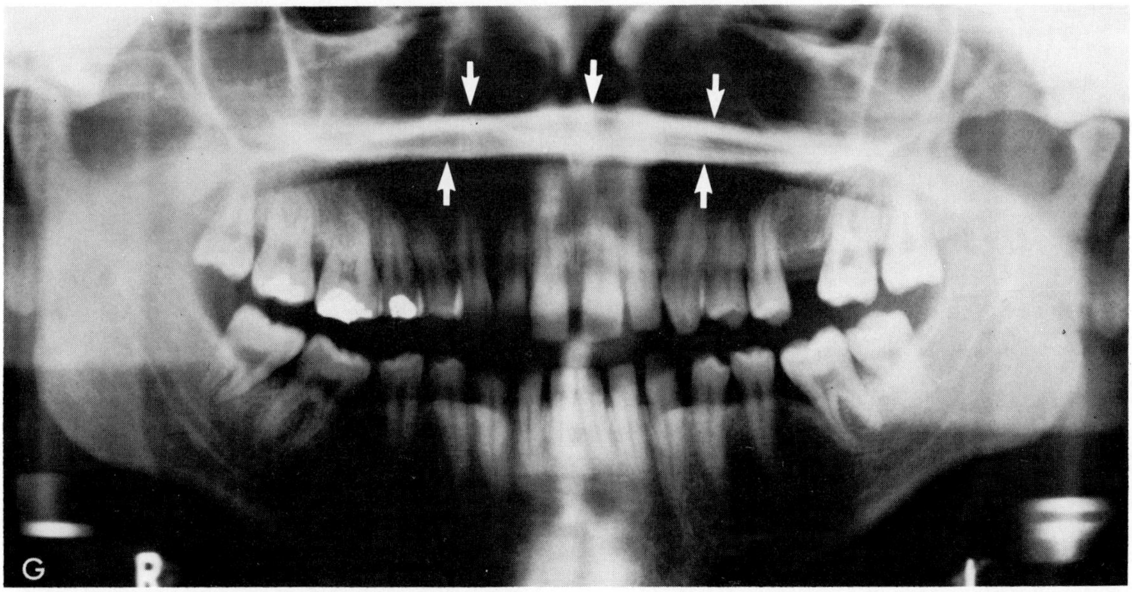

Figure 5–21 *Continued.* **F.** By placing the anterior teeth in the focal trough and positioning the occlusal plane slightly downward and forward, the maxillary palate will be projected superiorly and away from the roots of the maxillary teeth as shown in this diagram. **G.** Panelipse radiograph without undue distortion of images of the anterior teeth and with the maxillary palate projected superiorly away from the roots of the maxillary teeth.

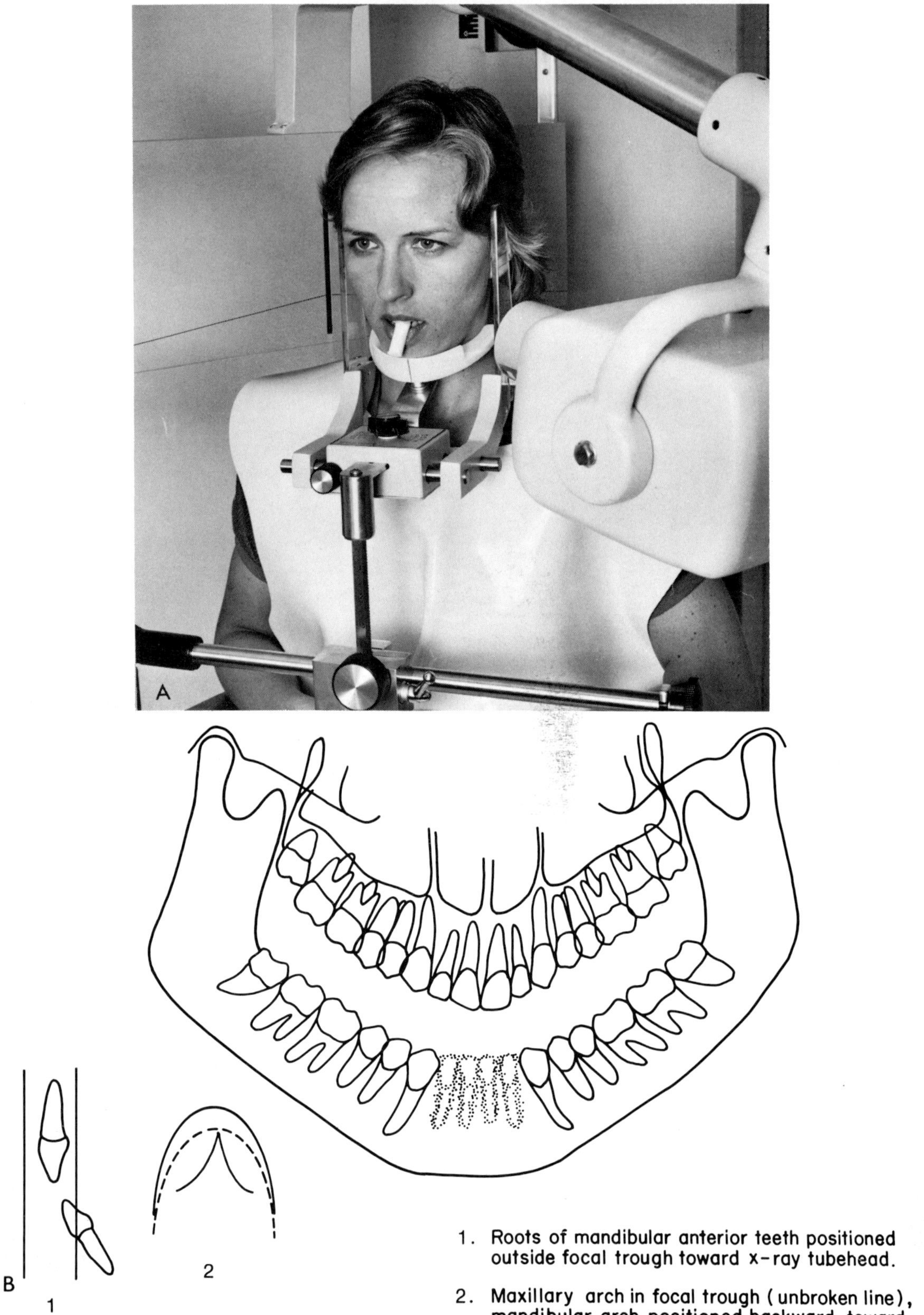

Figure 5–22. **A.** Patient positioned with chin too low in Panorex x-ray unit. Occlusal plane is overangulated downward from the correct position of placing tragus-ala line 5° downward and forward. **B.** Diagram illustrates the error of positioning the chin too low, resulting in a severe curvature of the occlusal plane and lack of definition of lower incisors.

Illustration continued on opposite page

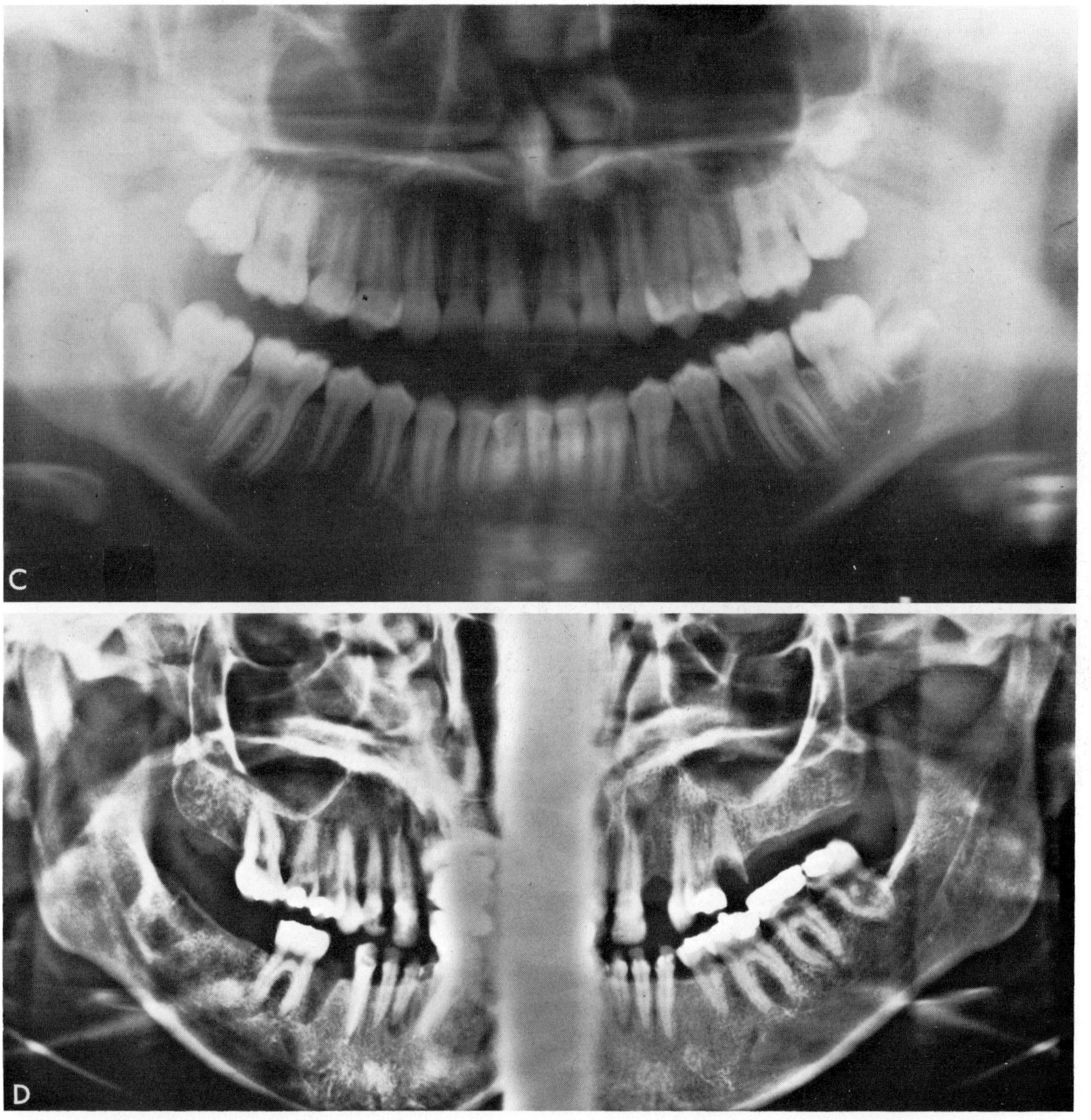

Figure 5–22 *Continued.* **C.** Chin positioned too low in a Panelipse x-ray machine, resulting in distortion of incisal edges of mandibular incisors. **D.** Panorex radiograph taken with patient's chin positioned too low, resulting in severe curvature of occlusal plane and lack of definition of crowns of mandibular incisors.

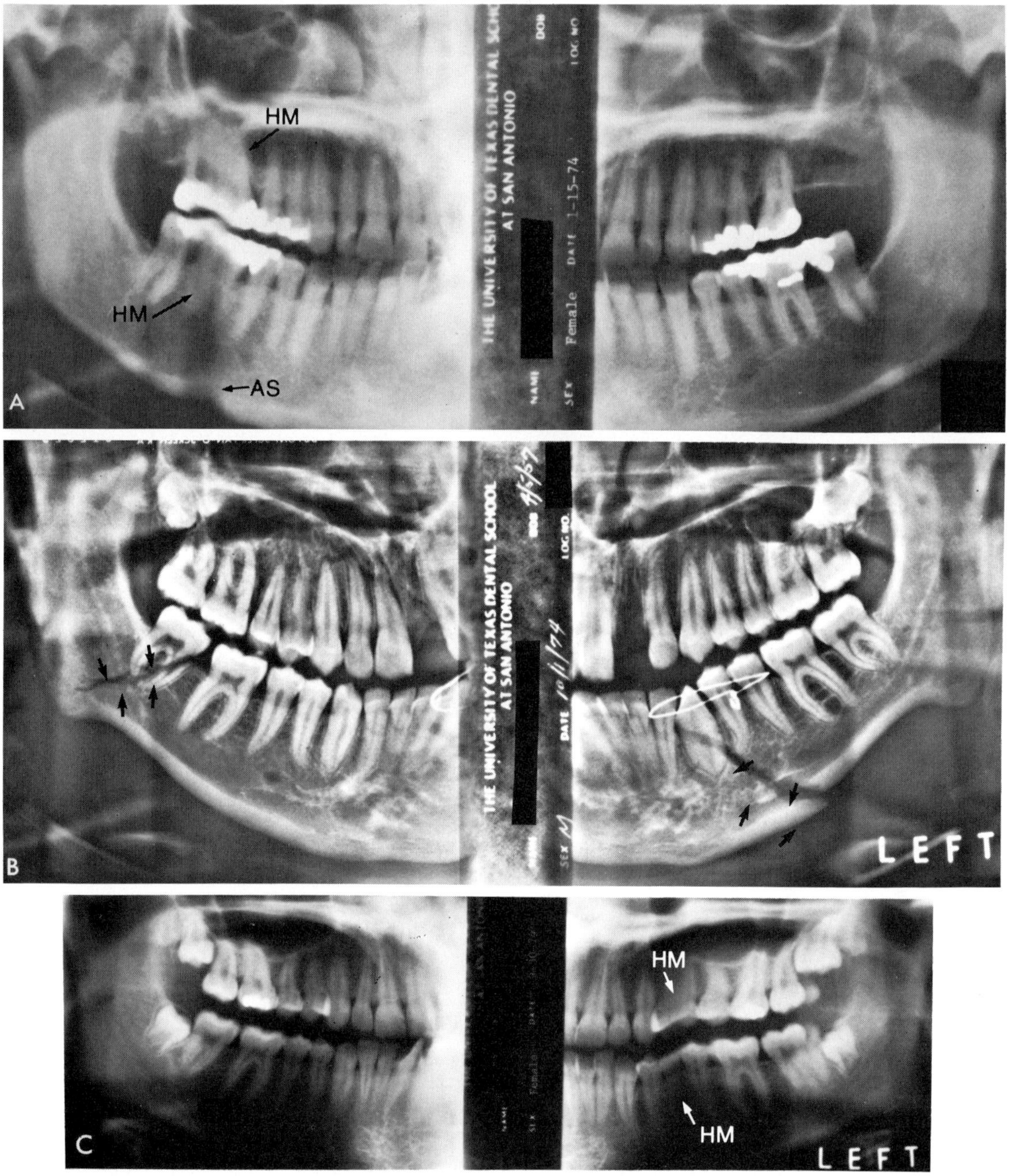

Figure 5–23. Distortion owing to patient movement. **A.** Panorex radiograph. Patient moved slowly in same direction as beam rotation causing the tooth to be horizontally magnified (HM). A sudden movement upward and downward caused the abrupt step (AS) in image mimicking a fracture. **B.** Panorex radiograph of patient with two fractures of the mandible (arrows). Compare with pseudofracture in **A** caused by patient movement during the exposure cycle. **C.** Panorex radiograph of patient who moved slowly in direction of beam rotation resulting in horizontal magnification (HM) of premolars (arrows).

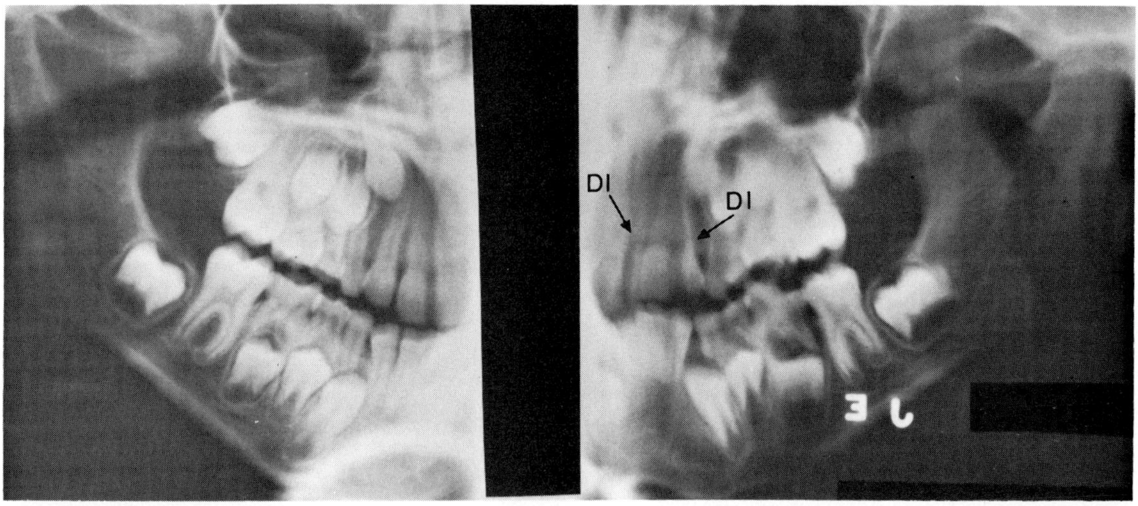

Figure 5–24. Double image (DI) produced in maxillary incisor region when patient made a sudden movement in the same direction as beam movement.

direction as the beam movement, the same area will be exposed for a prolonged time. All details in such a region will be stretched out in the image; the horizontal dimension will be increased (Fig. 5–23).

b. Should the patient move slowly in a direction opposite the beam movement, the horizontal dimension of the image in the region in which this movement occurred will be decreased.
c. Should the patient make a sudden move in the same direction as the beam movement, this region may be portrayed twice in the image (Fig. 5–24).
d. Should the patient make a sudden movement in a direction opposite the beam movement, a part of the object may be missing in the image.
e. Should the patient move up or down during the exposure, this will result (depending on how fast the patient moves) in an indentation in the lower border of mandible, which may mimic a fracture (see Fig. 5–23). Movement of any kind will decrease the definition of the radiographic image.

ERRORS IN FILM EXPOSURE AND PROCESSING

The image on the panoramic radiograph may be light (thin), dark (high density), blurred, or only partially visible owing to factors related to exposing the film to radiation. These factors interfere with the quality of the radiograph.

1. **Light or Thin Images.** These radiographs are especially difficult to interpret (Fig. 5–25). Low-density radiographs may be caused by any of the following:

a. kVp and/or mA not set high enough. The kVp and/or mA selection is dependent on the following patient variables: size and shape of head; skin pigmentation; thickness of soft tissue of face and neck; body structure; and whether or not patient has teeth.
b. X-ray beam not completely aligned with the slot in cassette holder.
c. Screen-film combination as recommended by manufacturer **not** used.
d. Weak developer solution (chemical replenishment cycle must be followed).
e. Inadequate developing time in manual processing.
f. Developer too cool for selected processing time (either manual or automatic processing).

2. **High-Density or Completely Black Images** (Fig. 5–26). This can be caused by several factors, such as:

a. Too high a kVp and/or mA selection.
b. Incorrect screen-film combination (usually too fast a film and/or screen for kVp and/or mA setting).
c. Developer too strong.
d. Developing time too long in manual processing.
e. Developer too hot for selected processing time (either manual or automatic processing).

3. **Fogged Film: Development of Unexposed Silver Halide Crystals in the Film Emulsion** (Fig. 5–27). This produces unwanted density,

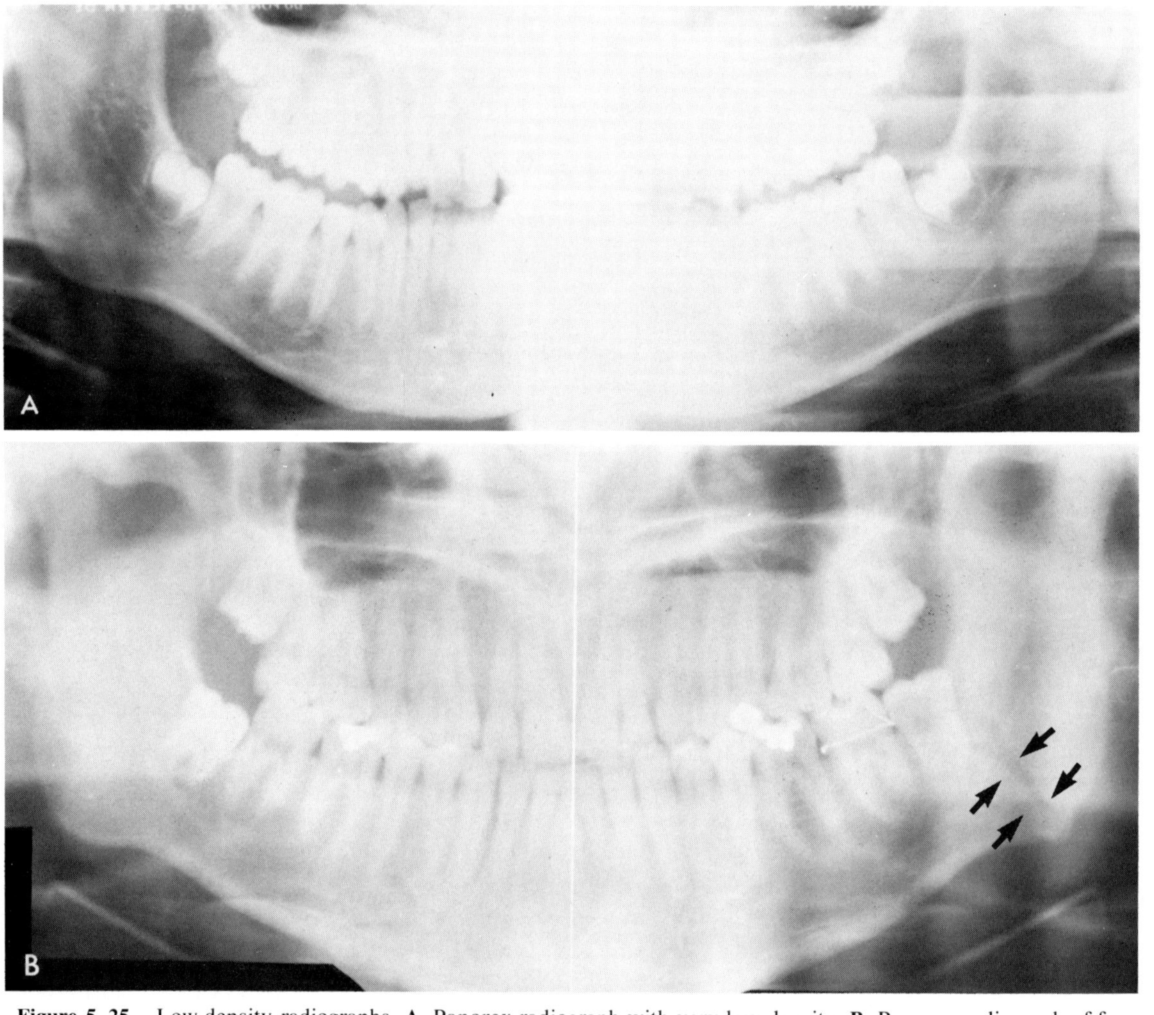

Figure 5–25. Low-density radiographs. **A.** Panorex radiograph with very low density. **B.** Panorex radiograph of fracture of mandible (arrows) with very low density.

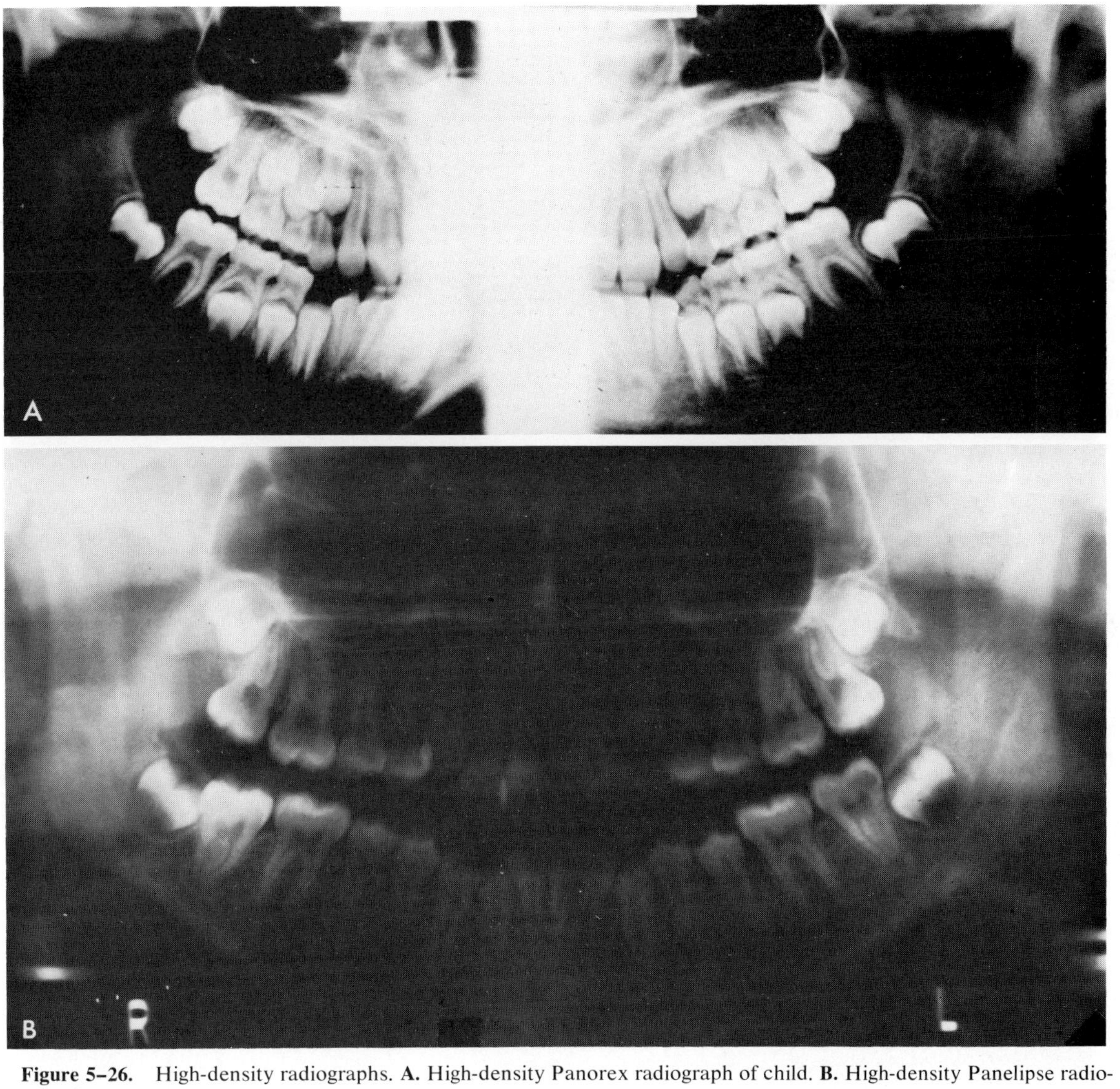

Figure 5–26. High-density radiographs. **A.** High-density Panorex radiograph of child. **B.** High-density Panelipse radiograph of teenager.

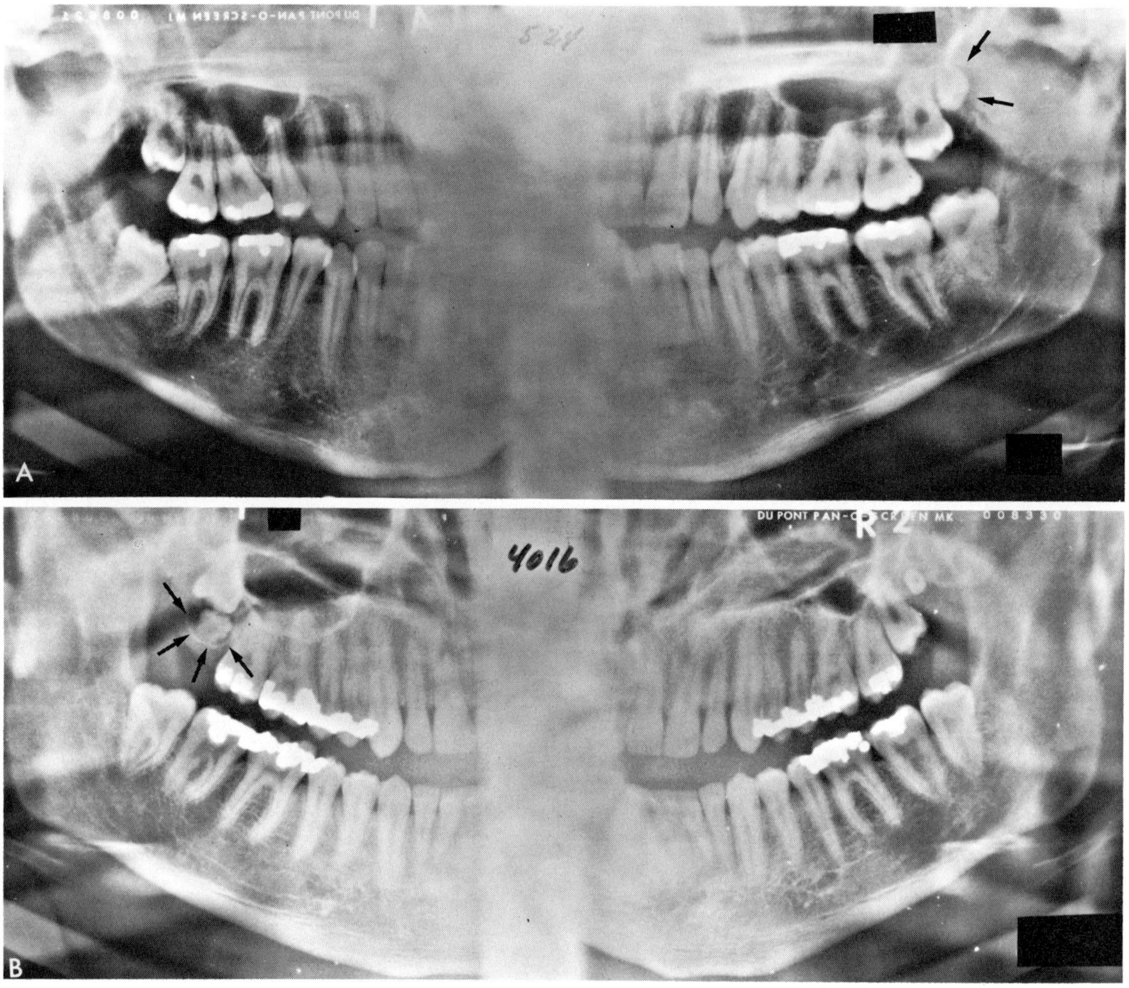

Figure 5–27. Fogged film. **A.** Panorex radiograph with fogging. Notice gray region in white band area. This was thought to be caused by inadequate safelight. Patient has a fourth maxillary molar (arrows). **B.** Panorex radiograph with fogging. Film lacks the proper contrast because of unwanted density from fogging. Possible follicular cyst of supernumerary tooth in maxillary third molar region (arrows). Also, small fourth molar can be seen in opposite maxillary third molar area.

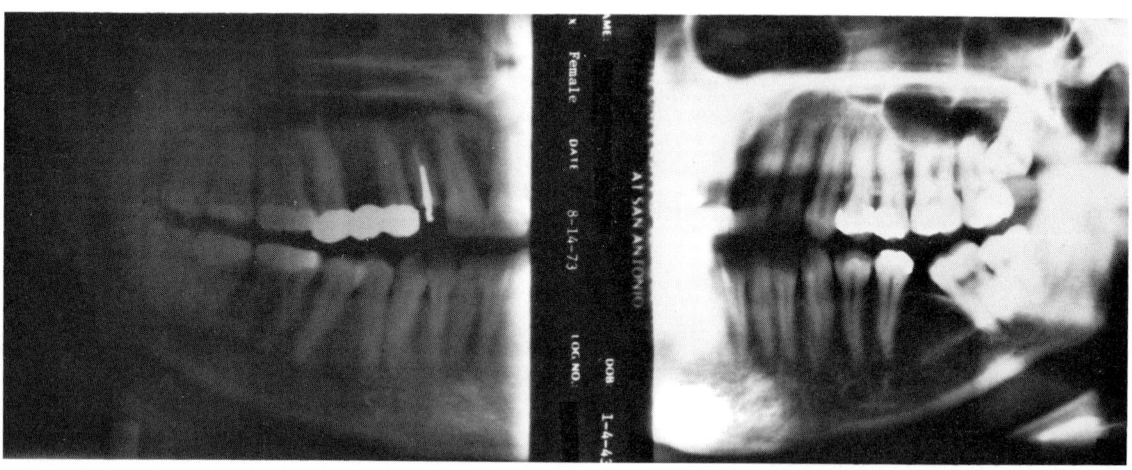

Figure 5–28. Fogging of film caused by accidentally turning on overhead light when film was halfway into the automatic processor.

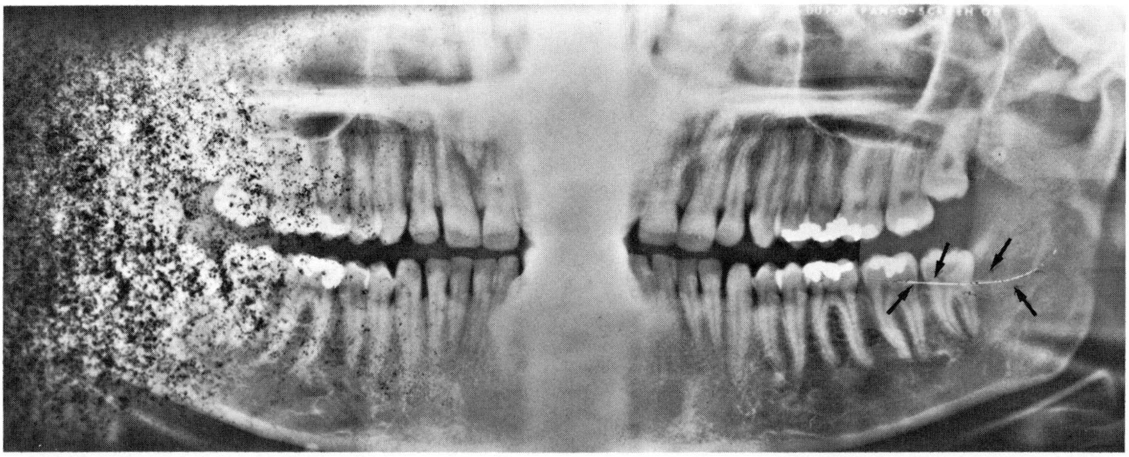

Figure 5–29. Panorex radiograph with white light paper mottled effect caused by light being accidentally turned on when film with protective paper on it was halfway out of box. White light penetrates the paper to produce a black mottled pattern on the radiograph. The white line is caused by breaking the emulsion by rough handling (arrows).

which lowers radiographic contrast. Fogged films may be caused by:

a. Improper film storage.
   (1) Storage of unexposed loaded cassettes in area of high temperature or humidity.
   (2) Storage of exposed and unprocessed films in the immediate vicinity of fumes from uncovered developer tanks.
   (3) Storage of unexposed loaded cassettes near source of x-radiation.
b. Use of outdated film.
c. Faulty processing solution selection (e.g., using a developing solution for replenishment or a manual developing solution in an automatic processor).
d. Accidental exposure to white light in darkroom.
   (1) Accidental white light exposure with half of film fogged (Fig. 5–28).
   (2) Paper-wrapped film accidentally exposed to light. If film with protective paper covering is accidentally exposed to white light in the darkroom, multiple small black spots or blotches (mottled effect) will result where the white light penetrated the paper (Fig. 5–29).
   (3) Unsafe safelight: improper wattage of bulb, improper filter, too short a distance between safelight and film, or too long a time under safelight (see Fig. 5–27).
   (4) Light leaks in a darkroom or through break in plastic cassette covering (Fig. 5–30).
   (5) Smoking in darkroom (Fig. 5–31).
e. Improper film-screen combination, especially if using high-speed film (highly sensitized emulsion). Use film-screen combination recommended by manufacturer.
f. Contaminated or exhausted developing solution.
g. Excessive development time or temperature.

4. **Only a Portion of the Film Exposed** (Fig. 5–32). This is usually caused by not correctly positioning the film cassette carriage or drum in the starting position or by not correctly placing cassette on drum.

5. **Random Artifacts on the Film.** Check screens inside the cassette for contaminants that may have collected. These contaminants (paper, felt, dust, and so on) will prevent light from reaching the film, resulting in less density on the film (Figs. 5–33 and 5–34).

6. **Vertical White Lines on Radiograph.** When the push button on the exposure switch is accidentally released and then pressed down for the remainder of the excursion, a blank space on the panoramic radiograph will result. Each time the button is released, the radiation to the film is cut off, resulting in a blank space or a vertical white line on the radiograph (Fig. 5–35).

7. **Automatic Processor Improperly Maintained.** Several faults may be seen on the processed radiograph.

a. Streaking (uneven density) (Figs. 5–36 to 5–38) may be caused by:
   (1) Developer and fixer replenishment low.
   (2) Rollers and crossovers encrusted with chemical deposits.
   (3) Dirty wash water.
   (4) Improper chemicals and/or film used.

Text continued on page 126

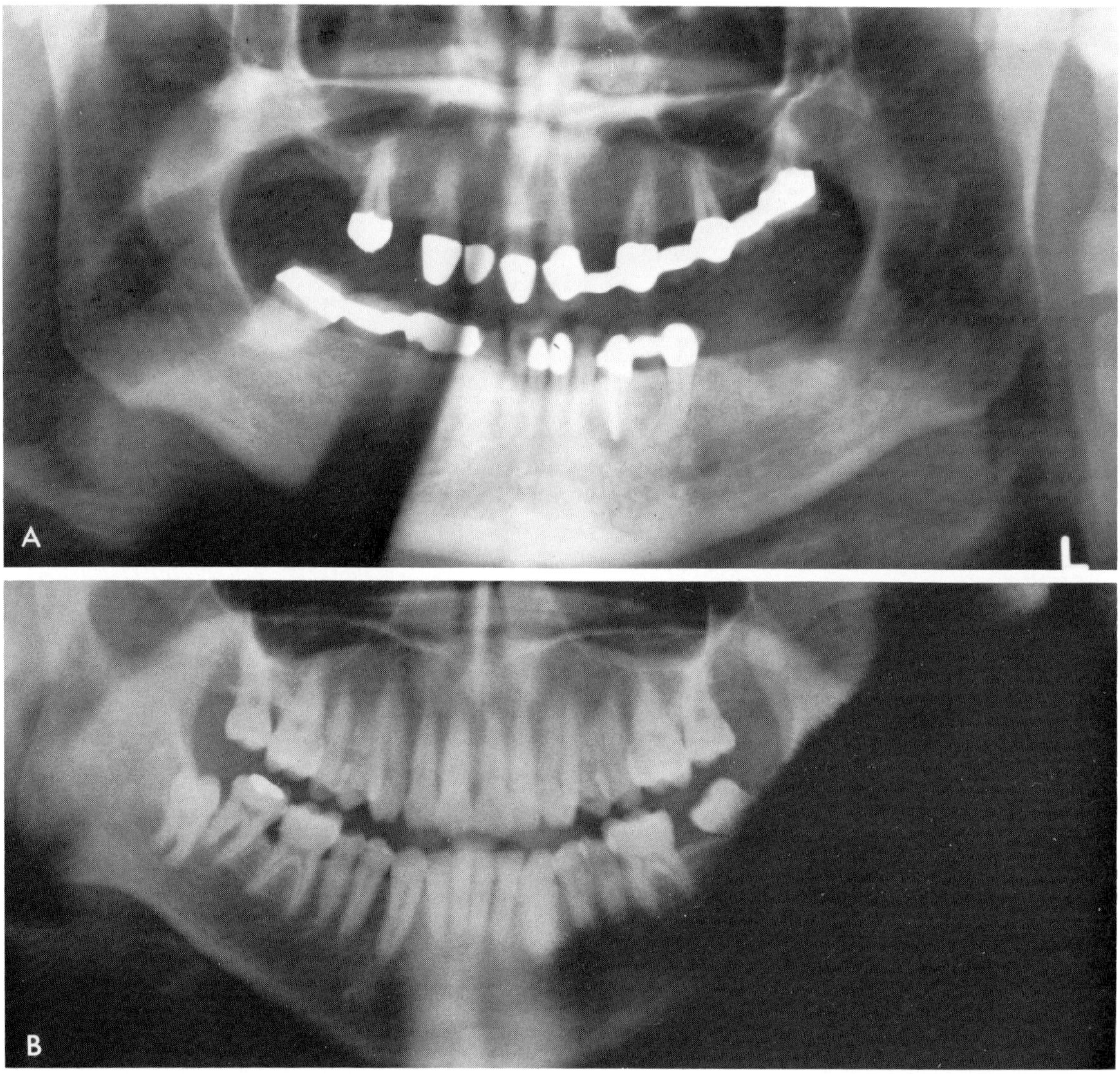

Figure 5–30. Light leaks through damaged Panoral cassettes. **A.** Small light leak. **B.** Large light leak.

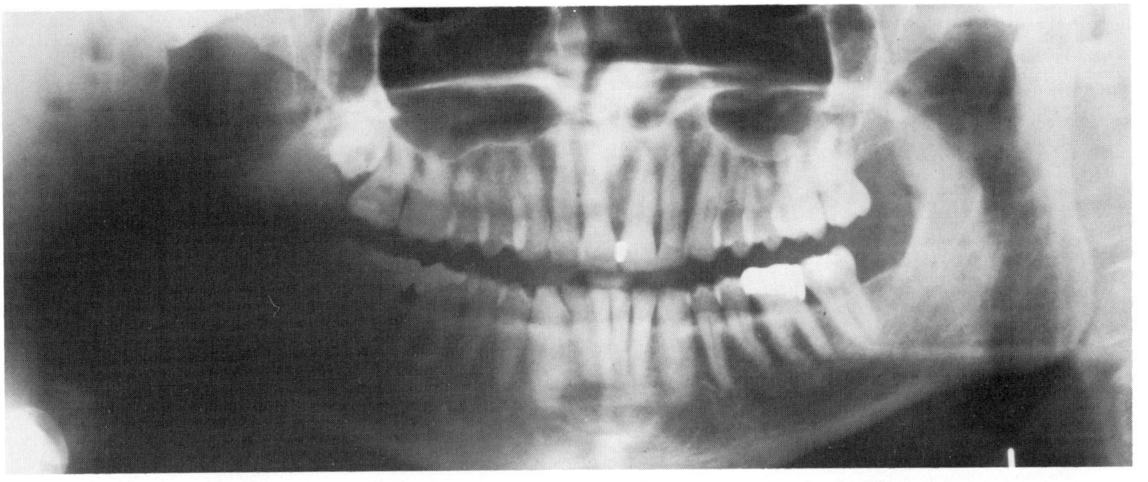

Figure 5–31. Light from cigarette has caused increased density on film.

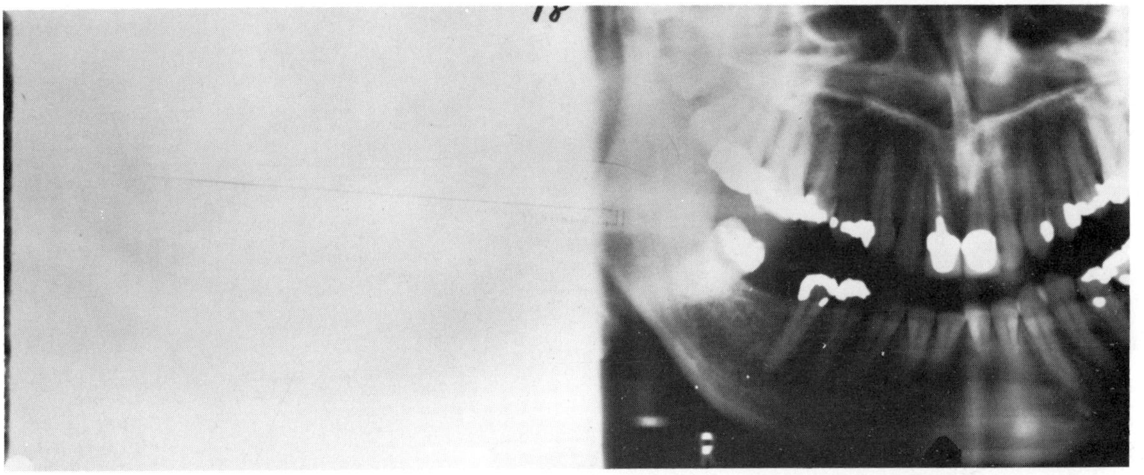

Figure 5–32. Panelipse radiograph shows a partial image because film cassette was positioned incorrectly.

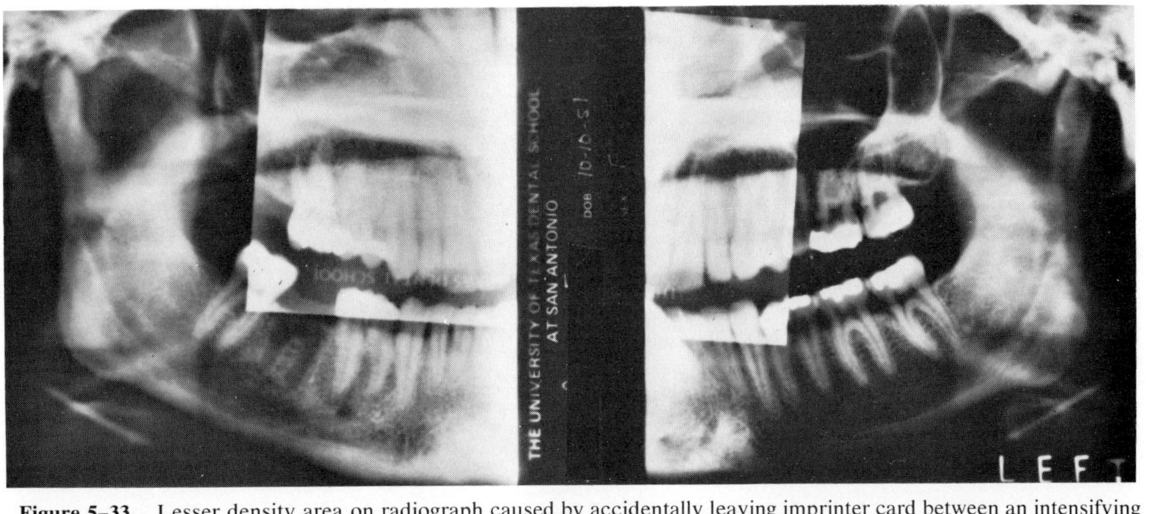

Figure 5–33. Lesser density area on radiograph caused by accidentally leaving imprinter card between an intensifying screen and film during exposure. The card prevented some of the light emitted by the screen to reach the film in this area.

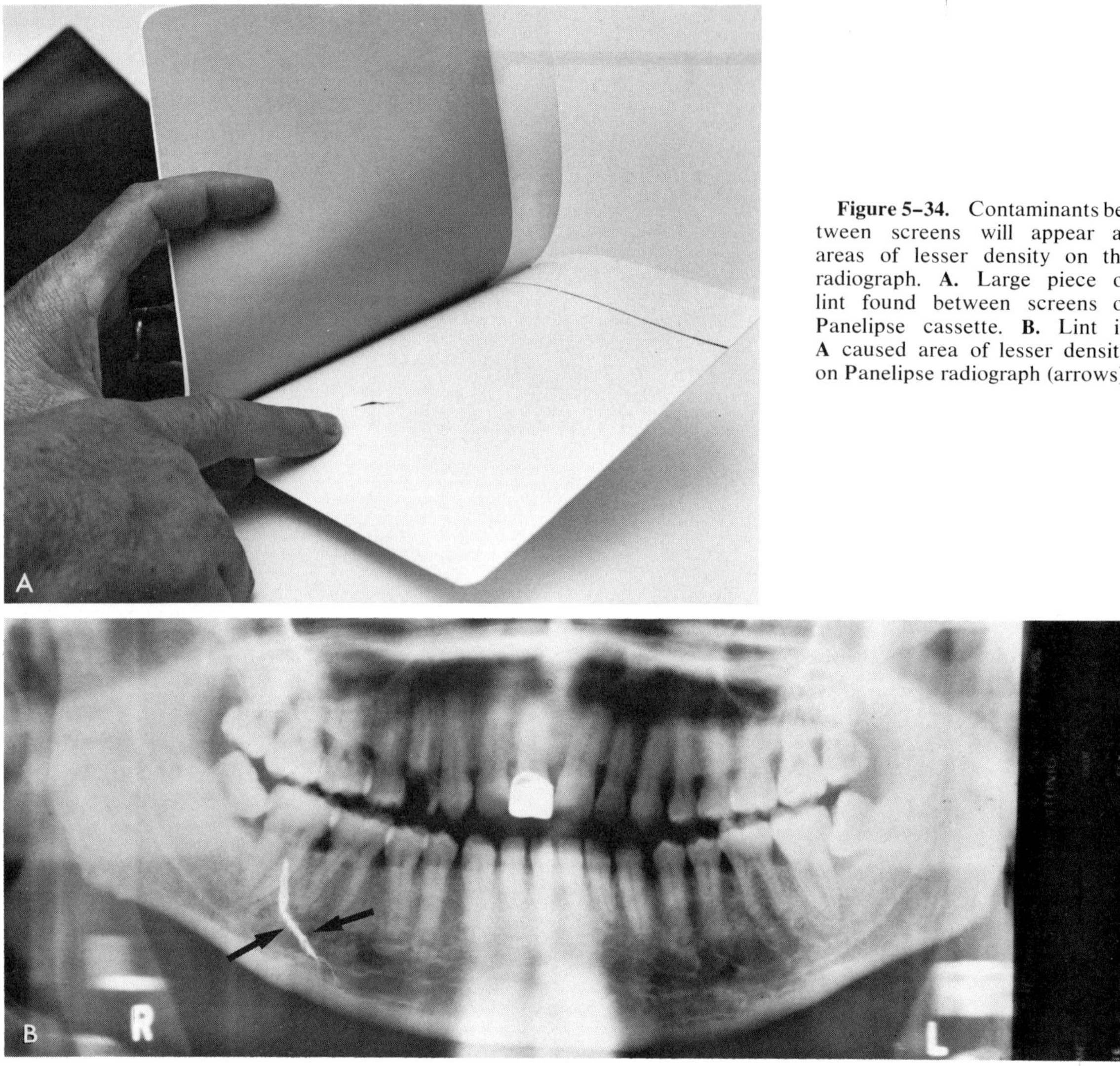

Figure 5–34. Contaminants between screens will appear as areas of lesser density on the radiograph. **A.** Large piece of lint found between screens of Panelipse cassette. **B.** Lint in **A** caused area of lesser density on Panelipse radiograph (arrows).

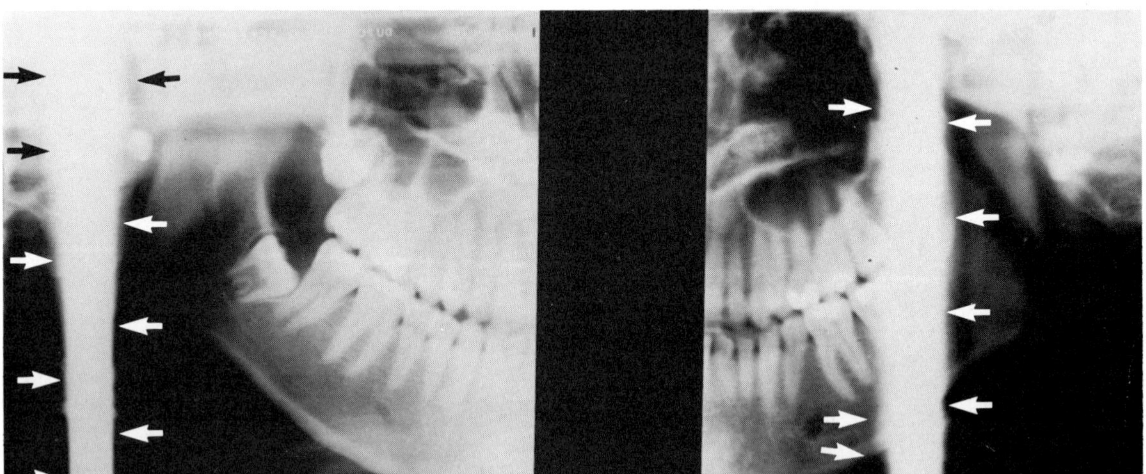

Figure 5–35. White vertical bands (arrows) appearing on processed Panorex radiograph as result of accidentally releasing the exposure switch and then pressing down for remainder of excursion.

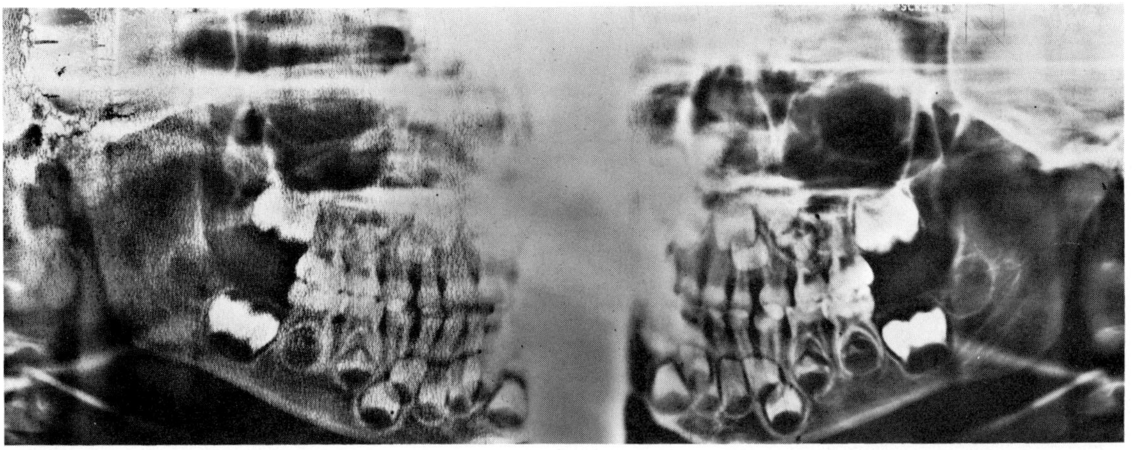

Figure 5–36. Streaking (uneven density) on Panorex radiograph caused by unclean rollers contaminated with chemical deposits.

Figure 5–37. Streaking (uneven density) on films caused by unclean rollers and crossovers. **A.** Panorex radiograph with alternate vertical black and white lines from unclean rollers. They are especially noticeable in region extending from maxillary molar to lateral incisor. **B.** Panelipse radiograph with alternate vertical black and white lines that will mimic those lines resulting from unclean rollers but that, in reality, are mechanical gear and cog lines seen only on Panelipse radiographs due to line voltage changes or a need for calibration of the mechanical movement of the film cassette–tubehead assembly.

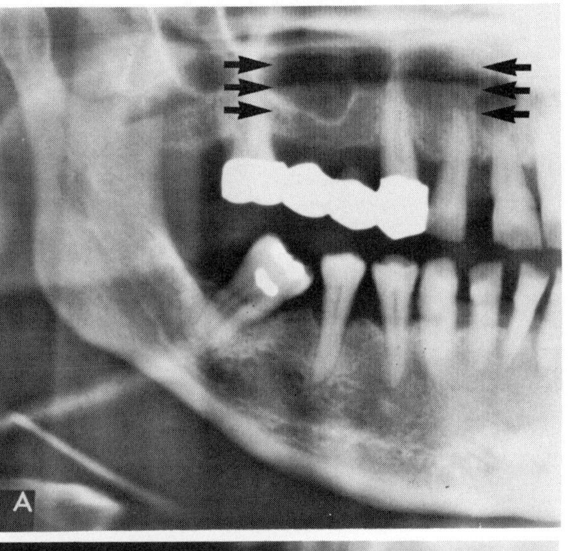

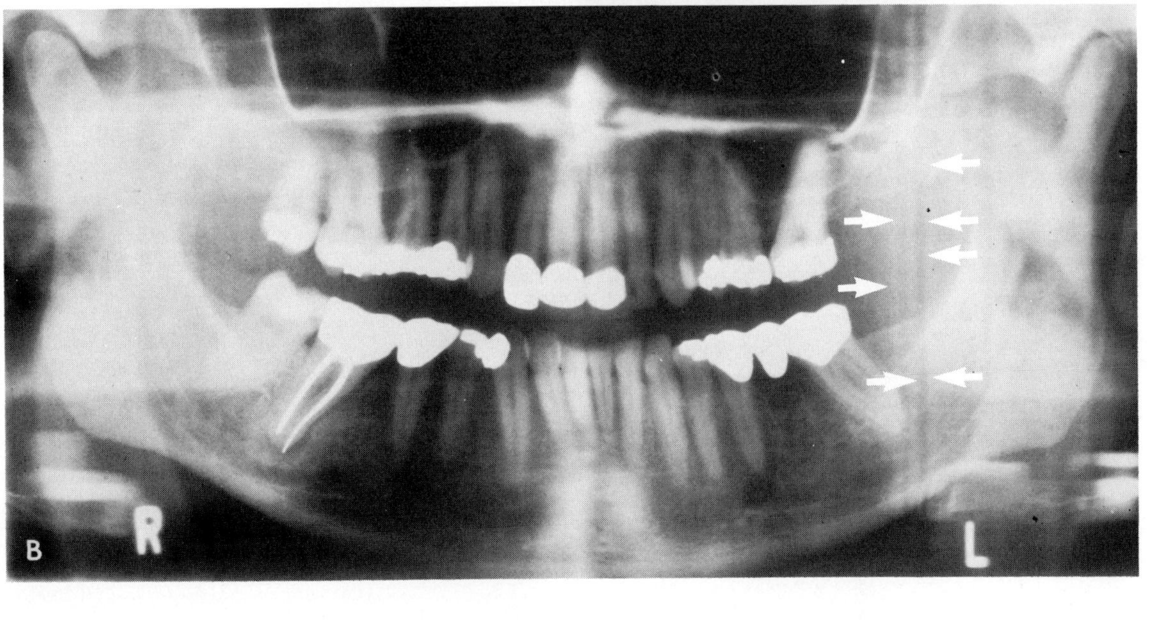

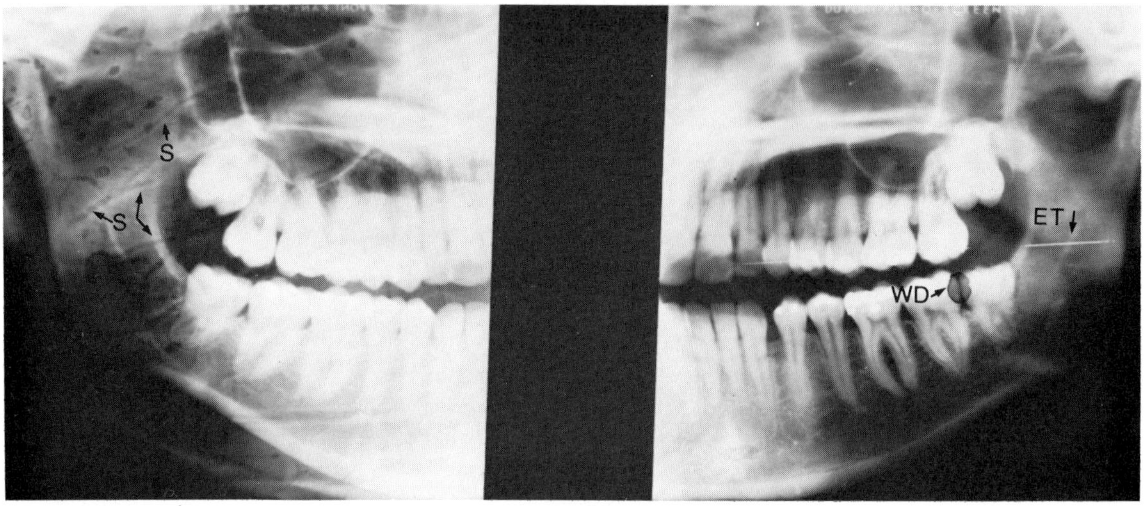

Figure 5–38. Panorex radiograph with streaking (S) (uneven density) from unclean wash water. Notice water droplet (WD) and emulsion tear (ET).

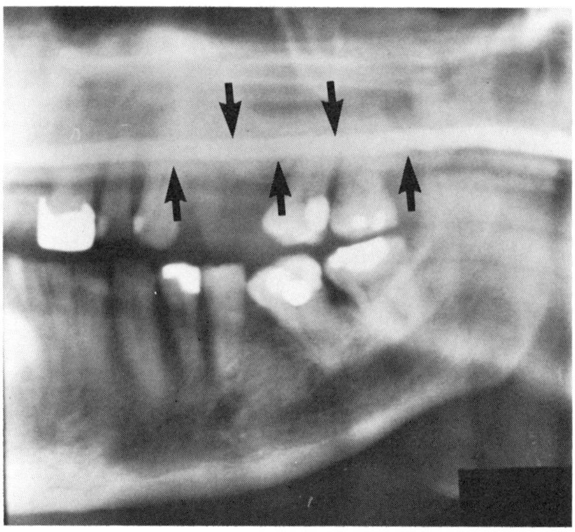

Figure 5–39. Panorex radiograph with broad horizontal white line on film as result of roller with an uneven surface (arrows).

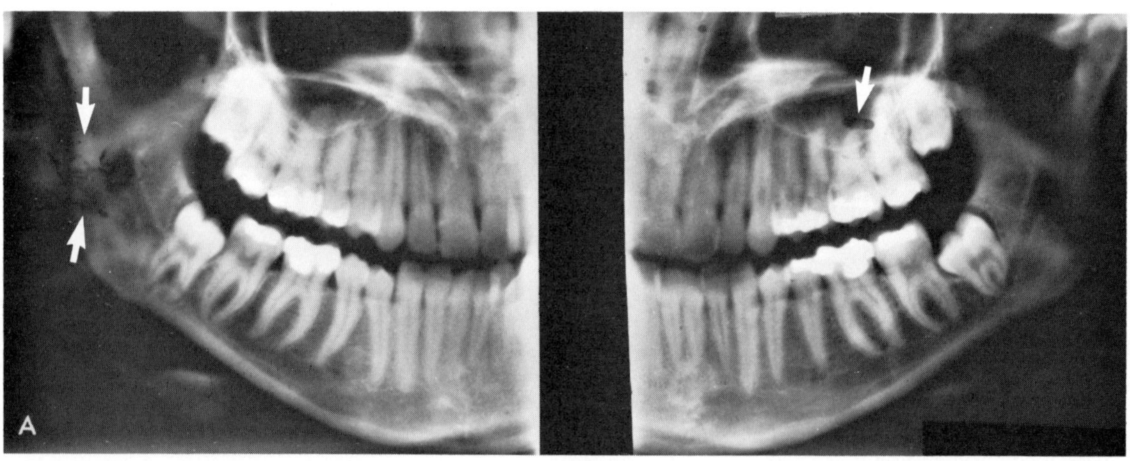

Figure 5–40. **A.** Panorex radiograph with black spots and lines from contaminated workbench (arrows).

Illustration continued on opposite page

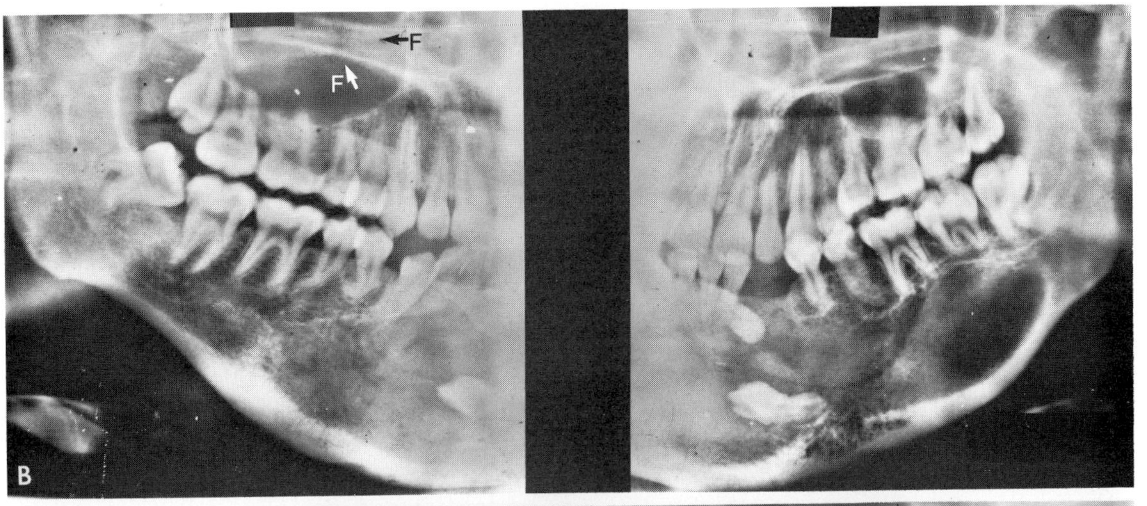

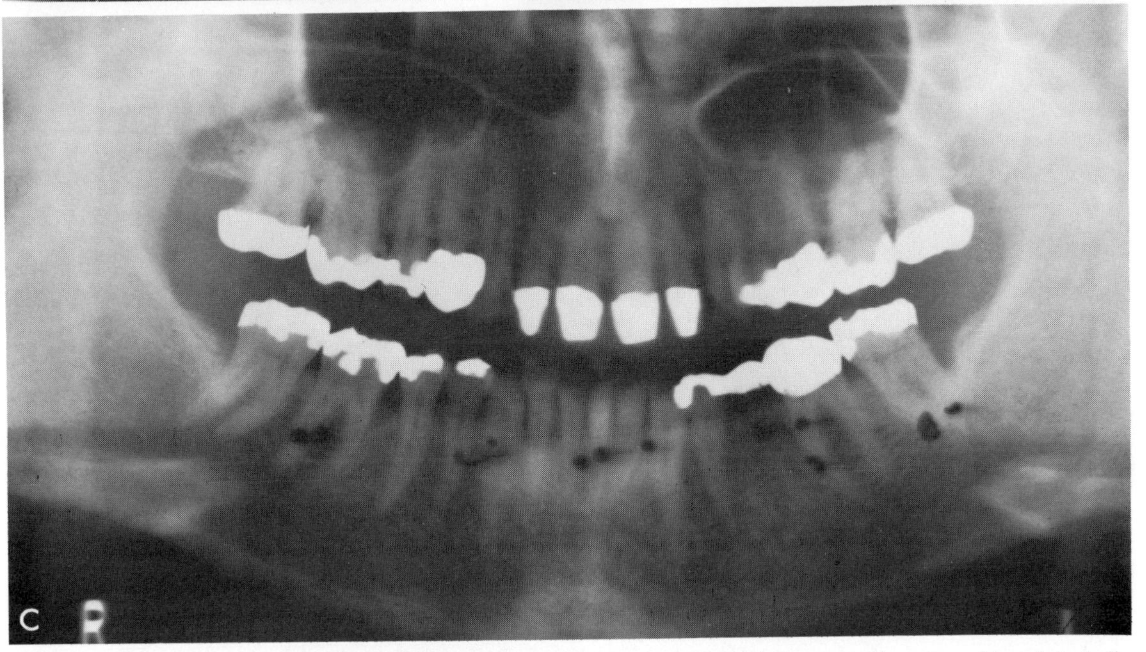

Figure 5–40 *Continued.* **B.** Fogged radiograph has many artifacts caused by a contaminated workbench including fingerprints (**F**). Patient has a large follicular cyst in the mandible. **C.** Panelipse radiograph with several black spots caused by water droplets on film prior to processing.

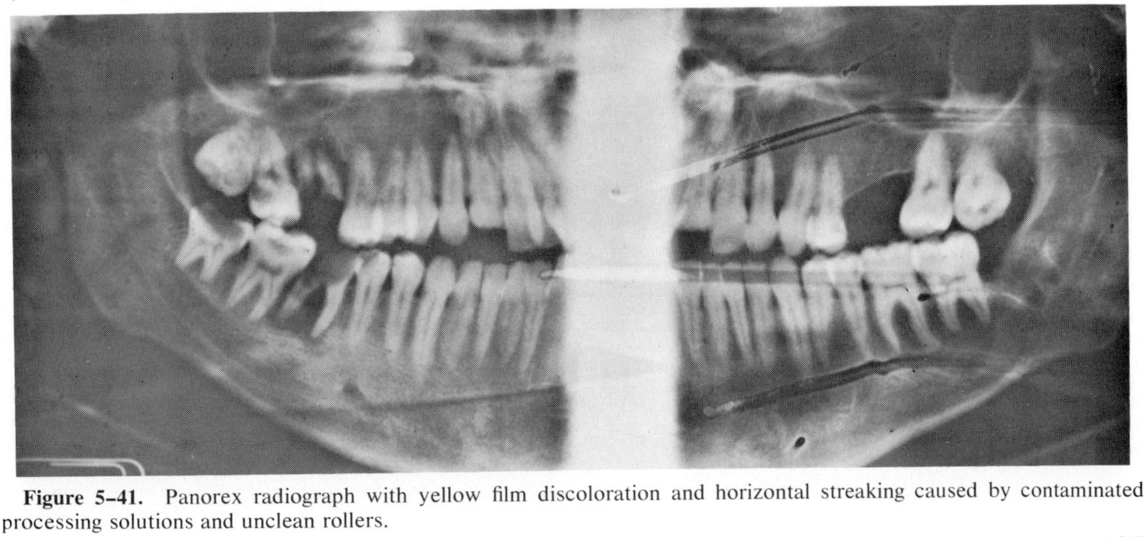

Figure 5–41. Panorex radiograph with yellow film discoloration and horizontal streaking caused by contaminated processing solutions and unclean rollers.

b. Surface marks on the radiograph may be caused by:
   (1) Irregularities on the surface of the rollers, causing a broad horizontal white line (Fig. 5–39).
   (2) Contamination of film by dirty workbench or water droplets (black spots and lines) (Fig. 5–40).

c. Film discoloration (Fig. 5–41) may be caused by:
   (1) Fixer in developer.
   (2) Processing too fast.
   (3) Exhausted fixer.

ERRORS IN HANDLING THE FILM

Many marks, streaks, and lines that appear on the film are the result of rough or careless handling of the film. They can be avoided by employing some care. Some of these handling errors are listed below.

1. **Static Electricity.** Black markings are actual points of static discharge, with black lines radiating from those points. The diagnostic information in these areas is destroyed. There are two common static markings: "naked tree" (lightning) static markings (Fig. 5–42), and

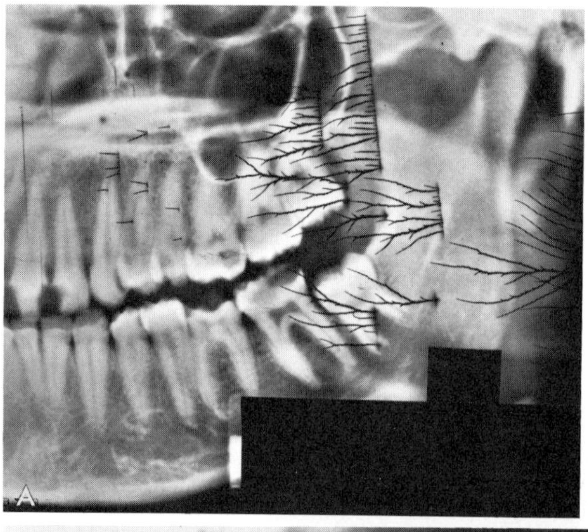

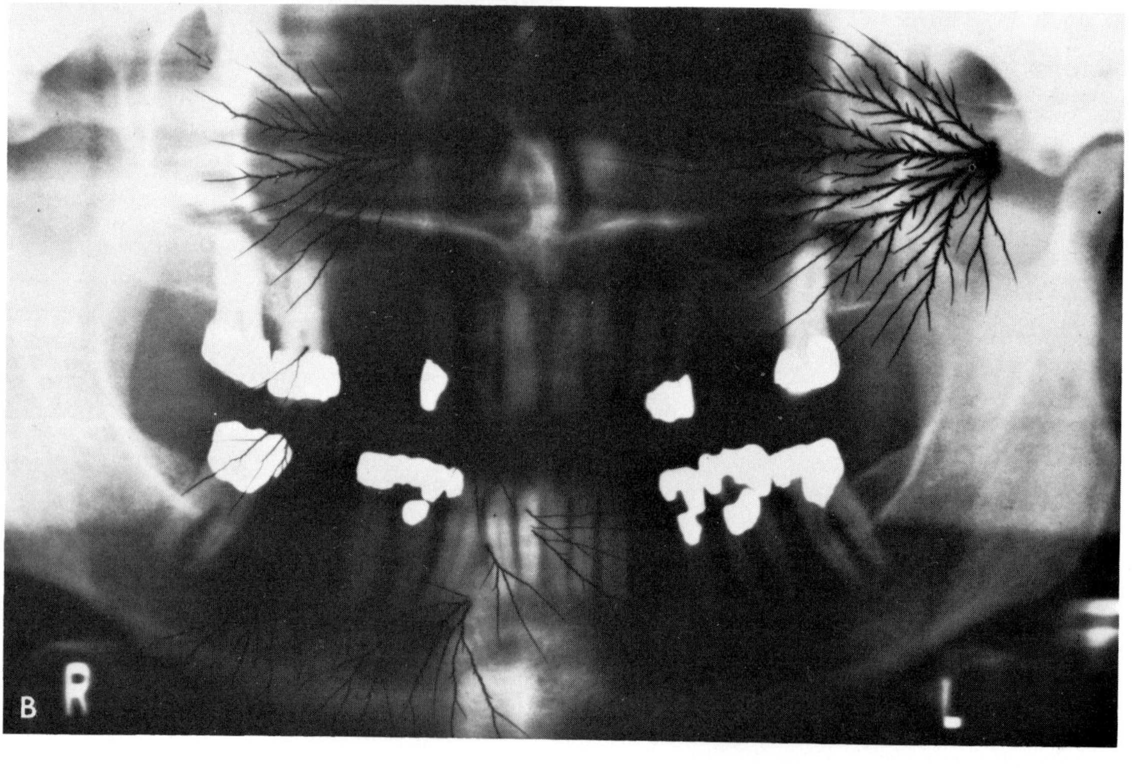

Figure 5–42. **A.** Panorex radiograph with naked tree static markings. **B.** Panelipse radiograph with naked tree static markings.

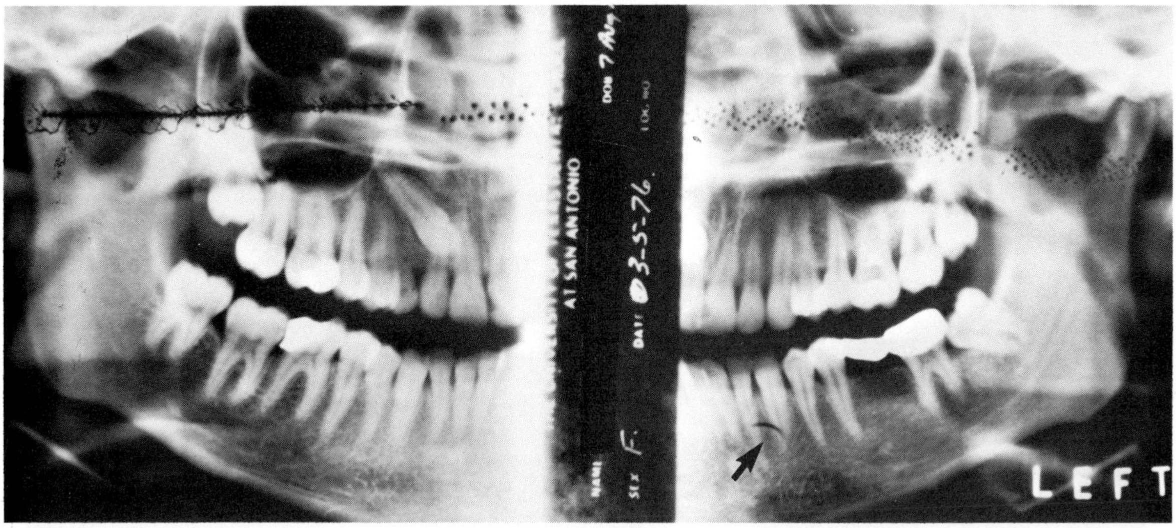

Figure 5–43. Smudge-type static electricity markings on Panorex radiograph caused by a low potential charge producing visible light from sparks. Notice crescent-shaped fingernail artifact caused by undue pressure on emulsion.

smudge static markings (Fig. 5–43). Naked tree markings are the result of electrical discharges that produce no visible light but occur on the surface of the emulsion. They are generally caused by very rapid movements in handling film and may occur when film is removed from the box, when film is removed from interleaving paper, or when film is touched by fingers of person processing film. Smudge markings may result from visible light produced by sparks caused by a relatively low potential electrical discharge in the air next to the film surface. The discharge follows a path induced by dust, lint, or a roughened intensifying screen. To overcome the most common causes of static, the following steps are recommended:

a. One of the more common causes of static electricity is the lack of moisture in the air. This occurs with greater frequency in the winter. There are several inexpensive electric humidifiers or cool vapor vaporizers on the market that can be installed in the darkroom. The relative humidity in the darkroom should be between 50 and 75 per cent.
b. If x-ray film has interleaving paper, handle the film gently. Let the paper fall away from the film, and place the film in the cassette gently.
c. Following x-ray exposure, remove the film carefully from the cassette.
d. Coat the intensifying screens in the cassette with an antistatic solution (usually available from a medical supply house).

2. **White Marks on Film as Result of Torn Emulsion** (Fig. 5–44; see Fig. 5–29). If films are handled roughly when they are mounted on the hangers or if the hangers are jammed against each other in the tank, the emulsion can be torn, leaving a clear area on the film. This decreases the diagnostic value of the film. Also, white marks on the film may be the result of a crack on the intensifying screen (Fig. 5–45).

3. **Fingerprints and Fluoride Artifacts.** Hands that have been contaminated with processing solutions or other chemicals will produce fingerprints on the film, which interfere with the diagnostic quality of the film. A dark gray fingerprint is caused by fingers contaminated by the developer, whereas white fingerprints are caused by fixer contamination. Some

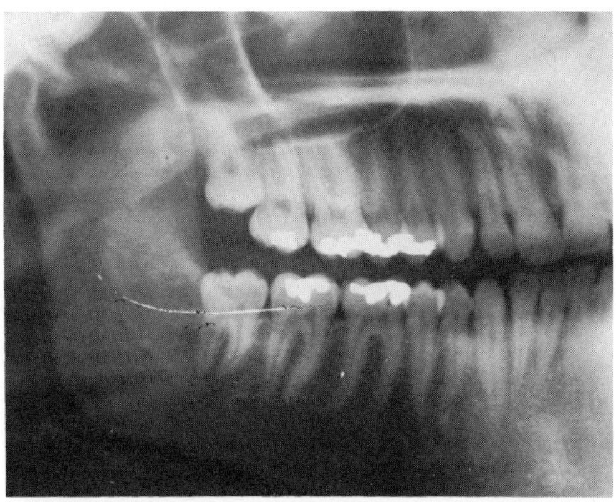

Figure 5–44. Panorex radiograph with a torn emulsion (long white line) that resulted when a film hanger was accidentally jammed against the film in the processing tank.

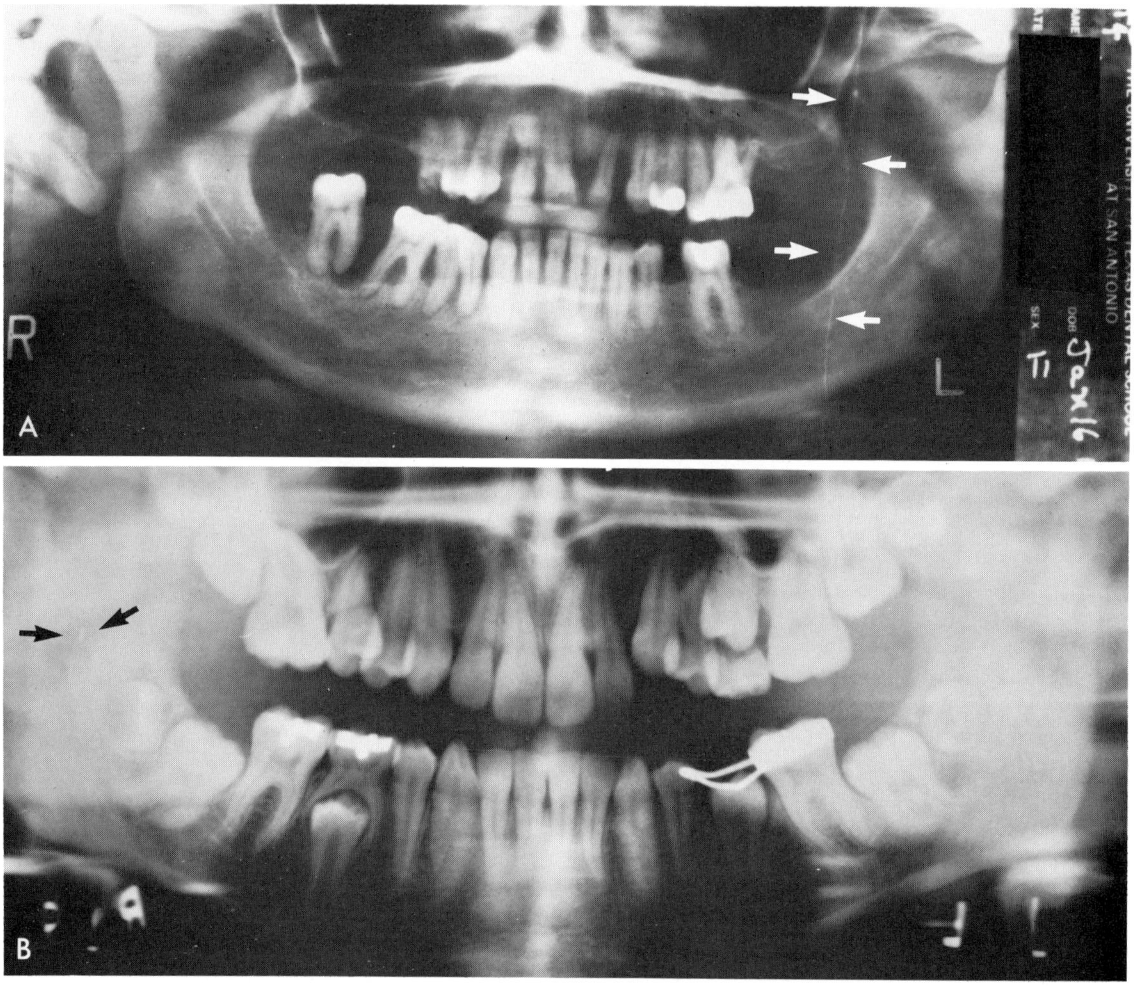

Figure 5–45. **A.** Panoral radiograph taken with cassette that had a crack in one of the intensifying screens, leaving a thin vertical white mark on the film (arrows). Patient has advanced destructive periodontitis. **B.** Panelipse radiograph of child with small radiopacity in shape of broken needle point located in right ramus (arrows). Surgery was contemplated to remove the object but was not done. Orthodontic treatment was started and radiographs **C** and **D** were taken two months later.

Illustration continued on opposite page

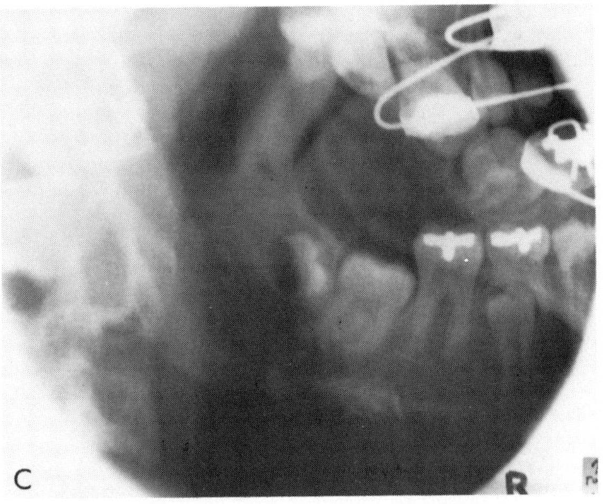

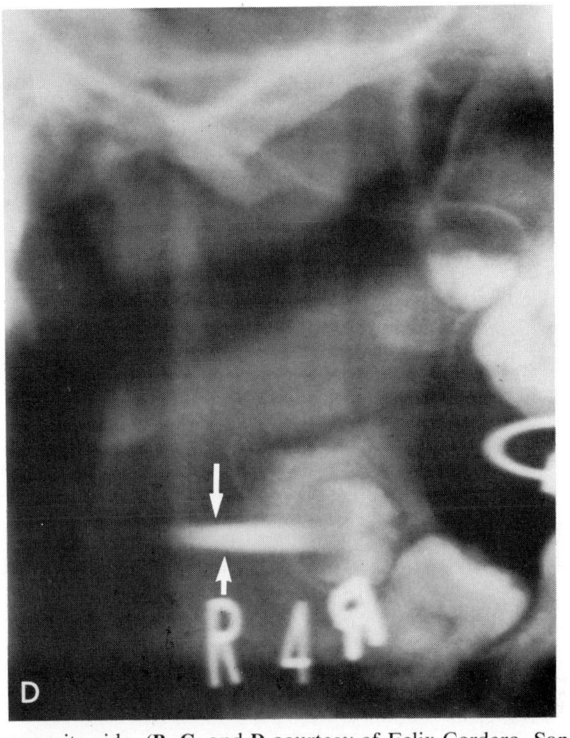

Figure 5–45 *Continued.* **C.** Right lateral jaw radiograph taken preoperatively two months later. Notice orthodontic appliances. No evidence of small radiopacity in right ramus can be noticed. **D.** Special temporomandibular joint Panelipse of right temporomandibular joint and ramus of same patient. The radiograph was taken with a different cassette than that used in **B.** Conclusion: there was a small defect in the intensifying screen used in **B,** causing a small radiopacity that mimicked a broken needle point. Arrows outline a radiopacity that is a ghost of the leaded letter "L" from the opposite side. (**B, C,** and **D** courtesy of Felix Cordero, San Antonio, TX.)

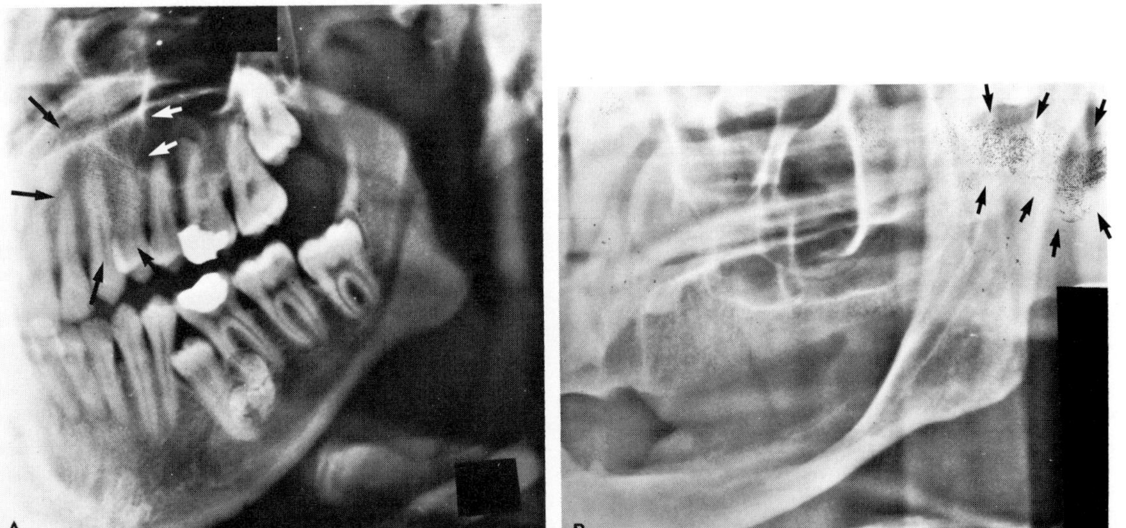

Figure 5–46. **A.** Panorex film with fingerprints in maxillary cuspid–first cuspid area (arrows). Patient had compound odontoma (confirmed after surgery) in area of impacted mandibular second bicuspid. **B.** Panorex of edentulous patient with fingerprints in temporomandibular joint region (arrows).

fluoride compounds, such as stannous fluoride, will produce black fingerprint marks on the film (Fig. 5–46). Even washing the hands with soap and water will not remove fluoride contamination. Wiping a mild acid such as vinegar or lemon juice on the hands prior to washing them with soap and water will effectively remove the fluoride contaminant.

REFERENCES

Ando, S.: **Orthopantomography.** Tokyo: Assoc. Oral Hygiene, 1971, pp. 31, 55 (Japanese).

Darkroom Technique. Wilmington, Delaware: DuPont Photo Products Department.

Gratt, B. M., Parks, C. R., Hall, G. L., and Sickles, E. A.: Use of an inclined footrest for panoramic dental radiography. **Oral Surg. 47**:568, 1979.

Lund, T. M., and Manson-Hing, L. R.: A study of the focal troughs of three panoramic dental x-ray machines. Part I, The area of sharpness. **Oral Surg. 39**:318, 1975a.

Lund, T. M., and Manson-Hing, L. R.: A study of the focal troughs of three panoramic dental x-ray machines. Part II, **Oral Surg. 39**:647, 1975b.

Lund, T. M., and Manson-Hing, L. R.: Relations between tooth positions and focal troughs of panoramic machines. **Oral Surg. 40**:285, 1975c.

Panorex Operator's Manual. Great Neck, New York: S. S. White Co. (Pennwalt Corp.).

Radiodontic Pitfalls. Rochester, New York: Eastman Kodak, Radiography Markets Division, 1977.

Samfors, K. A., and Welander, U.: Distortion in the pantomogram due to object movement. **Sven. Tandlak. Tidskr. 65**:211, 1972.

Updegrave, W. J.: The role of panoramic radiography in diagnosis. **Oral Surg. 22**:49, 1966.

Witcher, B. L., Gratt, B. M., and Sickles, E. A.: A leaded apron for use in panoramic dental radiography. **Oral Surg. 49**:467, 1980.

Chapter 6

Normal Panoramic Anatomy and Ghost Images

BRIEF OVERVIEW

This chapter is not meant to be an exhaustive treatise on the subject, since this would involve a volume of text equal to that found in any good anatomy book of the head and neck areas. Rather, it is the authors' intention to illustrate and identify as many structures as possible as they are seen on panoramic films. These include various bony landmarks as well as some of the soft tissue shadows and air spaces superimposed on the hard structures. Additionally, because of the unique nature of the panoramic projection, ghost images of structures from the contralateral side may be superimposed on the side being viewed.

Of further importance is the fact that some machines use devices to position the patient that are constructed of materials that are not completely radiotransparent. The shadow of these devices is superimposed on the hard tissue image, the soft tissue shadow, and the ghost image. Often the untrained eye or the novice will not be able to visualize all of these images on a given film when they are present. It is absolutely essential and of paramount importance that the observer become attuned to the presence of a great number of variations, all of which are normal, before the detection of an abnormality can be made with any conviction.

One further problem in interpreting panoramic radiographs is the manner in which the panoramic projection "spreads out" the structures being viewed. The shapes of structures and their interrelationships cannot be compared with what we see on ordinary films. For example, the mandible becomes a flat U-shaped structure, and we know that this is not the actual shape of this bone. Also, in the panoramic projection, the lateral pterygoid plate of the sphenoid bone is often superimposed over the coronoid process of the mandible. This superimposition causes the top of the coronoid process to become more opaque, thus mimicking a neoplasm. One last example is the torus palatinus. We know this to be a midline structure on the hard palate. In the panoramic view, it is projected as a bilateral radiopacity; paradoxically, the soft tissue shadow of the nose, which is also a midline structure, is projected in the midline on the panoramic film. Understanding these and many other peculiarities of the panoramic projection is the first step in learning to identify and interpret dental pathology.

Further details concerning the regional anatomy of the maxillary sinus and temporomandibular joint may be seen in Chapters 15 and 16, respectively.

The remainder of this chapter is presented in atlas form. First, try to learn the basic bony landmarks seen in Figure 6–1. Then go on to Figures 6–2, 6–3, and 6–4. Be sure that you really can see everything in the radiographs before going on. Next, see if you can identify these same landmarks in the edentulous case illustrated in Figures 6–5 and 6–6. The remainder of the figures are a selection of good examples of anatomic landmarks that may or may not have been illustrated and identified in the first six figures. In viewing these figures, try to identify the structure before reading the legend.

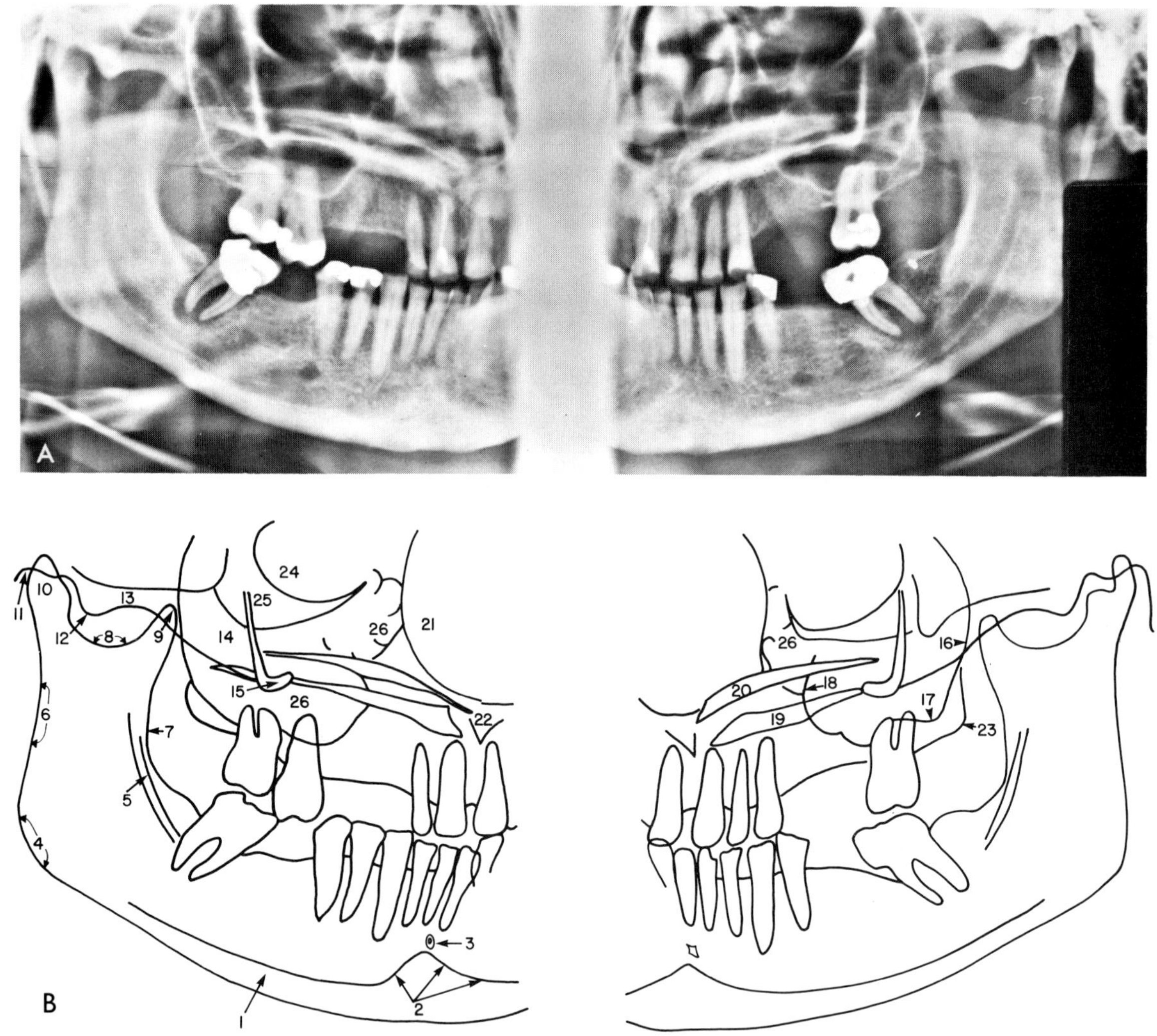

Figure 6–1. Basic bony landmarks. 1. Cortical bone lining inferior border of mandible. 2. Mental ridge. 3. Genial tubercles. 4. Angle of mandible. 5. External oblique ridge. 6. Posterior border of ramus. 7. Anterior border of ramus. 8. Sigmoid notch. 9. Coronoid process. 10. Mandibular condyle. 11. Glenoid fossa (condyle is superimposed). 12. Articular eminence. 13. Zygomatic arch (zygomatic proccess of temporal bone). 14. Zygomatic arch (temporal process of zygomatic bone). 15. Malar process (maxillary process of zygomatic bone). 16. Maxillary sinus (posterior wall). 17. Maxillary sinus (floor). 18. Maxillary sinus (anterior border). 19. Hard palate (actual image). 20. Hard palate (contralateral ghost image). 21. Nasal fossa. 22. Anterior nasal spine. 23. Maxillary tuberosity. 24. Orbit. 25. Inferior lateral border of orbit (frontal process of zygomatic bone). 26. Maxillary sinus.

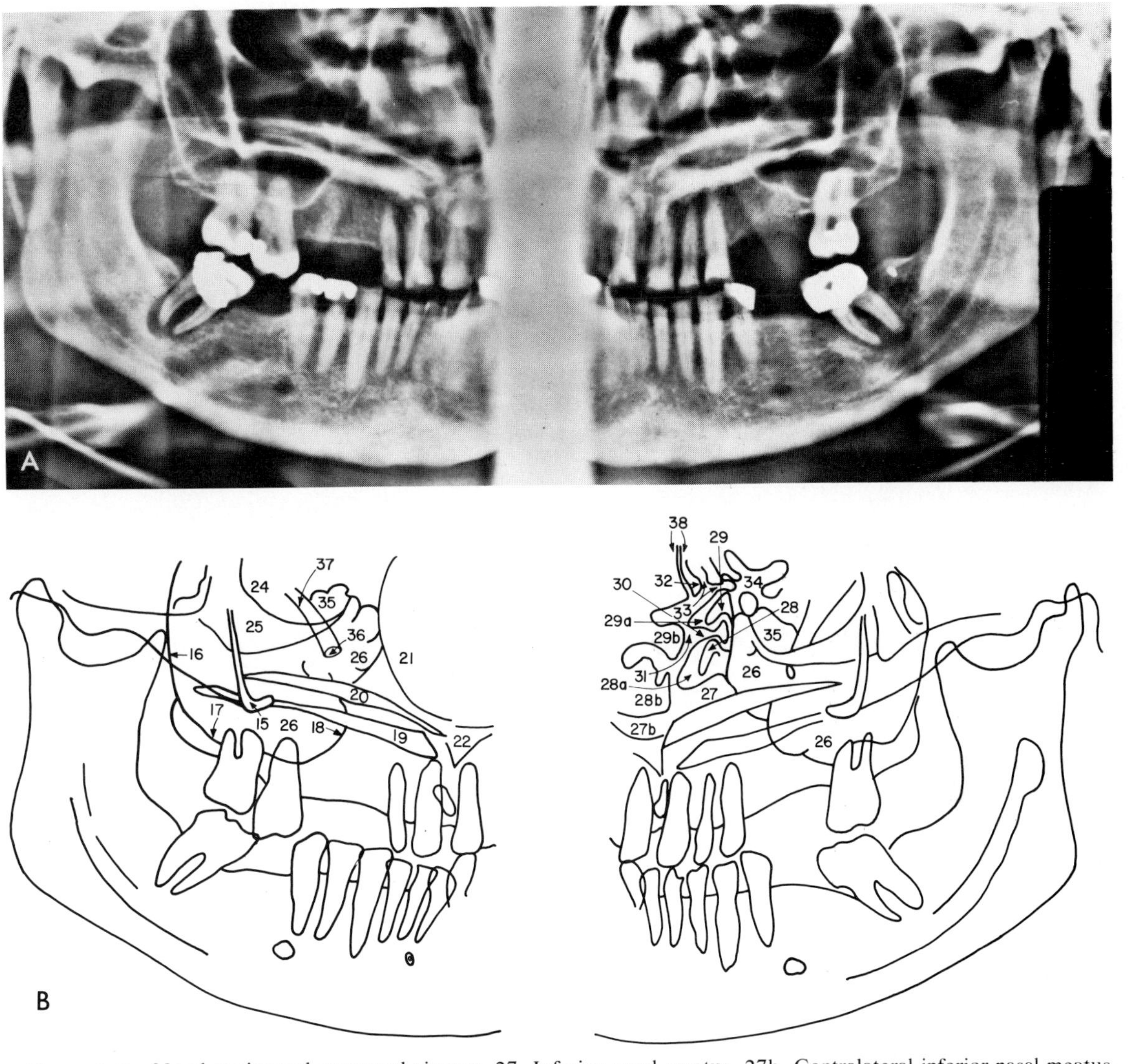

Figure 6–2. Nasal cavity and paranasal sinuses. 27. Inferior nasal meatus. 27b. Contralateral inferior nasal meatus. 28. Inferior nasal concha. 28a. Mucosal lining of inferior nasal concha. 28b. Contralateral inferior nasal concha and mucosal lining. 29. Middle nasal concha. 29a. Mucosal lining of middle nasal concha. 29b. Contralateral middle nasal concha and mucosal lining. 30. Middle nasal meatus. 31. Common nasal meatus. 32. Superior nasal concha. 33. Ethmoid sinus. 34. Frontal sinus. 35. Fossa for lacrimal sac. 36. Infraorbital foramen. 37. Infraorbital canal. 38. Cribriform plate.

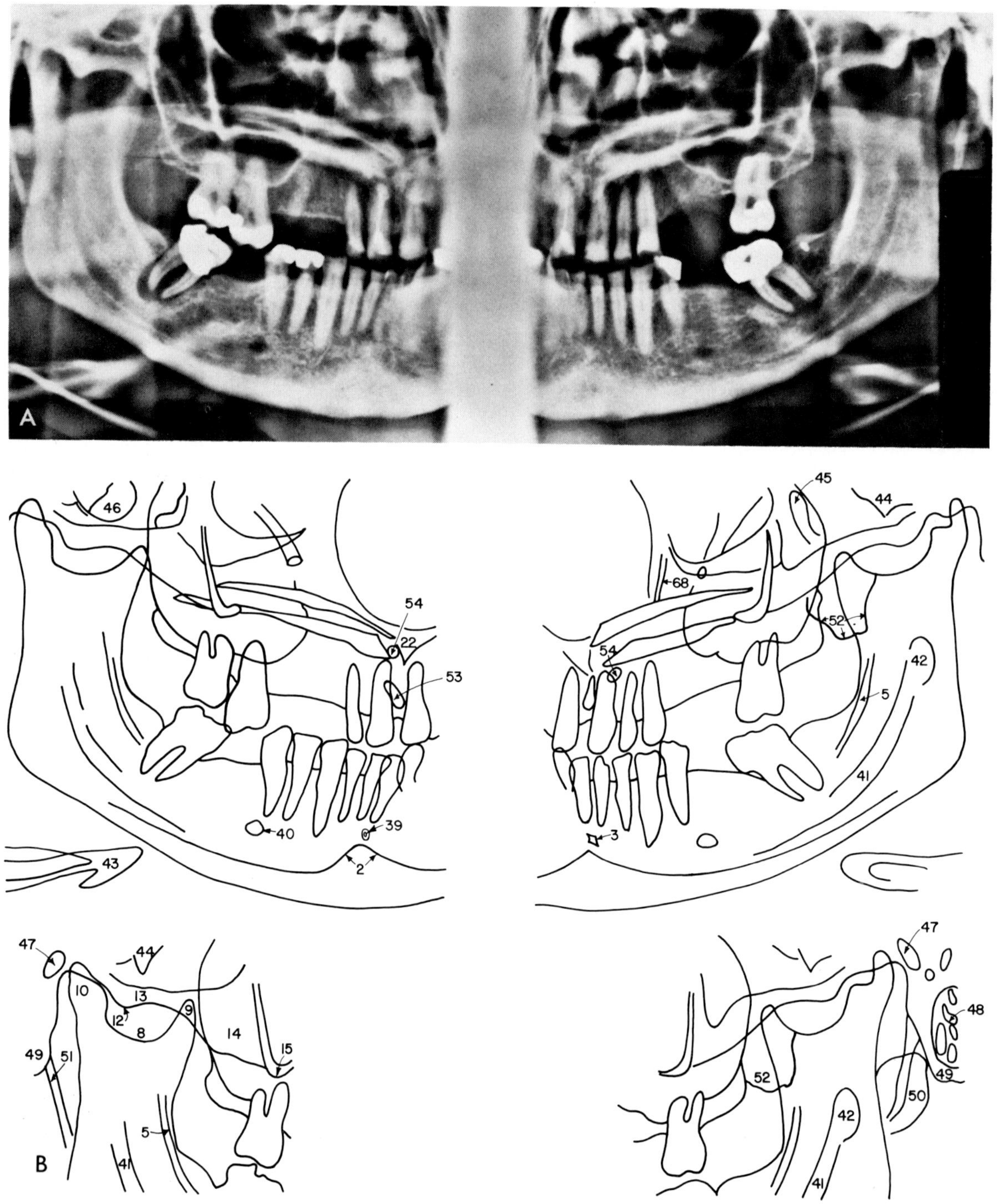

Figure 6–3. Other important landmarks. 39. Lingual foramen. 40. Mental foramen. 41. Mandibular canal (inferior alveolar canal). 42. Mandibular foramen. 43. Hyoid bone. 44. Infratemporal spine. 45. Pterygomaxillary fissure. 46. Inferior border of middle cranial cavity. 47. External auditory meatus. 48. Mastoid air cells. 49. Mastoid bone. 50. Soft tissue outline of ear lobe. 51. Styloid process (calcified stylomandibular ligament). 52. Lateral pterygoid plate. 53. Incisive foramen. 54. Superior foramen of incisive canal. 68. Lacrimal duct.

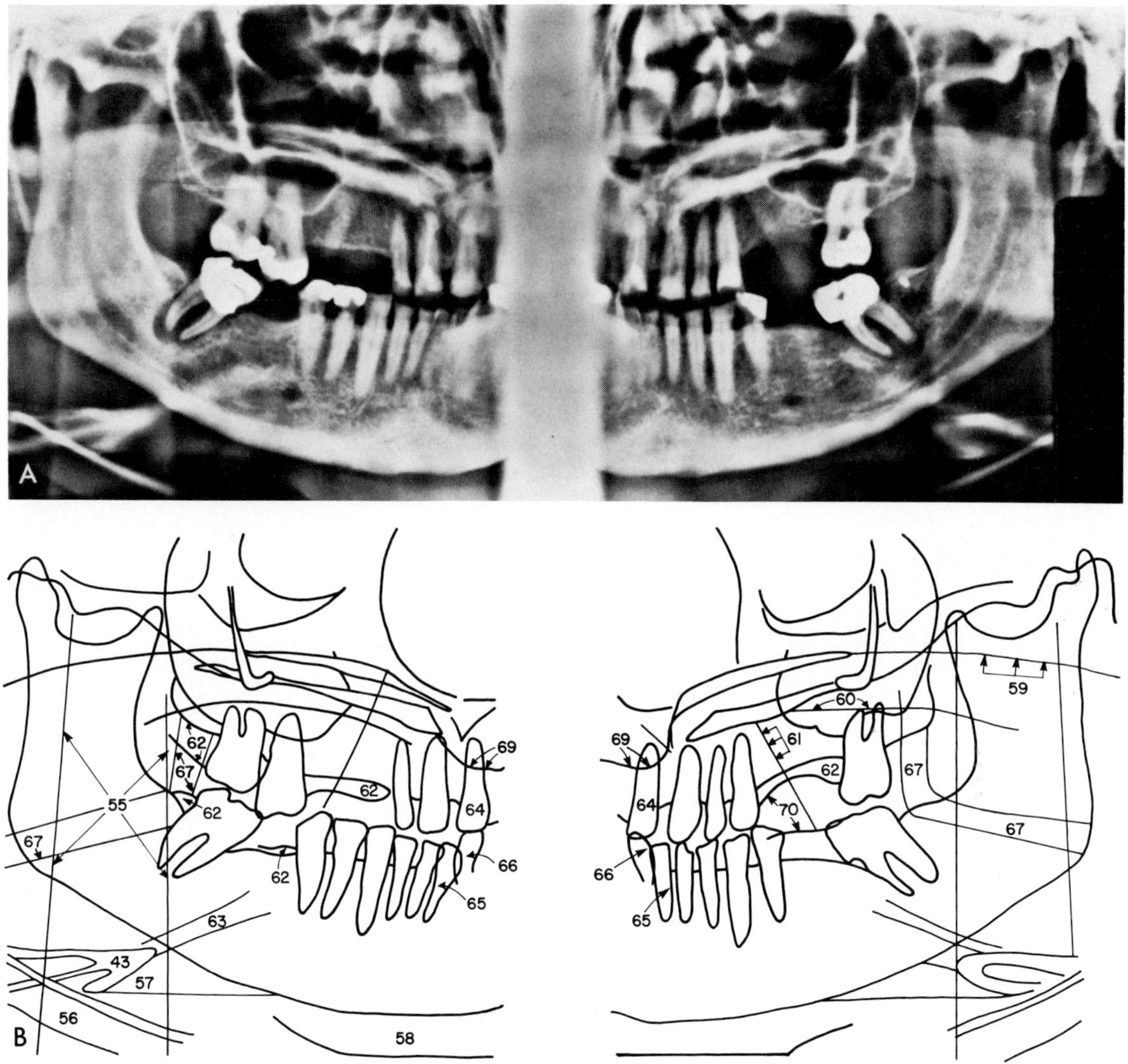

Figure 6–4. Soft tissue outlines, shadows, and ghosts. 55. Vertical head positioner (ipsilateral side). 56. Horizontal chin rest (ipsilateral side). 57. Shadow of contralateral hyoid bone. 58. Shadow of vertical wing extension of horizontal chin rest. 59. Soft palate. 60. Dorsum of tongue. 61. Nasolabial fold (ipsilateral side). 62. Soft tissue shadow of gingiva. 63. Horizontal chin rest (contralateral side). 64. Maxillary central incisor (contralateral). 65. Mandibular central incisor (contralateral). 66. Mandibular lateral incisor (contralateral). 67. Shadow of contralateral mandible (inferior border). 69. Soft tissue shadow of nose. 70. Soft tissue outline of lip.

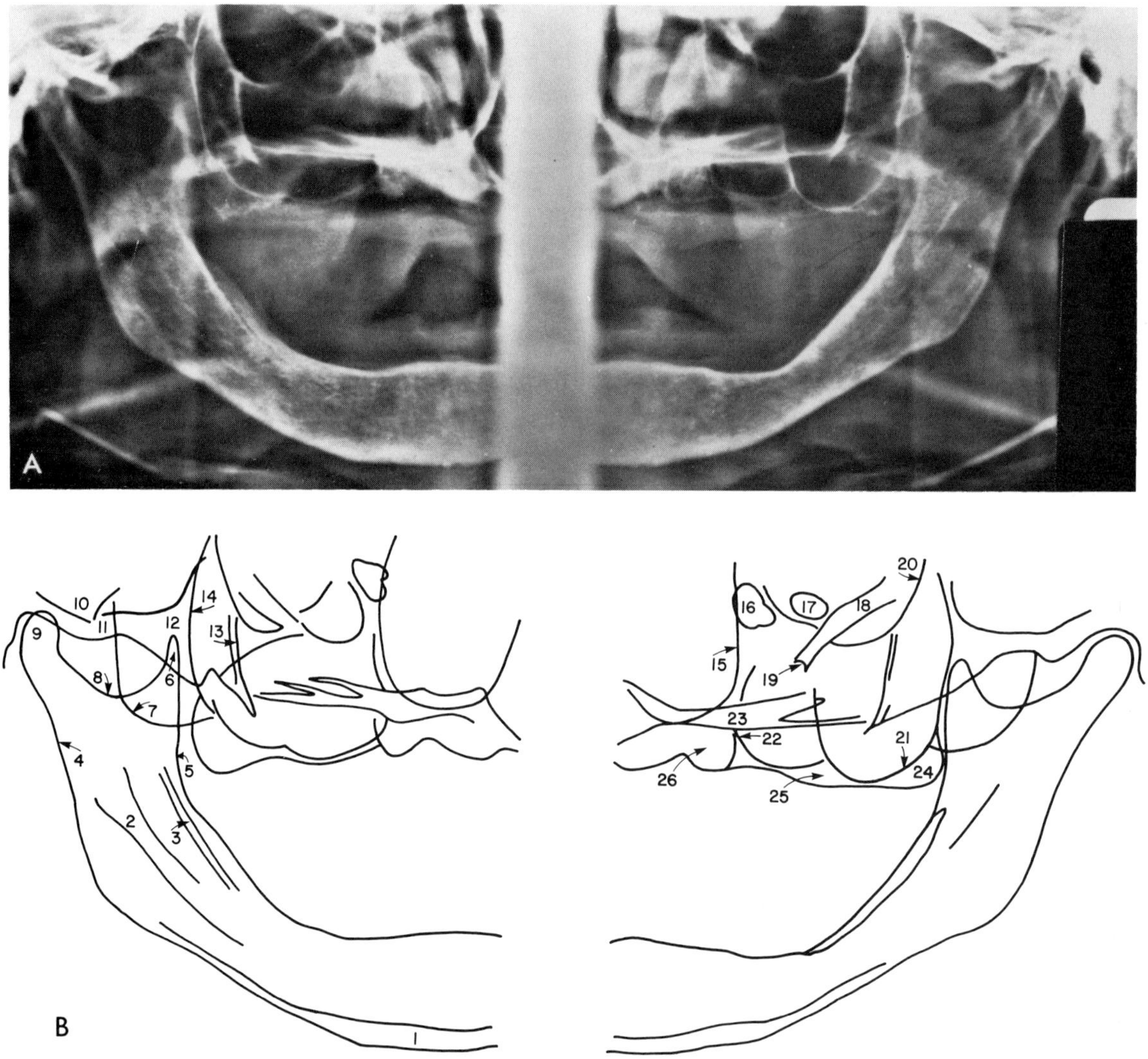

Figure 6–5. Basic bony landmarks. 1. Cortical bone lining inferior border of mandible. 2. Mandibular canal (inferior alveolar c.). 3. External oblique ridge. 4. Posterior border of ramus. 5. Anterior border of the ramus. 6. Coronoid process of mandible. 7. Lateral pterygoid plate. 8. Sigmoid notch. 9. Condylar process of mandible. 10. Infratemporal spine. 11. Temporal process of zygomatic bone. 12. Maxillary process of zygomatic bone. 13. Malar process of zygomatic bone. 14. Posterior wall of maxillary sinus (maxillary antrum). 15. Lateral wall of nasal fossa. 16. Ethmoid sinus. 17. Fossa for lacrimal sac. 18. Infraorbital canal. 19. Infraorbital foramen. 20. Superior half of panoramic innominate line (see Chapter 16). 21. Floor of maxillary sinus. 22. Anterior wall of maxillary sinus. 23. Hard palate. 24. Maxillary tuberosity. 25. Maxillary alveolar ridge. 26. Soft tissue of ala of nose.

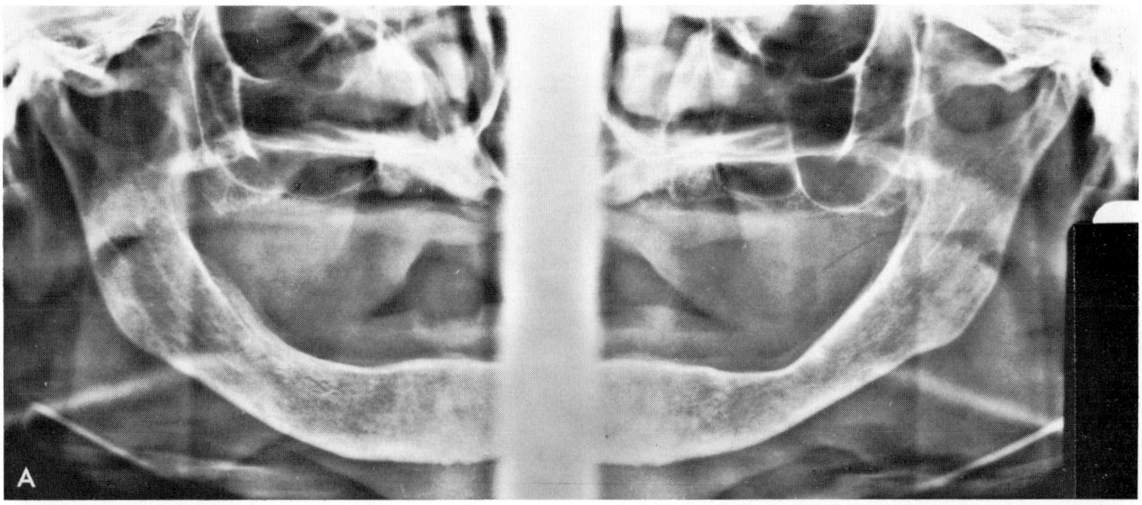

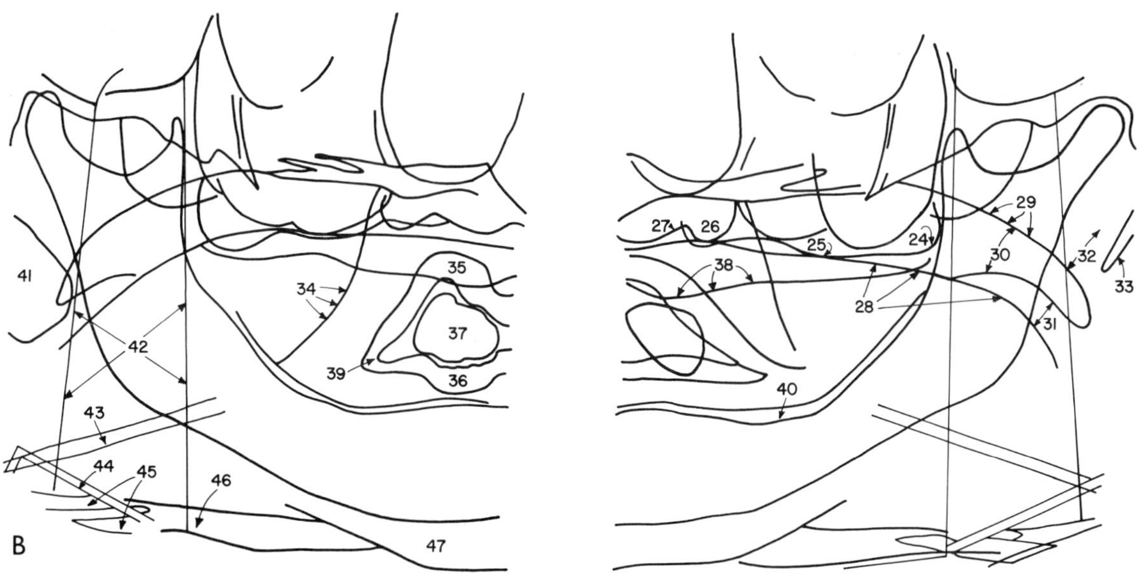

Figure 6–6. Soft tissue outlines, shadows, and ghosts. 27. Soft tissue shadow of tip of nose. 28. Dorsum of tongue. 29. Border of soft palate. 30. Soft tissue breadth of soft palate. 31. Oral pharynx (air space). 32. Nasopharynx (air space). 33. Styloid process. 34. Nasolabial fold. 35. Upper lip. 36. Lower lip. 37. Cotton roll. 38. Soft tissue of maxillary ridge (hyperplastic). 39. Commissure. 40. Soft tissue of mandibular ridge (normal). 41. Soft tissue of ear lobe. 42. Vertical head positioning bar (ipsilateral side). 43. Horizontal chin rest (contralateral side). 44. Horizontal chin rest (ipsilateral side). 45. Hyoid bone. 46. Shadow of hyoid bone. 47. Shadow of vertical wing extension (of horizontal chin rest).

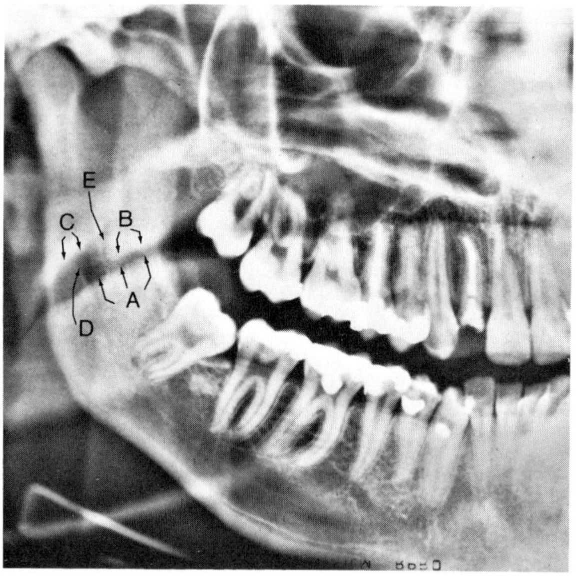

Figure 6–7. Soft tissue shadows and air spaces. A. Soft tissue shadow of dorsum of tongue. B. Shadow of soft palate. C. Shadow of posterior wall of pharynx. D. Oral pharynx air space. E. Beginning of inferior aspect of naso-pharyngeal air space.

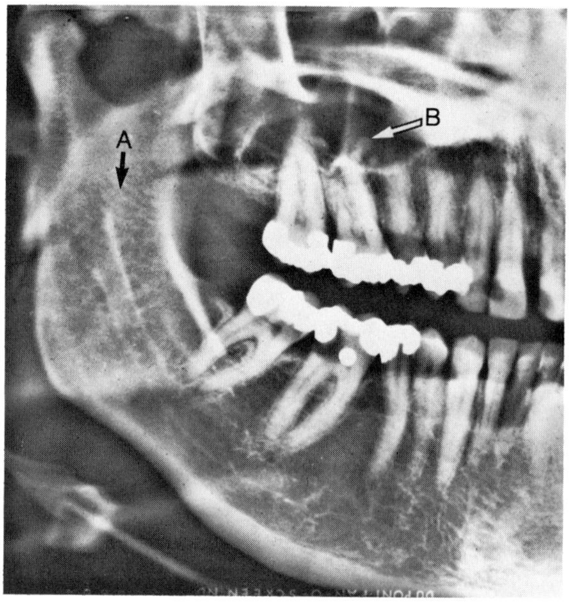

Figure 6–8. A. Air space between dorsum of tongue and soft palate mimics a fracture of the ramus. B. Note the small sinus opacities; these are antroliths.

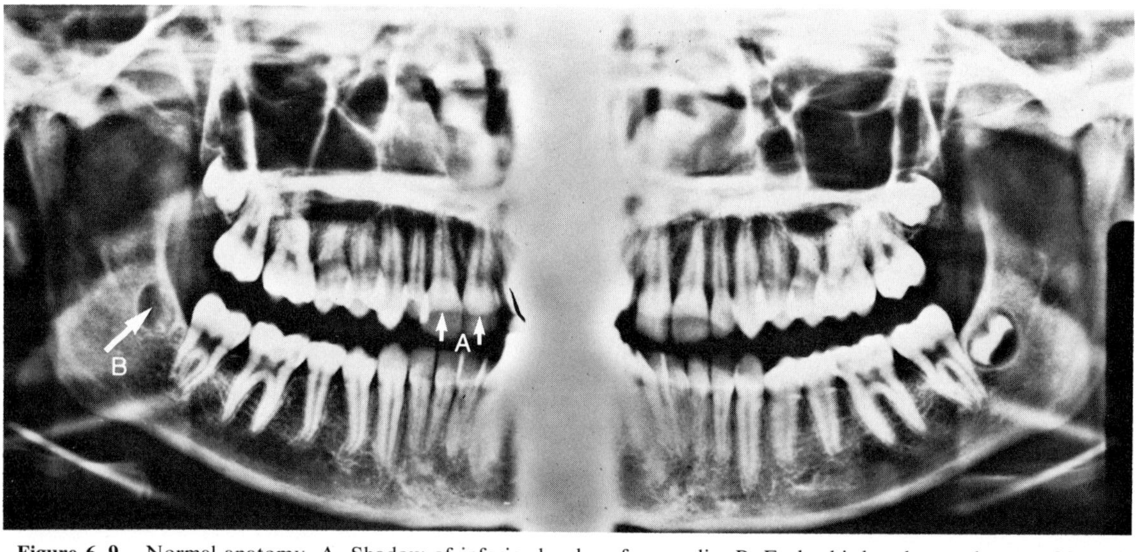

Figure 6–9. Normal anatomy. A. Shadow of inferior border of upper lip. B. Early third molar tooth crypt. Note the circumflex radiopacities representing the early cusp tips.

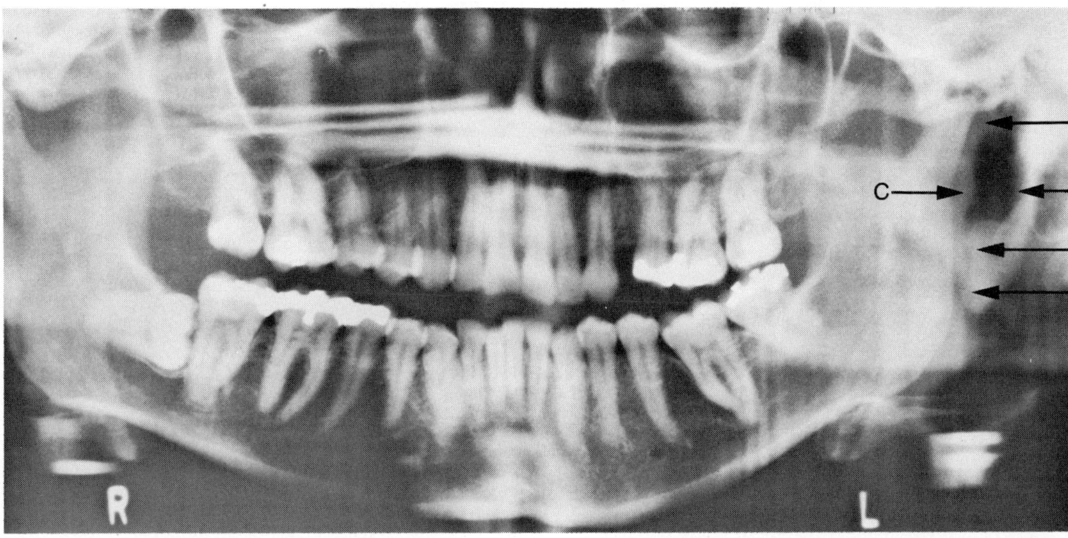

Figure 6–10. Soft tissue of the left ear. A. Ear lobe. B. Antitragus. C. Tragus. D. Antihelix. E. Helix.

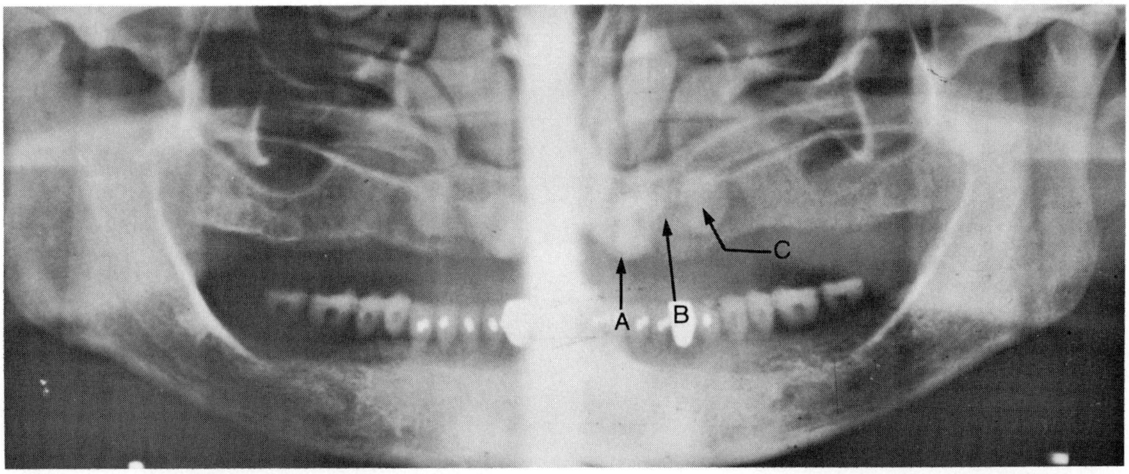

Figure 6–11. Soft tissue of the nose. A. Tip of the nose. B. Left naris. C. Left ala. This machine projects two partial images of the nose, but both are projected in the midline. This film illustrates the superimposition of the nasal turbinates, meati, and their ghost images on the maxillary sinuses.

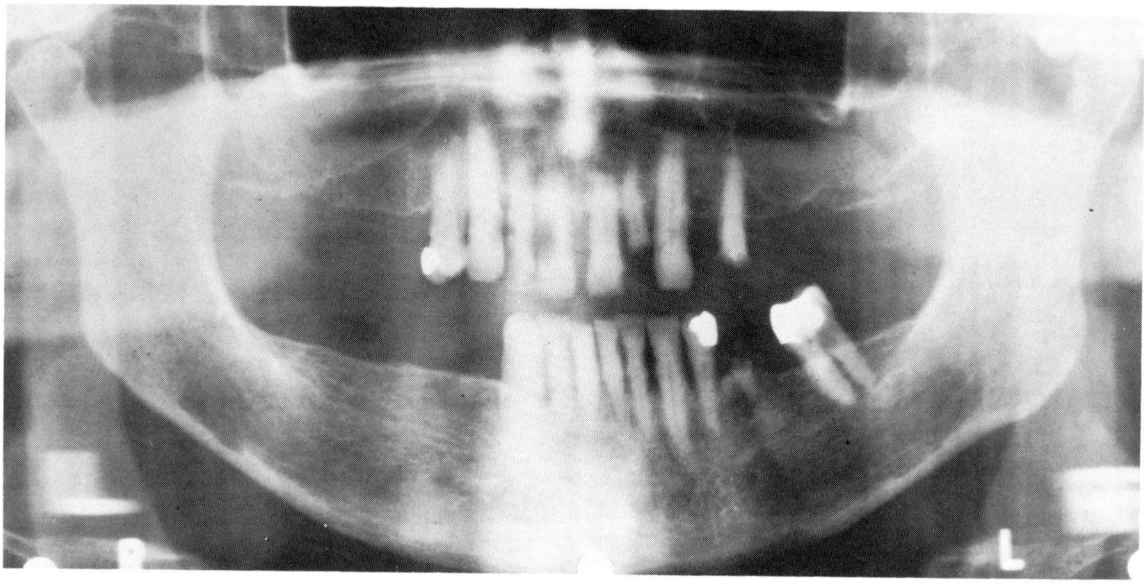

Figure 6–12. Soft tissue shadow of the nose. **A.** The nose is seen in the midline. **B.** Note the early lingual mandibular salivary gland depression in the right mandible.

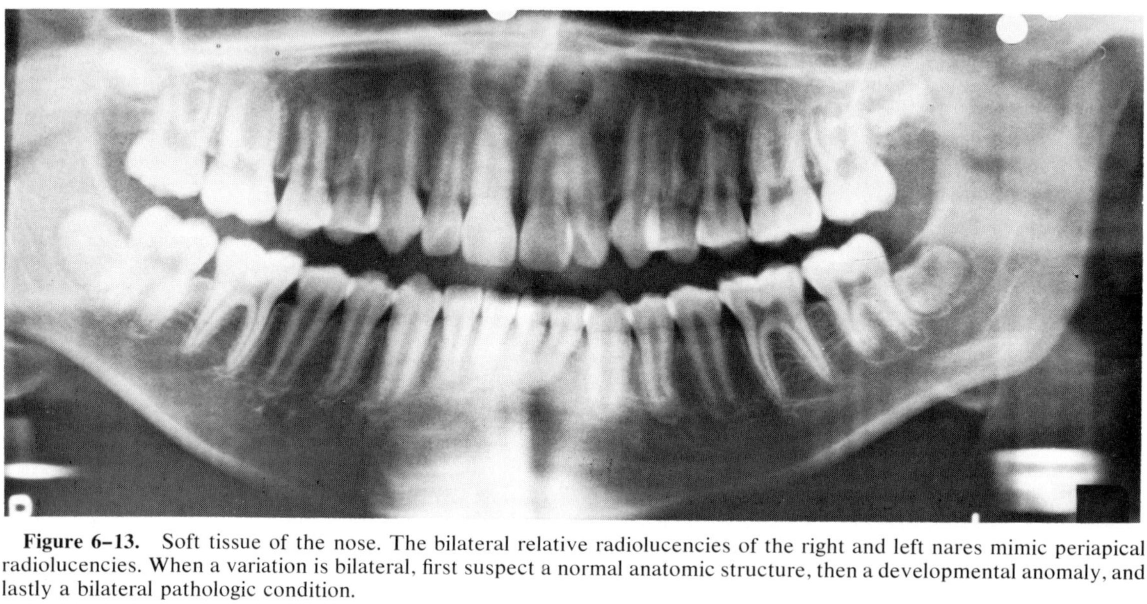

Figure 6–13. Soft tissue of the nose. The bilateral relative radiolucencies of the right and left nares mimic periapical radiolucencies. When a variation is bilateral, first suspect a normal anatomic structure, then a developmental anomaly, and lastly a bilateral pathologic condition.

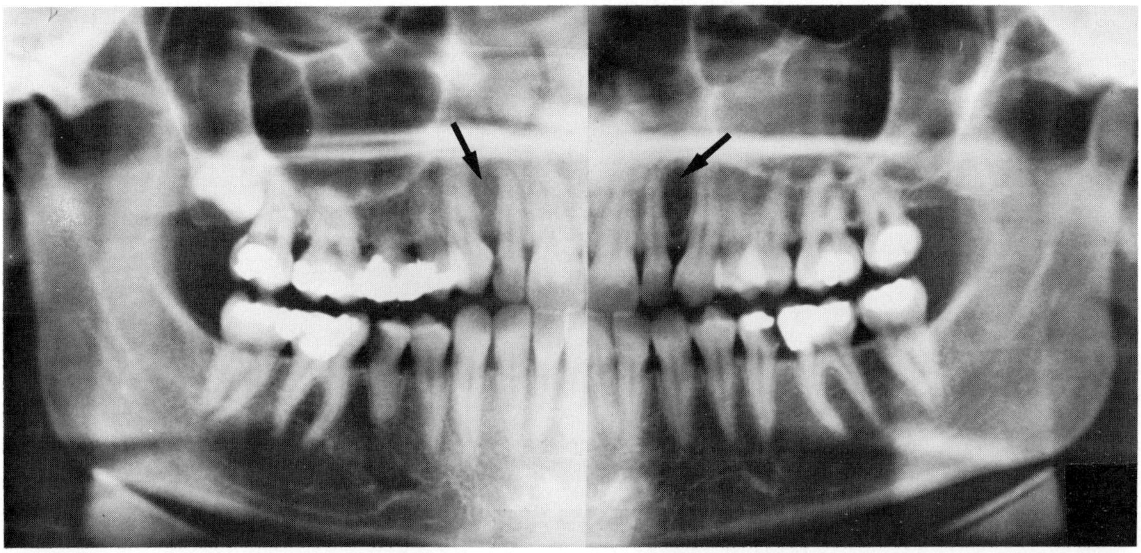

Figure 6–14. Lateral incisor fossae. These fossae represent depression and thinning of the alveolar bone in this area and mimic globulomaxillary cysts. The bilateralism of the condition suggests an anatomic variation.

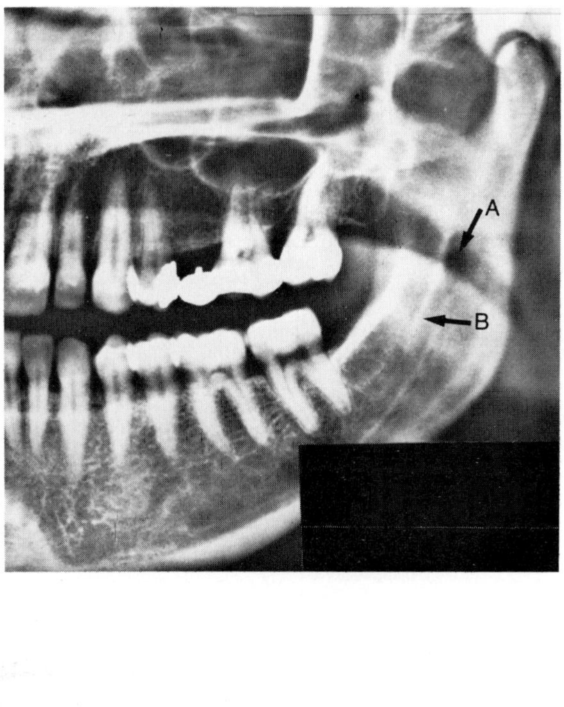

Figure 6–15. Normal anatomy. A. Mandibular foramen. B. Mandibular canal.

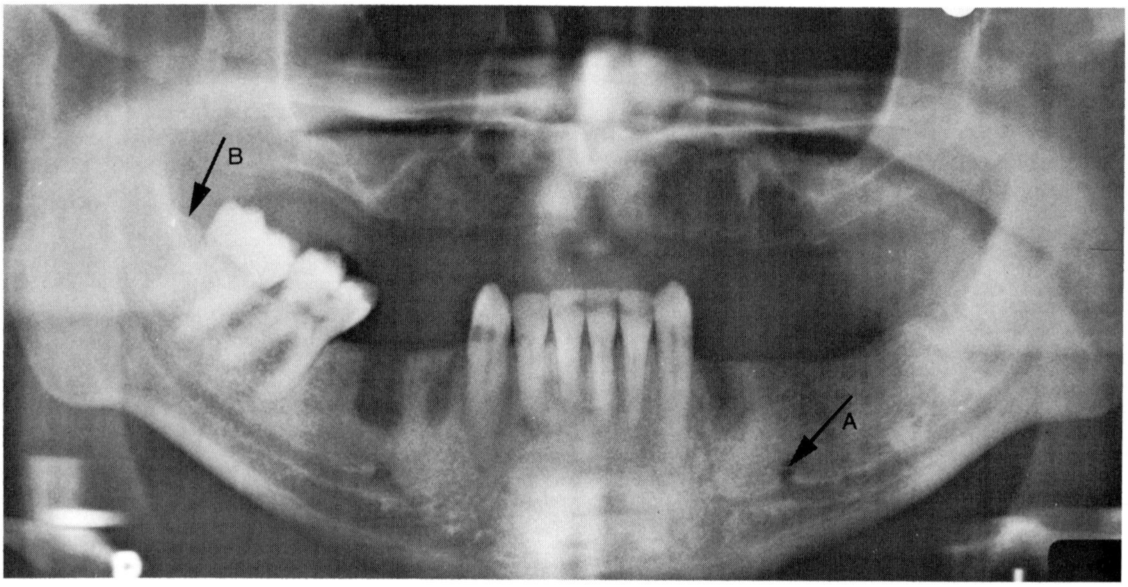

Figure 6–16. Normal anatomy. A. Mental foramen. Note the relationship of the mandibular canal to the mental foramen and the anterior extension of the canal beyond the foramen. B. Distal mandibular pseudohyperostosis. This apparently increased height of the alveolar bone occurs mainly on the distal aspect of mandibular molars, especially those that have tipped mesially.

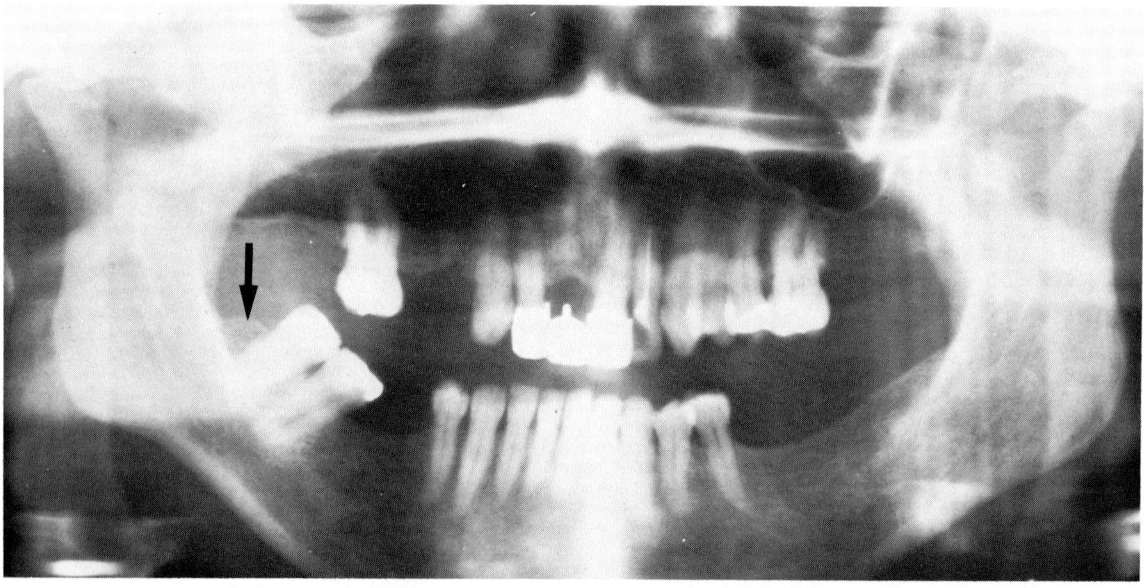

Figure 6–17. Distal mandibular pseudohyperostosis.

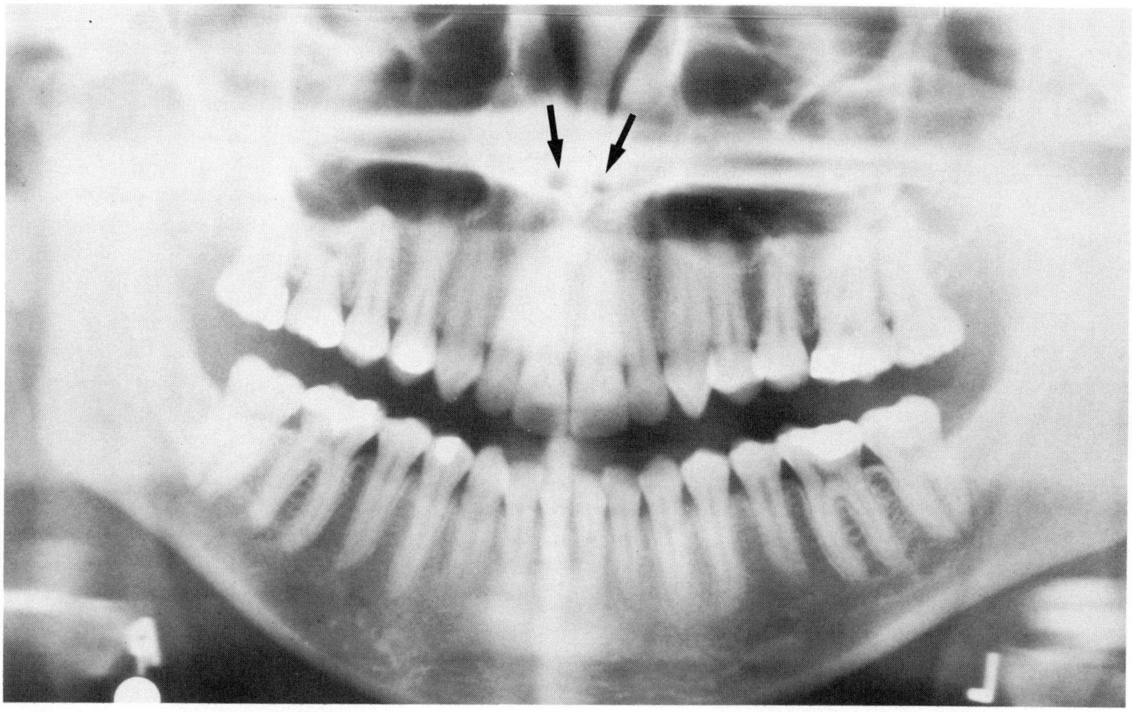

Figure 6–18. Normal anatomy. Superior foramina of the incisive canal. These open into the floor of the nose and are not patent in most individuals. When superimposed on the apices of the central incisors, they may mimic periapical pathology.

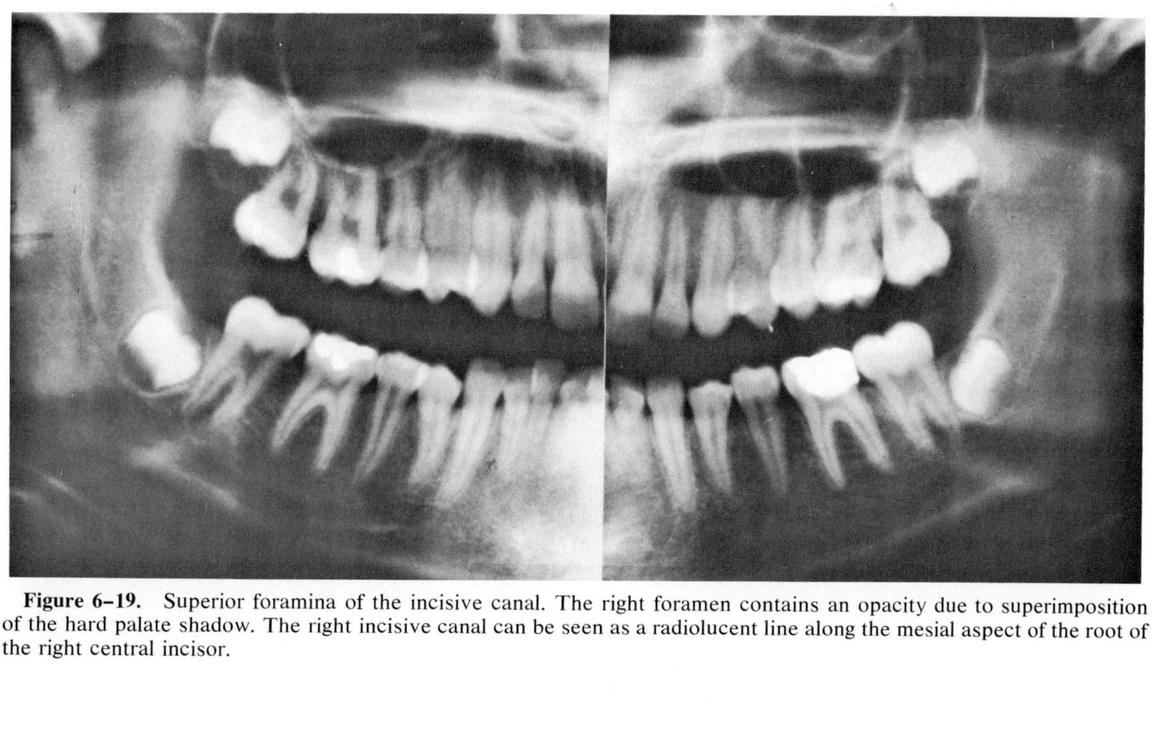

Figure 6–19. Superior foramina of the incisive canal. The right foramen contains an opacity due to superimposition of the hard palate shadow. The right incisive canal can be seen as a radiolucent line along the mesial aspect of the root of the right central incisor.

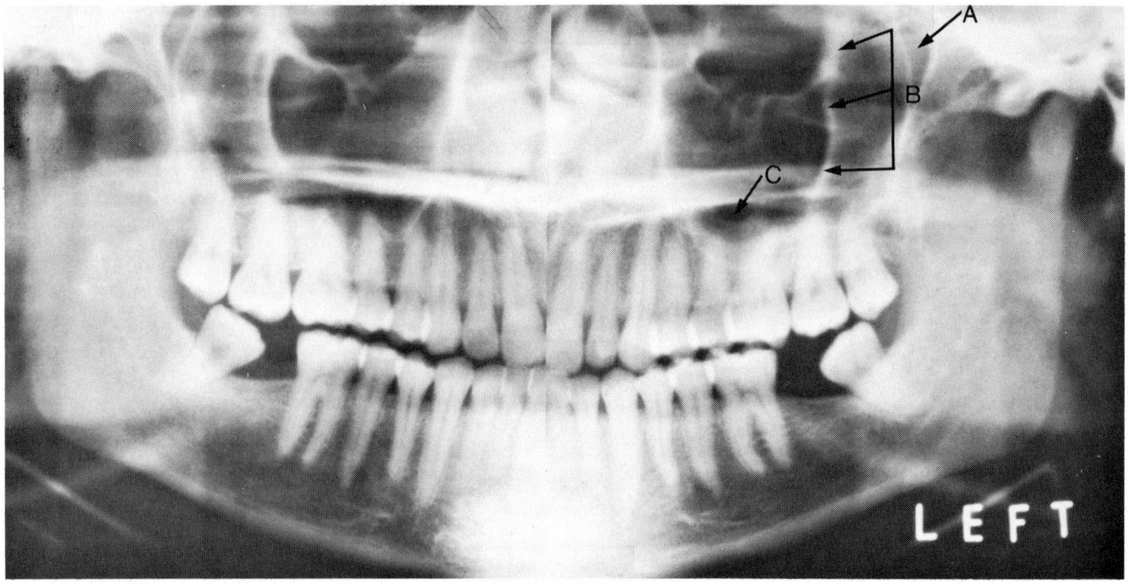

Figure 6–20. Normal anatomy. A. Pterygomaxillary grove (see Chapter 16). B. Panoramic innominate line (see Chapter 16). C. Sinus recess. This is a depression in the wall of the maxillary sinus.

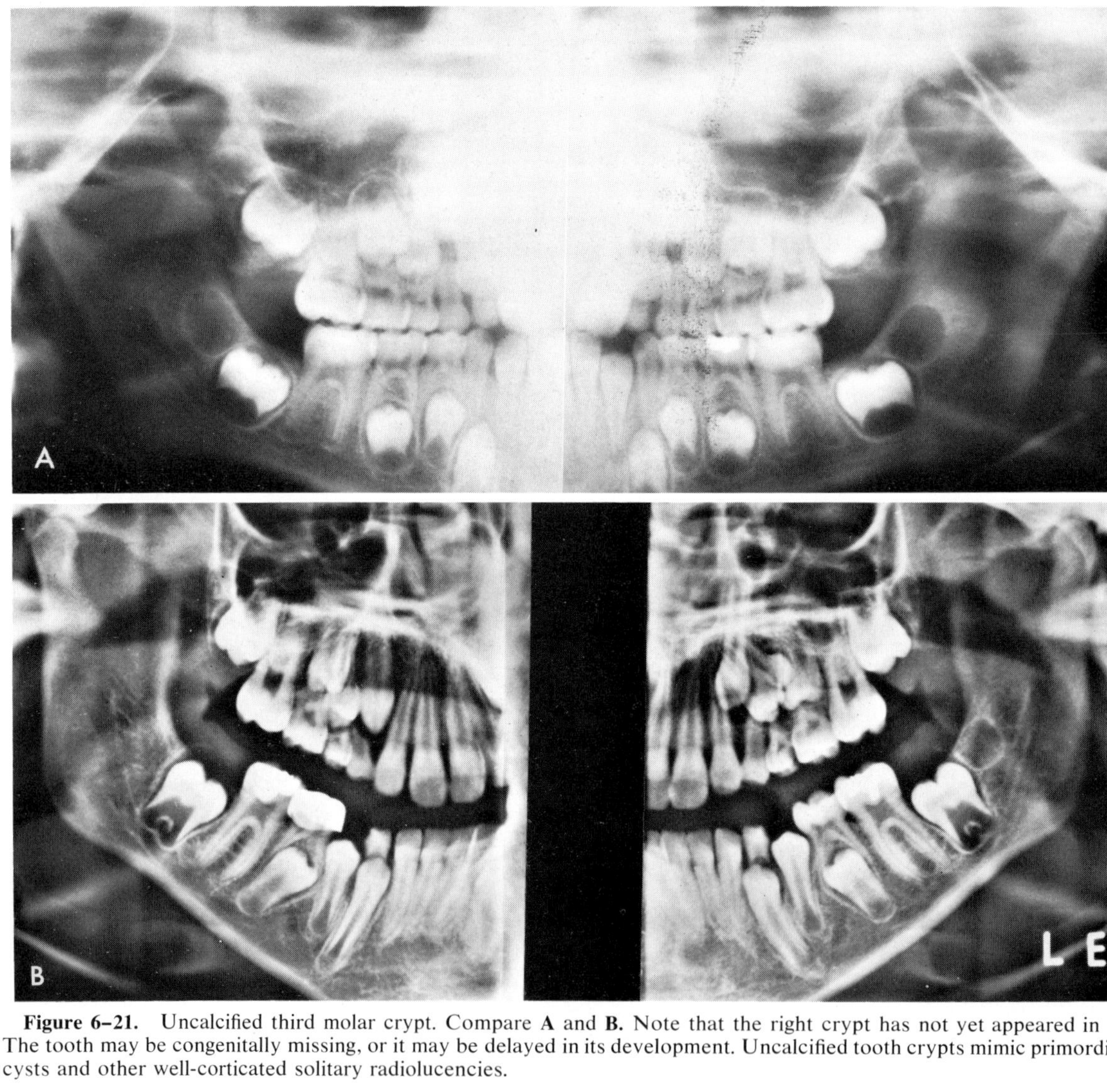

Figure 6–21. Uncalcified third molar crypt. Compare **A** and **B.** Note that the right crypt has not yet appeared in **B.** The tooth may be congenitally missing, or it may be delayed in its development. Uncalcified tooth crypts mimic primordial cysts and other well-corticated solitary radiolucencies.

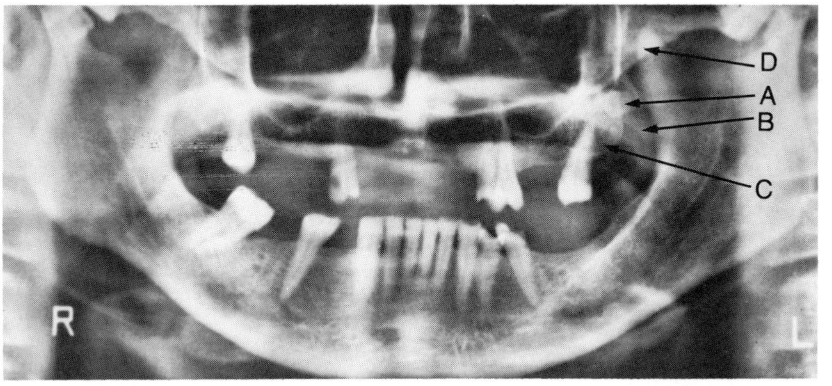

Figure 6–22. Normal anatomy. A. Lateral pterygoid plate. B. Hamular process. C. Maxillary tuberosity. D. The tip of the coronoid process is more opaque owing to superimposition by the zygomatic arch.

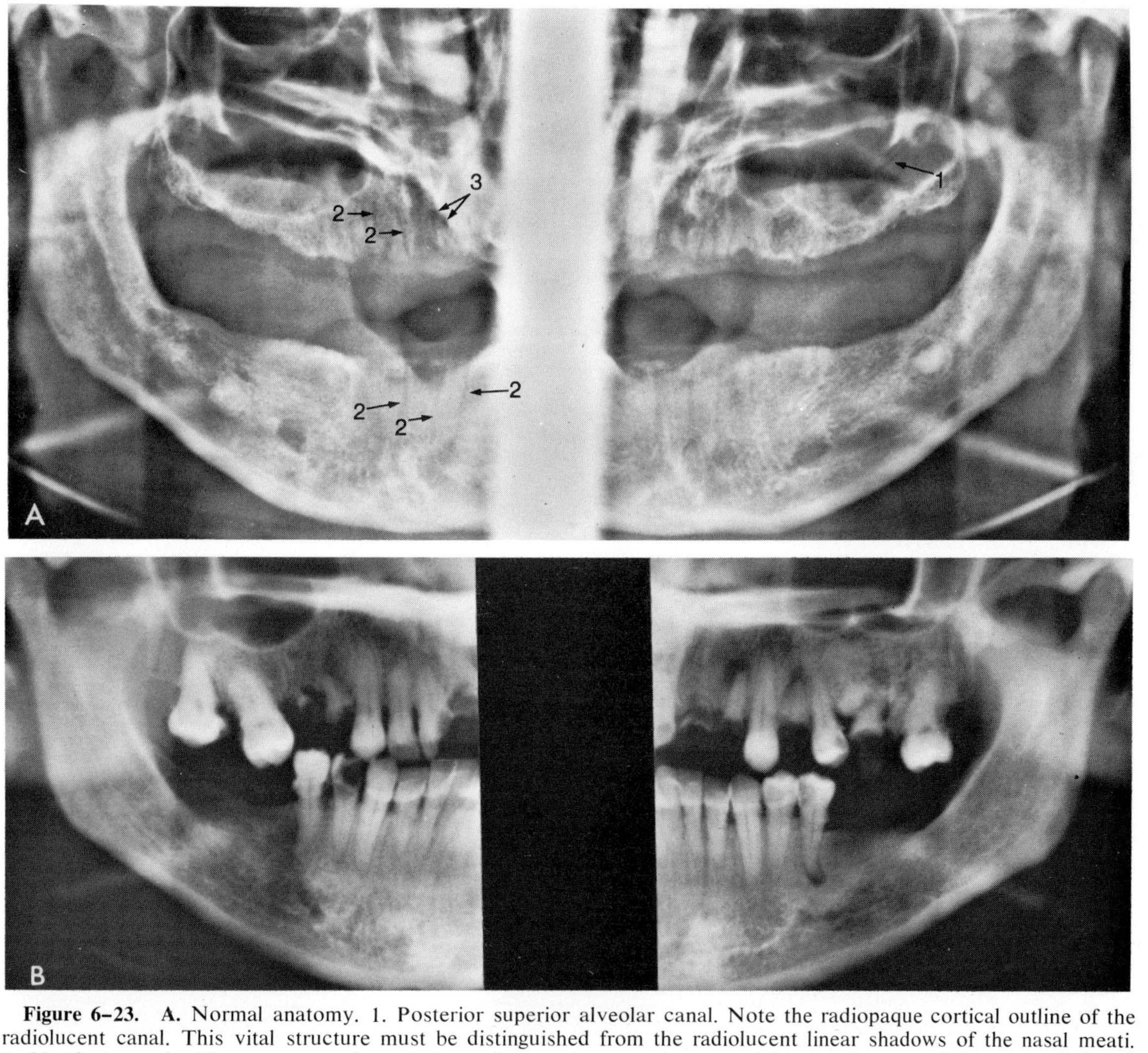

Figure 6–23. **A.** Normal anatomy. 1. Posterior superior alveolar canal. Note the radiopaque cortical outline of the radiolucent canal. This vital structure must be distinguished from the radiolucent linear shadows of the nasal meati. 2. Nutrient canals. The presence of nutrient canals may be an indication of increased susceptibility to periodontal disease. 3. Foraminae of nutrient canals. **B.** Note numerous nutrient canals.

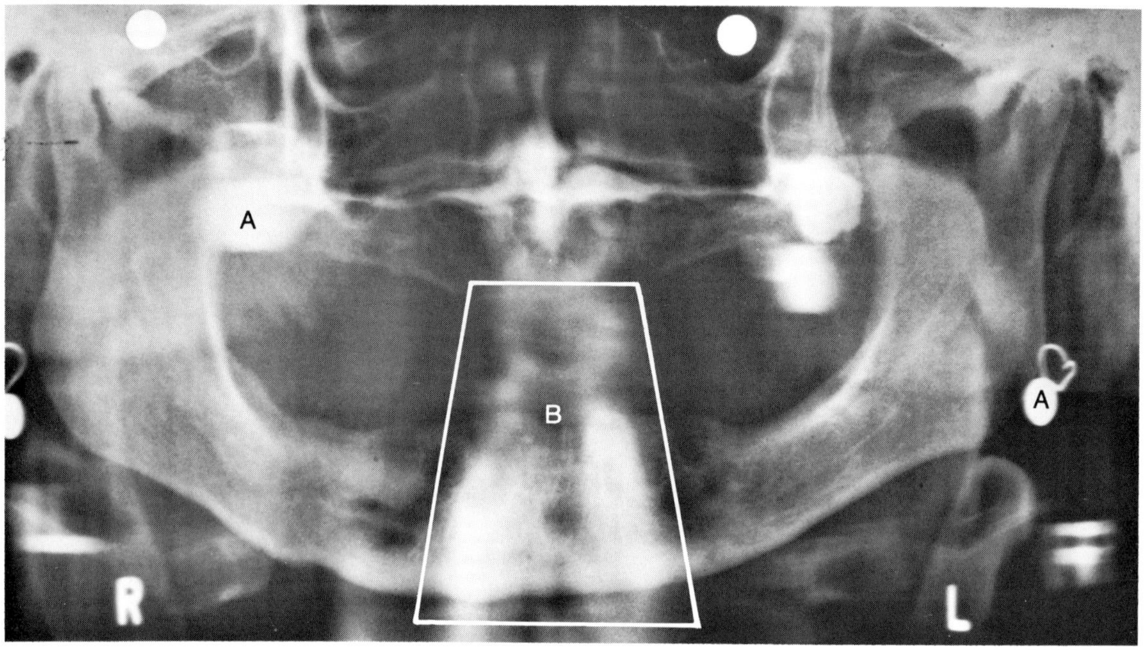

Figure 6–24. Ghost images. A. The left earring and its contralateral ghost image. The ghost image is superimposed on the right maxilla, possibly obliterating the presence of an impacted third molar as is the case in the left maxilla. B. Ghost image of the vertebral column.

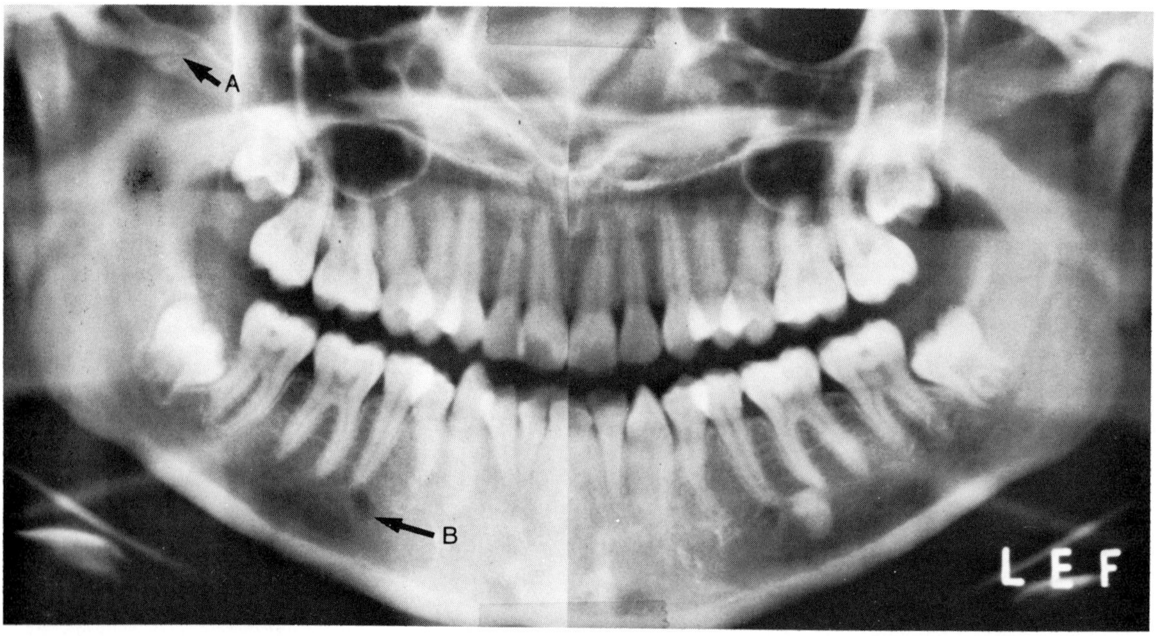

Figure 6–25. Normal anatomy. A. Zygomaticotemporal suture that mimics a fracture of the zygomatic arch. B. Mental foramen that mimics a periapical radiolucent lesion of the second bicuspid. Both A and B are bilateral findings, typical of normal anatomic landmarks.

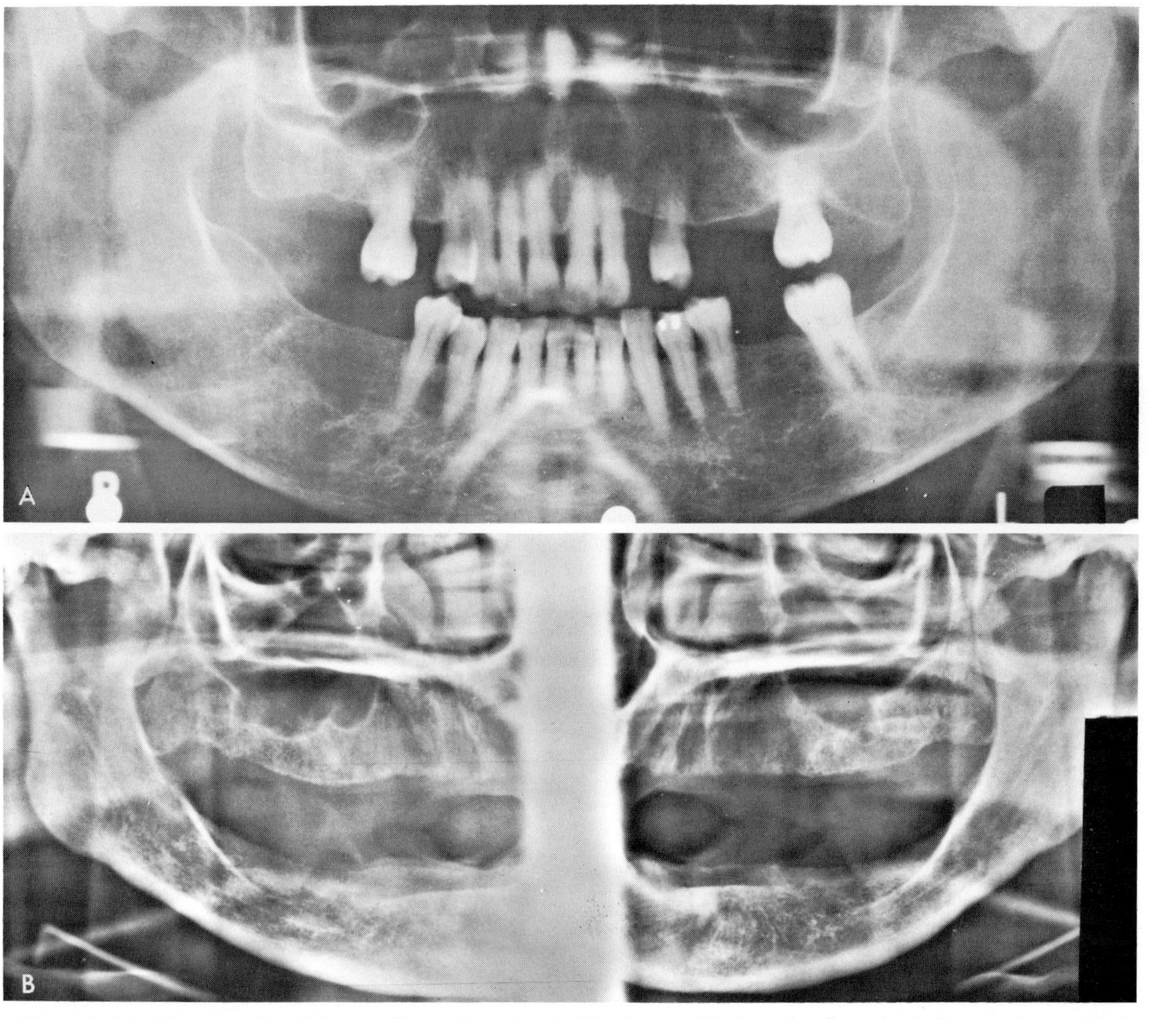

Figure 6–26. Hypertrophy of the maxillary tuberosity. **A.** The inverted V-shaped radiopacity in the anterior area is the ghost image of a neckchain or napkin chain. **B.** Note that the condition is bilateral, as it is in **A.**

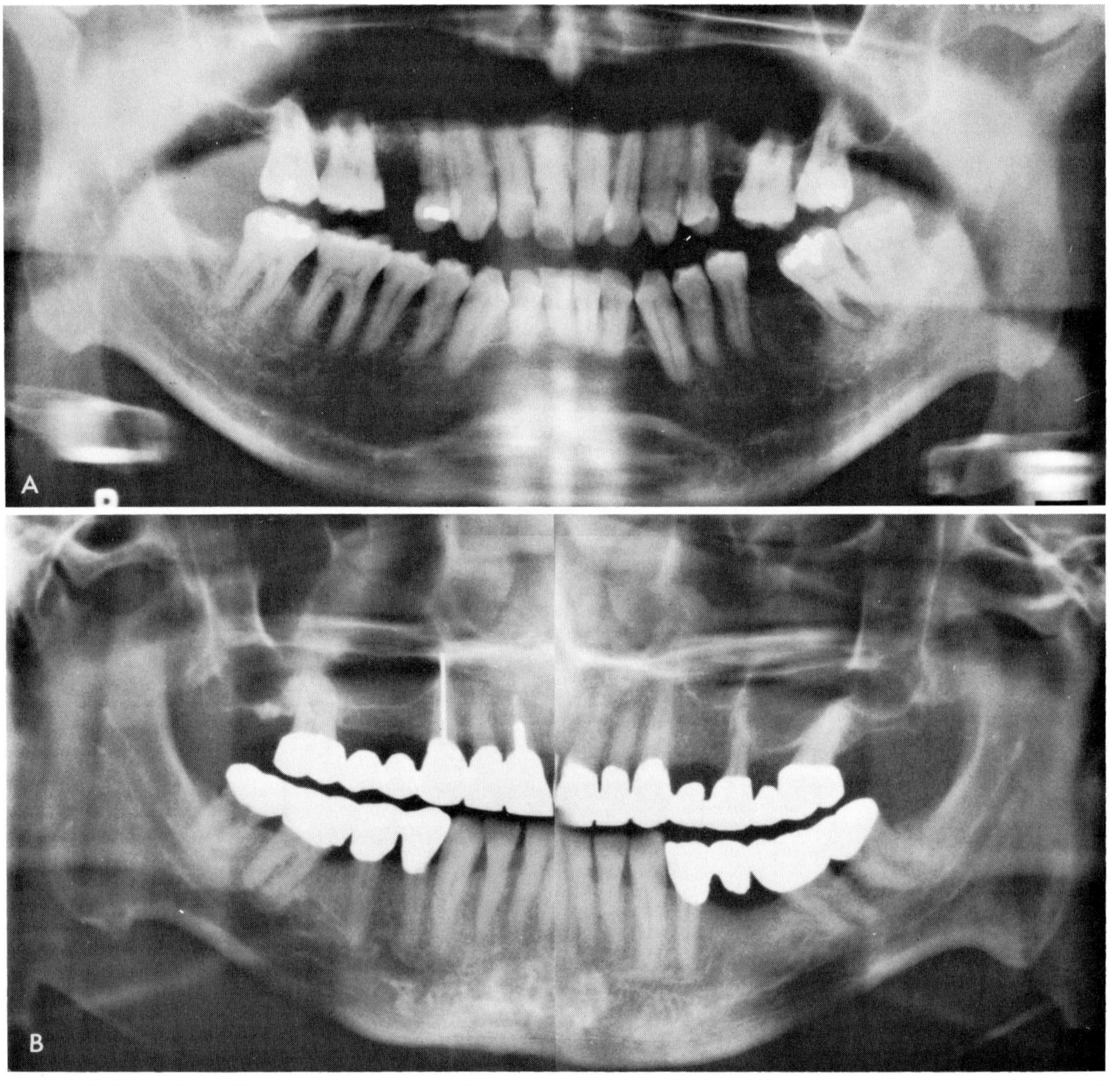

Figure 6–27A and **B.** Hypertrophy of the gonial angle and prominent gonial notch. Note that in both cases the condition is bilateral. In some instances the enlarged angle consists of thin cortical bone, which produces a relatively more radiolucent bone shadow in this area.

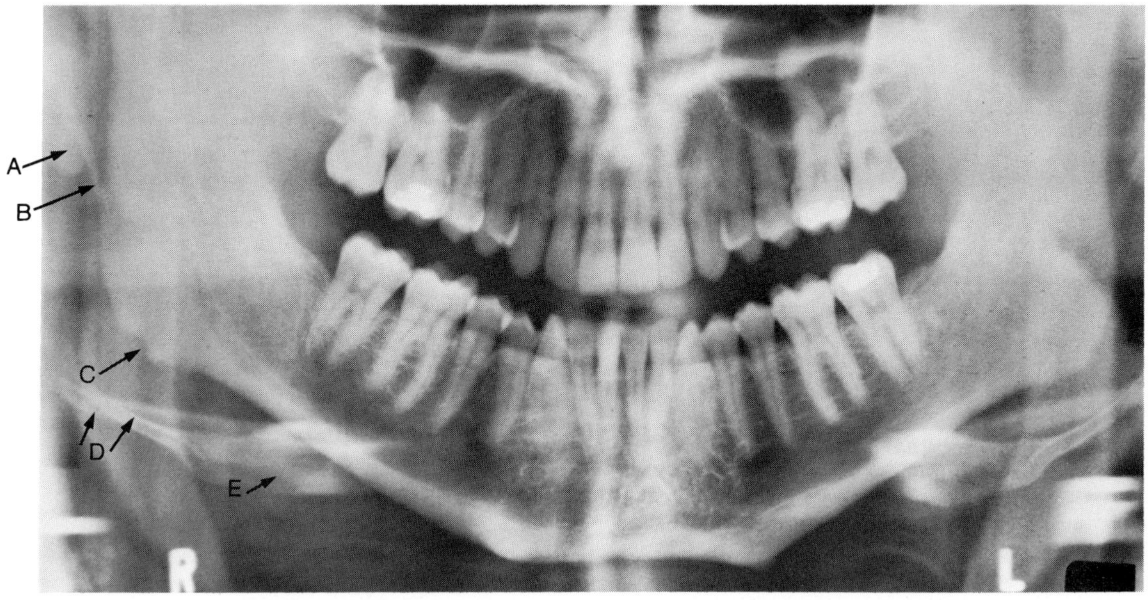

Figure 6–28. Square chin (thought to be due to anatomic variation rather than projection artifact). A. Ear lobe. B. Calcified stylomandibular ligament. C. Notch in gonial angle. D. Right and left greater horns of hyoid bone. E. Body of hyoid bone.

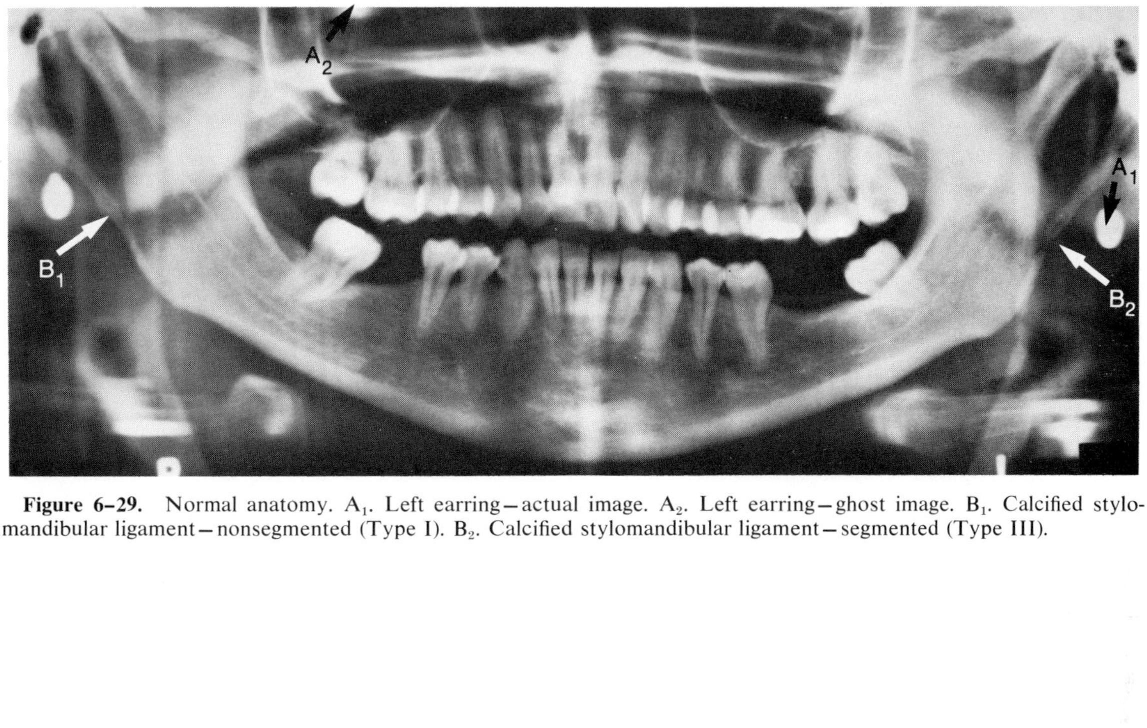

Figure 6–29. Normal anatomy. A_1. Left earring – actual image. A_2. Left earring – ghost image. B_1. Calcified stylomandibular ligament – nonsegmented (Type I). B_2. Calcified stylomandibular ligament – segmented (Type III).

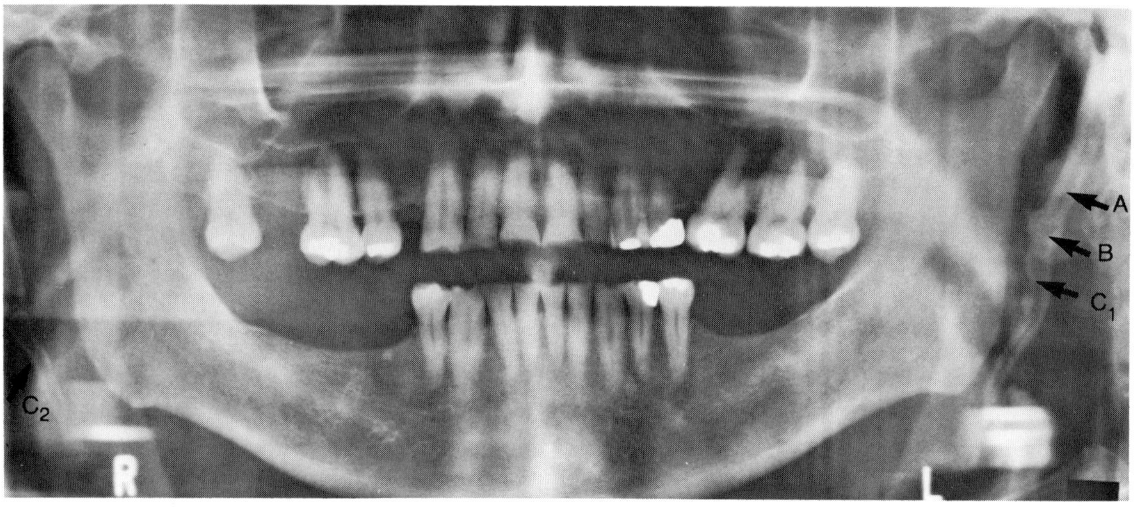

Figure 6–30. Calcified stylohyoid ligament. A. Styloid process. B. Pseudoarticulation between styloid process and calcified stylohyoid ligament. C_1. Calcified stylohyoid ligament—pseudoarticulated (Type II). Note the bonelike appearance of the calcified ligament with an outer cortex and inner radiolucent space. C_2. Calcified stylohyoid ligament—segmented (Type III). (Courtesy of Dr. Charles E. Cook, San Antonio, TX.)

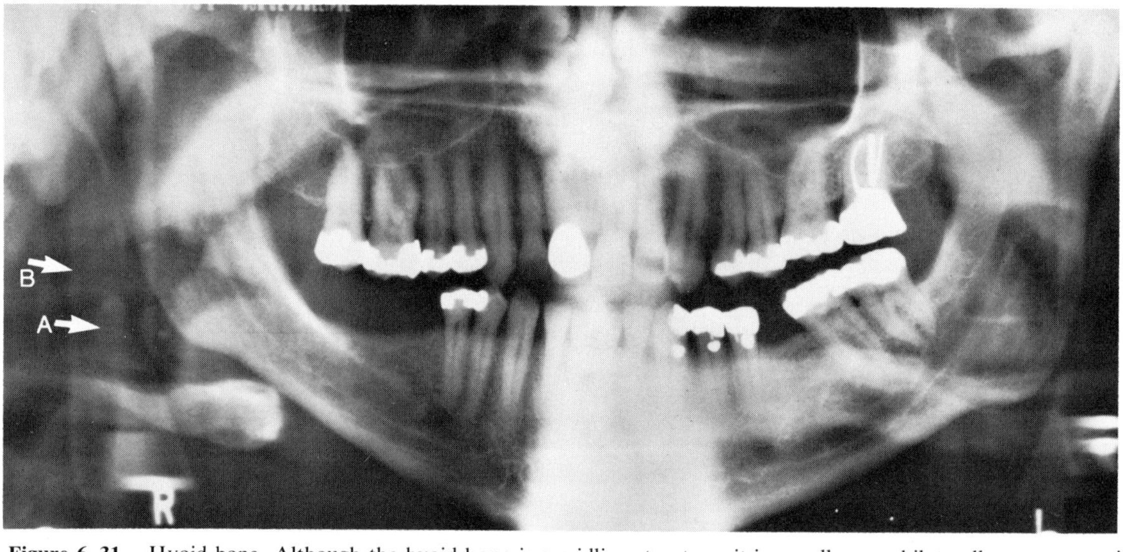

Figure 6–31. Hyoid bone. Although the hyoid bone is a midline structure, it is usually seen bilaterally on panoramic films. In this film the right side shows a good image of the body and right greater horn, whereas the left side was not within the sharply depicted layer. The radiopacity in the left body of the mandible is the ghost image of the right hyoid. The vertical opaque band in the anterior in the ghost image of the cervical spine. A. Epiglottis (crescent or semilunar shaped). B. Shadow of vertical head positioning device.

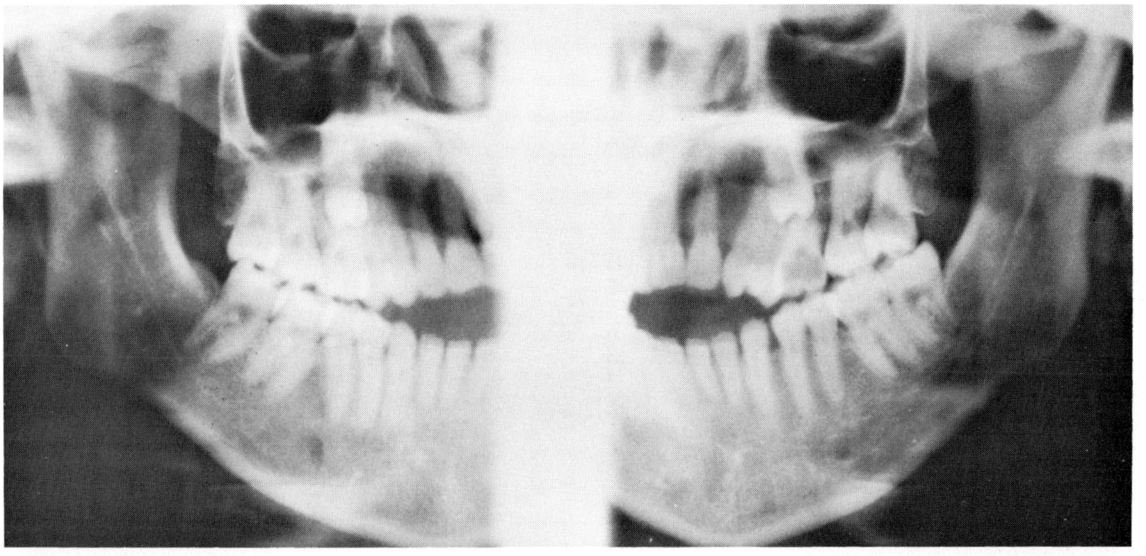

Figure 6–32. Anterior open bite. Panoramic information concerning the arrangement of teeth can be useful in post-trauma medico-legal cases and in forensic odontology.

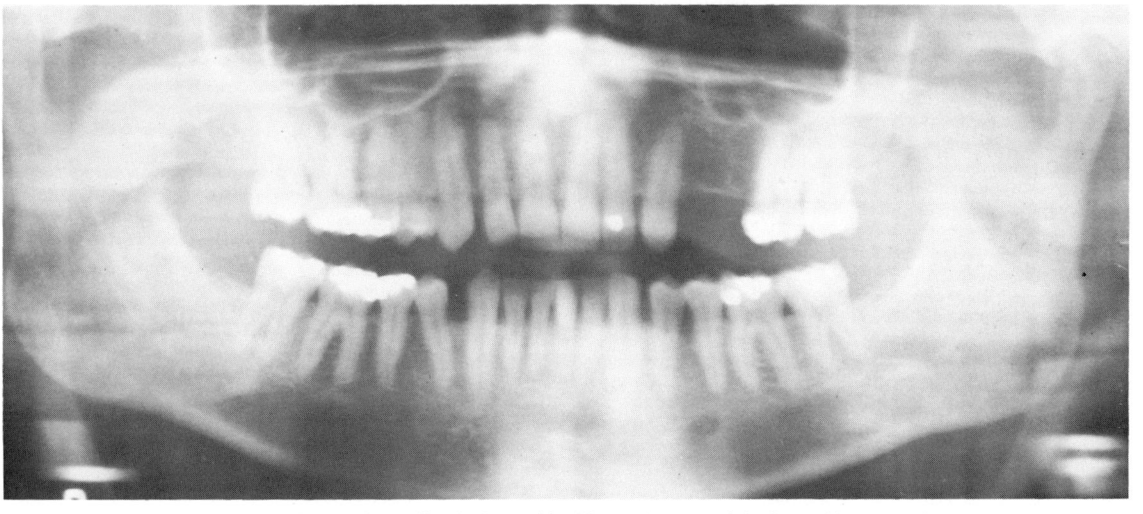

Figure 6–33. Primate space. Lower jaw: distal of cuspids. Upper jaw: mesial of cuspids. Note the bilateralism of these developmental spaces, a variation of normal seen in some individuals.

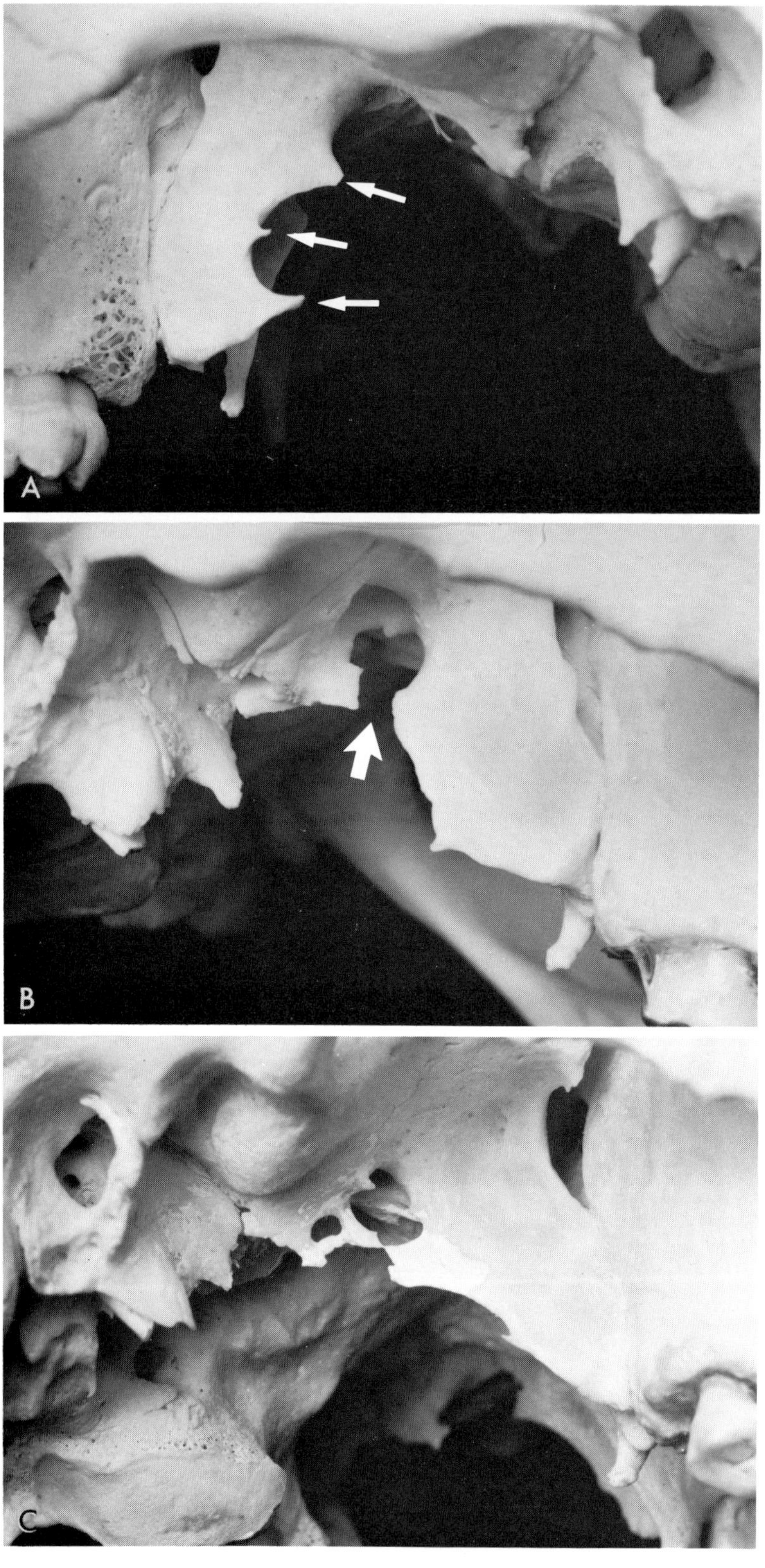

Figure 6–34. Pterygospinous bar. This is the completely ossified pterygospinous ligament that connects posterior margin of lateral pterygoid plate and base of spinous process of sphenoid bone. First described by Civinini, an Italian anatomist, in 1835. This ossification forms one or more foramina called the pterygospinous foramen or the foramen of Civinini.

Illustration continued on opposite page

Figure 6–34 *Continued.* A compilation of various studies of incidence of complete ossification of the pterygospinous ligament and formation of the foramina by Tebo (1968) indicates an average incidence of 4.3 per cent among 10,614 skulls. **A.** Type I. Civinini noted that the pterygospinous ligament could be more or less ossified, resulting in several variations: Type I consists of notching of the posterior border of the lateral pterygoid plate due to the formation of two or three spines. **B.** Type II. The attachment between the lateral pterygoid plate and the base of the spinous process is almost complete. **C.** Type III. In this rare instance, there is bony union between the lateral pterygoid plate and the base of the spinous process. **D.** Type III. Panoramic radiograph of dried specimen illustrated in **C.**

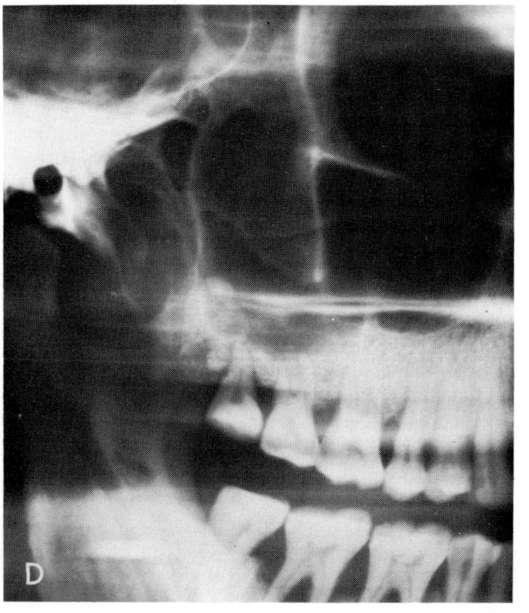

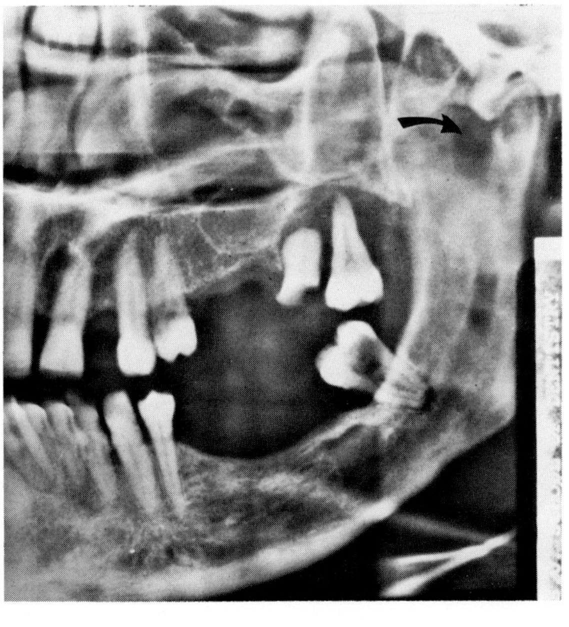

Figure 6–35. Pterygospinous foramen.

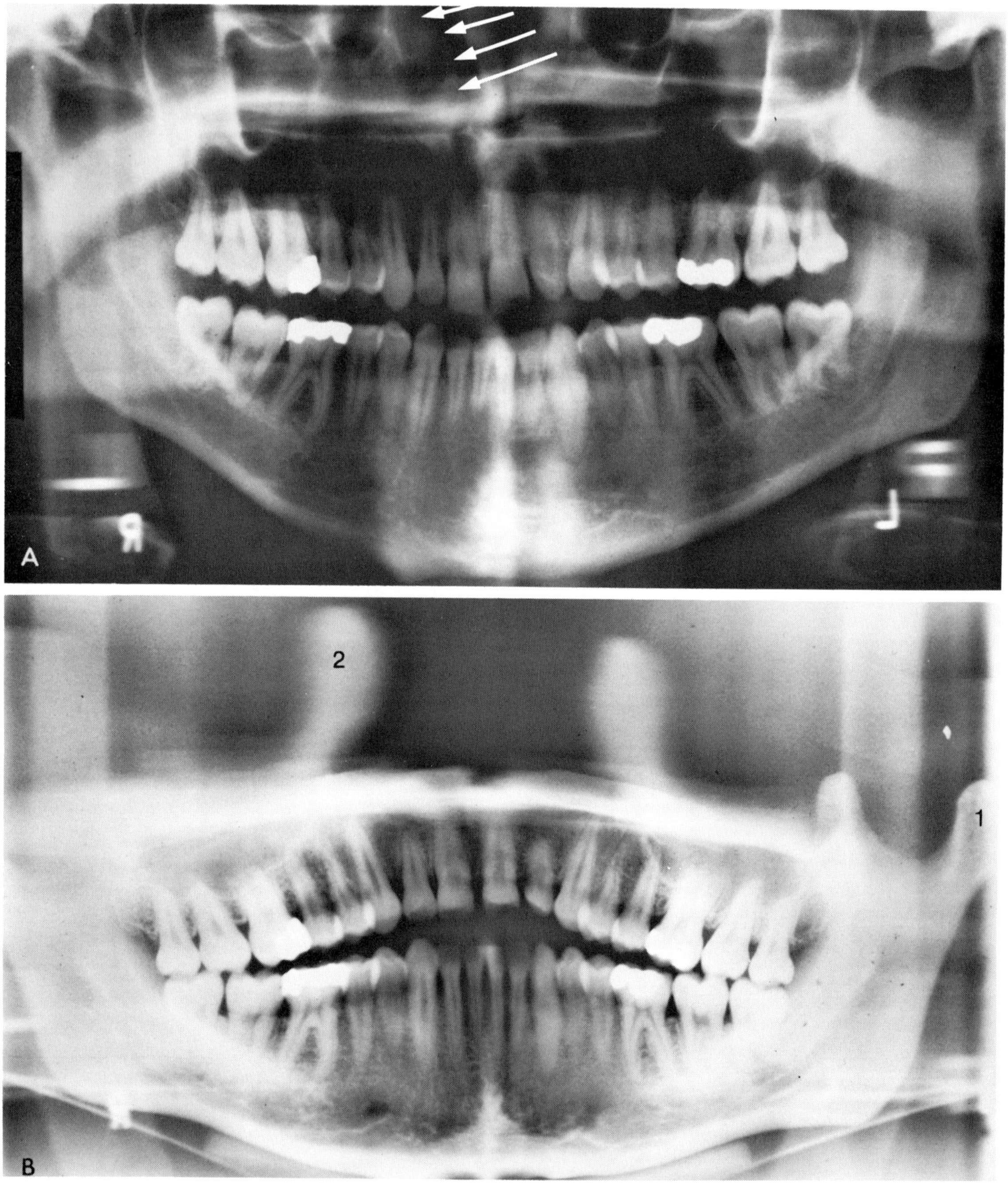

Figure 6–36. Ghost image of condyles. **A.** Antemortem panoramic radiograph. Arrows point to what is usually referred to as the inferior turbinate shadow. **B.** Postmortem radiograph. 1. Actual condyle. 2. Ghost image of condyle in **A.** Note also the ghost image of the contralateral condyle. (Courtesy of Dr. Doug Stoneman, Toronto, Ontario, Canada.)

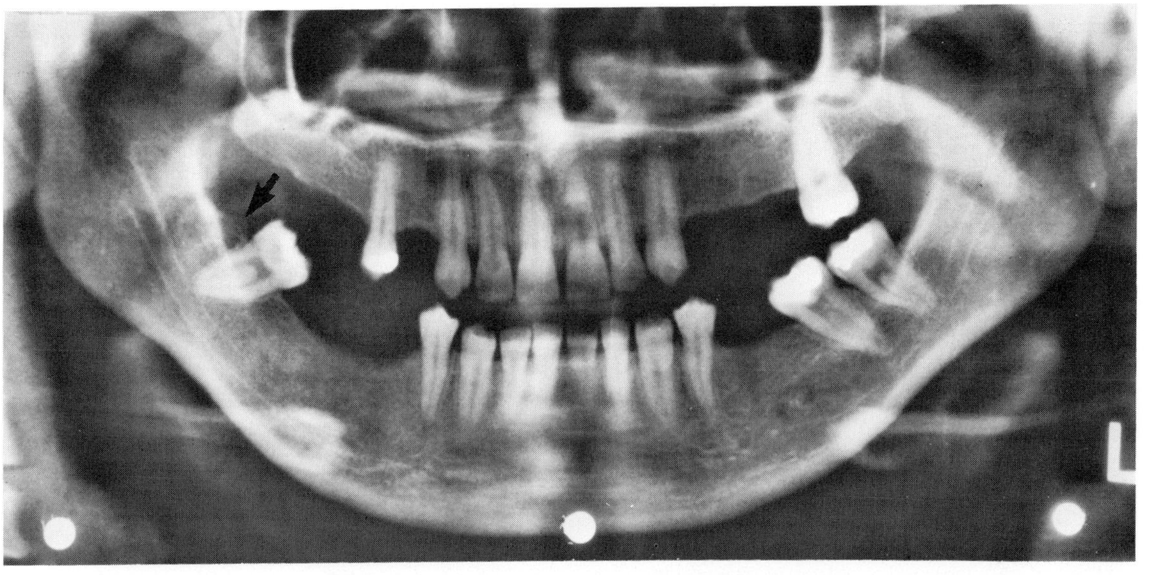

Figure 6–37. Distal mandibular pseudohyperostosis.

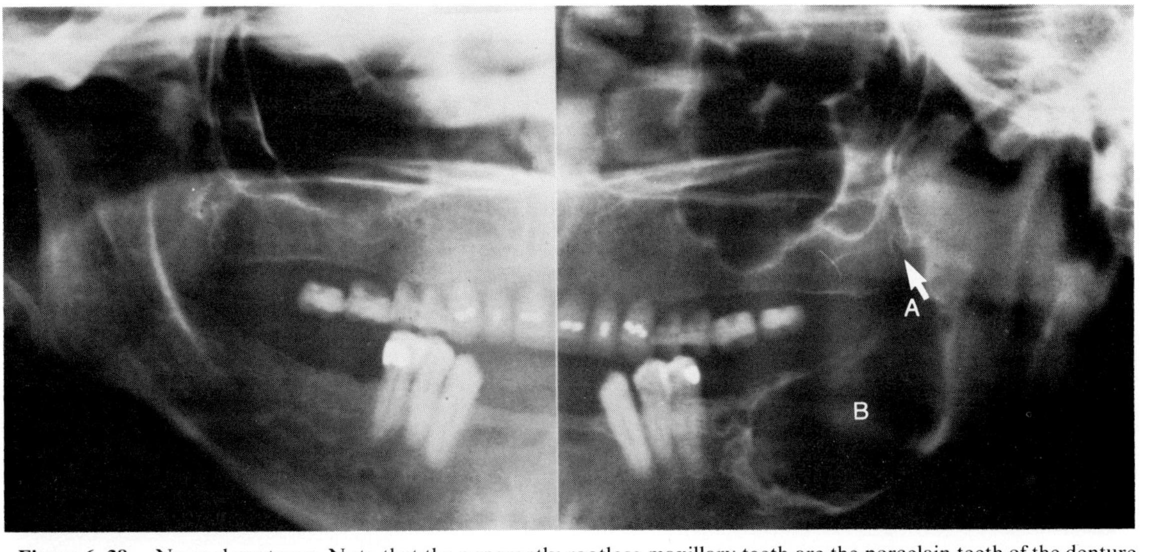

Figure 6–38. Normal anatomy. Note that the apparently rootless maxillary teeth are the porcelain teeth of the denture, which was left in during the taking of the radiograph. A. Hamular notch. B. Ameloblastoma. (Courtesy of Drs. Frank Sammis, Jr. and Carlos Portales, San Antonio, TX.)

REFERENCES

Chiles, J. L., and Gores, R. J.: Anatomic interpretation of the orthopantomogram. **Oral Surg. 35**:564, 1973.

Katayama, H., Qlba, T., and Ogawa, Y.: Panoramic innominate line and related roentgen anatomy of the facial bones. **Oral Surg. 37**:131, 1974.

Knight, N.: Anatomic structures as visualized on the panorex radiograph. **Oral Surg. 26**:326, 1968.

Knight, N.: Reverse images and ghosts of panorex radiography. **J.O.S.P.D. 3**:53, 1973.

Langlais, R. P., and Kasle, M.: **Exercises in Dental Radiology**, Vol. 1, Intra-Oral Radiographic Interpretation. Philadelphia: W. B. Saunders, 1978, pp. 82, 138.

Langland, O. E., and Sippy, F. H.: Anatomic structures as visualized on the orthopantomogram. **Oral Surg. 26**:475, 1968.

Nortjé, C. J., Farman, A. G., and Grotepass, F. W.: Variations in the normal anatomy of the inferior dental (mandibular) canal: A retrospective study of panoramic radiographs from 3,612 routine dental patients. **Br. J. Oral Surg. 15**:55, 1977.

O'Carroll, M. K.: Interpretation of panorex radiographs. **J. Oral Med. 26**:86, 1971.

Pernkopf, E.: **Atlas of Topographical and Applied Human Anatomy**, Vol. 1, Head and Neck. Philadelphia: W. B. Saunders, 1963, pp. 123–130.

Perrelet, L. A., and Garcia, L. F.: The identification of anatomical structures on orthopantomographs. **Dent.-Max.-Fac. Radiol. 1**:11, 1972.

Smith, C. J., and Fleming, R. D.: A comprehensive review of normal anatomic landmarks and artifacts as visualized on panorex radiographs. **Oral Surg. 37**:291, 1974.

Tebo, H. G.: The pterygospinous bar in panoramic roentgenography. **Oral Surg. 26**:654, 1968.

Turvey, T. A., and Fonseca, R. J.: The anatomy of the internal maxillary artery in the pterygopalatine fossa: Its relationship to maxillary surgery. **J. Oral Surg. 38**:92, 1980.

Chapter 7

Developmental and Acquired Defects of the Teeth and Jaws

ALTERATIONS IN TOOTH MORPHOLOGY

MICRODONTIA AND MACRODONTIA

BRIEF OVERVIEW

Although these conditions may affect all of the teeth, usually only one or several teeth are involved. Microdontia is much more common than macrodontia, and the most common microdontic teeth are the maxillary permanent lateral incisors, often referred to as peg laterals, followed by the third molars. Paramolars are supernumerary molars (fourth molars) that sometimes erupt buccal or palatal to the molars, usually the maxillary molars. Distomolars or retromolars are supernumerary molars that develop distal to the third molars, usually in the maxilla. Peg lateral incisors are often bilateral and are familial in occurrence. In the clinical experience of the authors, an idiopathic generalized shortening and/or tapering of the roots of any or all of the teeth has been noted among Mexican Americans, the lower bicuspids being the most commonly affected. The crowns are normal except that there are prominent marginal ridges in the maxillary central and lateral incisors, often referred to as shovel-shaped incisors. This combination of findings has been loosely named the shovel-shaped incisor syndrome.

RADIOGRAPHIC FEATURES (Figs. 7–1 to 7–6)

As the names imply, an alteration in size is noted in one tooth or several teeth. When macro- or microdontia affects one tooth or a few teeth, the condition is generally considered

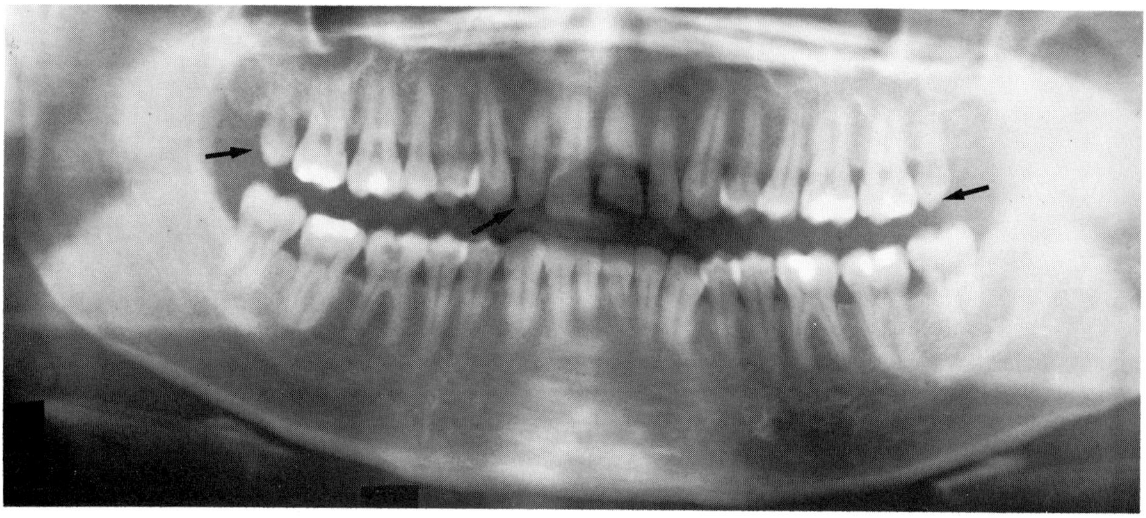

Figure 7–1. Microdontia. Peg lateral incisor and bilateral microdontic third molars. (Courtesy of Dr. Birgit Junfin Glass, San Antonio, TX.)

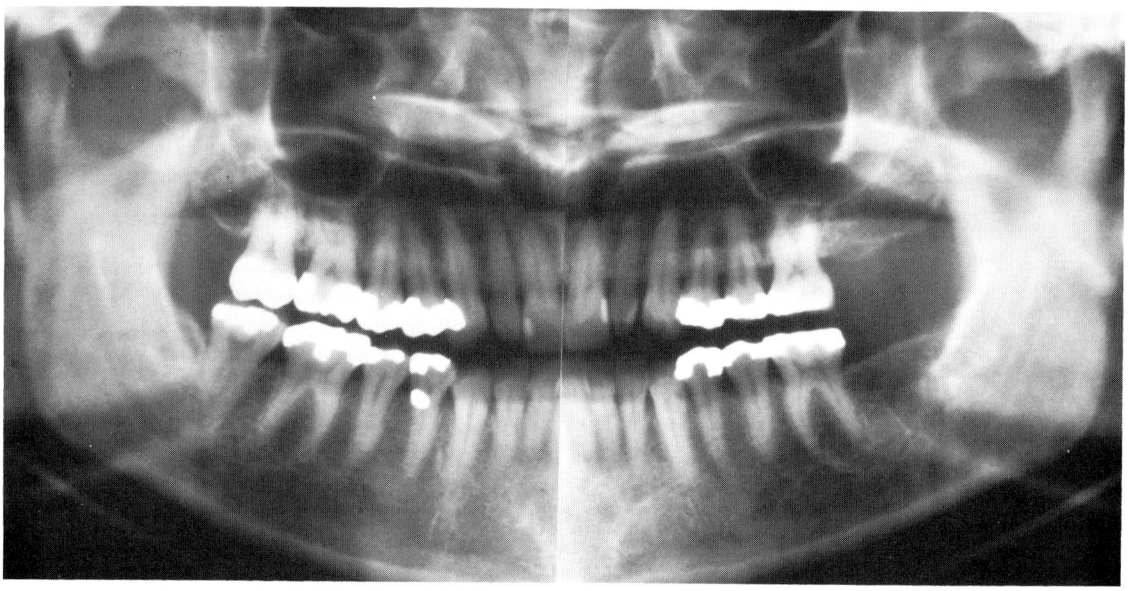

Figure 7–2. Microdontia. Bilateral peg lateral incisors. (Courtesy of Dr. Birgit Junfin Glass, San Antonio, TX.)

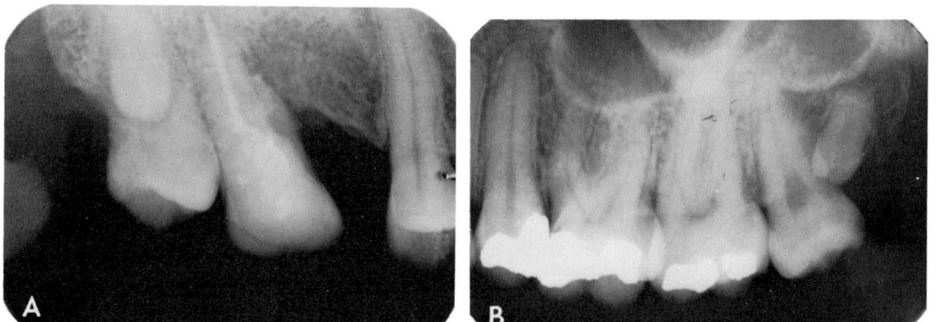

Figure 7–3. **A.** Paramolar. **B.** Distomolar.

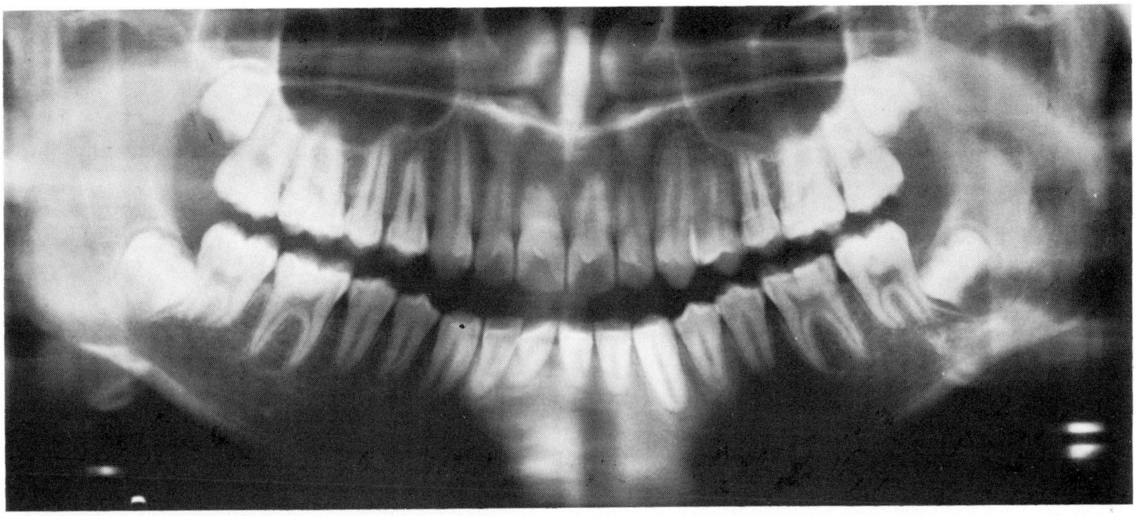

Figure 7–4. Microdontia. Many small teeth and shovel-shaped incisors in a Mexican American. (Courtesy of Dr. Jack Hartley, San Antonio, TX.)

to be of no clinical significance, and treatment would only be an esthetic or restorative consideration. When the condition is generalized, however, there may be some significant underlying systemic or developmental disorder such as pituitary dwarfism or giantism.

When the shovel-shaped incisor syndrome is suspected, the clinician should look for the following abnormalities in the maxillary incisors: interproximal caries, lingual pit caries, and periapical lesions of pulpal origin. Additionally, the presence of shortened or tapered roots is of significance in planning treatment. Also, generalized shortening of the roots must be distinguished from dentinal dysplasia and orthodontic root resorption.

GEMINATION (Schizodontism)

BRIEF OVERVIEW

Gemination is an aborted attempt by a single tooth bud to divide. Clinically, the crown may be widened, notched, or grooved. Gemination is more common in the primary teeth than in the

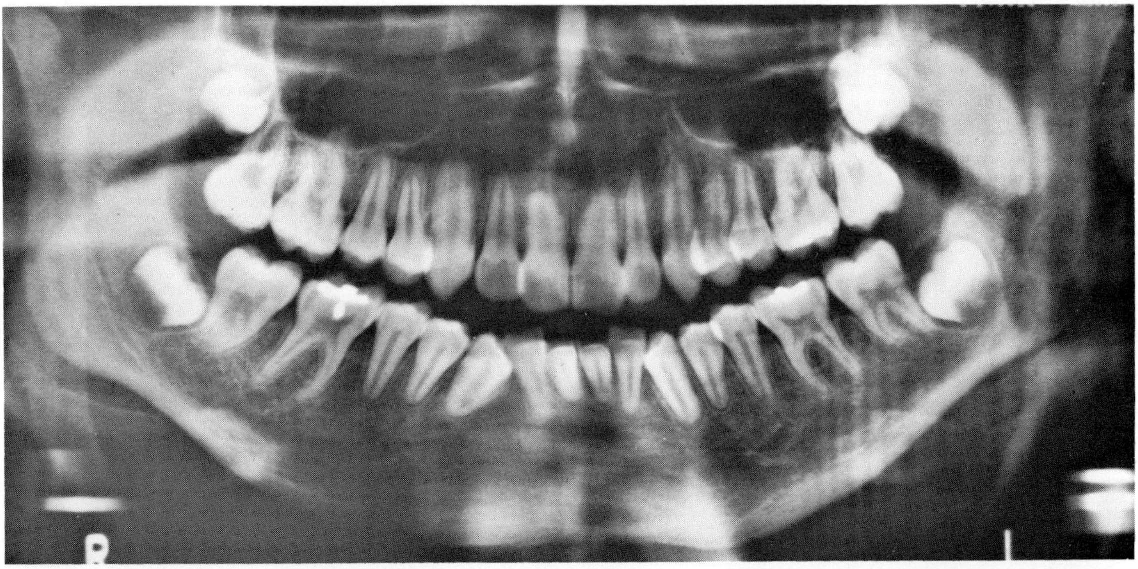

Figure 7–5. Microdontia. Multiple shortened roots and shovel-shaped incisors in a Mexican American. (Courtesy of Dr. Jack Hartley, San Antonio, TX.)

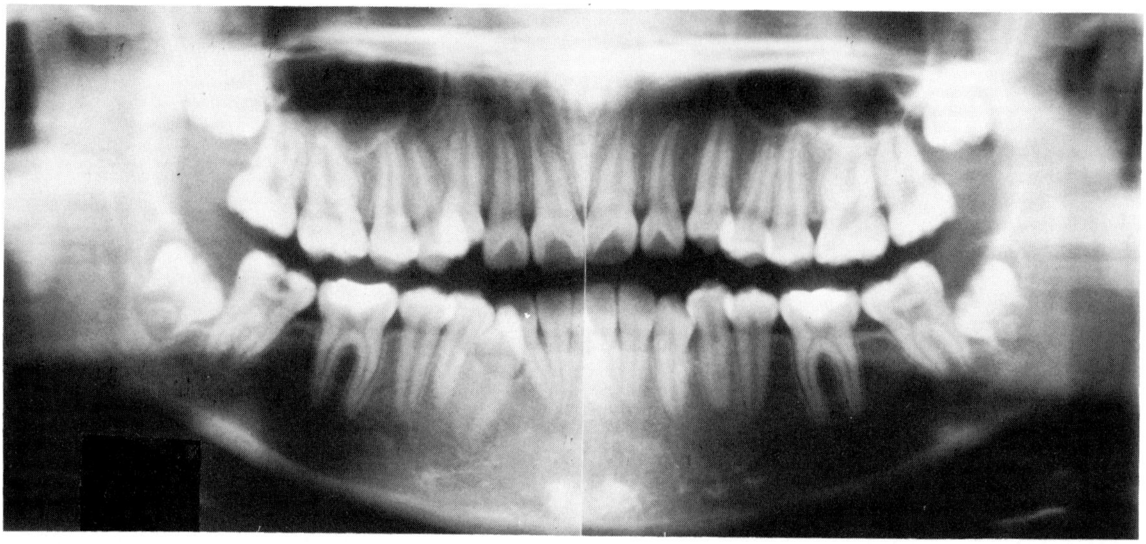

Figure 7–6. Shovel-shaped incisor syndrome of Hartley. Note the prominent marginal ridges on the maxillary anterior teeth and the slightly shortened, tapered, or blunted roots of the bicuspids in this 13-year-old Mexican American. (Courtesy of Dr. Jack Hartley, San Antonio, TX.)

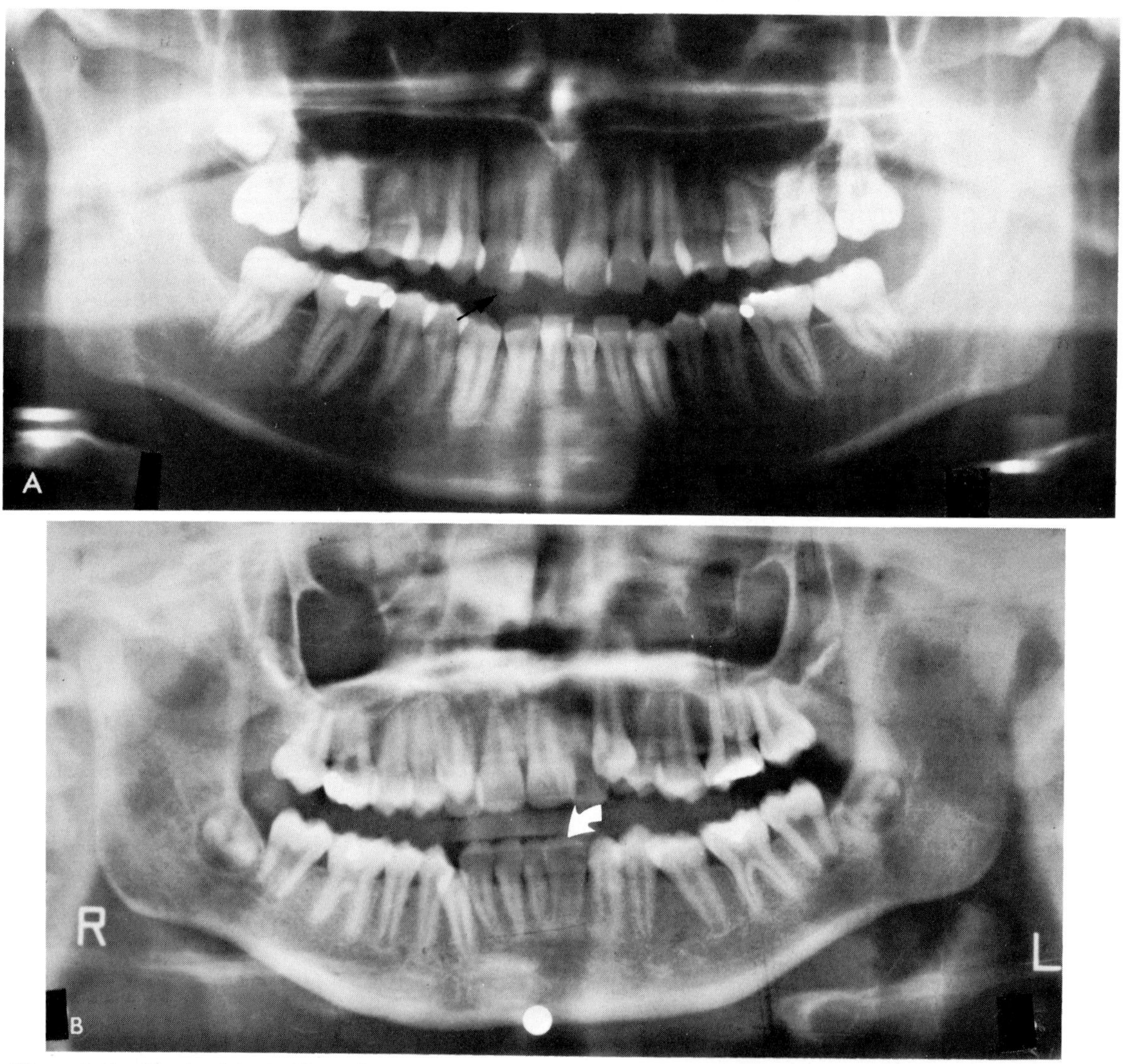

Figure 7–7. Gemination. **A.** Note the enlarged, notched crown (arrow). (Courtesy of Dr. Birgit Jungin Glass, San Antonio, TX.) Gemination. **B.** Note the enlarged crown (arrow), single pulp chambers, and two root canal spaces.

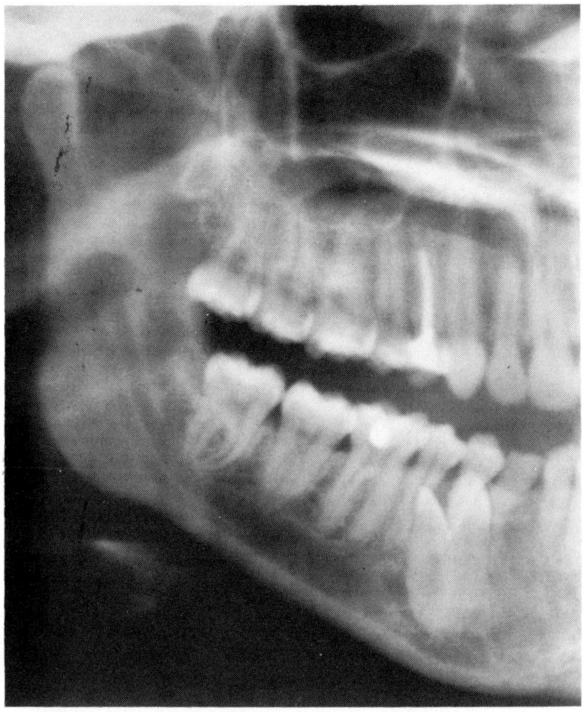

Figure 7–8. Fusion. Note the fusion between the permanent cuspid and what appears to be a supernumerary incisor.

permanent dentition, and in both cases the incisor canine region is the most common location.

RADIOGRAPHIC FEATURES (Fig. 7–7)

The panoramic radiographs are especially helpful here. To distinguish gemination from fusion, a normal complement of teeth must be established, confirmed by an accurate history. Often an enlarged notched crown with two pulp chambers and a single root and pulp canal is noted.

FUSION (Synodontism)

BRIEF OVERVIEW

Fusion is the union of two separate tooth buds, usually by dentin and enamel and rarely by enamel only. The fusion may be between two normal tooth buds or between a normal tooth bud and a supernumerary tooth bud. It is often impossible to distinguish the latter situation from gemination. Fusion of the primary teeth may be followed by hypodontia of the permanent teeth. Fusion is more common in the primary dentition, and the most common location is the incisor region.

RADIOGRAPHIC FEATURES (Fig. 7–8)

It is important to count the teeth. If one tooth appears to be missing, fusion may be suspected. Usually the anomalous tooth will look like two teeth stuck together, and often the dentin is confluent. The diagnosis is easier when there are two separate pulp chambers and root canals. A single, confluent pulp chamber and root canal in an oversized tooth may also be seen.

DILACERATION

BRIEF OVERVIEW

Dilaceration refers to a curved or bent tooth. It may involve the crown or, more frequently, the root. It is usually caused by trauma.

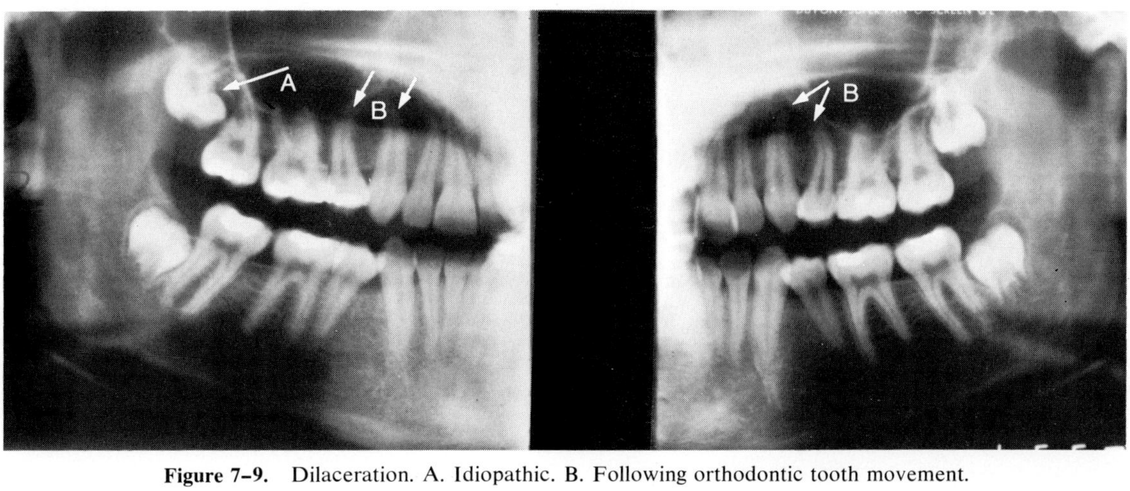

Figure 7–9. Dilaceration. A. Idiopathic. B. Following orthodontic tooth movement.

RADIOGRAPHIC FEATURES (Fig. 7–9)

Dilacerated teeth should always be noted radiographically. Both erupted and unerupted dilacerated teeth may present problems in removal or orthodontic difficulties. Unerupted dilacerated teeth may indicate the sight of previous surgery, may erupt ectopically, or may not erupt at all.

TAURODONTISM

BRIEF OVERVIEW

This is a term given to a tooth morphology in which the pulp chambers are abnormally large, with reduced roots. The word taurodontism means bull-like tooth. The animal has a disproportionately large body and relatively short but powerful legs, hence the name for these large teeth. The finding of taurodontism is usually of no significance. It has been shown to be associated with tricho-dento-osseous and Felty's syndromes.

RADIOGRAPHIC FEATURES (Fig. 7–10)

In the experience of the authors, the condition often involves a molar. The crown is of normal size, but the pulp chamber appears to be much larger than normal, and the portion of the roots beyond the furcation is much shorter than normal. The overall length of the tooth is normal. The shape of the enlarged pulp chamber is usually rectangular, with a flat, boxlike floor, which does not tend to taper at the beginning of the root canal space.

SUPERNUMERARY ROOTS

BRIEF OVERVIEW

Supernumerary roots may occur on any tooth, particularly the mandibular cuspids and bicuspids. Their detection is of significance in endodontics, oral surgery, orthodontics, and crown and bridge procedures.

RADIOGRAPHIC FEATURES (Figs. 7–11 and 7–12)

When supernumerary roots are not superimposed on other roots, they are easier to detect. An extra root canal or double periodontal membrane space may be a clue. When supernumerary roots are suspected, an off-angle periapical film may be helpful. Supernumerary roots

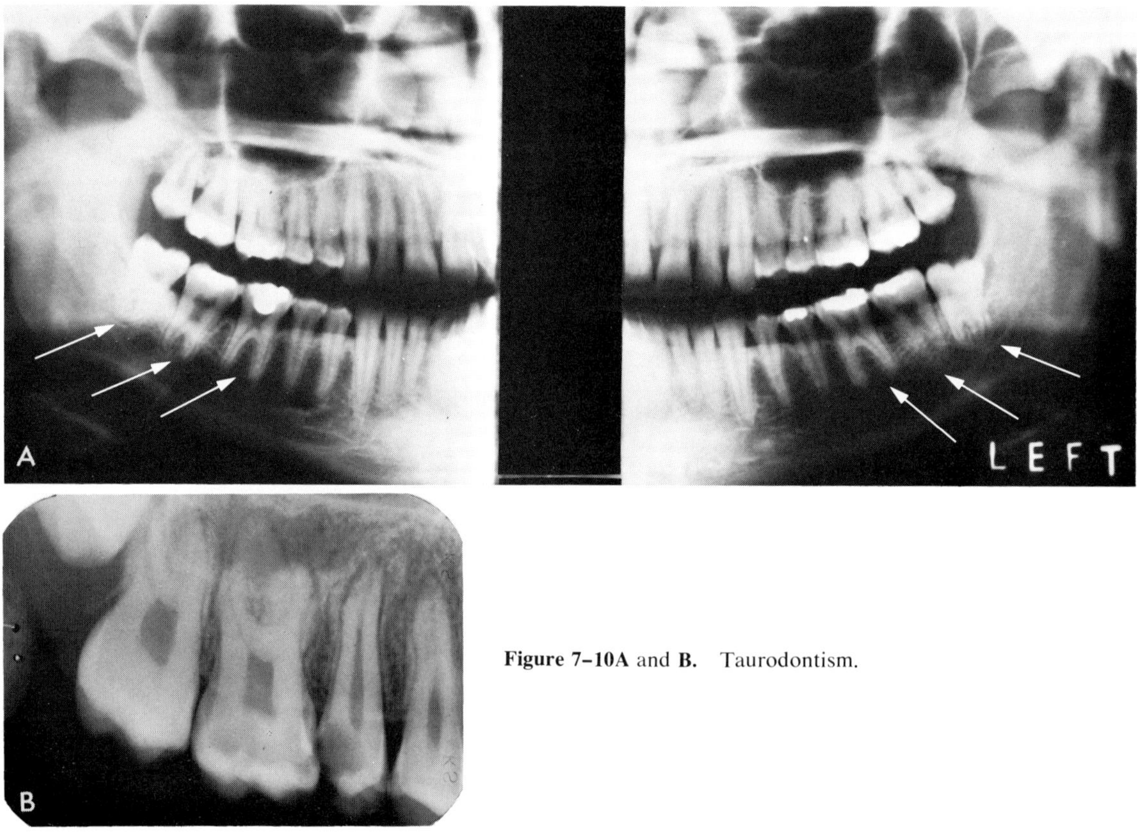

Figure 7–10A and **B.** Taurodontism.

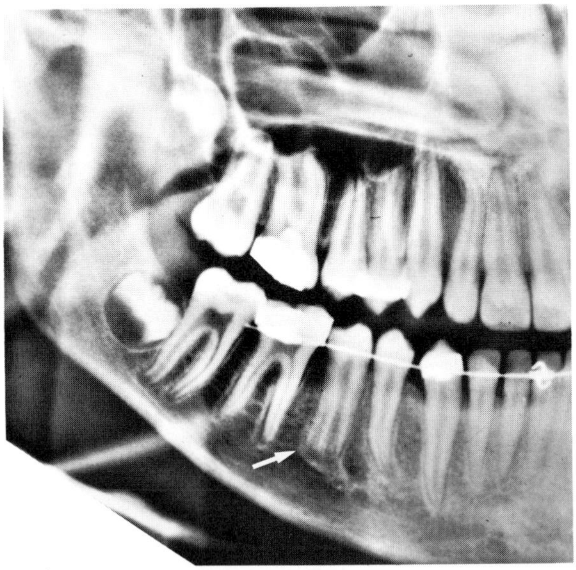

Figure 7–11. Developing supernumerary root.

may be suspected when there is a sudden diminution in the size of the root canal space or when it appears to divide into several smaller root canal spaces (see Fig. 7–12**B**).

ENAMEL PEARL (Enameloma)

BRIEF OVERVIEW

The enamel pearl is usually a round or ovoid droplet of enamel at the furcation of the maxillary and mandibular molars. An enameloma at an interproximal location, especially on the upper molars, can interfere with scaling, root planing, and flossing; at a buccal location, especially on the lower molars, it can interfere with furcal hygiene. When excessive vertical angulation is used on the periapical film, the enamel pearl may be superimposed on the pulp chamber and may be mistaken for a pulp stone.

Lesions detected on panoramic films and those located on teeth to be treated endodontically should be further examined preoperatively with the following intraoral views: a bitewing view, a straight-on standard periapical view, and an off-angle periapical view. In differentiations between an enamel pearl and a pulp stone, the enamel pearl will probably move out of the pulp chamber in the bitewing view, whereas the pulp stone or denticle will remain within the pulp chamber in all views.

RADIOGRAPHIC FEATURES (Figs. 7–13 and 7–14)

Enamel pearls can usually be identified by their smooth, generally round outline. In contrast to the dentin and cementum in the furcation area, the enamel pearl stands out with a radiodensity comparable to other enamel structures such as cusp tips. The condition may be bilateral and may involve all the molars of a quadrant.

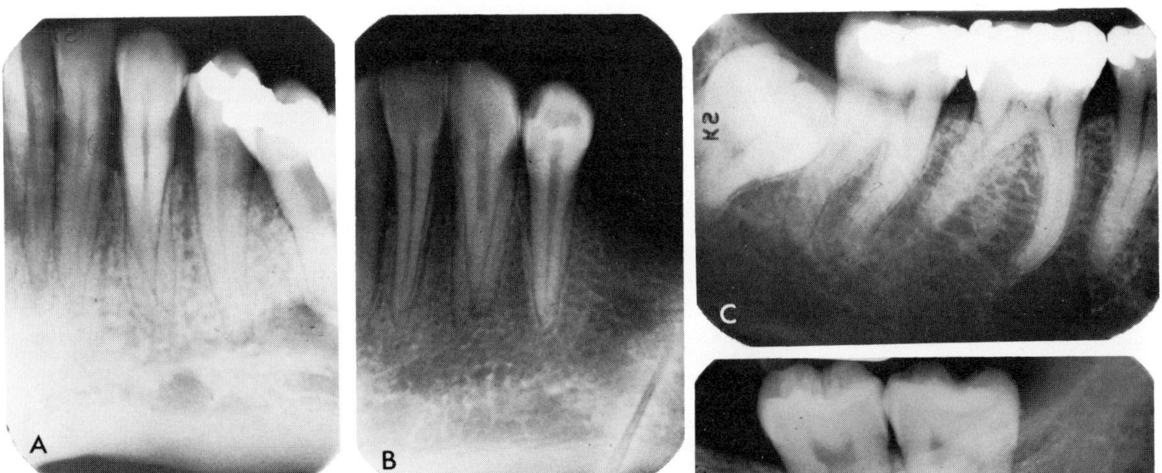

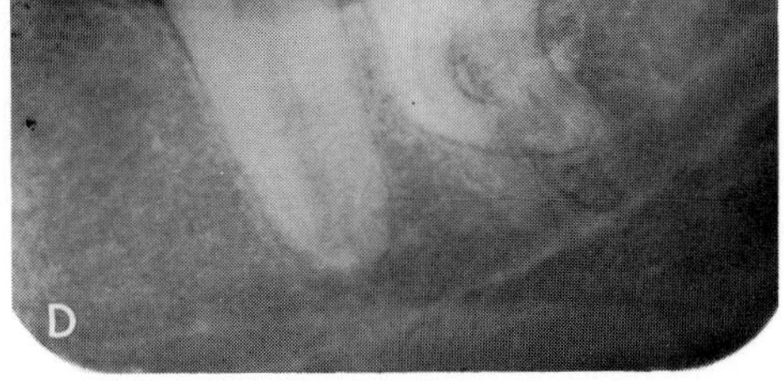

Figure 7–12A, B, C, and **D.** Supernumerary roots.

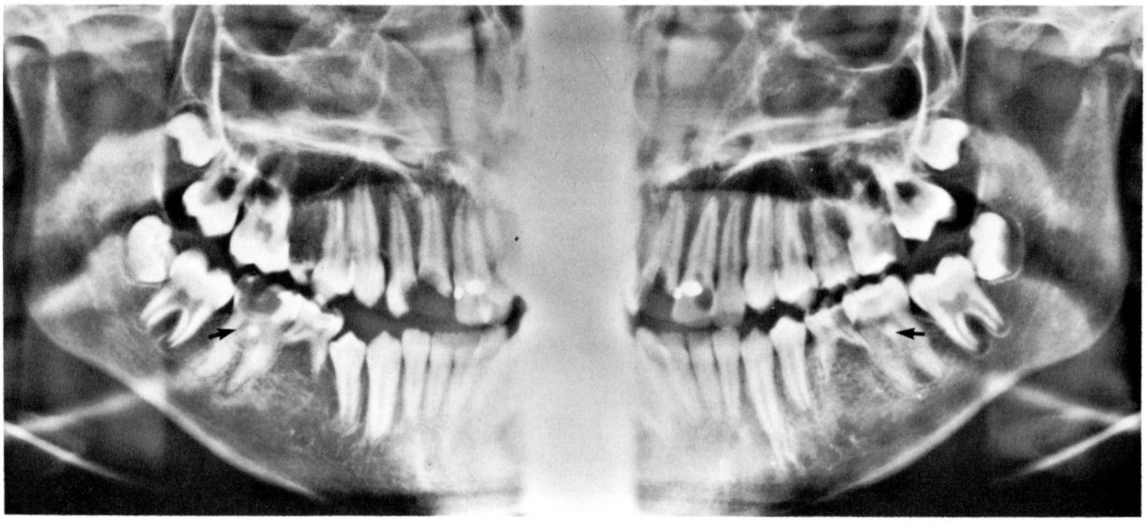

Figure 7–13. Bilateral enamel pearls.

DENS INVAGINATUS (Dens in Dente)

BRIEF OVERVIEW

Dens invaginatus is an invagination or ingrowth of coronal enamel and dentin into the pulp chamber of the tooth. The tooth most commonly involved is the maxillary lateral incisor, and the condition may be bilateral. Dens in dente is rare in mandibular and primary teeth. When recognized, the tooth should be pulp tested and, if vital, prophylactically restored. Since the enamel invagination into the pulp is thin, early pulpal involvement often occurs as a result of minimal carious activity. Preparation should be extremely conservative in prophylactic restoration, as accidental mechanical pulp exposure can occur as a result of perforation of the thin enamel and dentin. Endodontic treatment of these teeth may be difficult.

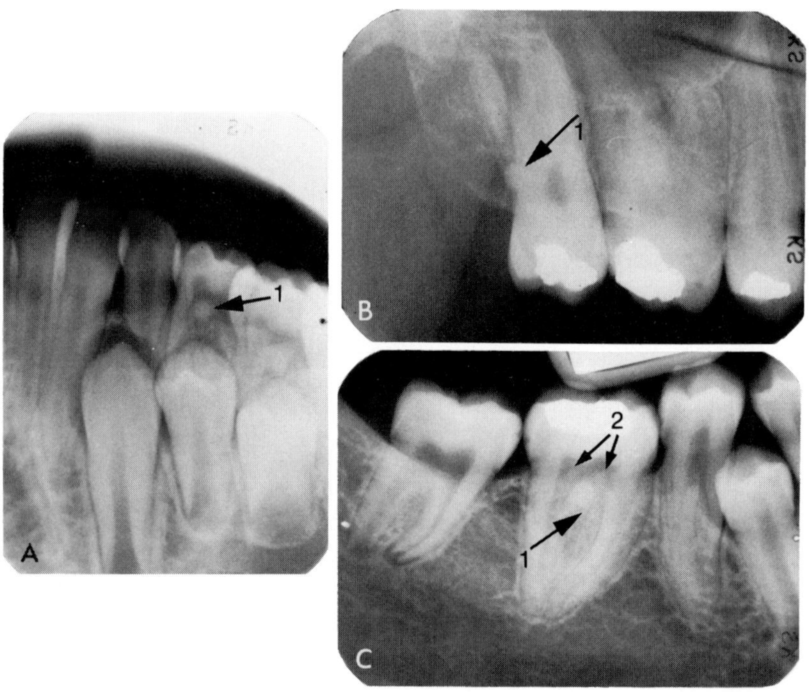

Figure 7–14A, B, and **C.** Enamel pearls. 1. Enamel pearl. 2. Pulp stones.

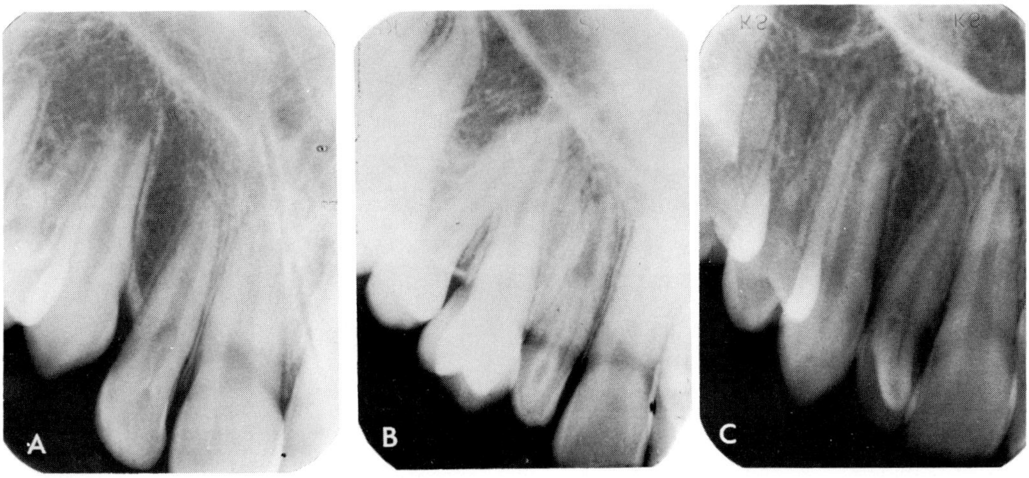

Figure 7–15A, B, and **C.** Dens in dente.

RADIOGRAPHIC FEATURES (Fig. 7–15)

A teardrop- or hourglass-shaped distinct radiopaque line can be seen within the pulp chamber of the involved tooth. Close examination will show a minute opening into the lingual cingulum area, and further examination may show a break or discontinuity in the apical portion of the invaginated enamel. The latter will usually be associated with a periapical radiolucency of pulpal origin and may be completely asymptomatic. In its minimal presentation, dens invaginatus may be difficult to visualize on panoramic radiographs.

DENS EVAGINATUS (Leong's Premolar)

BRIEF OVERVIEW

Dens evaginatus is an evagination or outgrowth of enamel, dentin, and pulp that forms a tubercle on the occlusal surface of the mandibular premolars in persons of Mongoloid extraction. A pinpoint pulp exposure may occur with attrition. Mechanical exposure of the pulp during operative procedures is a possibility.

RADIOGRAPHIC FEATURES

In dens evaginatus, a tubercle on the occlusal surface of a mandibular premolar may be quite evident (Fig. 7–16**A** and **B**).

ALTERATIONS IN NUMBERS OF TEETH

ANODONTIA AND HYPODONTIA (Oligodontia)

BRIEF OVERVIEW

Anodontia means no teeth; this condition is a rare occurrence. It is sometimes seen in hereditary anhidrotic ectodermal dysplasia. Idiopathic hypodontia is much more common and refers

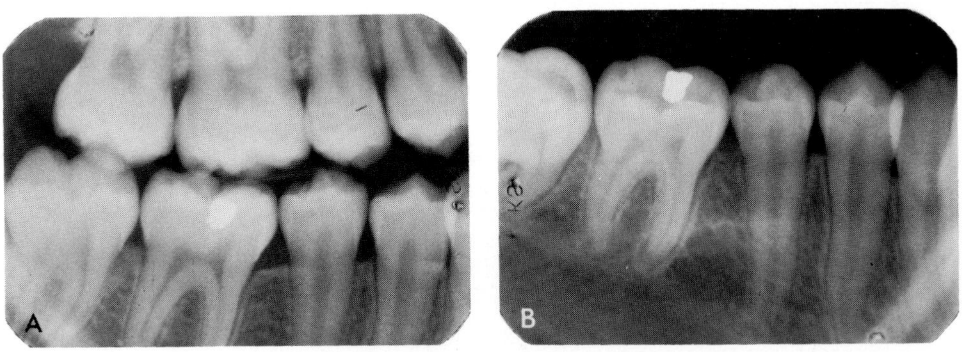

Figure 7–16A and **B.** Dens evaginatus.

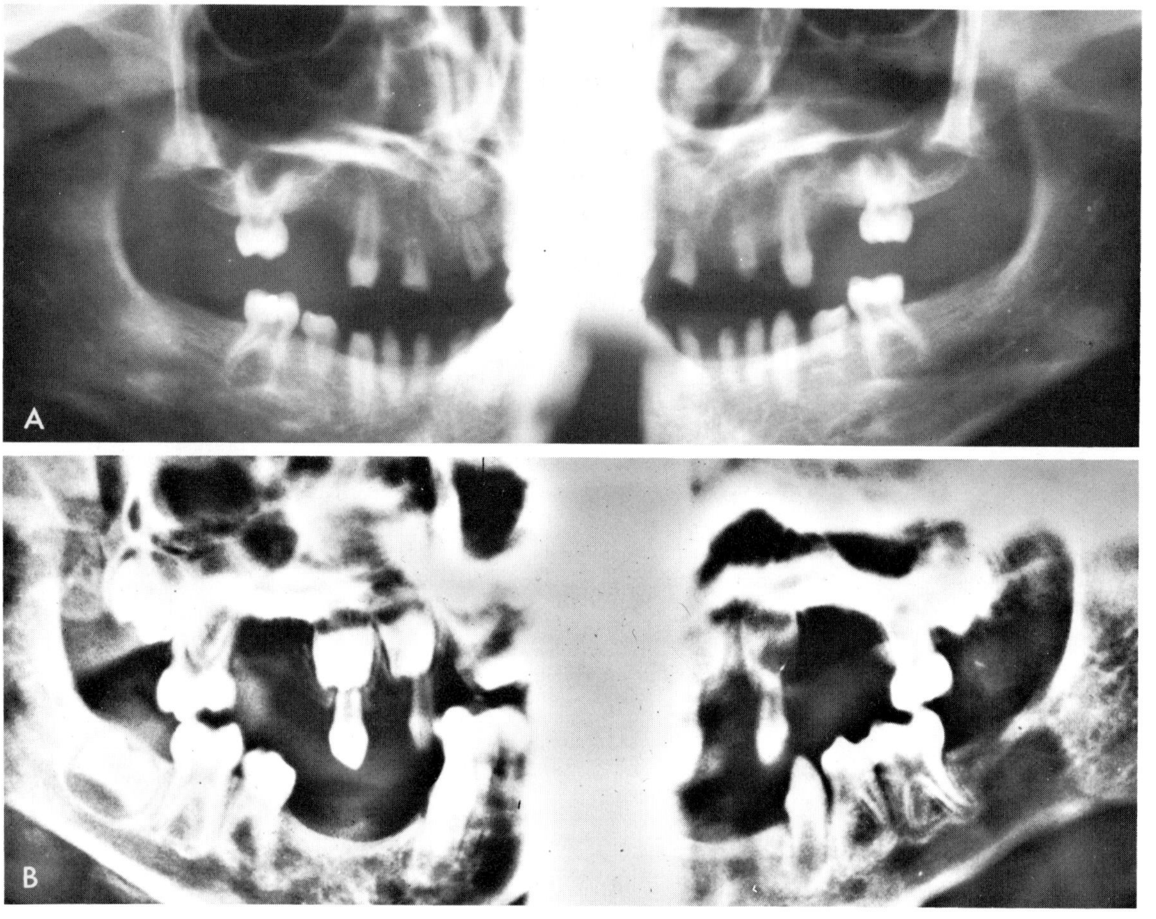

Figure 7–17. Hereditary anhidrotic ectodermal dysplasia. **A.** Note the anodontia of the permanent dentition. **B.** Hypodontia of many permanent teeth and hypoplastic conical tooth forms of many existing teeth.

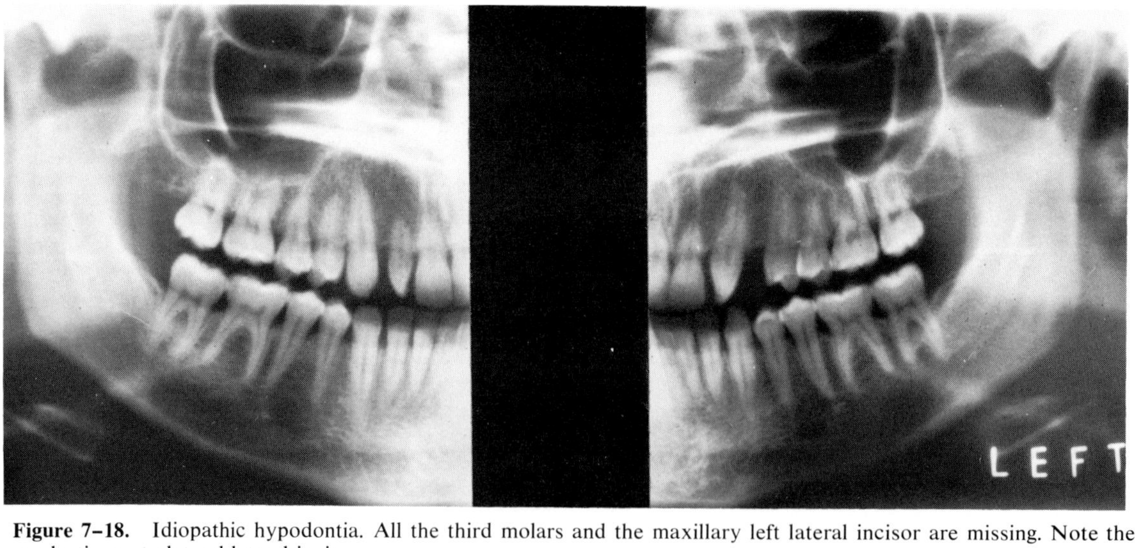

Figure 7–18. Idiopathic hypodontia. All the third molars and the maxillary left lateral incisor are missing. Note the hypoplastic contralateral lateral incisor.

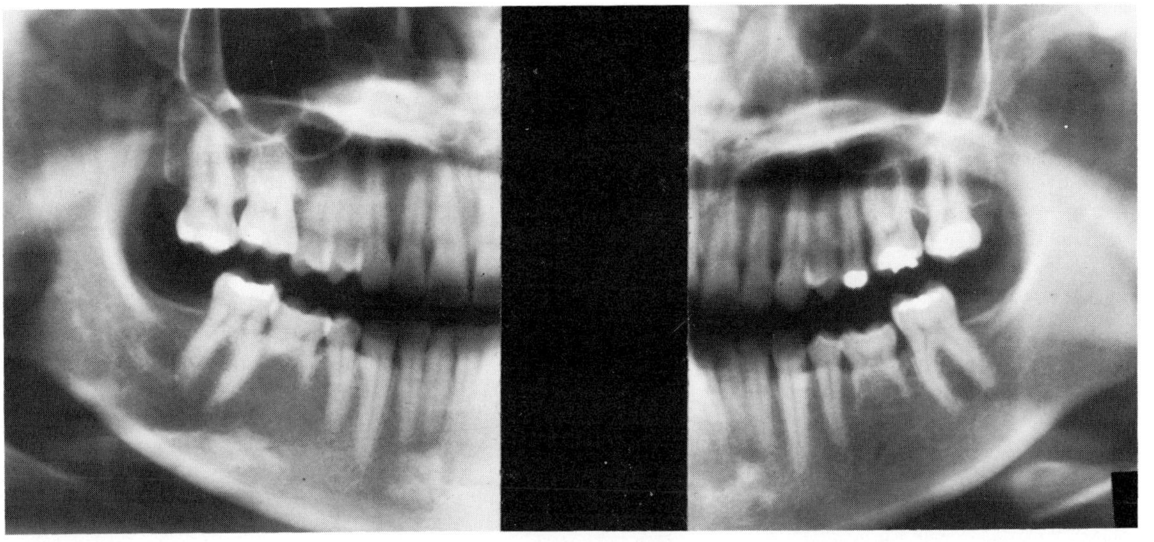

Figure 7–19. Idiopathic hypodontia. The mandibular second bicuspids, second molars, and all third molars are missing.

to one or several missing teeth. The most common congenitally missing teeth are the third molars, followed by the mandibular second bicuspids, maxillary second bicuspids, and maxillary lateral incisors. The condition may be bilateral when these teeth are missing. A sequela of congenitally missing second premolars is the ankylosed, submerged, second primary molar. If this condition is present, the submerged tooth makes the involved arch more susceptible to periodontal disease owing to its altered interproximal contact. Additionally, its antagonist, especially in the case of a maxillary second bicuspid, may extrude and is also more susceptible to periodontal disease because of its altered interproximal contact.

Hypodontia is associated with the following conditions: hereditary anhydrotic ectodermal dysplasia, incontinentia pigmenti, and chondroectodermal dysplasia. Rieger's syndrome should be suspected in any case of hypodontia, particularly when the permanent maxillary central and lateral incisors are missing. This syndrome is associated with congenital glaucoma, which may produce blindness by age 6 or 8.

RADIOGRAPHIC FEATURES (Figs. 7–17 to 7–20)

Panoramic radiographs are particularly useful in evaluating the number of missing teeth and the collapse of the arches, which may occur as a consequence.

The dental findings of hereditary anhidrotic ectodermal dysplasia, incontinentia pigmenti, and chondroectodermal dysplasia are radiographically identical and consist of hypodontia and a mixture of normal and conical tooth shapes. The teeth also show delayed eruption in incontinentia pigmenti and chondroectodermal dysplasia. Incontinentia pigmenti is seen only in females, as it is lethal in males.

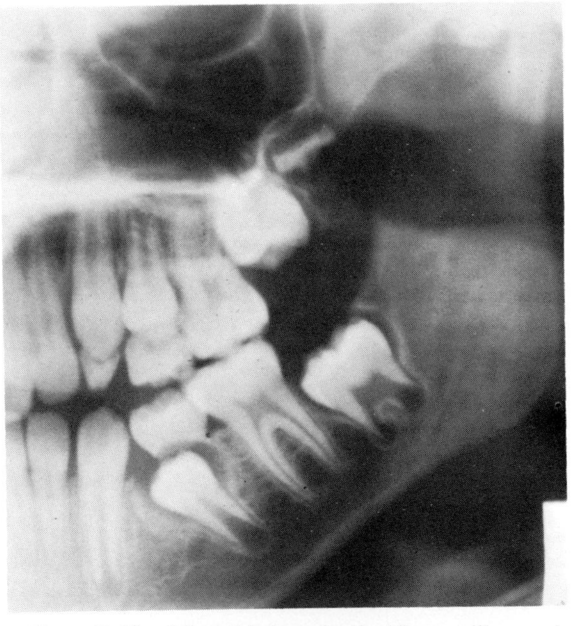

Figure 7–20. Idiopathic hypodontia. The maxillary and mandibular second premolars are missing.

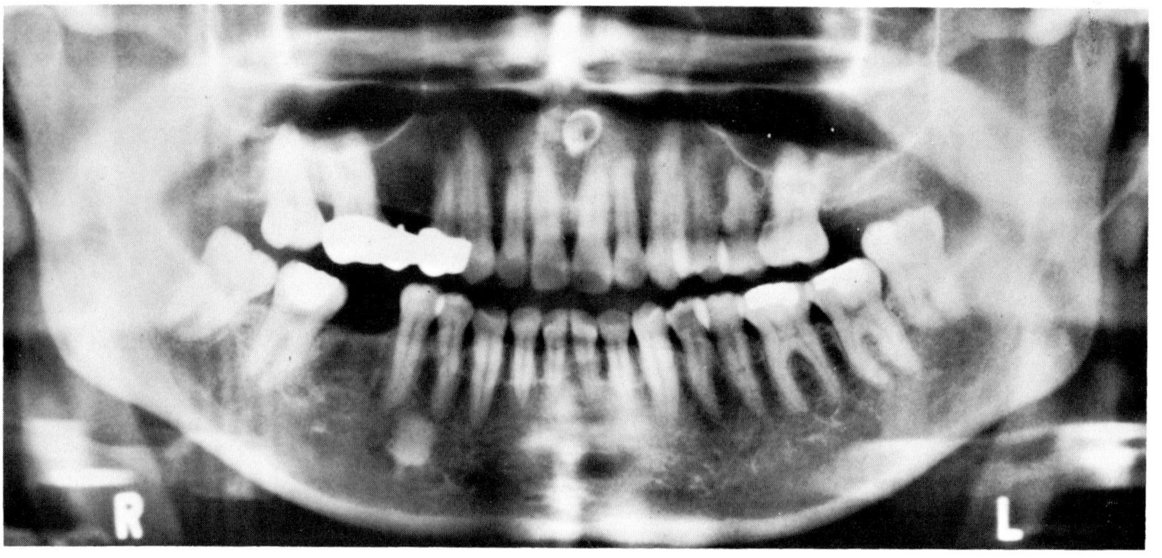

Figure 7–21. Hyperdontia. This mesiodens greatly resembles a phlebolith owing to its round shape and radiolucent center. (Courtesy of Dr. Steven Bricker, San Antonio, TX.)

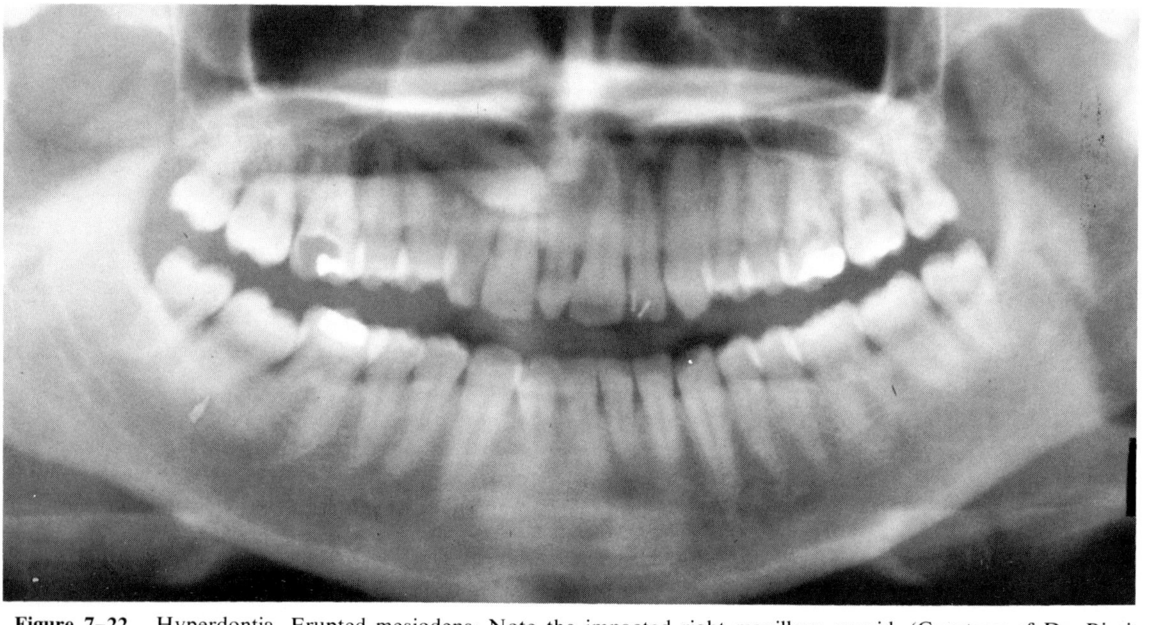

Figure 7–22. Hyperdontia. Erupted mesiodens. Note the impacted right maxillary cuspid. (Courtesy of Dr. Birgit Junfin Glass, San Antonio, TX.)

HYPERDONTIA (Supernumerary Teeth)

BRIEF OVERVIEW

Idiopathic hyperdontia is a fairly common condition and consists of one or more supernumerary teeth. The most common supernumerary tooth is the maxillary mesiodens, followed by maxillary fourth molars, maxillary fourth paramolars, and mandibular premolars. Supernumerary teeth in extreme lingual or buccal version may be outside the focal trough in panoramic radiography and may sometimes not be visualized on the radiograph. Supernumerary teeth may also be seen in cleidocranial dysplasia and Gardner's syndrome.

RADIOGRAPHIC FEATURES (Figs. 7–21 to 7–26)

Supernumerary teeth are easily detected in the absence of superimposition of other structures. The paramolar is often difficult to detect because it may be superimposed on the molars and may resemble an odontoma or gemination.

Cleidocranial Dysplasia (Fig. 7–27). The following features may be seen in cleidocranial dysplasia: prolonged retention of the primary teeth, multiple unerupted supernumerary teeth, and delayed eruption of the permanent teeth. The maxillary sinus is often small. Other features include frontal bossing, hypertelorism, high arched palate, and deficient or missing clavicles that allow the patient's shoulders to be brought together (cleidocranial dysostosis).

Gardner's Syndrome (Fig. 7–28). The following features may be seen in this syndrome: retention of several primary teeth, with delayed eruption of their permanent successors; multiple unerupted supernumerary teeth and odontomas; and osteomas of the jaws, sinuses and facial bones. The osteomas in the jaws may be distinct, well-delineated radiopaque lesions or they may be diffuse sclerotic masses that appear to affect the entire jaw. Other features of Gardner's syndrome include multiple skin lesions consisting of epidermoid and sebaceous cysts and fibrous (desmoid) tumors. The most significant feature is a tendency to develop polyps in the colon and rectum, which usually undergo malignant transformation. Since this is a hereditary disorder, siblings and other family members should be investigated and should receive genetic counseling.

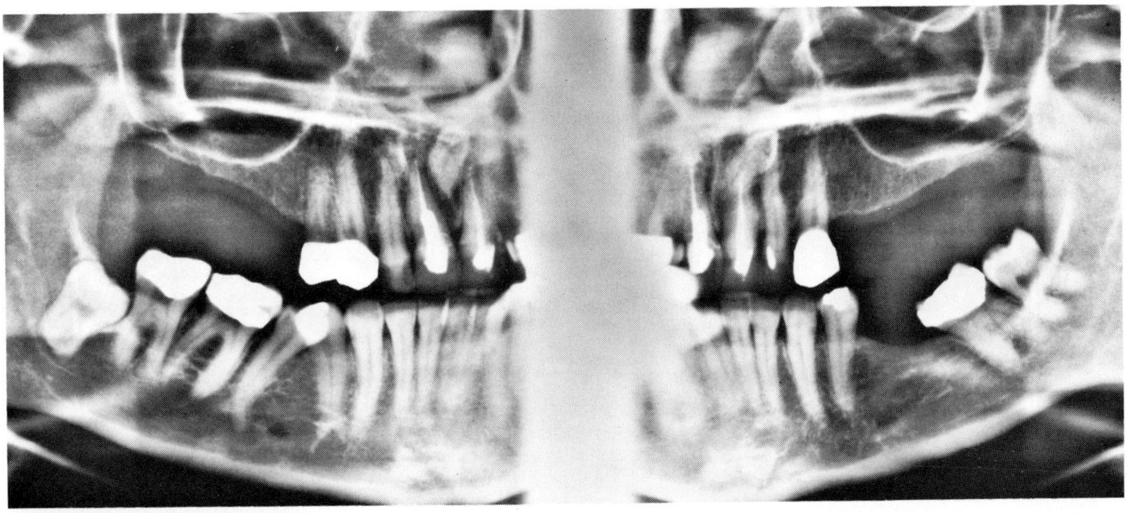

Figure 7–23. Hyperdontia. This mesiodens can be located to the palatal side in the following manner. The left-hand image (patient's right) moves further to the right in the right-hand image (patient's left). The mesiodens moves in the same direction as the observer's eye. As the SLOB rule states, "same on lingual, opposite on buccal." Therefore, this mesiodens is located on the lingual or palatal side, and no further films are necessary to localize it. Localization of some anterior objects is possible only with the split–image type machine.

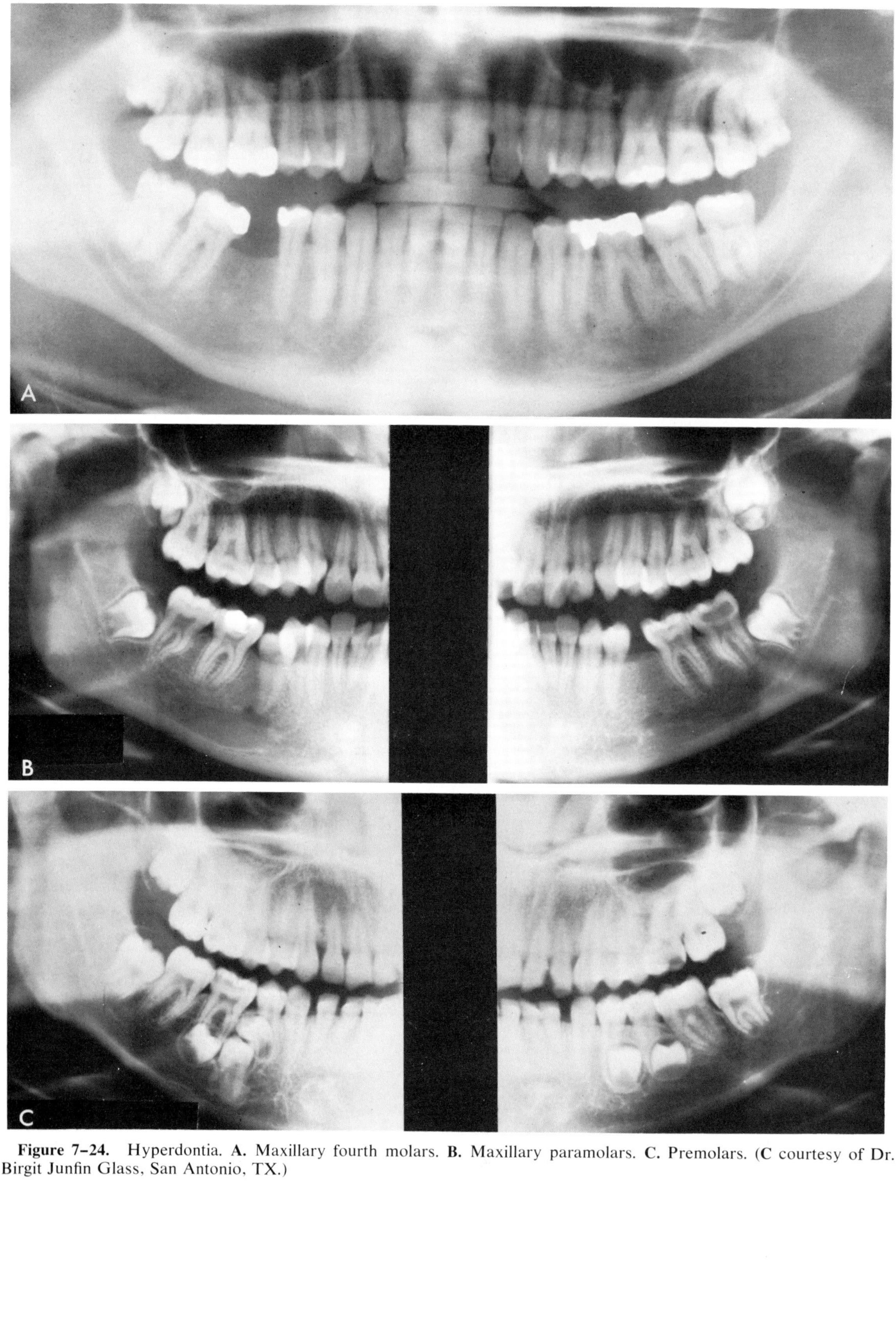

Figure 7–24. Hyperdontia. **A.** Maxillary fourth molars. **B.** Maxillary paramolars. **C.** Premolars. (C courtesy of Dr. Birgit Junfin Glass, San Antonio, TX.)

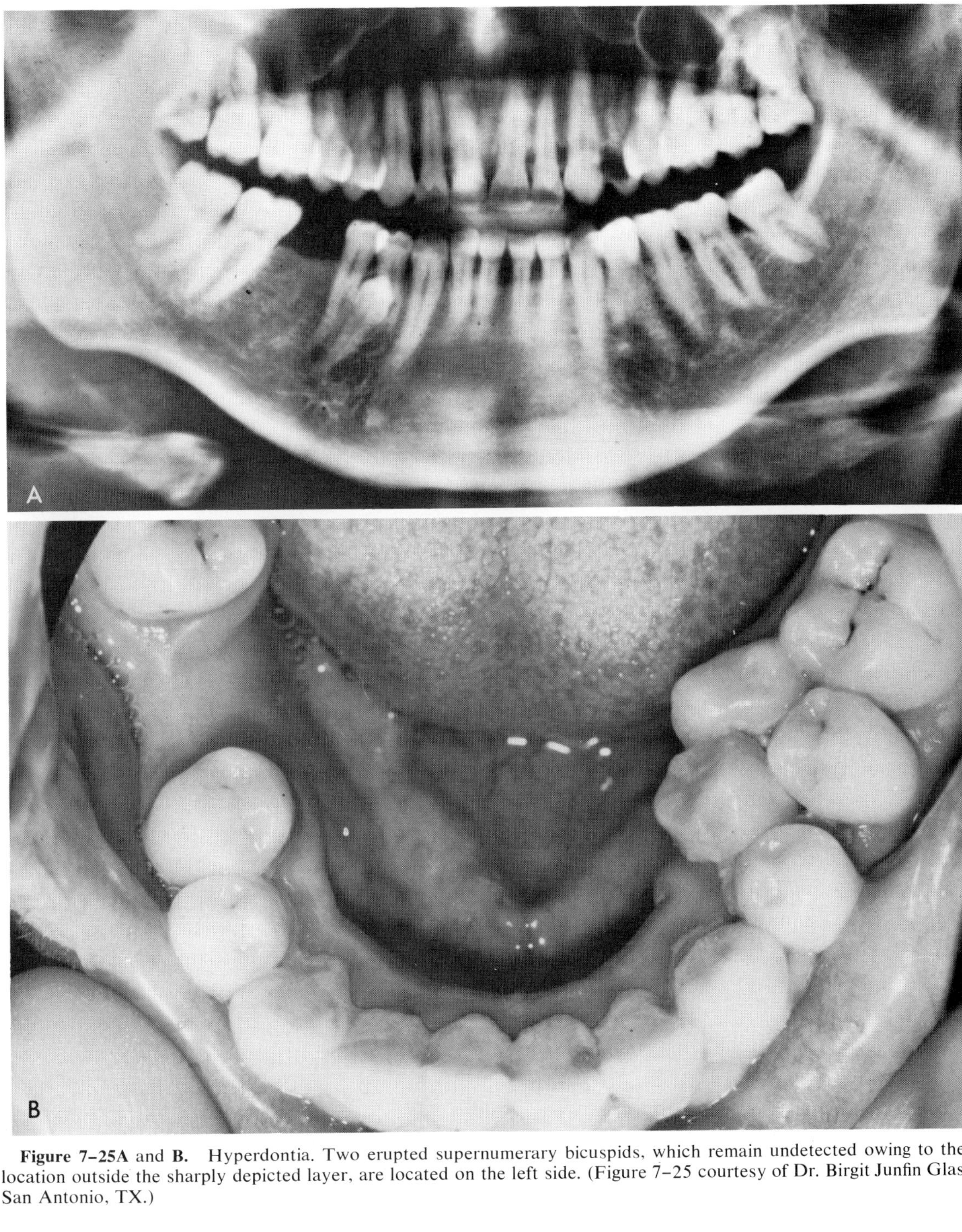

Figure 7–25A and **B.** Hyperdontia. Two erupted supernumerary bicuspids, which remain undetected owing to their location outside the sharply depicted layer, are located on the left side. (Figure 7–25 courtesy of Dr. Birgit Junfin Glass, San Antonio, TX.)

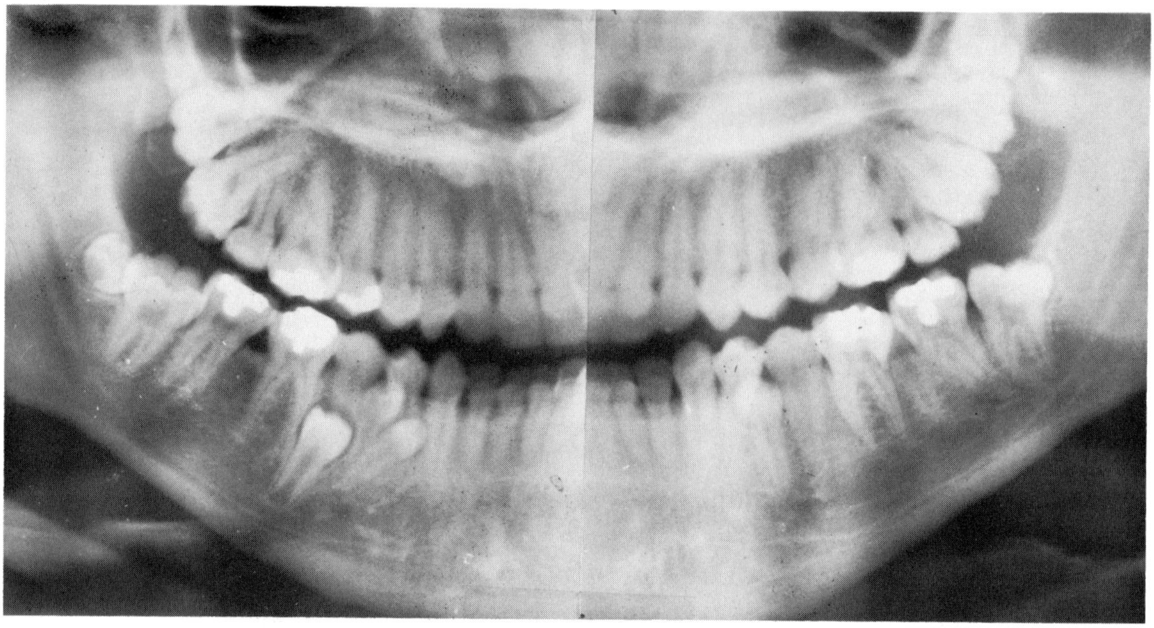

Figure 7–26. Multiple idiopathic hyperdontia.

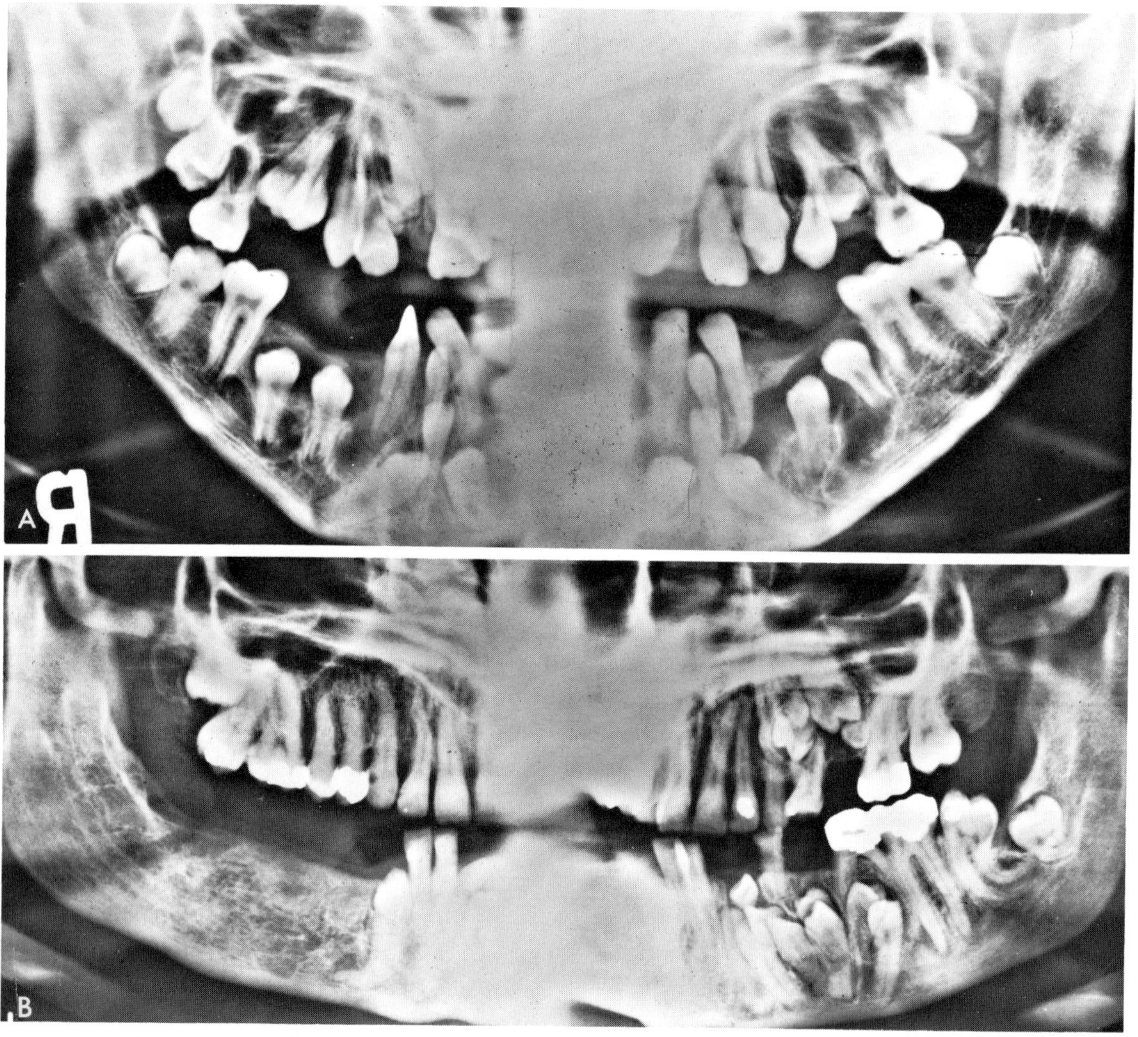

Figure 7–27A and **B.** Hyperdontia. Cleidocranial dysplasia.

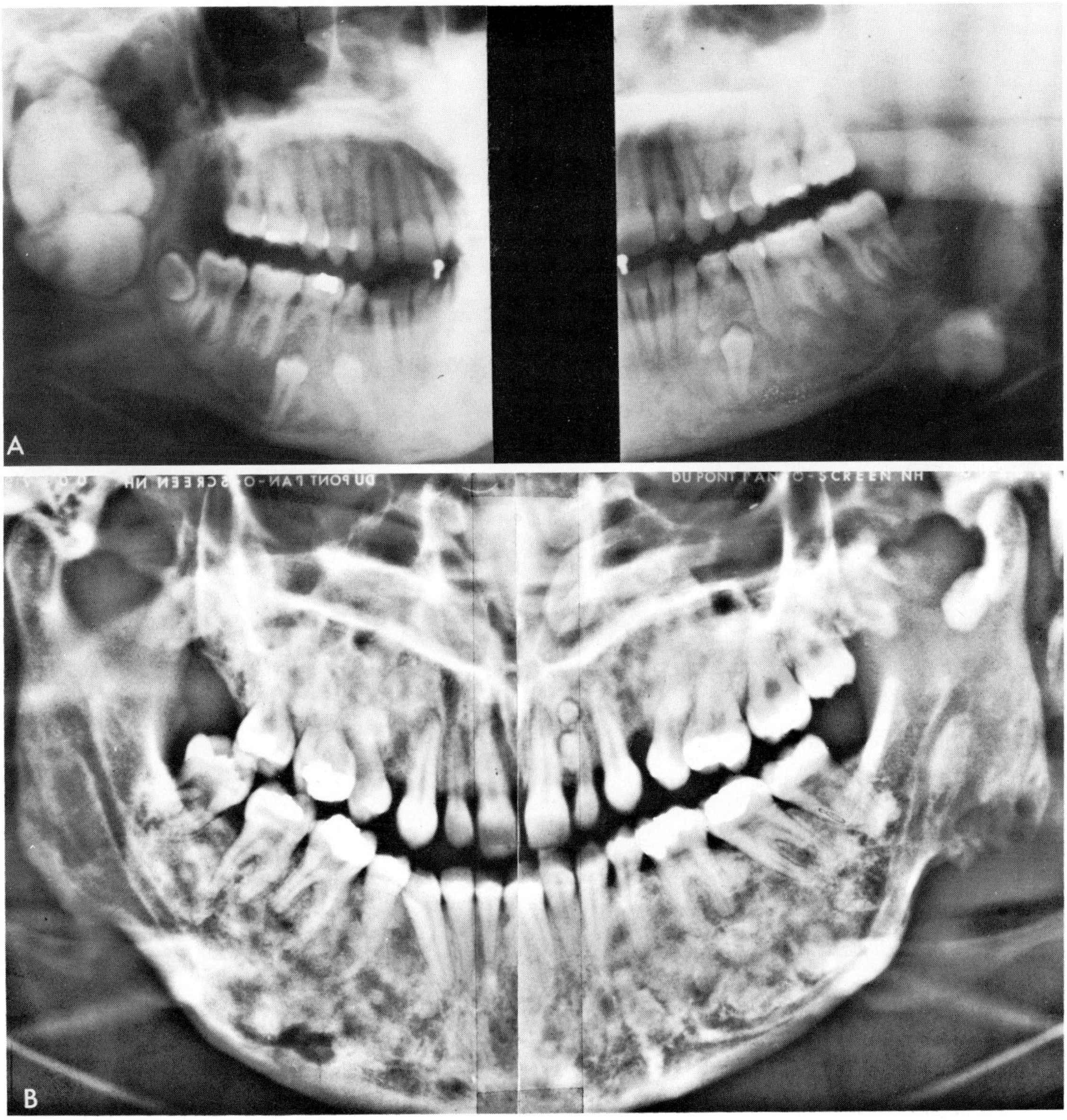

Figure 7–28A and **B.** Hyperdontia. Gardner's syndrome. Note the peripheral and diffuse central osteomas.

ALTERATIONS IN TOOTH STRUCTURE

ENAMEL HYPOPLASIA

BRIEF OVERVIEW

Enamel hypoplasia may result from a variety of influences that interfere with the activity of the ameloblasts during tooth formation. The condition may be inherited or may be the result of high fevers associated with childhood diseases; birth injuries; local factors such as periapical or furcal inflammation of the primary tooth; direct trauma by intrusion of the primary tooth; and specific conditions such as fluorosis and congenital syphilis (Hutchinson's incisors and mulberry molars). Enamel hypoplasia may also occur idiopathically.

The pattern of enamel deficiency depends on the nature of the influencing factor and the period of time during which the ameloblasts were affected. If the influence occurred over the entire period of amelogenesis, such as a genetic predisposition or fluorosis, the entire tooth of the whole dentition will be affected, thus producing mottled enamel or a generalized yellowish, rough, pitted pattern. If the influence occurred over a relatively short period, only the

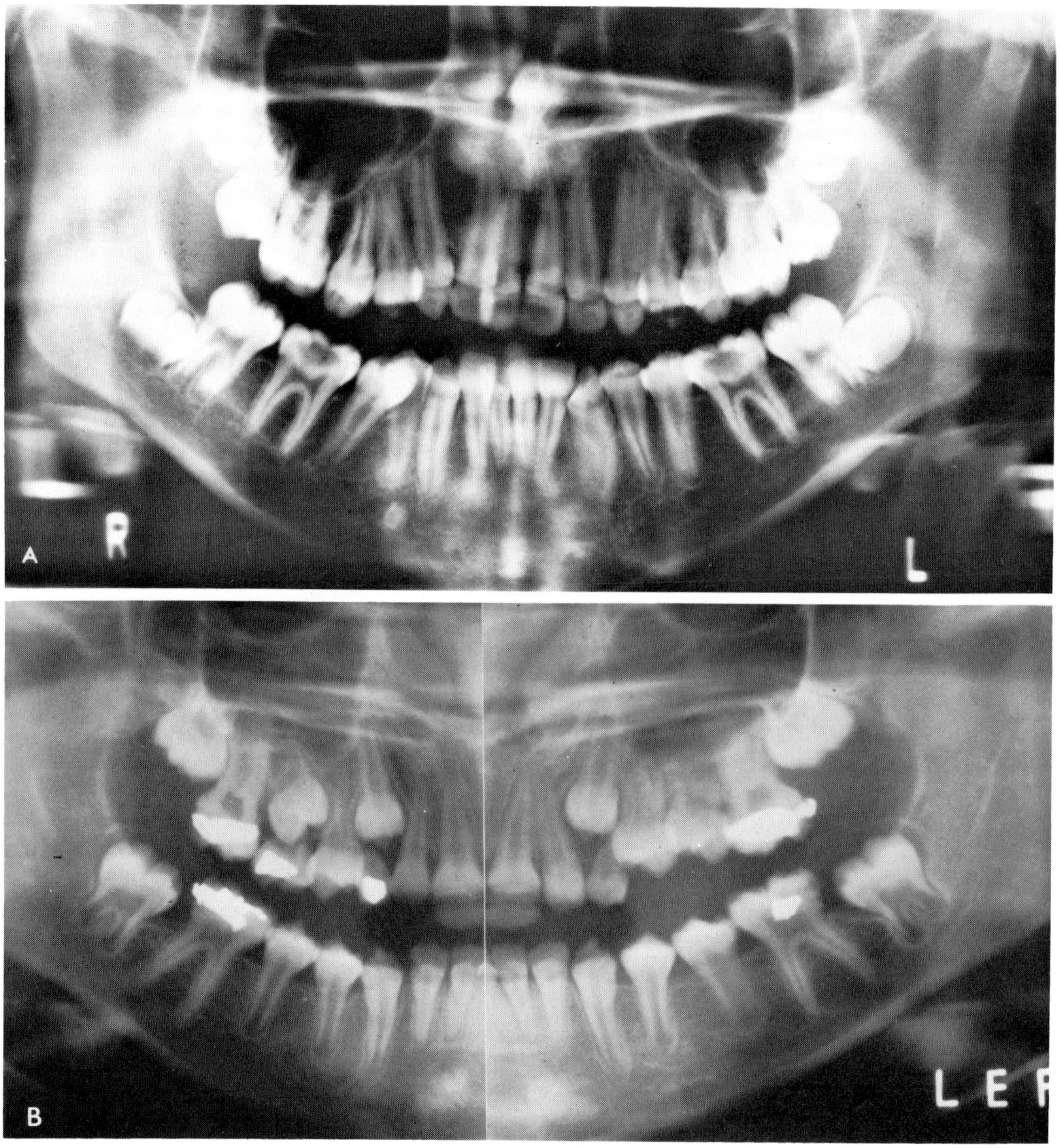

Figure 7–29A and **B.** Enamel hypoplasia. Linear pattern, affecting many teeth. (Fig. 7–29 courtesy of Dr. Birgit Junfin Glass, San Antonio, TX.)

enamel formed during that time will be affected, thus producing a horizontal linear pattern, the degree of severity of which may vary from discoloration to pitting to a distinct groove in the affected tooth. If the injury was local, such as inflammation or trauma, then only that part of the tooth is affected. Intruded primary anterior teeth may affect the labial surface of the permanent successors, and Turner's teeth occur as a result of inflammation.

RADIOGRAPHIC FEATURES (Figs. 7–29 to 7–31)

Only severely involved teeth will be detected in panoramic radiography, and there may be difficulty in distinguishing enamel hypoplasia from other disorders that affect the enamel such as erosion, certain patterns of abrasion, and unusual carious patterns. When enamel hypoplasia is suspected from panoramic radio-

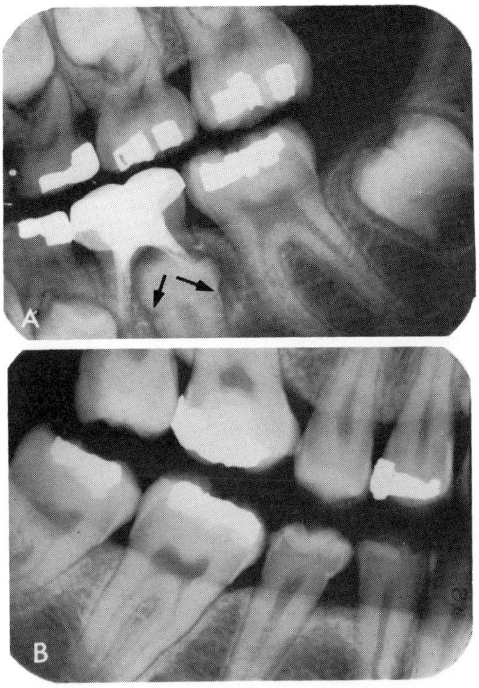

Figure 7–30A and **B.** Enamel hypoplasia. Turner type.

graphs, it is best to confirm the finding with clinical studies and intraoral radiography.

AMELOGENESIS IMPERFECTA

BRIEF OVERVIEW

Amelogenesis imperfecta is a hereditary disorder and is divided into two subtypes: the hypoplastic type, in which there is quantitatively less qualitatively normal enamel; and the hypomineralized type, in which there is a quantitatively normal amount of enamel that is qualitatively poorly mineralized. In the latter type, the chalky enamel tends to fracture off after eruption, leaving a rough discolored surface. In both types, the primary and permanent dentitions may be affected.

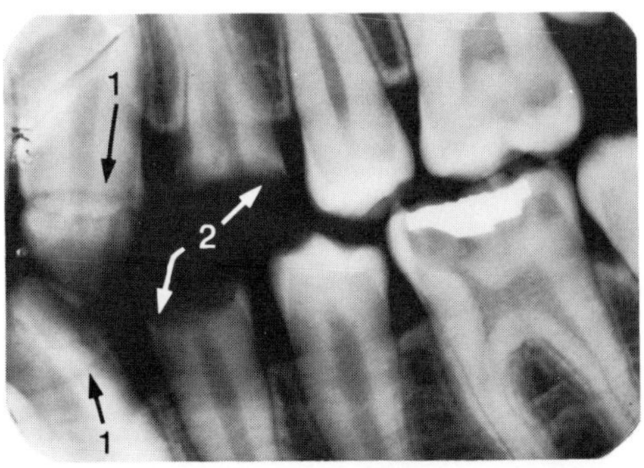

Figure 7–31. Enamel hypoplasia. 1. Linear type. 2. Turner type.

RADIOGRAPHIC FEATURES (Fig. 7–32)

The hypoplastic type of amelogenesis imperfecta is characteristic radiographically. At first glance, the crowns of both erupted and developing teeth appear to have no enamel and almost look as though they had been prepared for full crown restorations. Closer examination usually reveals a thin band of enamel covering the crown. In the hypomineralized type, the unerupted teeth may look fairly normal, whereas the erupted teeth may have varying amounts of missing enamel. Surprisingly, both types are more resistant to caries than normal teeth, and there is sometimes delayed eruption or impaction of the permanent teeth.

DENTINOGENESIS IMPERFECTA (Hereditary Opalescent Dentin)

BRIEF OVERVIEW

Dentinogenesis imperfecta is a hereditary disorder that can affect either sex. Both the primary and permanent teeth are involved, and the condition is generalized. Dentinogenesis imperfecta is sometimes associated with osteogenesis imperfecta. In milder cases, the presence of blue sclera and a history of fractures may be the only indications of an accompanying osteogenesis imperfecta.

The teeth may look normal when they first erupt. Shortly thereafter, they become translucent and develop a grayish to brownish opalescent sheen. Although the defect is limited to the dentin, the dentinoenamel junction is also affected. Thus, the enamel, especially at the incisal and occlusal surfaces, chips away, leaving exposed dentin that is generally neither sensitive nor more susceptible than normal to caries.

RADIOGRAPHIC FEATURES (Fig. 7–33)

The radiographic features of dentinogenesis imperfecta are characteristic. The crowns appear bulbous owing to a constriction of the

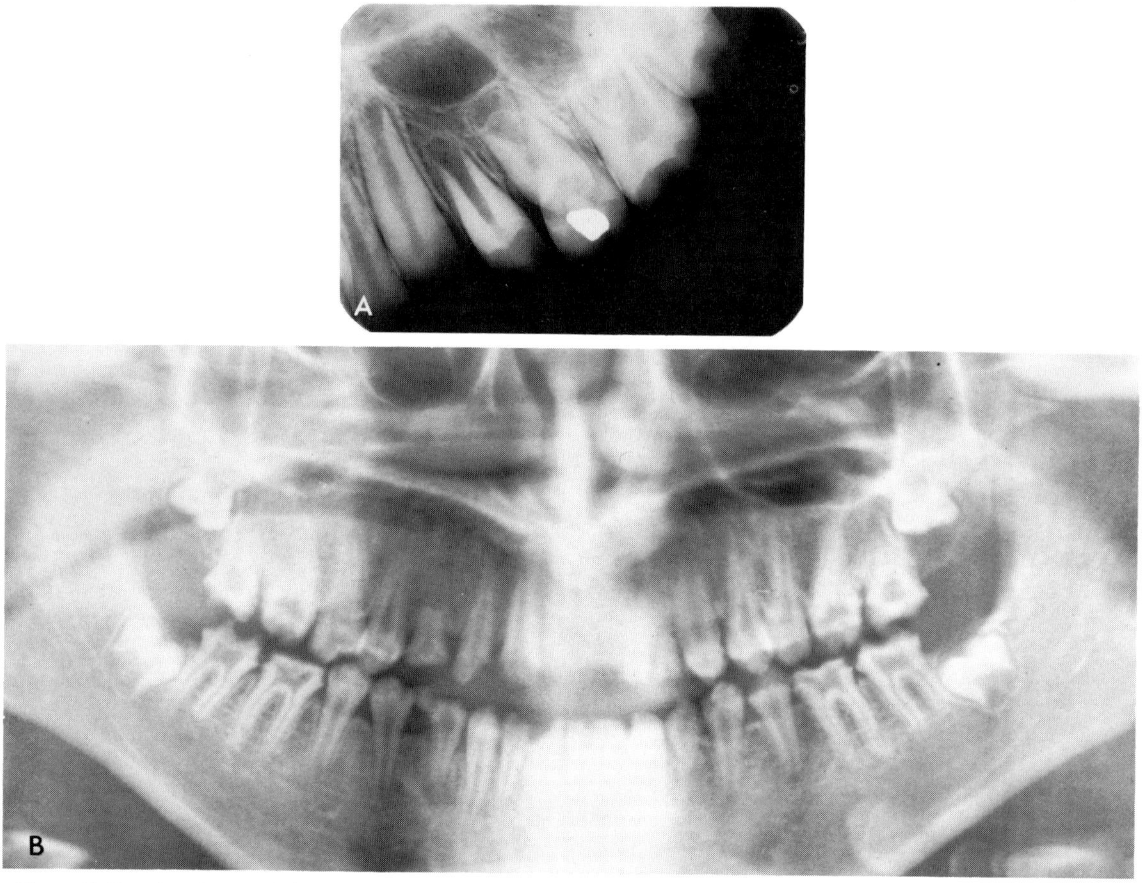

Figure 7–32. Amelogenesis imperfecta. **A.** Hypoplastic type. **B.** Hypomineralized type. (**B** courtesy of Dr. Gus Pappas, Columbus, OH.)

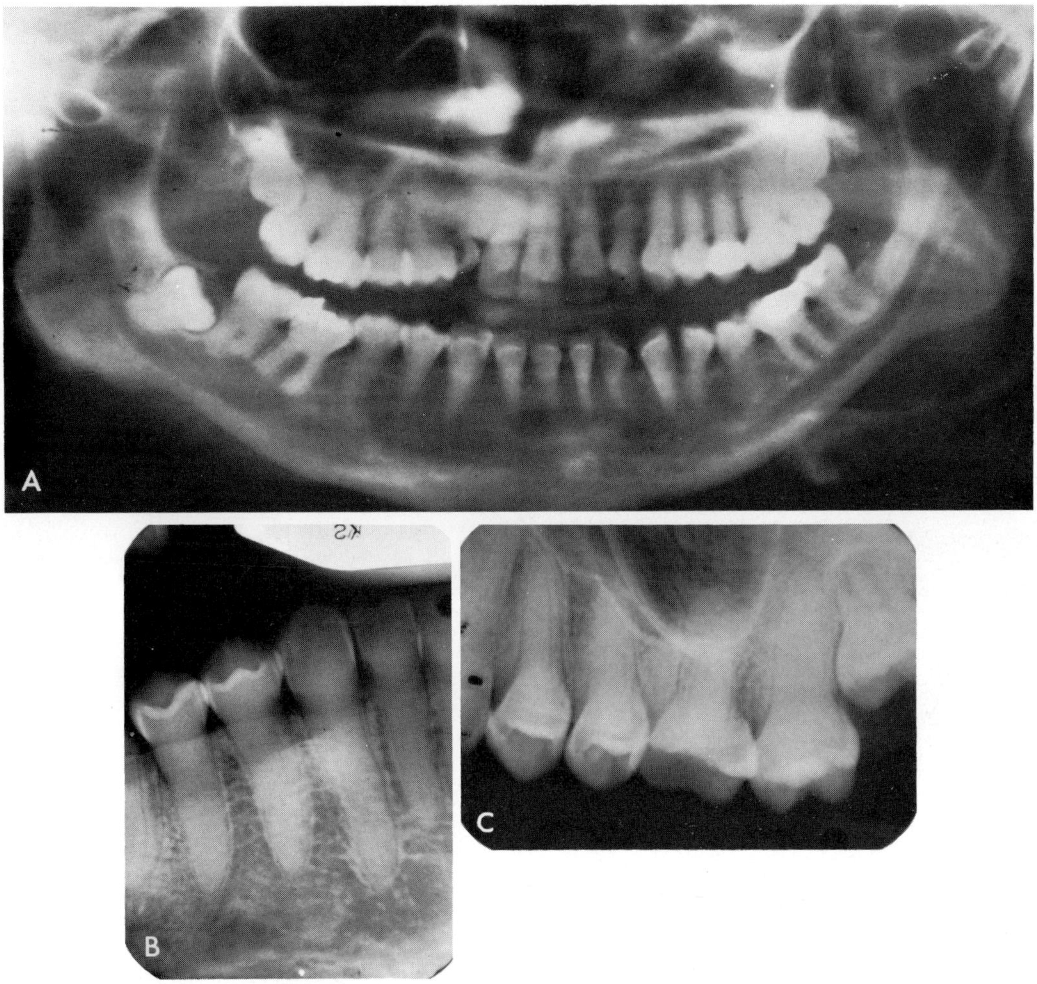

Figure 7–33A, B, and **C.** Dentinogenesis imperfecta.

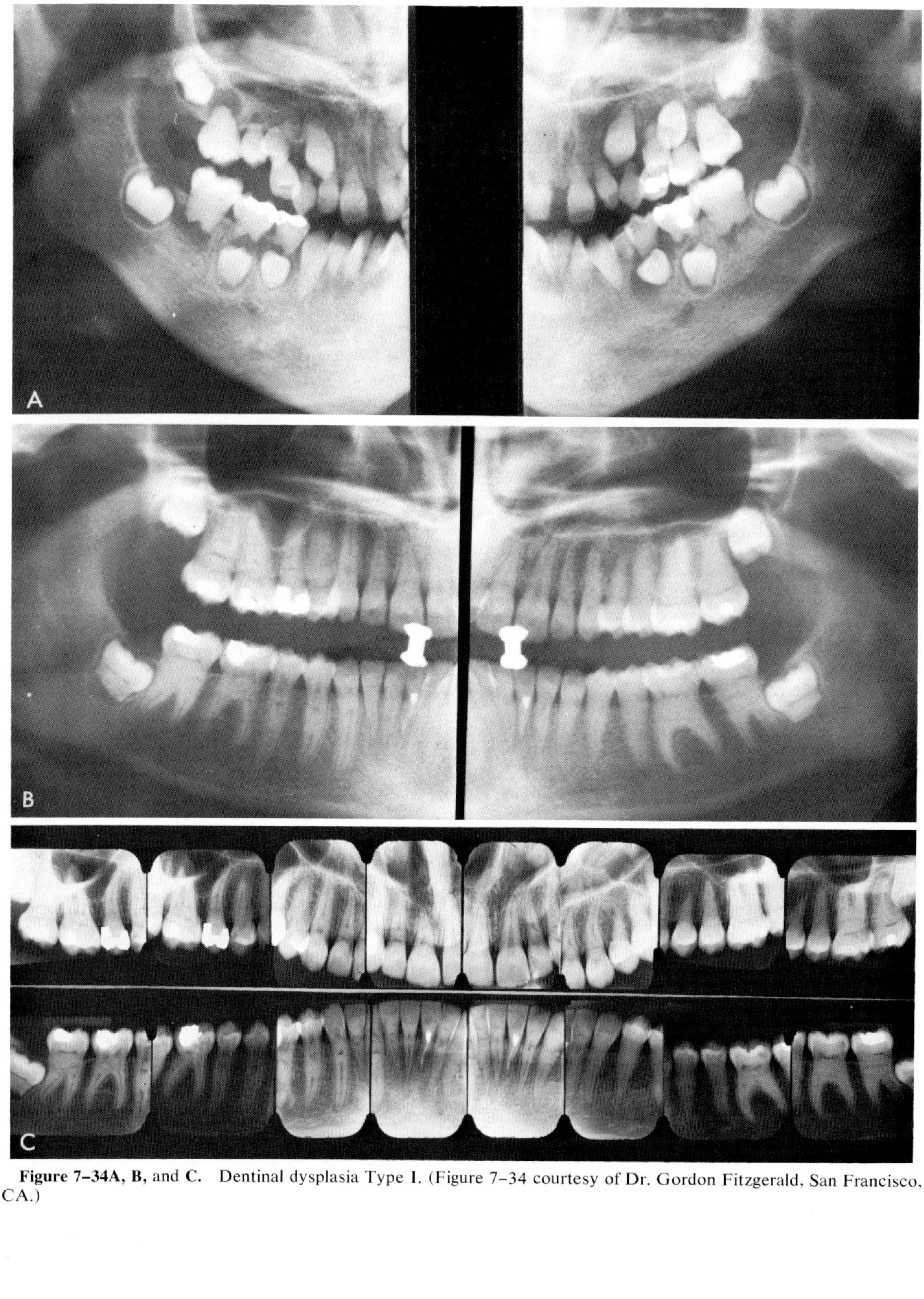

Figure 7–34A, B, and **C.** Dentinal dysplasia Type I. (Figure 7–34 courtesy of Dr. Gordon Fitzgerald, San Francisco, CA.)

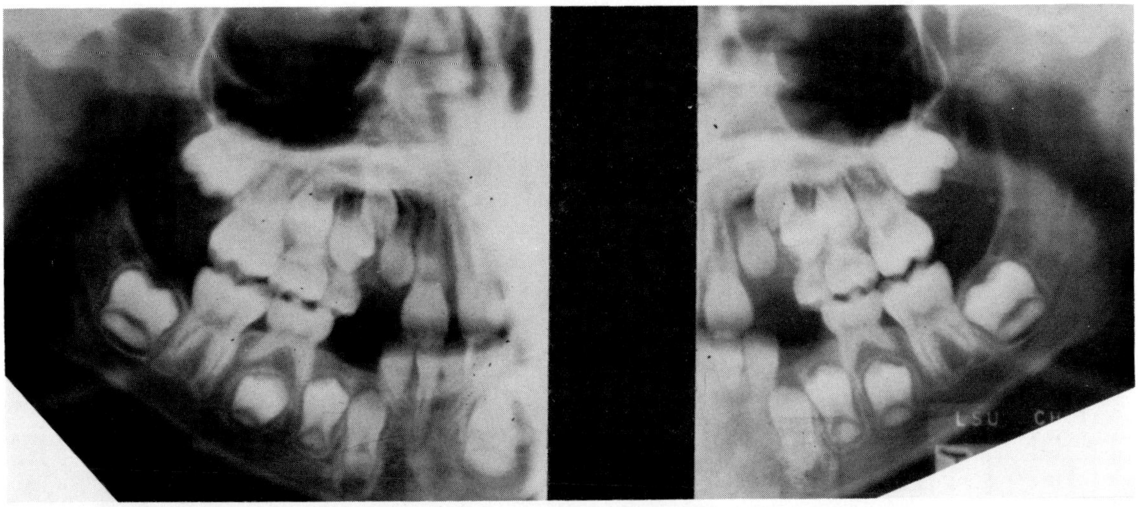

Figure 7–35. Possible dentinal dysplasia Type I. Note the unusual radiopaque dental papillae.

cervical portion of the root. The roots tend to be shorter and more tapered than normal. Like the long bones in osteogenesis imperfecta, the roots of these teeth tend to fracture. The pulp and root canal spaces are usually obliterated, with dentin as an early and striking feature once eruption has occurrred. There may be normal caries susceptibility and mild to severe incisal or occlusal attrition due to the fractured-off enamel. The teeth are no more susceptible to periodontal disease than normal.

DENTINAL DYSPLASIA

BRIEF OVERVIEW

Dentinal dysplasia has been subclassified by Shields, Bixler, and El-Kafrawy into **Type I** and **Type II.** Both types are hereditary and may affect both the primary and permanent dentitions. In Type I the teeth look clinically normal, whereas in Type II the primary teeth may look like those affected by dentinogenesis imperfecta but the permanent teeth look normal. The preliminary diagnosis of dentinal dysplasia and the distinction between Types I and II are based on the radiographs. If a tooth is available for histopathological study, the findings are characteristic.

RADIOGRAPHIC FEATURES (Figs. 7–34 to 7–36)

In dentinal dysplasia Type I, the primary and permanent teeth have a similar appearance. The features include normal sized crowns with normal enamel and dentin; very short, blunted molar roots; and short, tapered bicuspid and incisor roots. Pulp obliteration is a very early feature, often prior to eruption. Large pulp stones are often present. Sometimes the roots show horizontal radiolucent lines, making them appear carrotlike. These teeth are susceptible to early loosening, exfoliation, and idiopathic periapical radiolucencies. Idiopathic early loosening and exfoliation of the permanent teeth is characteristic of hypophosphatasia, but the pulp chambers are enlarged and the roots are normal in size.

In dentinal dysplasia Type II, the primary teeth resemble those affected by dentinogenesis imperfecta both clinically and radiographically.

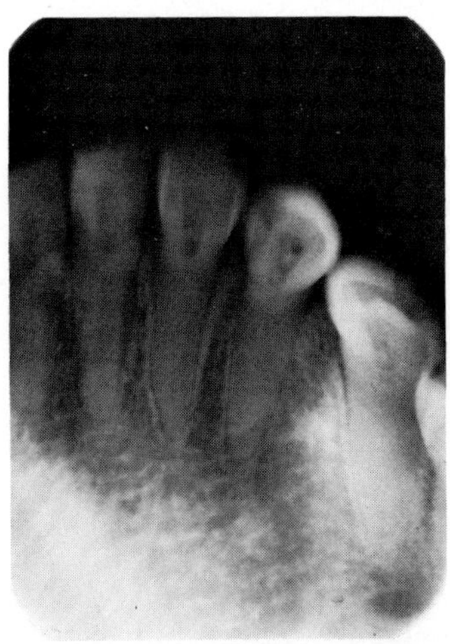

Figure 7–36. Dentinal dysplasia Type II. (Courtesy of Dr. Monique Michaud-Shields, Montreal, Quebec, Canada.)

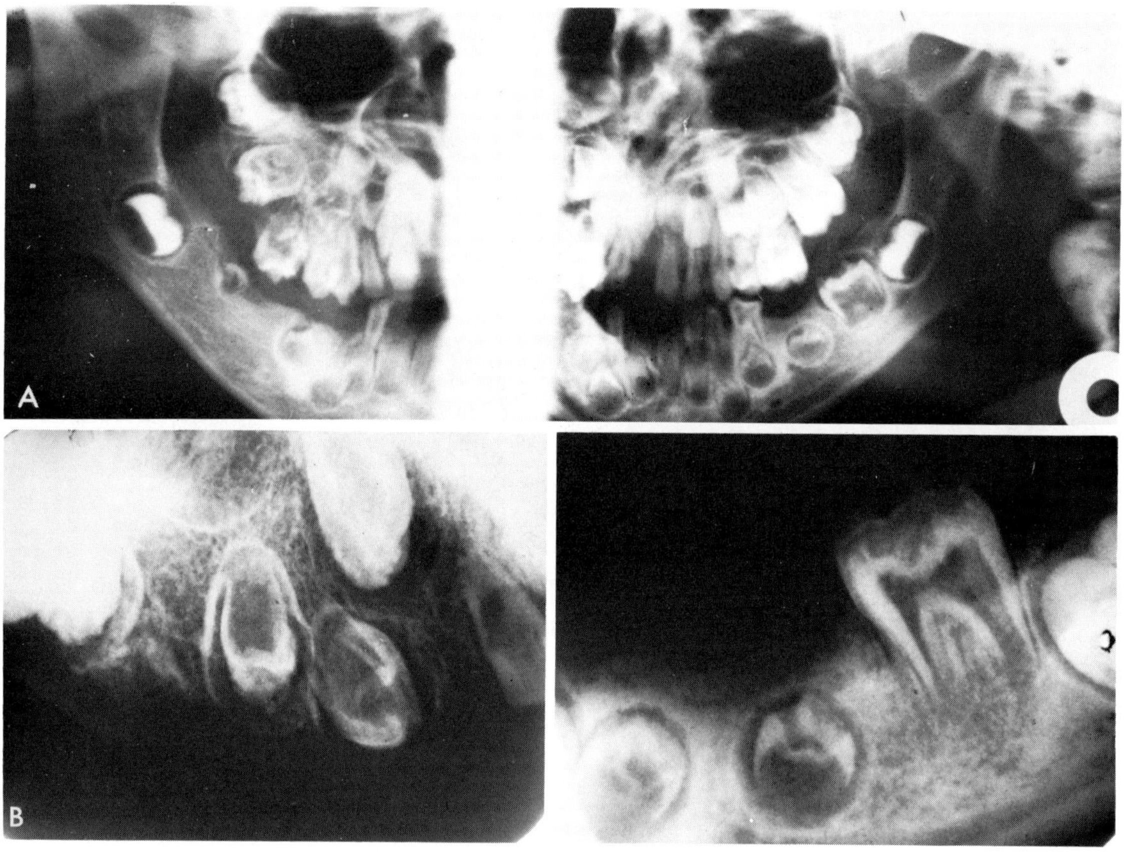

Figure 7–37A and **B.** Regional odontodysplasia.

The permanent teeth look clinically normal but have a large pulp chamber with a relatively narrower but visible root canal, thus resembling a thistle tube. The enlarged pulp chambers usually contain pulp stones.

REGIONAL ODONTODYSPLASIA (Ghost Teeth)

BRIEF OVERVIEW

Regional odontodysplasia is a poorly understood idiopathic entity involving one or several teeth. Clinically, the teeth are distorted and yellow in appearance.

RADIOGRAPHIC FEATURES (Fig. 7–37)

The radiographic features are characteristic. The ghostlike appearance is due to the large pulp and root canal space with meager amounts of enamel and dentin. It is sometimes difficult to distinguish between the enamel and dentin. Eruption may be delayed, sometimes permanently. The authors have observed ghostlike teeth radiographically in one case of pseudo-pseudohypoparathyroidism and in one case of focal dermal hypoplasia (Gorlin-Goltz-syndrome). Both cases involved multiple quadrants and delayed eruption.

ACQUIRED DEFECTS OF THE TEETH

ATTRITION

BRIEF OVERVIEW

Attrition is the physiologic wearing away of tooth structure as a result of normal mastication. It affects the incisal, occlusal, and interproximal surfaces. It begins as a small, polished, wear facet and may advance to a degree whereby the occlusal and incisal edges are completely flattened with cupped-out areas of shiny, stained, exposed dentin. In patients with mandibular prognathism, an unusual form of attrition occurs on the incisal-labial surface of the maxillary anterior teeth, whereas persons having an angle Class II Division 2 malocclusion with a deep overbite develop a similar form

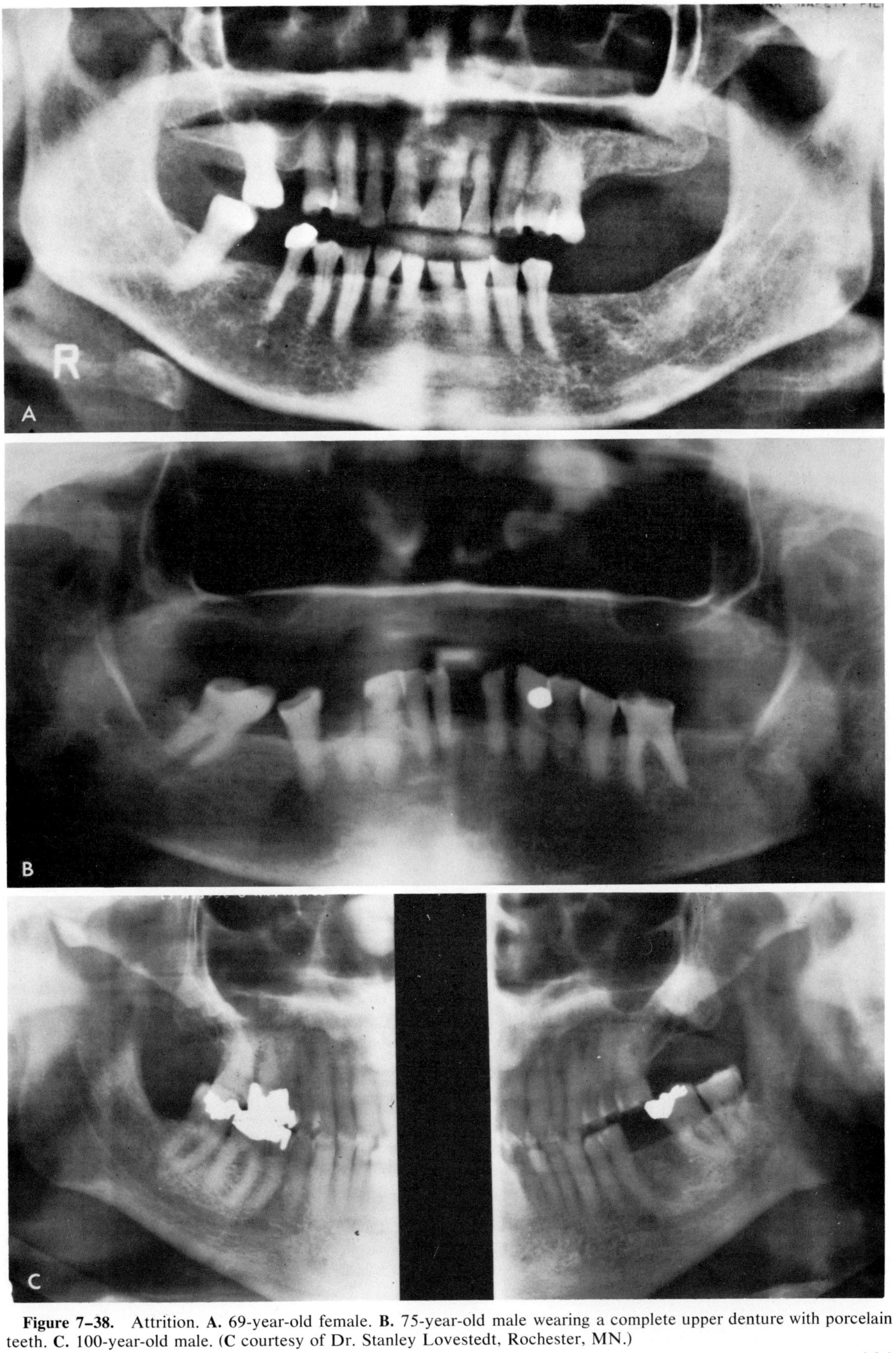

Figure 7–38. Attrition. **A.** 69-year-old female. **B.** 75-year-old male wearing a complete upper denture with porcelain teeth. **C.** 100-year-old male. (**C** courtesy of Dr. Stanley Lovestedt, Rochester, MN.)

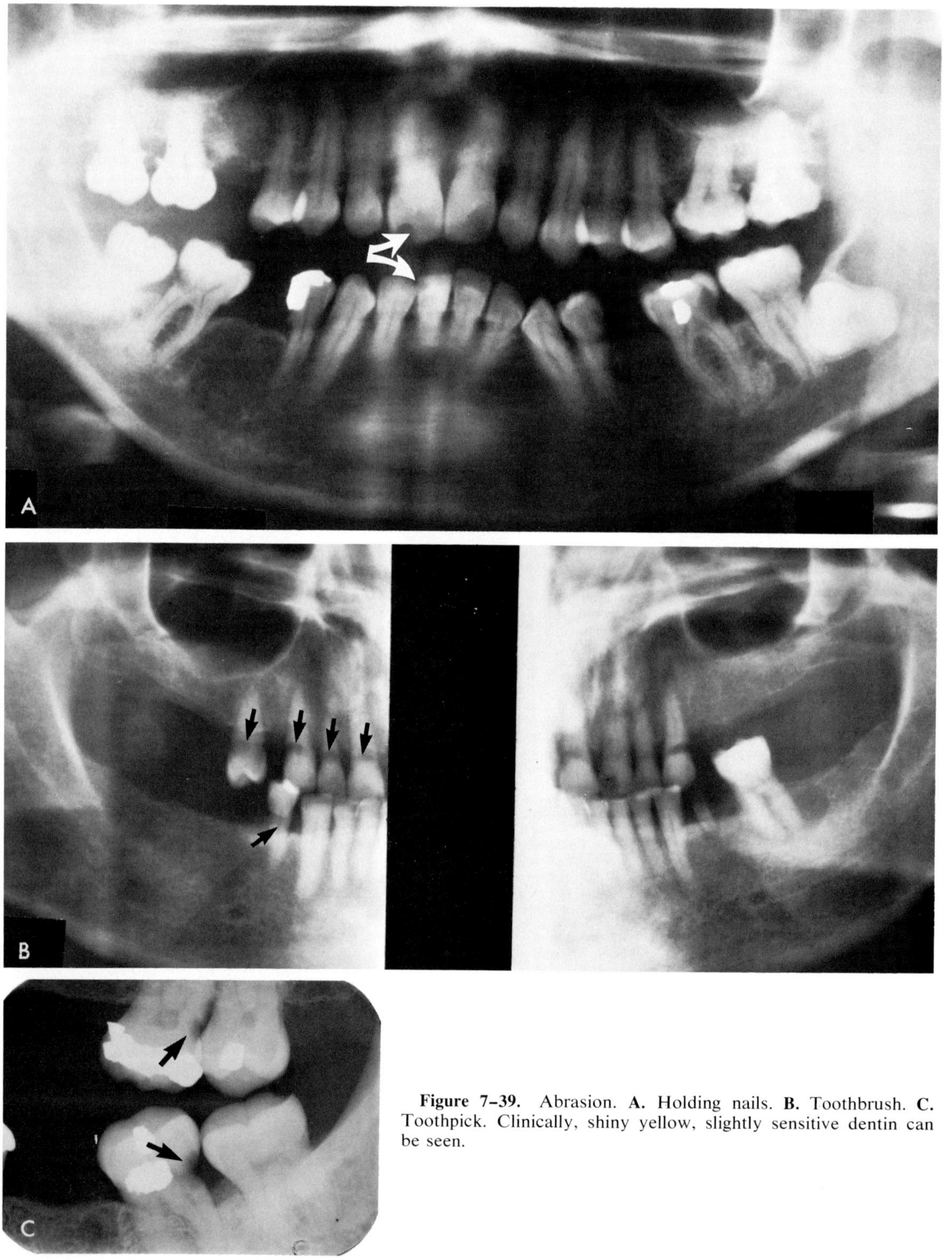

Figure 7–39. Abrasion. **A.** Holding nails. **B.** Toothbrush. **C.** Toothpick. Clinically, shiny yellow, slightly sensitive dentin can be seen.

of attrition on the incisal-labial surfaces of the mandibular anterior teeth. Both the primary and permanent teeth may be affected by attrition. The teeth are usually not sensitive.

RADIOGRAPHIC FEATURES (Fig. 7–38)

Only more advanced cases of attrition will be seen on panoramic radiographs. Once noted, a careful history will be required to rule out abrasion. Prior to complete flattening of the occlusal plane, the cuspid inclines may be worn flat but may still form inclined planes. Because of these straight lines, the occlusal surfaces take on an angular, geometric appearance, with markedly thinner enamel.

ABRASION

BRIEF OVERVIEW

Abrasion is the pathologic wearing away of tooth structure by a mechanical process. The occlusal surfaces may be severely worn, mimicking advanced attrition in a person who, for example, is a sand blaster. Probably the most common form of abrasion is toothbrush abrasion, caused by improper brushing. This produces a V-shaped notch in the buccal-cervical portion of the tooth and may eventually lead to pathologic pulp exposure and tooth fracture. Although dentinal sensitivity is common, caries is usually absent. The most common area affected is the cuspid-bicuspid region, owing to the prominence of these teeth and the curvature of the arch. Right-handed persons may show more toothbrush abrasion on the left side and vice versa for left-handed persons, a fact often used in forensic odontology. Other forms of abrasion occur with pipe smoking, improper flossing, improper home use of scalers, improper utilization of toothpicks, opening bobby pins with the teeth, holding nails in the mouth, and so on. Abraded teeth may be sensitive, and treatment is aimed at removal of the physical source of wear. Restorative procedures may be required for esthetics, function, and comfort.

RADIOGRAPHIC FEATURES (Fig. 7–39)

Localized areas of abrasion often show an unusual pattern of wear, which may alert the practitioner that further clinical investigation is necessary. Toothpick abrasion may be suspected if a circular defect in the enamel and/or dentin is seen, usually below the unaffected contact point. When more advanced, toothbrush abrasion will show a well-demarcated, horizontal radiolucent line in the cervical area of the tooth. If the tooth is slightly rotated or if the radiation is directed at the tooth from slightly off-angle, a V-shaped radiolucency may be noted, with one side of the V highly angular and well demarcated and the other side seen as a fuzzy, indistinct outline. Other forms of wear will show similar, unusual patterns depending on the source.

EROSION

BRIEF OVERVIEW

Erosion is the loss of tooth substance by a chemical process, usually involving an acid. Clinically, the teeth appear smooth and shiny, and there may be exposed, sensitive dentin. With chronic vomiting or regurgitation and with chronic intake of acidic carbonated soft drinks, the most involved area will usually be the palatal aspect of the maxillary teeth. The occlusal, mandibular lingual, and buccal surfaces may be involved, in descending order of frequency. When the buccal surfaces mainly are involved, especially the maxillary anterior teeth, lemon sucking may be suspected. Erosion may also occur idiopathically.

RADIOGRAPHIC FEATURES (Fig. 7–40)

Only severe, advanced cases of erosion will show up radiographically. The findings are vague and nonspecific. Basically, the crown looks vaguely more radiolucent than it should. What is believed to be a peculiar but charac-

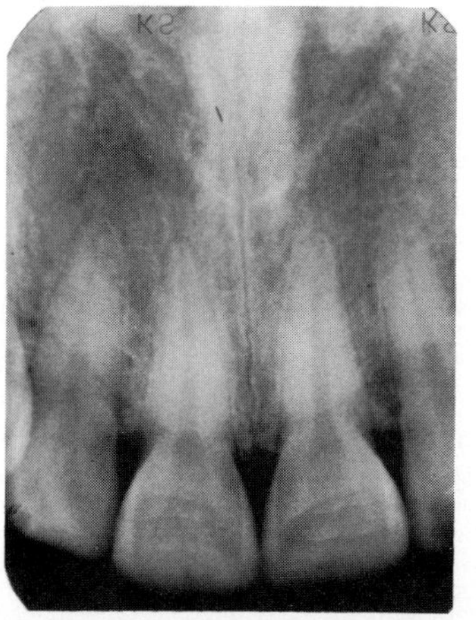

Figure 7–40. Erosion. The horizontal radiolucent lines are caused by toothbrush wear of the exposed dentin in this 23-year-old lemon sucker.

teristic form of toothbrush abrasion may be due to lemon-sucking erosion. Tooth brushing produces characteristic horizontal radiolucent lines mesiodistally across the crowns of the maxillary anterior teeth. These vague changes may be difficult to see on panoramic films.

EXTERNAL RESORPTION

BRIEF OVERVIEW

External resorption is the loss of tooth material from the outer surface of any part of any tooth that is surrounded by bone. The apices of the teeth may be resorbed in association with some periapical granulomas, neoplasms, impacted teeth, or excessive orthodontic forces. The crowns of long-standing embedded teeth are also prone to external resorption. The roots of endodontically treated and reimplanted teeth may eventually completely resorb over a period of years. Additionally, external root resorption may be idiopathic. Physiologic resorption of the primary teeth occurs in association with the eruption of the succedaneous permanent teeth. The root of the primary tooth may or may not resorb in the absence of its successor. This is an important consideration in treatment planning. Further discussion of external resorption may also be found in Chapter 8.

RADIOGRAPHIC FEATURES
(Figs. 7–41 to 7–43)

In the case of orthodontics and in the reimplantation of an avulsed or extracted tooth, the radiographs are a helpful follow-up procedure.

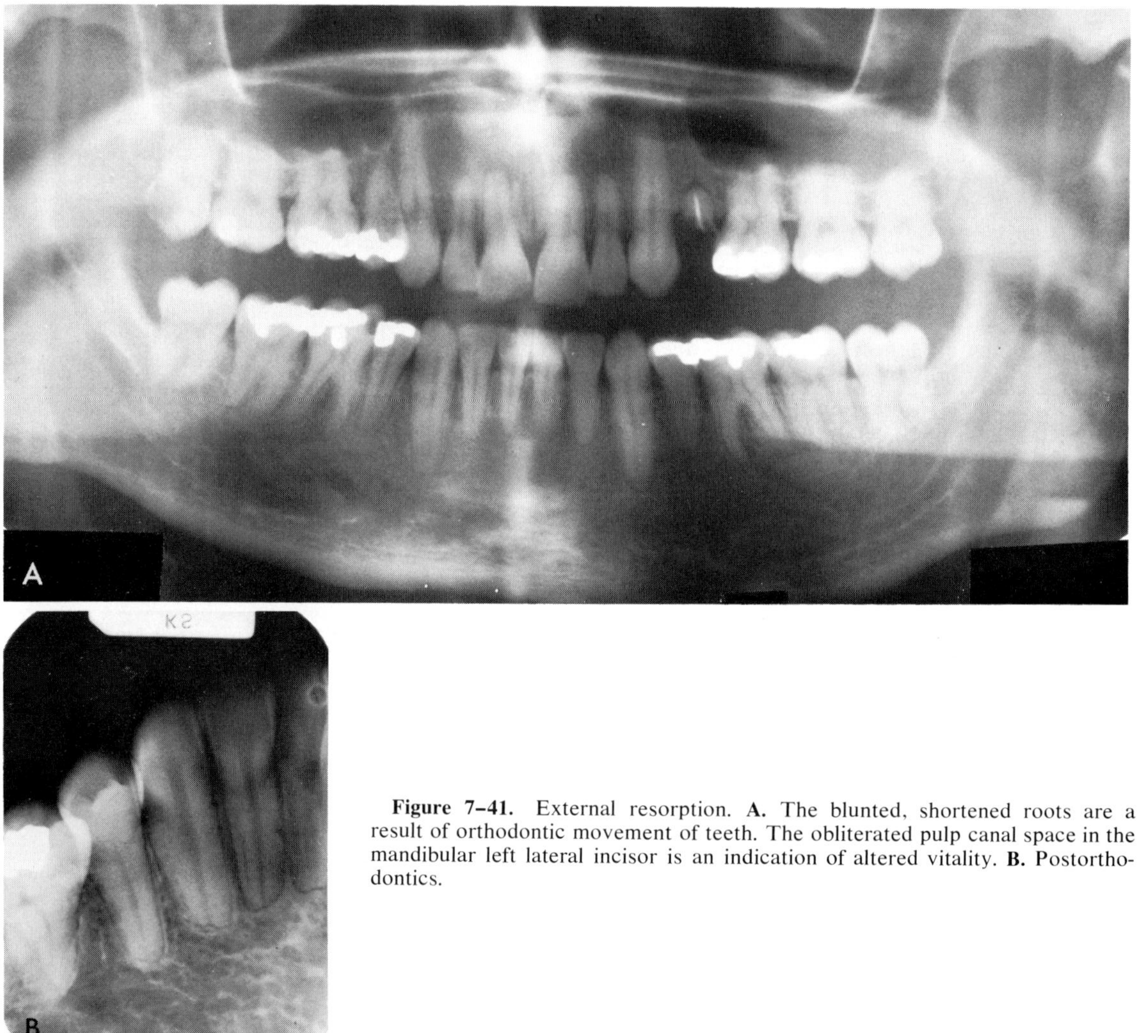

Figure 7–41. External resorption. **A.** The blunted, shortened roots are a result of orthodontic movement of teeth. The obliterated pulp canal space in the mandibular left lateral incisor is an indication of altered vitality. **B.** Postorthodontics.

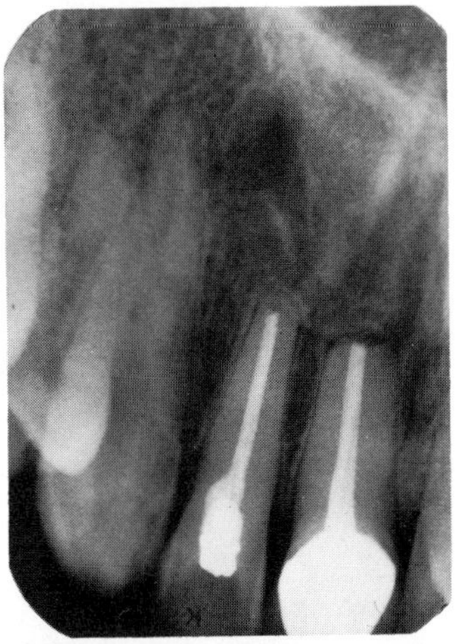

Figure 7–42. Blunted apices following apicoectomy. Not to be confused with resorption.

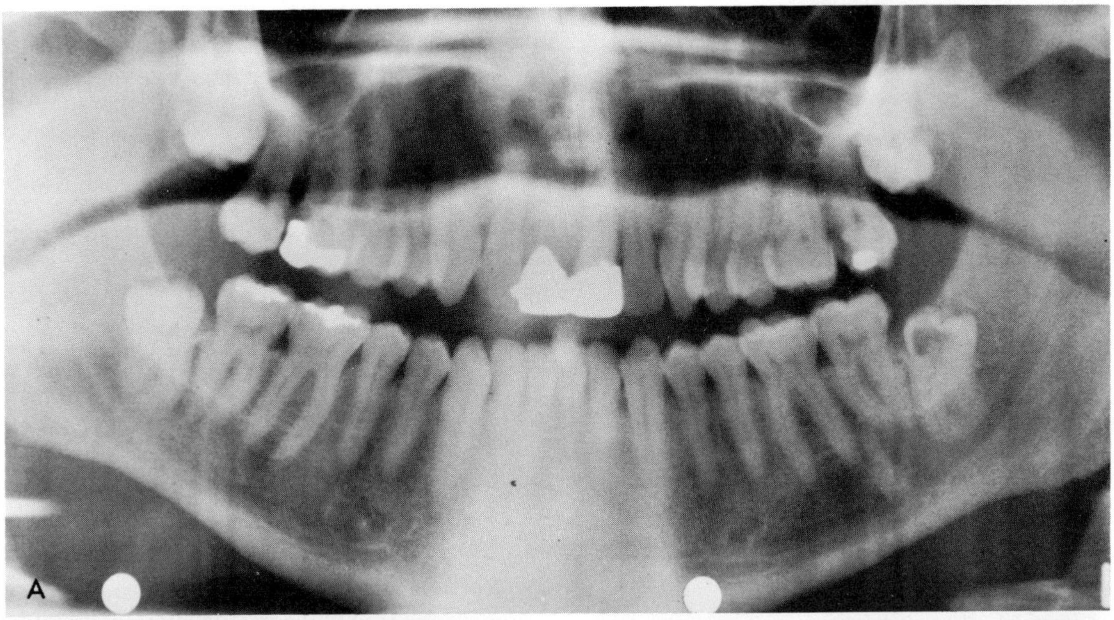

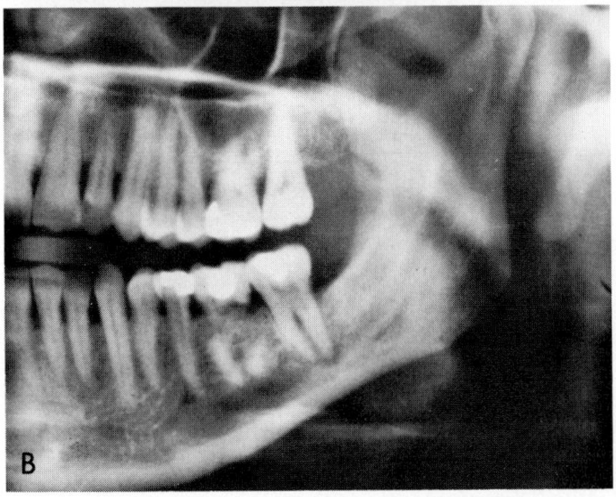

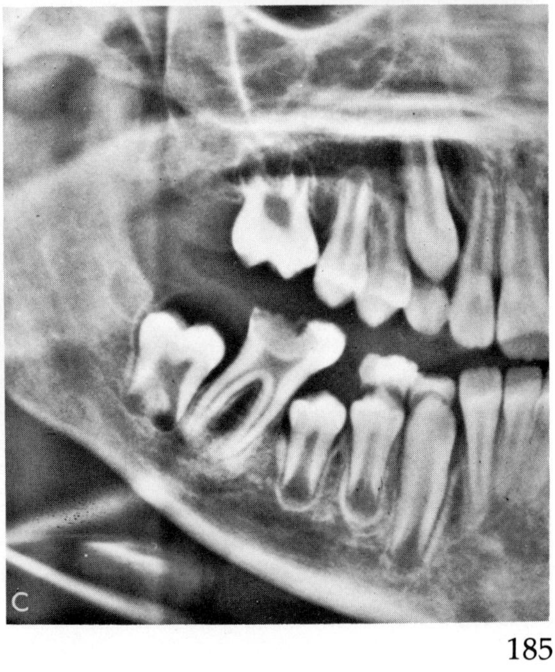

Figure 7–43. External resorption. **A.** Affecting an unerupted tooth. This should not be referred to as pre-eruptive caries. **B.** Affecting the roots of an erupted tooth. **C.** Physiologic resorption of primary teeth.

A finding of root resorption with any pathologic process is neither an indication of a benign process nor conclusive evidence of a malignancy. When root resorption is found, further investigation and treatment are usually necessary. External resorption of embedded teeth, especially in the crown portion, should not be referred to as pre-eruptive caries. Such teeth are often ankylosed and may require no further treament other than periodic radiographic observation.

INTERNAL RESORPTION

BRIEF OVERVIEW

Internal resorption is a process that begins inside the tooth. The pulp is usually hyperplastic, but inflammation (caries) is apparently not a prerequisite for its development. When this process is advanced, the coronal portion of the tooth may look pink clinically (pink tooth of Mummery).

To arrest the resorption process, an attempt should be made to remove the pulp and complete endodontic therapy. If the affected area is in the root portion of the tooth and appears to have been internally resorbed, close radiographic follow-up is required for signs of buccal or lingual perforation. If such a perforation is suspected, the affected area should be surgically exposed and sealed with amalgam or the tooth should be extracted. Further discussion of internal resorption may also be found in Chapter 8.

RADIOGRAPHIC FEATURES (Fig. 7–44)

A round or ovoid enlargement will occur somewhere within the pulp chamber, which may eventually hollow out the whole tooth and break through to the outside. Once this happens, it is difficult to determine if the resorption is external or internal. External resorption on the buccal or lingual aspect of a root is difficult, if not impossible, to distinguish from internal resorption. Often a root that has been perforated laterally by a post will show either internal or external resorption.

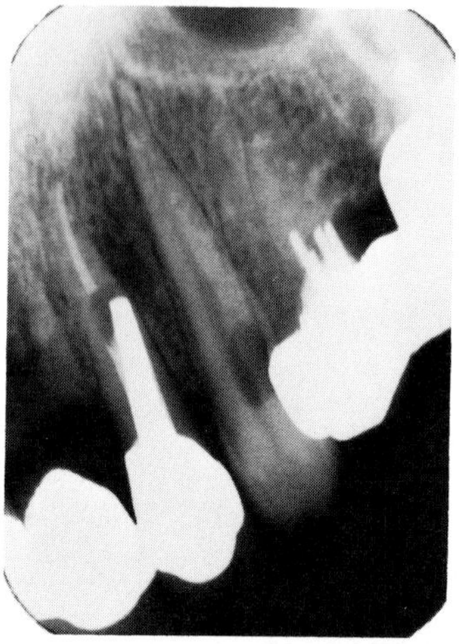

Figure 7–44. Internal resorption with perforation associated with a cast post. Contrast this with the caries in the adjacent cuspid tooth.

PULP OPACITIES

BRIEF OVERVIEW

Pulp stones or pulp calcifications appear with age in some individuals and, other than the endodontic considerations, are of no significance. A further discussion of pulpal opacities may be found in Chapter 8.

RADIOGRAPHIC FEATURES (Figs. 7–45 to 7–47)

Pulp stones may consist of dentin or a ball of calcified tissue. Additionally, they may be free within the pulp chamber or root canal, or they may be attached to the wall. They may also be singular or multiple. Diffuse calcification consists of varying degrees of dystrophic calcification, usually generalized throughout the pulp.

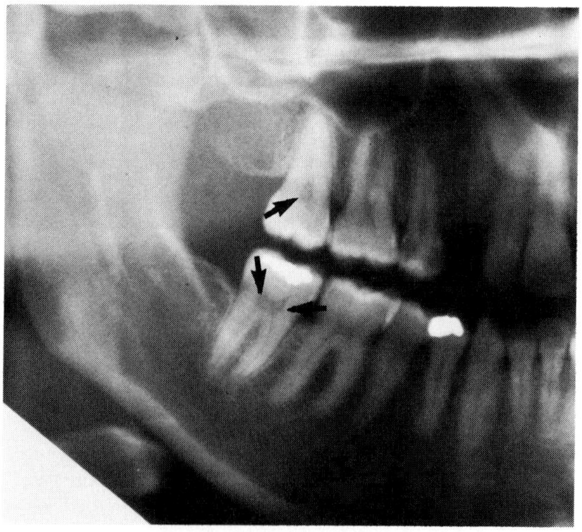

Figure 7–45. Pulp stones.

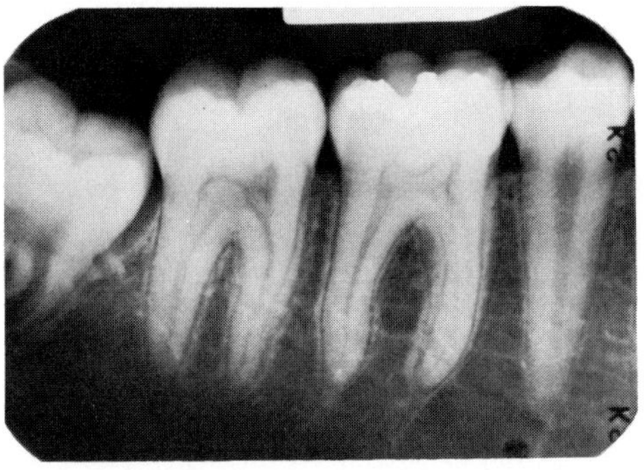

Figure 7–46. Diffuse pulp calcification.

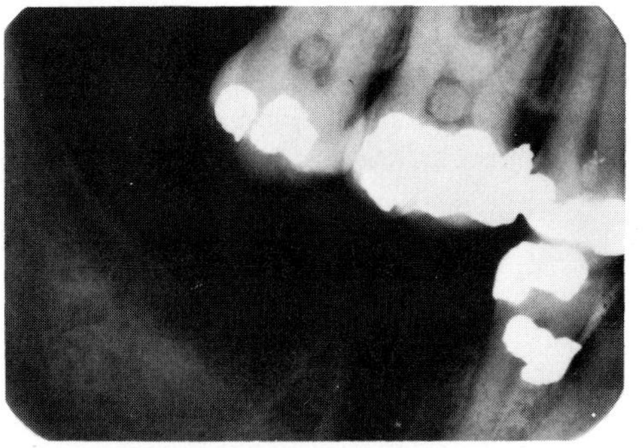

Figure 7–47. Pulp stones. Note the resemblance to enamel pearls and the density, which resembles dentin rather than enamel.

PULP OBLITERATION

BRIEF OVERVIEW

This phenomenon may be found in two forms: generalized pulp obliteration and localized pulp obliteration. In the absence of other tooth deformities, the generalized form is probably a part of the aging process and is usually seen in older individuals. If only one tooth is involved, especially in a younger individual, it is usually a sign of altered vitality of the pulp. This may be seen following trauma to a tooth that did not fracture and may be analogous to internal resorption. However, in this case the stimulus, possibly anachoretic inflammation, causes the injured pulp to lay down odontoblasts at an accelerated rate, thus attempting "self-" or natural endodontia. Generalized pulp chamber obliteration and an enlarged root canal space in a younger individual, along with a ground-glass trabecular pattern and loss of the lamina dura, are suggestive of secondary hyperparathyroidism (renal osteodystrophy).

RADIOGRAPHIC FEATURES (Figs. 7–48 to 7–50)

In the generalized form, the pulp chamber may be completely obliterated or hairline thin in most teeth. It is often accompanied by attrition.

In the localized form, a single tooth is affected. The tooth often tests nonvital to electric and other pulp tests such as percussion, hot, cold, and a test cavity. Periapical disease, deep caries, a large restoration, recurrent caries, secondary dentin, or other radiographic signs of pulp inflammation may or may not be present.

PULP ENLARGEMENT

BRIEF OVERVIEW

Relative pulp enlargement is a normal finding in newly erupted teeth. If only one tooth is affected, the clinician should suspect an altered

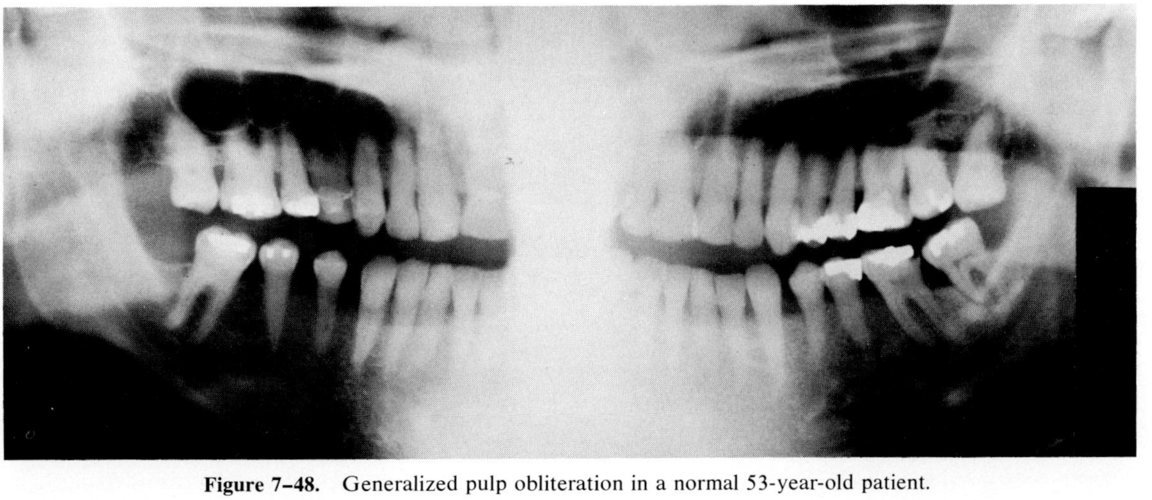

Figure 7–48. Generalized pulp obliteration in a normal 53-year-old patient.

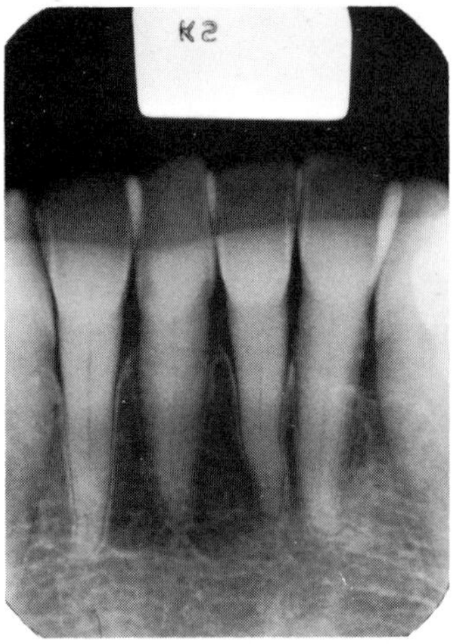

Figure 7–49. Generalized pulp obliteration.

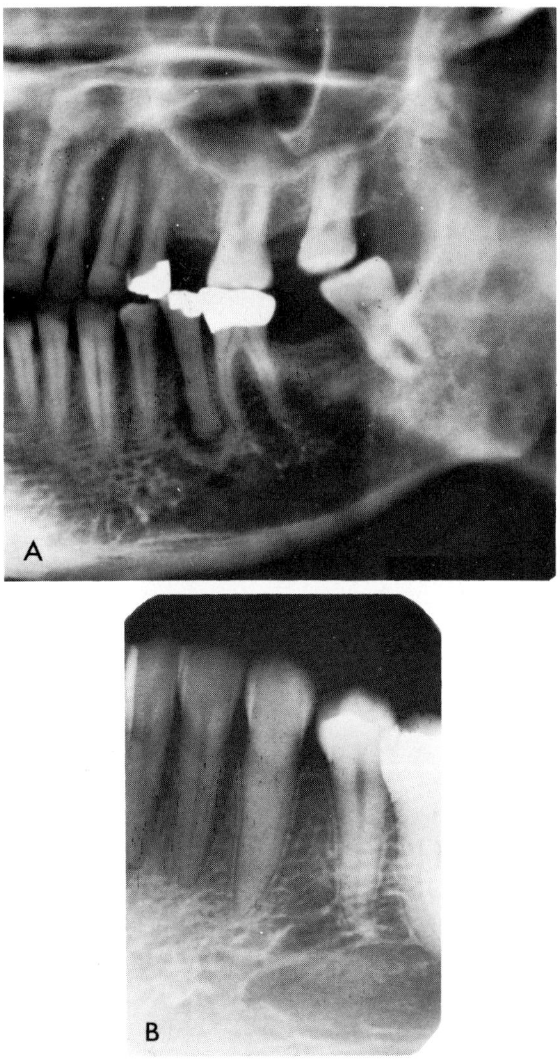

Figure 7–50A and **B.** Localized pulp obliteration.

vitality that has caused the tooth to cease development. A clue to this situation is the blunderbuss or wide-open apex of the involved tooth. Endodontic treatment may consist of a pulpotomy initially to stimulate apex closure (apexification), followed by routine endodontic treatment.

Localized pulp enlargement may also be seen with internal resorption. The objective of endodontic treatment in this situation is to remove the hyperplastic pulp tissue to prevent further internal destruction of the tooth. Localized pulp enlargement is also seen in taurodontism and regional odontodysplasia.

The classic cause of generalized pulp enlargement is vitamin D–resistant rickets (hypophosphatemia). Another cause is hypophosphatasia (low phosphatase rickets). Pulp enlargement is also seen as an idiopathic finding. When the pulp enlargement is idiopathic, the pulp lacks the ability to lay down secondary dentin and remains enlarged well into adulthood. In all instances, these teeth are susceptible to early pulp involvement by caries and accidental mechanical exposure during routine operative procedures.

RADIOGRAPHIC FEATURES (Fig. 7–51)

The identification of enlarged pulps is of clinical significance because of the factors previously discussed. Panoramic radiographs are especially useful in classifying the condition as either localized or generalized. The localized form is obvious when advanced. Minimal manifestations are best identified by comparing the tooth with its neighbors or with its opposite member on the other side of the arch. Generalized pulp enlargement may be suspected when the size of the pulp is either unusual or inconsistent with the patient's age. This may be a clinical sign of systemic disease. A peculiarity of hypophosphatasia is that the walls of the enlarged pulp spaces are parallel to each other, thus producing a characteristic picture.

ALTERATIONS IN ERUPTION OF TEETH

ERUPTION SEQUESTRUM

BRIEF OVERVIEW

An eruption sequestrum is an anomalous spicule of bone associated with the occlusal

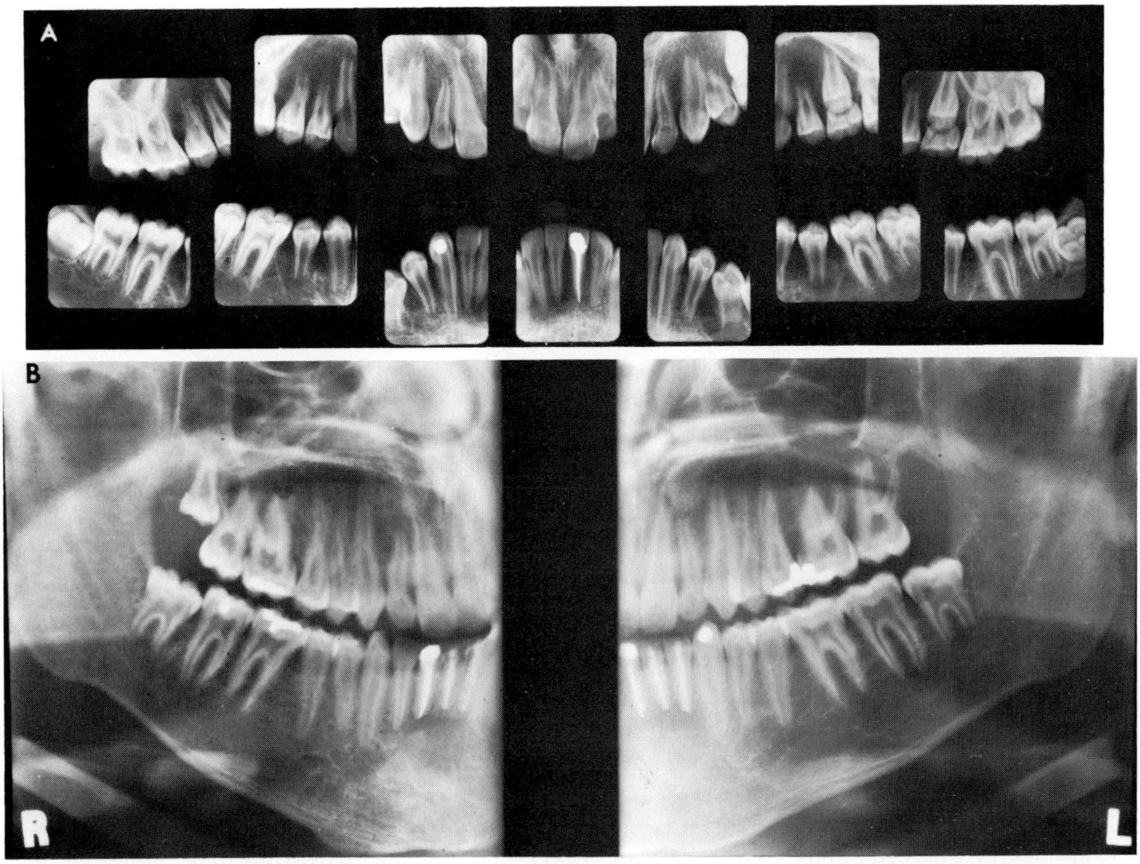

Figure 7–51A and **B.** Pulp enlargement. Vitamin D-resistant rickets at ages 13 and 18, respectively. (Figure 7–51 courtesy of Dr. Stanley Lovestedt, Rochester, MN.)

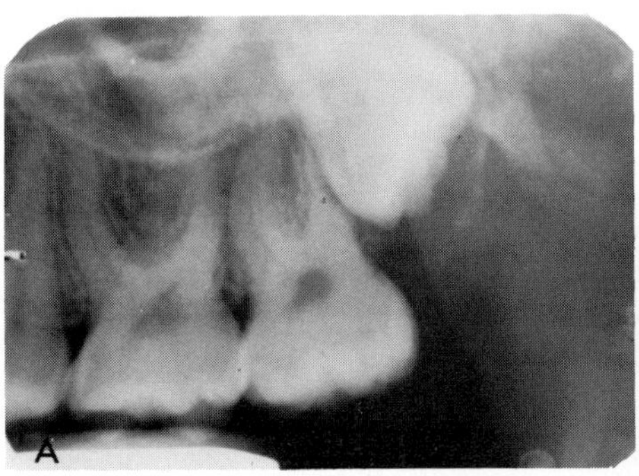

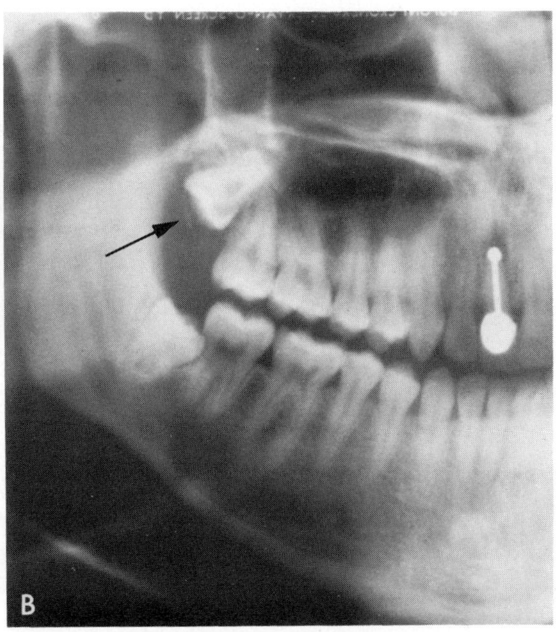

Figure 7–52A and **B.** Eruption sequestrum.

surface of some erupting teeth, mainly molars. Normally, an erupting molar will break into soft tissue and the intervening bone will have been resorbed. When an eruption sequestrum occurs, there may be mild discomfort, and the small piece of bone may sometimes be seen breaking through the gingiva. The condition is temporary and self-limiting.

RADIOGRAPHIC FEATURES (Fig. 7–52)

The bony spicule is seen as apparently floating in the soft-tissue overlying the crown of the erupting tooth. It is most frequently seen as a narrow radiopaque band that may be pencil thin, crescent shaped, figure-eight shaped, round, or ovoid.

SUPRAERUPTION

BRIEF OVERVIEW

Supraeruption is the eruption of teeth beyond the normal occlusal plane. This phenomenon may occur when the opposing tooth is missing. Supraeruption is more apt to occur with maxillary teeth and in the presence of periodontal disease. Mandibular teeth may also supraerupt. Additionally, the altered interproximal contact of a supraerupted tooth contributes to the collapse of the occlusion and to the development of localized periodontal disease. In planning treatment for restoration of the missing teeth, the antagonistic supraerupted teeth should be restored first to reestablish a proper plane of occlusion and the proper interproximal contact. During restoration it may be possible to reduce the supraerupted tooth or teeth to create a space to accommodate the prosthesis for the missing tooth or teeth. Supraeruption must be distinguished from vertical tooth displacement by a tumor mass. The distinction between these two conditions is based on the radiographs.

RADIOGRAPHIC FEATURES (Fig. 7–53)

Radiographically, a tooth is seen without an antagonist in the opposite arch, and the affected occlusal plane, usually the upper, is stepped or out of line with the other occluding teeth. Occasionally, supraerupted teeth may be seen occluding with the opposing ridge. The clinician should be on the alert for periodontal disease, especially in association with the supraerupted teeth.

DRIFT AND MIGRATION

BRIEF OVERVIEW

Drift refers to movement of an erupted tooth once either mesial or distal contact is lost. When mesial contact is lost, mesial drift, or more commonly mesial tipping, occurs because of the mesial inclination of the occlusion forces. Paradoxically, when distal contact is lost, one does not usually expect distal drift or tipping of the tooth. When distal drift does occur, it is of

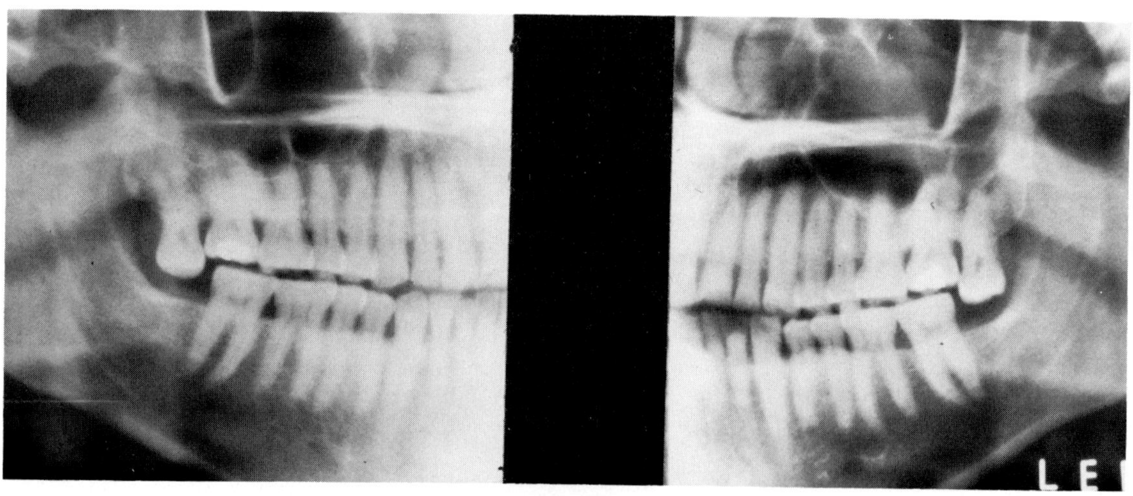

Figure 7–53. Supraeruption. Note the maxillary third molars.

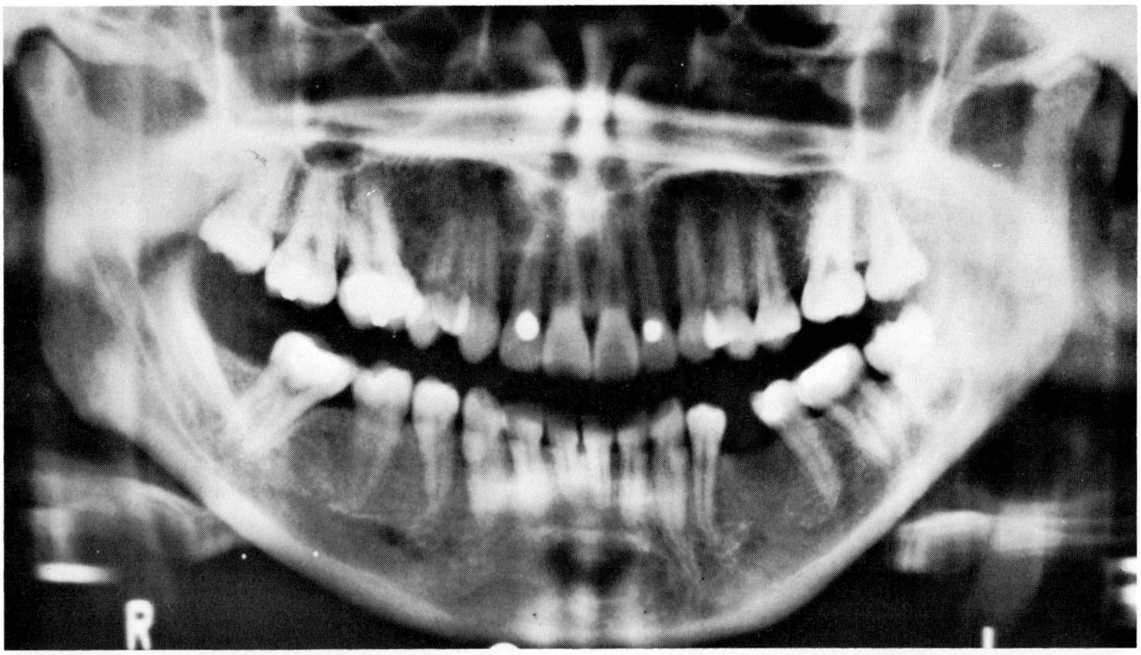

Figure 7–54. Distal drift. Note the mandibular left second bicuspid. (Courtesy of Dr. Steven Bricker, San Antonio, TX.)

clinical significance, especially with respect to treatment planning.

The term **migration** indicates the abnormal movement of an unerupted tooth, usually in a mesial direction. This is perhaps due to the mesial inclination of some erupting teeth, especially the cuspids and third molars. Distal migration may also occur. Whenever migration is noted, an attempt should be made to identify an underlying cause, such as congenitally or otherwise missing teeth or displacement by a tumor mass or cyst. Migration may occur idiopathically, but when a cause is present, it may be more important to recognize and treat the cause than to remove or treat the migrated tooth. Some authors use the terms drift and migration interchangeably with respect to erupted and unerupted teeth.

RADIOGRAPHIC FEATURES (Figs. 7–54 and 7–55)

In distal drift, the involved tooth occupies a position distal to where it should be. The tooth distal to the involved tooth is usually missing. The authors have observed this phenomenon most frequently in the mandibular second bicuspid.

Although migrating teeth may erupt, an unerupted migrated tooth of long standing may show signs of external resorption and ankylosis. In the absence of abnormal clinical and radiographic findings, periodic radiographic observation is recommended.

TRANSLOCATION (TRANSPOSITION) AND ECTOPIC ERUPTION

BRIEF OVERVIEW

Translocation or transposition is a term indicating that a tooth has erupted into the normal place of another. It also refers to the interchange in position of two adjacent teeth. When a migrating tooth erupts it may occupy a translocated position. Since translocated teeth occupy the normal position of another tooth, they are usually positioned within the normal curvature of the arch. **Ectopic eruption** refers to a tooth that is not translocated and that does not erupt into its normal position. It may be crowded or located buccal or lingual to the curvature of the arch. Translocation is often associated with a missing tooth. The most common situation, in the experience of the authors, is for the maxillary permanent lateral incisor to be missing and the permanent cuspid to erupt into the position of the missing lateral incisor, leaving the primary cuspid in place of the permanent cuspid.

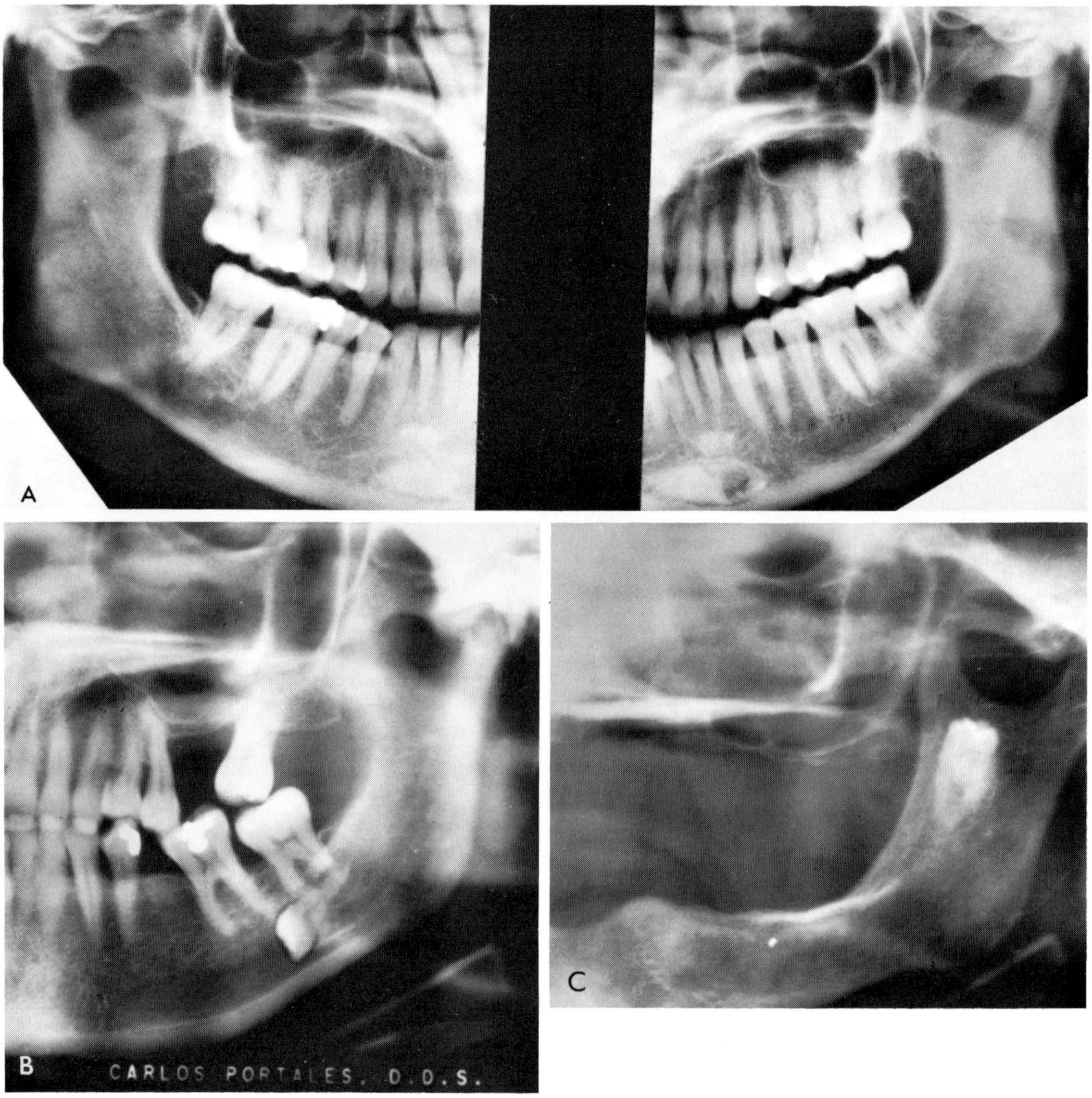

Figure 7–55A, B, and **C.** Migration. (Figure 7–55 courtesy of Drs. Frank Sammis Jr. and Carlos Portales, San Antonio, TX.)

RADIOGRAPHIC FEATURES (Figs. 7–56 and 7–57)

With translocated teeth, it is important to note any signs of abnormal occlusal stress such as heavy wear facets on the inclined planes or a localized widening of the periodontal membrane space. It is especially important to note these findings in the teeth adjacent to the translocated tooth, as when a first bicuspid or primary cuspid is functioning as a cuspid.

The degree of root resorption of any retained primary tooth is an important treatment-planning consideration. Idiopathic resorption of the root of a retained primary tooth may occur at any time or not at all.

If ectopically erupted teeth are to be extracted or treated orthodontically, a dilacerated root may sometimes be seen radiographically in association with these teeth and may be an important treatment-planning consideration.

ANKYLOSIS

BRIEF OVERVIEW

Ankylosis is a continuity between the tooth and the alveolar bone. This rare condition may affect primary or permanent teeth and any erupted or unerupted tooth. According to Shafer, Hine, and Levy, there is resorption of

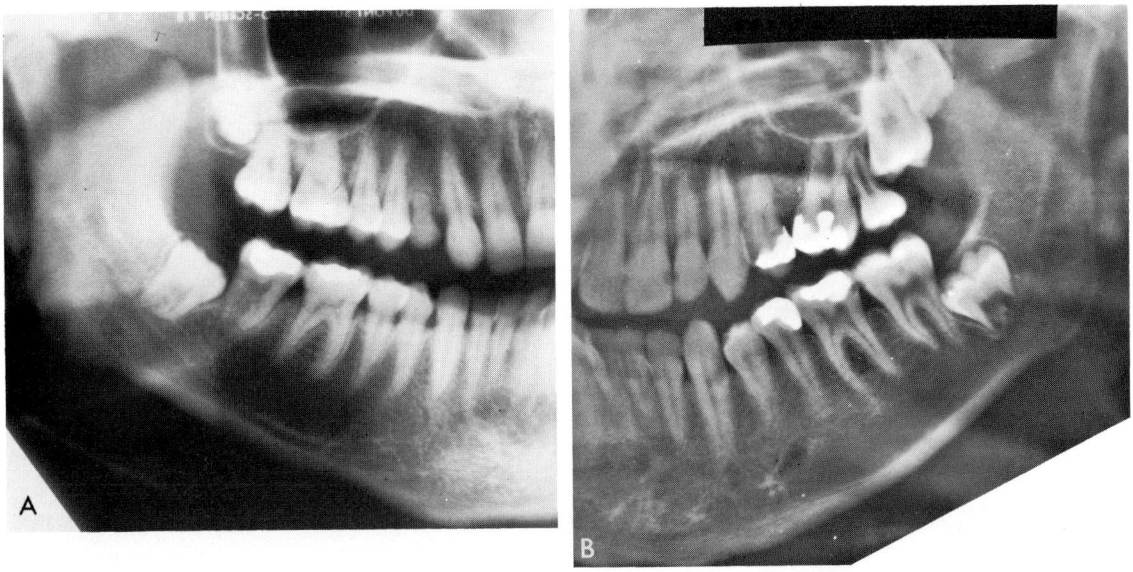

Figure 7–56. Translocation. **A.** Note the maxillary cuspid. **B.** Note the maxillary second bicuspid.

the root and replacement by bone. Worth refers to this bony replacement as inostosis. Ankylosis is most commonly seen in some cases of retained, submerged second primary molars.

Ankylosis may also be seen in association with an erupted permanent tooth and embedded teeth of long standing. There may be external resorption of the crown associated with the embedded teeth. The ankylosis may involve all or part of the affected root. It is important to recognize ankylosis if the tooth is to be removed, since ankylosed teeth are more difficult to extract.

RADIOGRAPHIC FEATURES (Figs. 7–58 and 7–59)

The periodontal membrane space is completely lost in the affected area, and the root surface appears to be continuous with the adjacent bone. The exact outline of the root may be

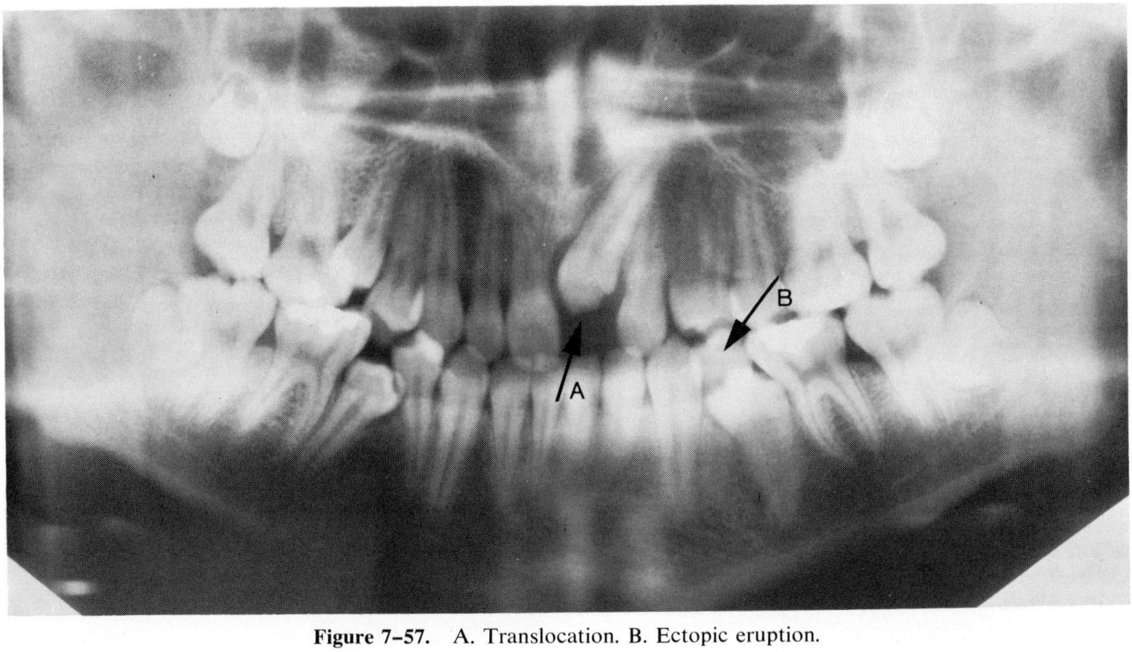

Figure 7–57. A. Translocation. B. Ectopic eruption.

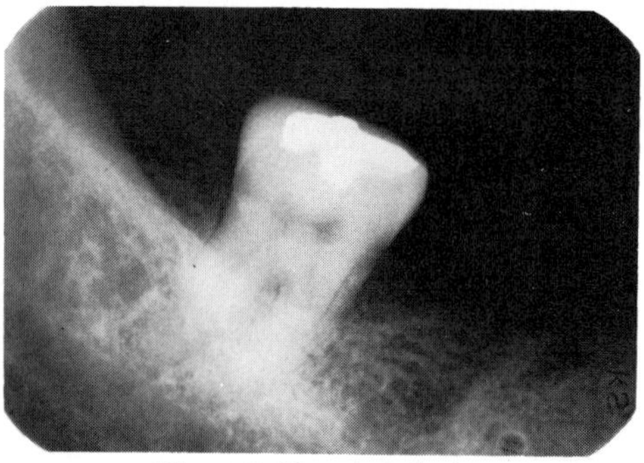

Figure 7–58. Ankylosis.

difficult to see. Partial or complete ankylosis should be suspected in retained primary teeth, embedded teeth of long standing, and some endodontically treated teeth.

EMBEDDED AND IMPACTED TEETH

BRIEF OVERVIEW

An **embedded tooth** is one that has failed to erupt and remains buried in bone. An **impacted tooth** is one in which some physical entity has prevented its eruption. The most commonly impacted teeth, in descending order of frequency, are the mandibular third molars, maxillary third molars, maxillary cuspids, bicuspids, and supernumerary teeth.

RADIOGRAPHIC FEATURES (Figs. 7–60 to 7–72)

In evaluating impacted and embedded teeth, it is extremely helpful to determine the eruptive potential of the tooth. The earliest sign of an impending impaction may be radiographic evi-

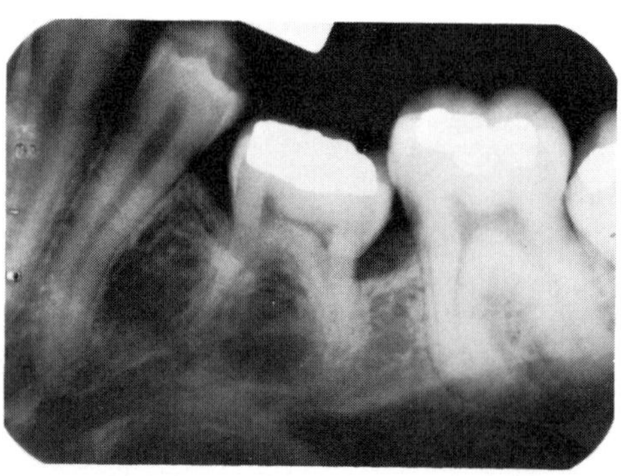

Figure 7–59. Submerged, ankylosed, retained second primary molar.

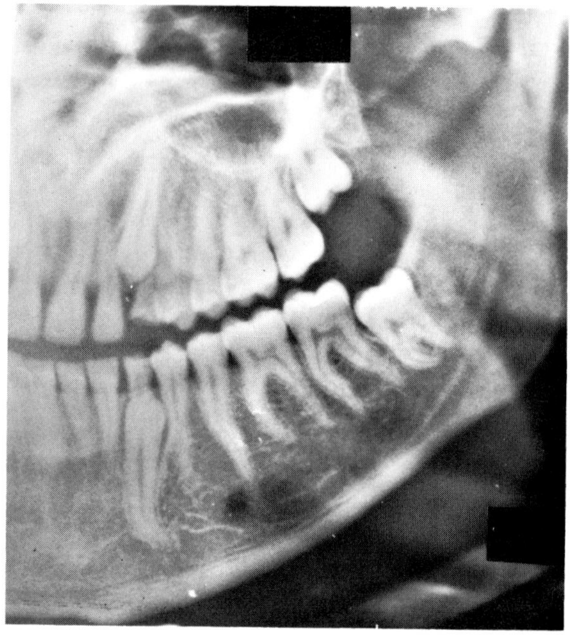

Figure 7–60. Embedded cuspids and third molars.

dence of delayed eruption. Barring the presence of obvious physical barriers, missing teeth, or systemic disorders such as hypopituitarism, delayed eruption may not be obvious in its early stages. Generally, if the tooth is behind its contralateral twin or if root formation has exceeded crown length, delayed eruption may exist. Delayed eruption is more obvious when the contralateral twin has erupted or when root formation and apex closure are complete. In the latter instance, the eruptive potential of the tooth is markedly reduced and may be the most important factor distinguishing a normally erupting third molar from one that is impacted. (Delayed eruption will be discussed separately.)

If the impacted tooth is a third molar, the impaction should be classified. Most classifications are based on the radiographic position of the tooth. Impacted teeth as seen on the panoramic film should sometimes be further examined with intraoral periapical views if buccal or lingual localization is necessary. In this instance, Clark's rule or the buccal-object rule of Richards may be used. Occlusal, right-angle, and maxillary crossfire views are also helpful. In some panoramic radiographs, impacted and embedded anterior teeth can be localized towards the buccal or lingual side with the panoramic film alone. In the latter instance, the lingual object moves in the same direction as the observer's eye movement. Therefore, if the

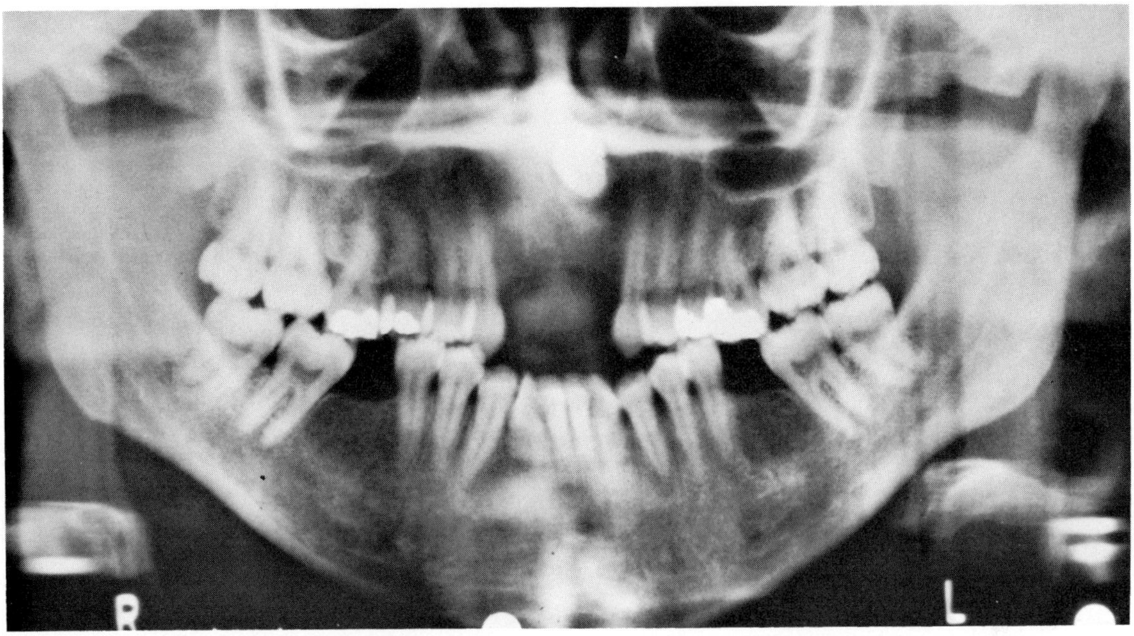

Figure 7–61. Embedded supernumerary mesiodens.

tooth involved is a maxillary cuspid and it can be visualized on both sides of the blank area in the center of the film, it will be located on the palatal side if the image on the left side moves more to the right on the right side, i.e., it has moved in the same direction as the observer's

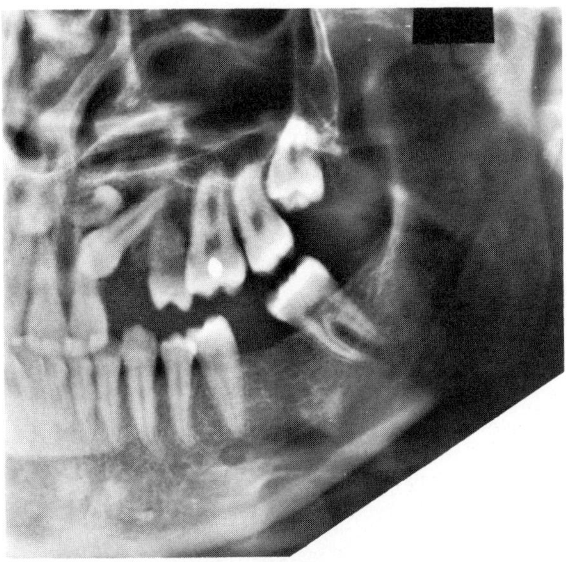

Figure 7–62. Embedded cuspid. This is probably owing to the missing lateral incisor, which normally guides the cuspid into position. Impaction owing to interference by the supernumerary mesiodens is unlikely. This illustrates the distinction between embedded and impacted teeth.

eye. The opposite holds true for buccally positioned teeth (see Fig. 7–23).

Mandibular impacted third molars are classified as follows (based on the classifications of Pell and Gregory and Winters):

Factor 1 — Distance Between Distal Aspect of Second Molar and Ramus.

Class I. Space between distal aspect of second molar and ramus is equal to or larger than the mesiodistal diameter of the crown of the third molar.

Class II. Space between distal aspect of second molar and ramus is less than the mesiodistal diameter of the crown of the third molar.

Class III. All or most of the third molar is located within the ramus.

Factor 2 — Depth of Third Molar in Bone.

Position A. Most superior aspect of third molar is level with or above the occlusal plane of the second molar.

Position B. Most superior aspect of third molar is below occlusal plane but above cervical line of the second molar.

Position C. Most superior aspect of third molar is below cervical line of the second molar.

Factor 3 — Position of Long Axis of Third Molar Relative to Long Axis of Second Molar.

This can be: Vertical, horizontal, inverted, mesioangular, distoangular, buccoangular, lingoangular.

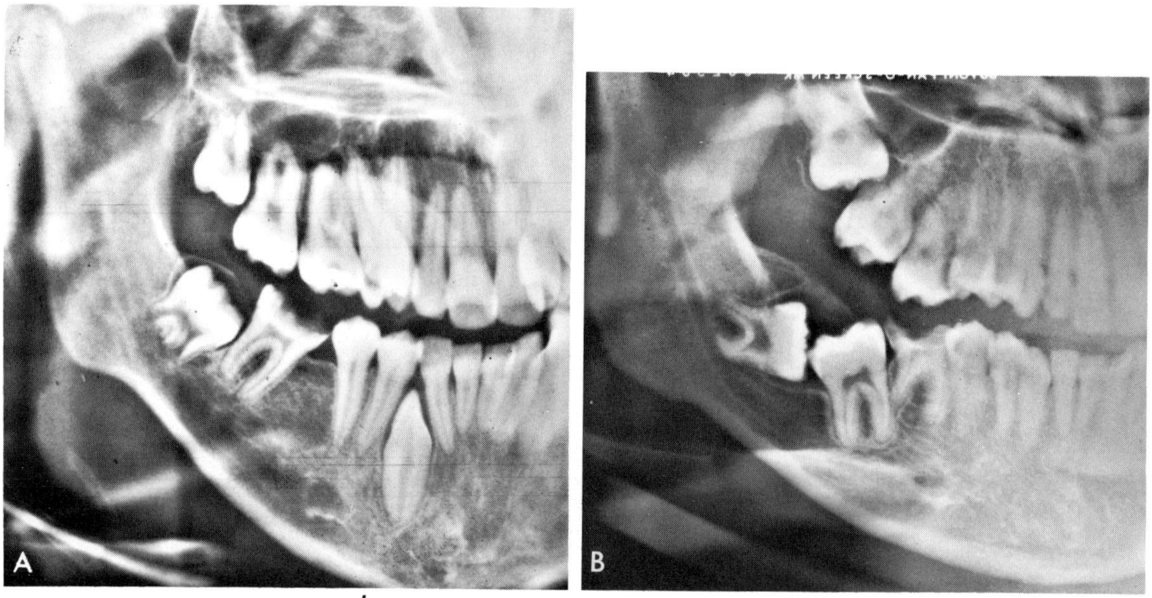

Figure 7–63. Impacted teeth. **A.** Impacted mandibular cuspid and ectopic eruption of the maxillary bicuspid. **B.** Maxillary and mandibular second and third molars.

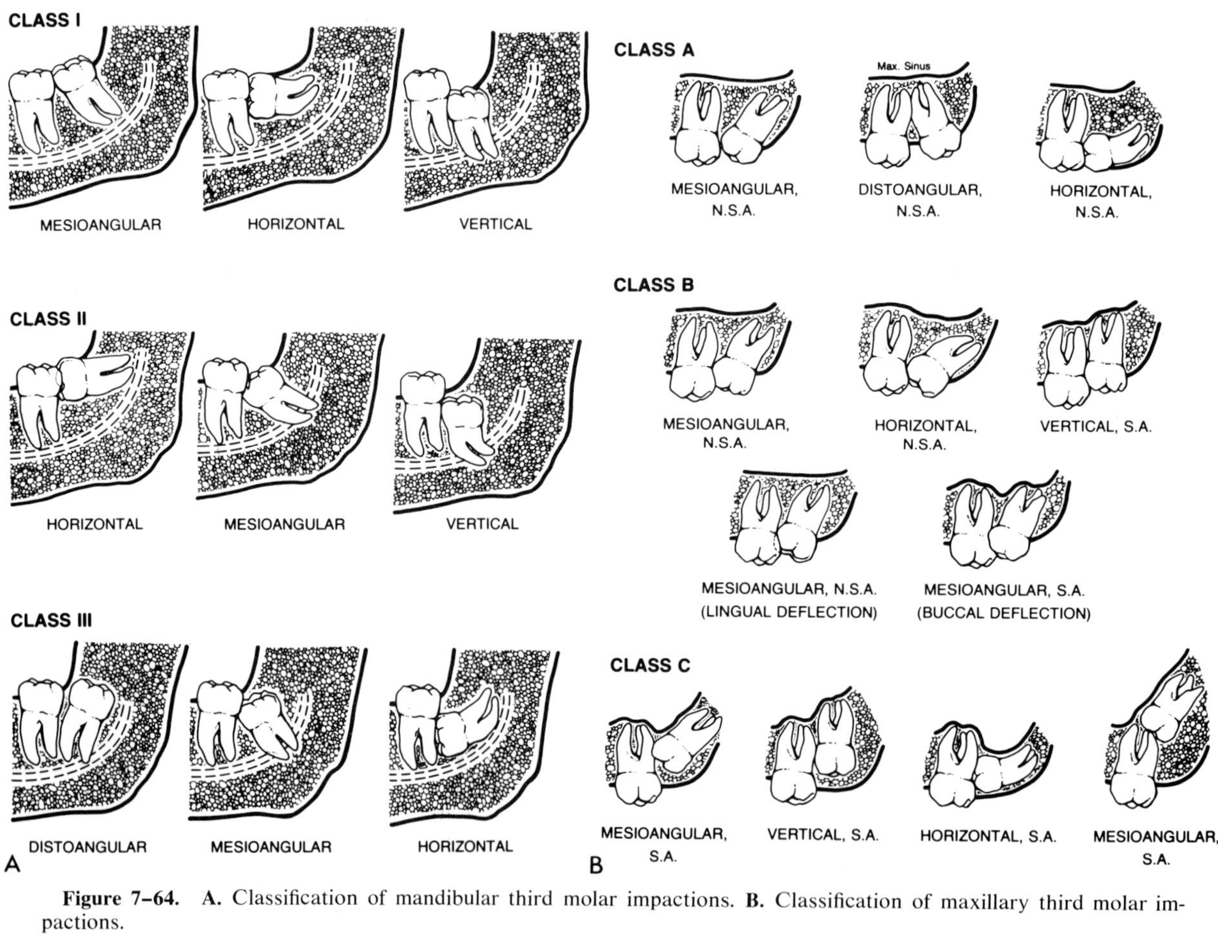

Figure 7–64. **A.** Classification of mandibular third molar impactions. **B.** Classification of maxillary third molar impactions.

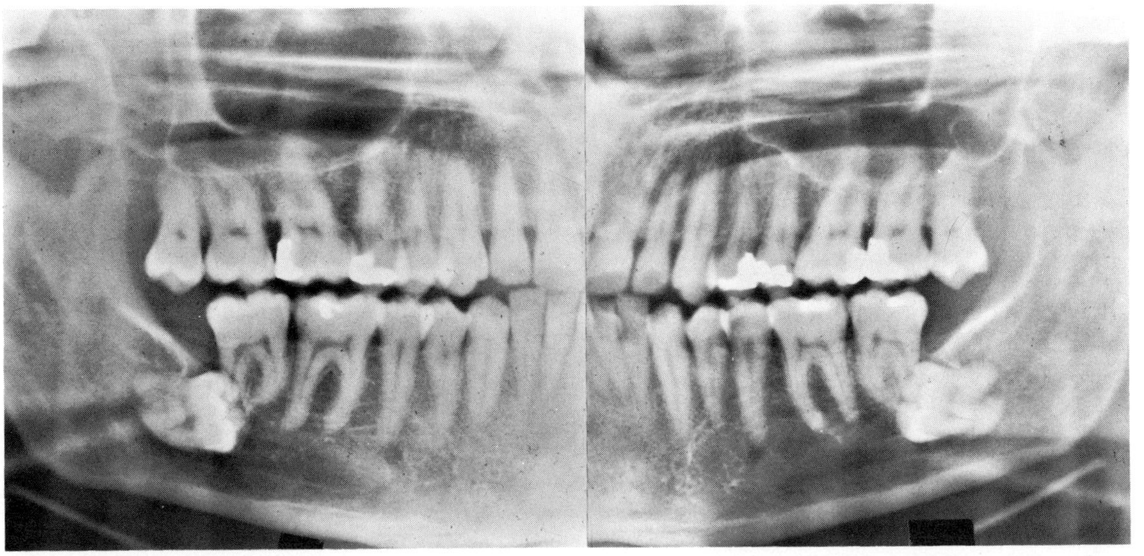

Figure 7–65. Classification of mandibular third molar impactions. Class III, position C, horizontal. (Courtesy of Dr. E. A. Scott, Garden Grove, CA.)

This may also be: Deflected buccally, deflected lingually, torsioned.

Other Factors to Note Radiographically. Dilaceration, bulbous roots, supernumerary roots, hypercementosis, ankylosis, external resorption, relationship to the mandibular canal, and the presence of associated lesions or cysts.

Maxillary impacted third molars are classified in the following manner (based on the classification of Archer).

Factor 1 — Depth of Third Molar in Bone.

CLASS A. Most inferior aspect of crown is level with or below the occlusal plane of the second molar.

CLASS B. Most inferior aspect of crown is

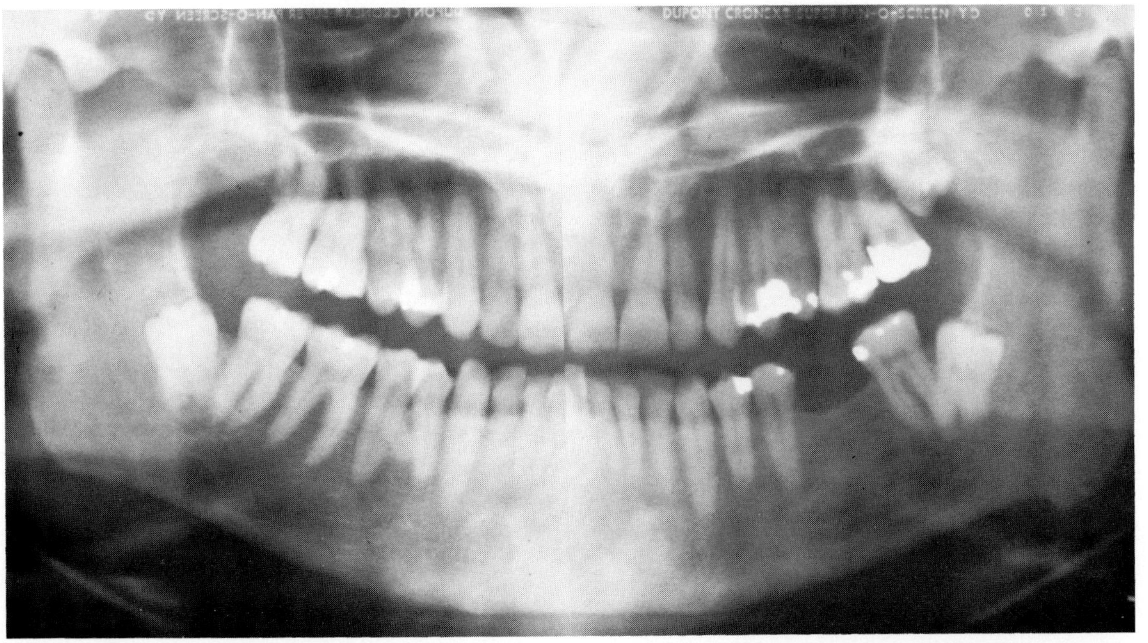

Figure 7–66. Classification of mandibular third molar impactions. Class II, position B, distoangular.

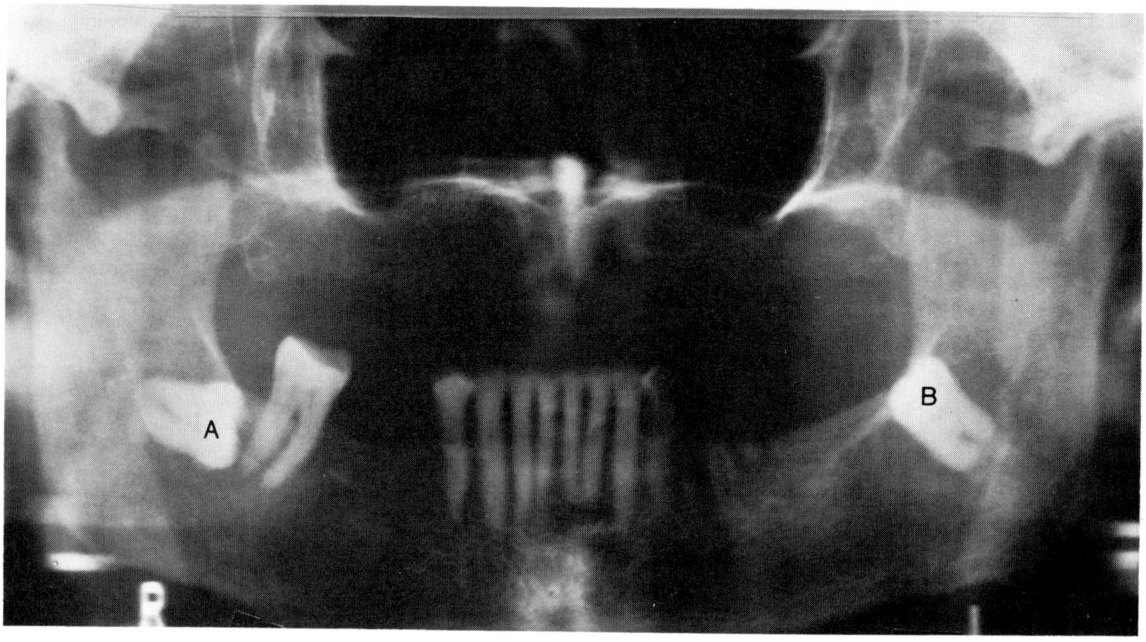

Figure 7–67. Classification of mandibular third molar impactions. A. Class III, position C, horizontal. B. Class III, mesioangular.

between the occlusal plane and cervical line of the second molar.

CLASS C. Most inferior aspect of crown is at or above the cervical line of the second molar.

Factor 2 — Position of Long Axis of Third Molar Relative to Long Axis of Second Molar.

This can be: Vertical, horizontal, mesioangular, distoangular, inverted, buccoangular, lingoangular.

This may also be: Deflected buccally, deflected lingually, torsioned.

Factor 3 — Relationship of Third Molar to Maxillary Sinus.

SINUS APPROXIMATION (SA). Thin bone or no bone between third molar and maxillary sinus.

NO SINUS APPROXIMATION (NSA). Two mm or more of bone between third molars and maxillary sinus.

Other Factors to Note Radiographically.

Dilaceration, bulbous roots, supernumerary roots, hypercementosis, ankylosis, external re-

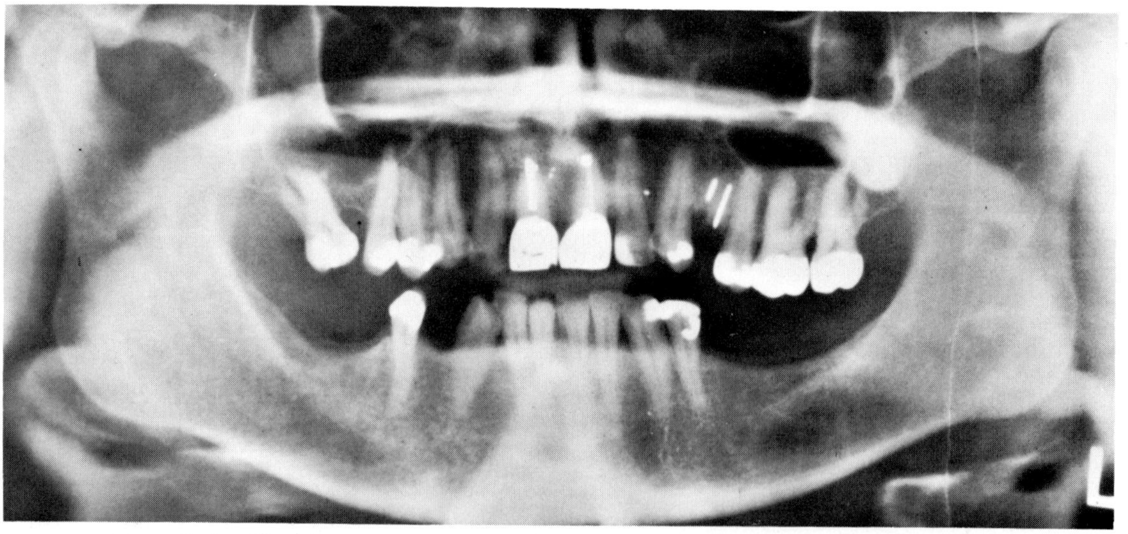

Figure 7–68. Classification of maxillary third molar impactions. Class C, distoangular, S.A.

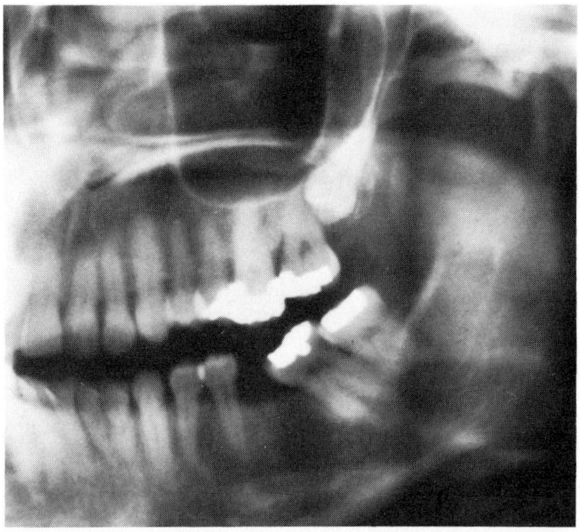

Figure 7-69. Classification of maxillary third molar impactions. Class C, mesioangular, torsioned, S.A.

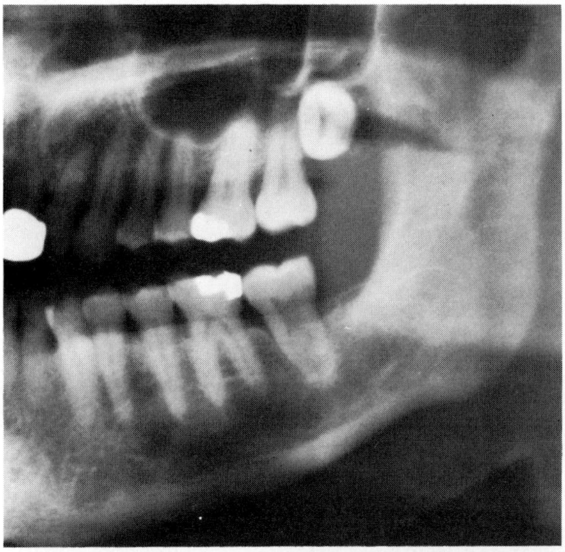

Figure 7-70. Classification of maxillary third molar impactions. Class C, buccoangular, and deflected bucally, S.A. (Further films and localization techniques were required to classify this impaction.)

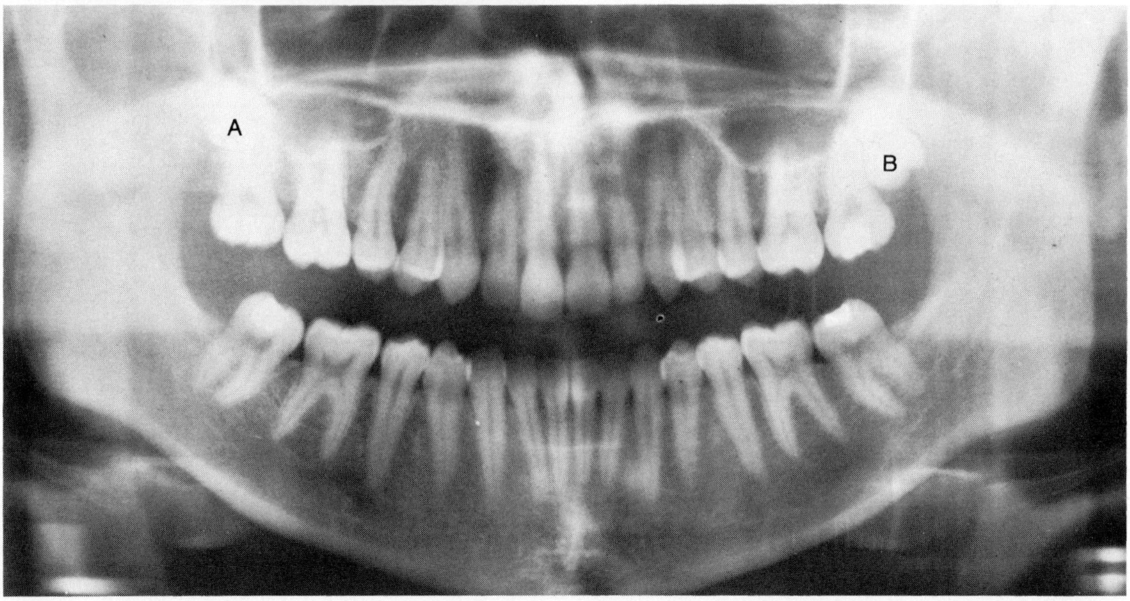

Figure 7-71. Classification of maxillary third molar impactions. A. Class C, buccoangular, S.A. B. Class C. vertical, S.A.

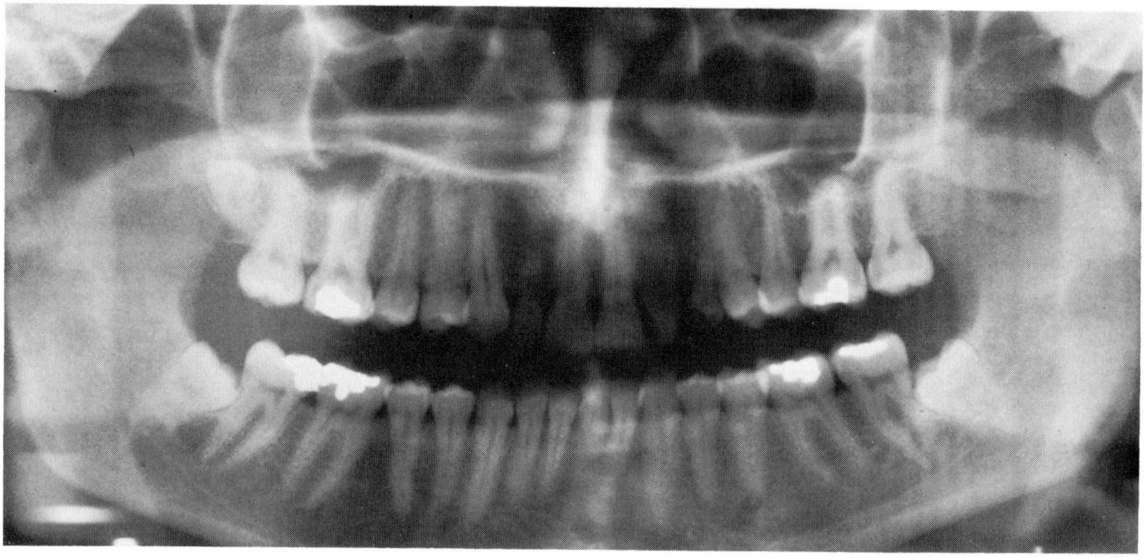

Figure 7–72. Classification of third molar impactions. Maxillary third molar: Class C, inverted, S.A., dilacerated root. Mandibular third molars: Class II, position B, mesioangular.

sorption, fusion or concrescence with roots of second molar, and the presence of associated lesions or cysts.

The radiographic description of any impacted or embedded tooth should include its position relative to adjacent teeth, its relationship to other anatomic structures, alterations in morphology, and the presence of other pathologic conditions. Some conditions that tend to be associated with impacted teeth include Pindborg tumor; odontoma; squamous odontogenic tumor; adenomatoid odontogenic tumor; follicular (dentigerous) cyst and its sequelae, such as ameloblastoma, squamous cell carcinoma, and mucoepidermoid carcinoma; odontogenic keratocyst; and the Gorlin cyst.

DELAYED ERUPTION

BRIEF OVERVIEW

Delayed eruption occurs when a tooth or teeth fail to erupt on time. Eruption tables are helpful but not diagnostic. The diagnosis of delayed eruption is based on the findings of clinically missing teeth and the radiographic evidence. One or several teeth may be affected, or the condition may be generalized. Delayed eruption may be associated with the following:

1. Local Conditions. These include crowding; impacted and embedded teeth; supernumerary teeth; the presence of local pathologic conditions, particularly Pindborg tumor, odontomas, squamous odontogenic tumor, adenomatoid odontogenic tumor, follicular cyst, odontogenic keratocyst, Gorlin cyst, and monostotic fibrous dysplasia; and therapeutic irradiation of the jaws during odontogenesis.

2. Defective or Anomalous Teeth Associated with Delayed Eruption. These include permanent teeth in amelogenesis imperfecta and regional odontodysplasia.

3. Syndromes, Dysplasias, or Conditions with Delayed Eruption as a Feature. Delayed eruption may be idiopathic, or it may be due to the presence of lesions, the absence of some teeth, or a variety of other known or postulated causes including Gardner's syndrome, cleidocranial dysplasia, cherubism, neurofibromatosis, osteopetrosis, craniometaphyseal dysplasia, mongolism, progeria, focal dermal hypoplasia syndrome, hereditary anhidrotic ectodermal dysplasia, incontinentia pigmenti, and chondroectodermal dysplasia.

4. Systemic or Metabolic Disorders Associated with Generalized Delayed Eruption. These include vitamin D–deficient rickets, vitamin D–resistant rickets, and hypoparathyroidism and its variants, hypopituitarism and hypothyroidism.

RADIOGRAPHIC FEATURES (Fig. 7–73)

These include inconsistent degree of eruption relative to the child's age, inconsistent pattern of eruption, significant difference between the affected tooth and its contralateral twin, root

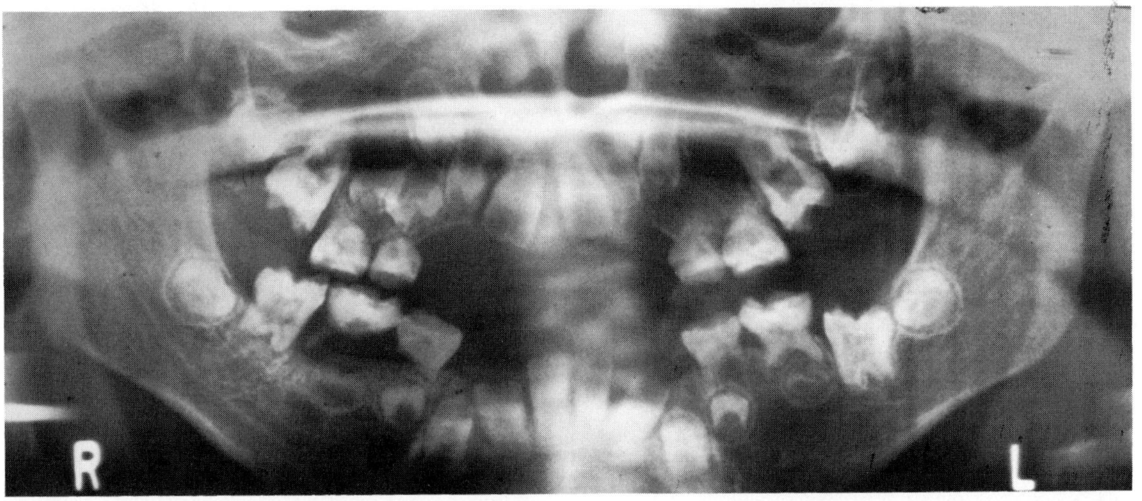

Figure 7–73. Delayed eruption. This 10-year-old girl presented with delayed eruption as her only complaint and was found to have pseudo-pseudohypoparathyroidism. Note the hypoplastic, ghostlike teeth.

formation that exceeds two-thirds of its length prior to eruption, and complete root formation with apex closure prior to eruption. Additionally, the presence of physical barriers should be noted as well as any of the conditions previously outlined, which may be either diagnosed or suspected on the basis of the radiographic findings.

ERUPTION PROBLEMS THAT ARE EARLY RADIOGRAPHIC INDICATIONS OF CROWDING IN THE PERMANENT ARCH

BRIEF OVERVIEW

These inconspicuous radiographic signs have been discussed in some detail by Berlocher and Mueller. The findings are seen on the radiographs and may indeed be the first signs of impending crowding problems. Some of the changes indicate a genetic space deficiency, whereas others indicate an acquired space loss. Once recognized, these problems are managed by space supervision, serial extraction, or space regaining. Mixed dentition analysis (space analysis) and cephalometric analysis should precede treatment.

RADIOGRAPHIC FEATURES

The radiographic signs of a genetic space deficiency include relatively larger tooth size; moderate to severe crowding of the permanent incisors; ectopic resorption of the primary cuspid roots on eruption of the permanent lateral incisors; ectopic eruption with lack of resorption of the primary root, especially in the mandibular anterior area; ectopic eruption with resorption of the adjacent tooth, especially the permanent first molars, which causes resorption of the distal root of the primary second molars; and ectopic eruption. The radiographic signs of an acquired space loss include gross interproximal caries with loss of space and premature extraction of primary teeth.

ALTERATIONS OF THE JAWS AND FACIAL BONES

BRIEF OVERVIEW

There are a number of conditions in this category. Owing to the clinical features of most of these disorders or their development at an early age, they are not usually discovered on panoramic films. Panoramic films are excellent when the relative size of structures is to be studied or when a comparison of the right and left sides is desirable. Some of these conditions include **facial hemihypertrophy, facial hemiatrophy, micrognathia, macrognathia, cleft palate,** and **unusual defects** such as **agenesis** or **twinning of the jaws.** A common condition whose only clinical manifestation may be a large diastema between the maxillary central incisors is the **median maxillary anterior alveolar cleft,** which is unrelated to cleft palate and is of no significance, except that orthodontics may be contraindicated.

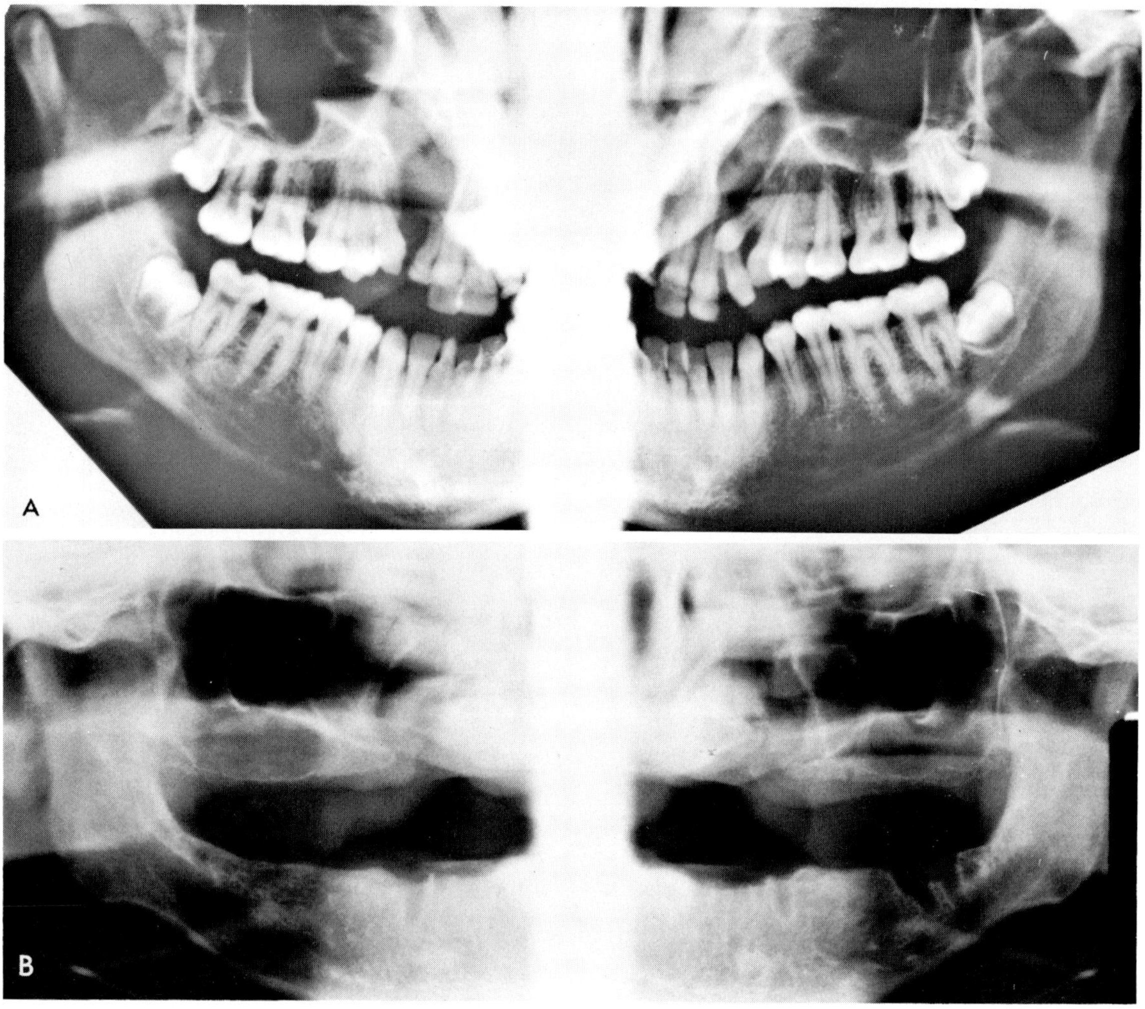

Figure 7–74A and **B.** Bilateral cleft palate.

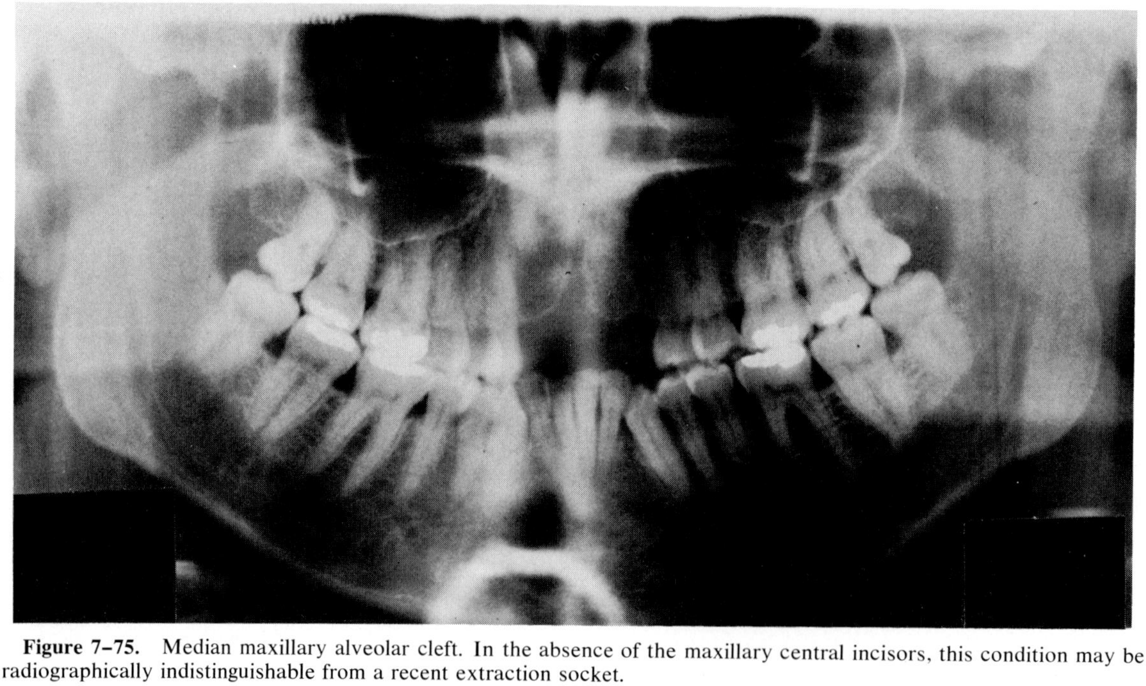

Figure 7–75. Median maxillary alveolar cleft. In the absence of the maxillary central incisors, this condition may be radiographically indistinguishable from a recent extraction socket.

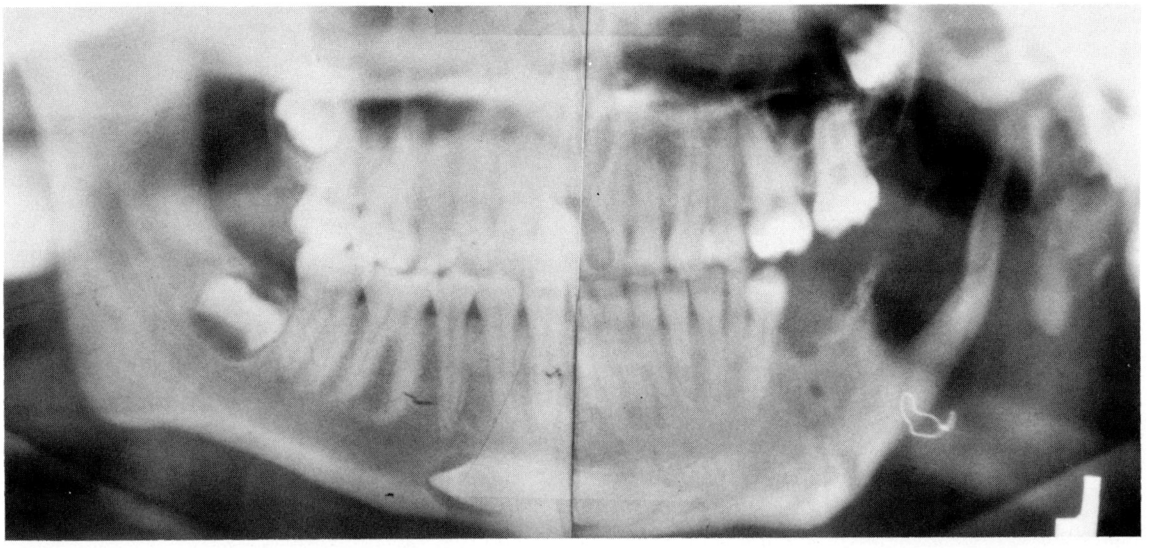

Figure 7–76. Hypoplasia of the left ramus; agenesis of the left condyle; hypodontia of the permanent teeth in the region.

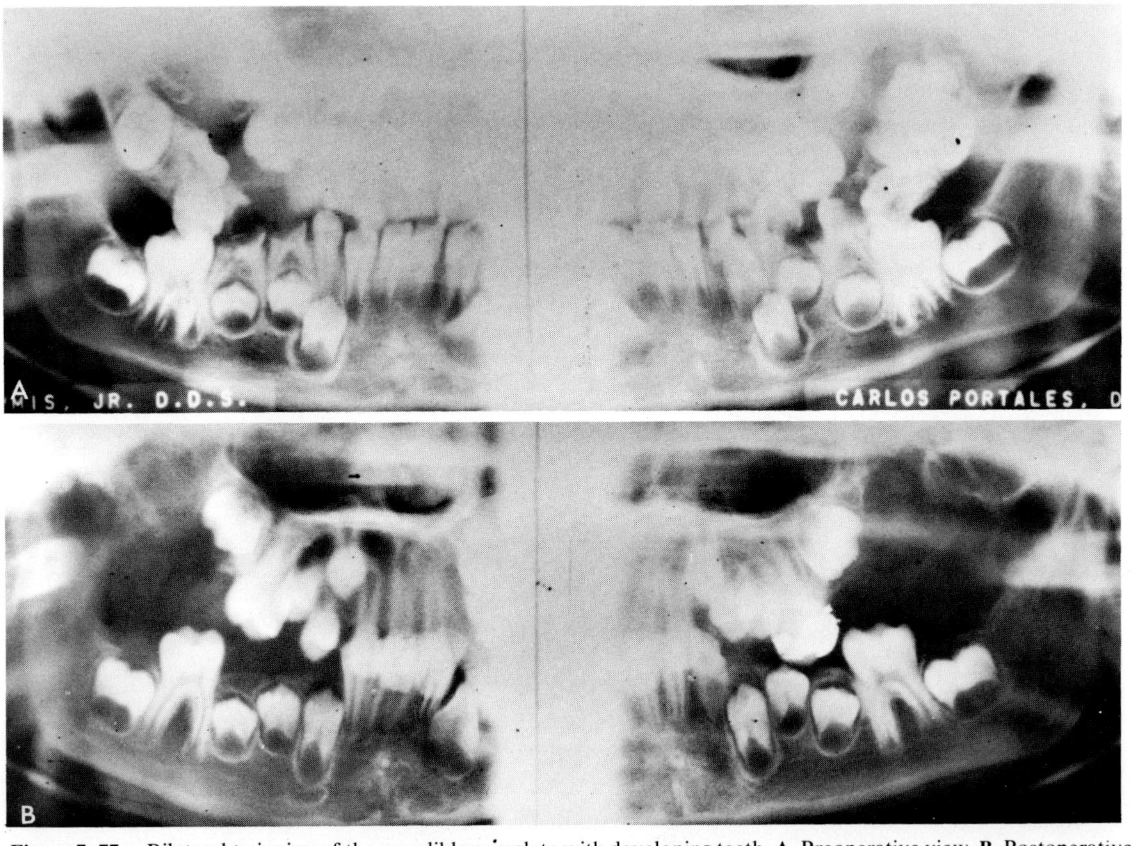

Figure 7–77. Bilateral twinning of the mandible complete with developing teeth. **A.** Preoperative view. **B.** Postoperative view. (Figure 7–77 courtesy of Drs. Frank Sammis Jr. and Carlos Portales, San Antonio, TX.)

RADIOGRAPHIC FEATURES (Figs. 7–74 to 7–77)

Palatal clefts may be unilateral or bilateral and may also involve the lip, soft palate, and uvula. Although the cleft may have been corrected surgically, it may be visible on the panoramic film and should not be mistaken for a pathologic lesion or fracture. Radiographically, cleft palate may be associated with a very tiny lateral incisor, a larger peg lateral incisor, a deformed lateral incisor, or a supernumerary tooth.

The median maxillary anterior cleft may be difficult to visualize on panoramic films, as the anterior area on these films is not particularly sharp. The presence of a diastema between the maxillary central incisors should alert the clinician that such a defect may be present. A diastema may, however, not always be present. This defect should be distinguished from an extraction socket or an incisive canal cyst.

REFERENCES

Reference Texts

Dixter, C., Langlais, R. P., and Lichty, G. C.: **Exercises in Dental Radiology,** Vol. 3, Pediatric Radiographic Interpretation. Philadelphia; W. B. Saunders, 1980, pp. 63–70, 216–221, 260.

Eversole, L. R.: **Clinical Outline of Oral Pathology.** Philadelphia; Lea & Febiger, 1978, pp. 255–277.

Gorlin, R. J., and Goldman, H. M.: **Thoma's Oral Pathology,** 6th Edition. St. Louis; C. V. Mosby, 1970, pp. 112–120.

Pindborg, J. J.: **Pathology of the Dental Hard Tissues.** Philadelphia; W. B. Saunders, 1970, pp. 51–54, 65, 77–94.

Shafer, W. G., Hine, M. K., and Levy, B. M.: **A Textbook of Oral Pathology,** 3rd Edition. Philadelphia; W. B. Saunders, 1974, pp. 14–17, 34–66, 493.

Stafne, E. C., and Gibilisco, J. A.: **Oral Radiographic Diagnosis,** 4th Edition. Philadelphia, W. B. Saunders, 1975, pp. 16–38.

Worth, H. M.: **Principles and Practice of Oral Radiologic Interpretation.** Chicago; Year Book Medical Publishers, 1963, pp. 206–207.

Selected References

Congleton, J., and Burkes, E. J., Jr.: Amelogenesis imperfecta with taurodontism. **Oral Surg. 48**:540, 1979.

Gardner, D. G., and Girgis, S. S.: Talon cusps: A dental anomaly in the Rubinstein-Taybi syndrome. **Oral Surg. 47**:519, 1979.

Gier, R. E., and Fast, T. B.: Median maxillary anterior alveolar cleft. **Oral Surg. 24**:496, 1967.

Gotoh, T., Kawahara, K., Imai, K., Kishi, K., and Fujiki, Y.: Clinical and radiographic study of dens invaginatus. **Oral Surg. 48**:88, 1979.

Gotoh, T., Kawahara, K., Kondo, T., Imai, K., and Fujiki, Y.: Clinical and radiographic study of dens evaginatus. **J. Dent.-Max.-Fac. Radiol. 8**:78, 1969.

Jedrychowski, J. R., and Duperon, D.: Childhood hypophosphatasia with oral manifestations. **J. Oral Med. 34**:18, 1979.

Jorgenson, R. L., Levin, L. S., Cross, H. E., Yoder, F., and Kelly, T. E.: The Rieger s
Gen. **2**:307, 1978.

Jorgenson, R. J., and Warsaw, R. W.: Dental abnormalities in the tricho-dento-osseous syndrome. **Oral Surg. 36**:693, 1973.

Koch, P. E., and Hammer, W. B.: Cleidocranial dysostosis: Review of the literature and report of a case. **J. Oral Surg. 36**:39, 1978.

McLarty, E. L., Giansanti, J. S., and Hibbard, E. D.: X-linked hypomaturation type of amelogenesis imperfecta exhibiting lyonization in affected females. **Oral Surg. 36**:678, 1973.

Melnick, M., Eastman, J. R., Goldblatt, L. I., Michaud, M., and Bixler, D.: Dentin dysplasia, Type II: A rare autosomal dominant disorder. **Oral Surg. 44**:592, 1977.

Morris, C. R., Marano, P. D., Swinley, D. C., and Runco, J. G.: Abnormalities noted on panoramic radiographs. **Oral Surg. 28**:772, 1969.

Nortjé, C. J., Farman, A. G., Thomas, C. J., and Watermeyer, C. J. J.: X-linked hypohydrotic ectodermal dysplasia—An unusual prosthetic problem. **J. Pros. Dent. 40**:137, 1978.

Perl, T., and Farman, A. G.: Radicular (Type I) dentin dysplasia. **Oral Surg. 43**:748, 1977.

Shields, E. D., Bixler, D., and El-Kafrawy, A. M.: A proposed classification for heritable human dentine defects with a description of a new entity. **Arch. Oral Biol. 18**:543, 1973.

Shifman, A., and Buchner, A.: Taurodontism: Report of sixteen cases in Israel. **Oral Surg 41**:400, 1976.

Shifman, A., and Chanannel, I.: Prevalence of taurodontism found in radiographic dental examination of 1200 young adult Israeli patients. **Community Dent. Oral Epidemiol. 6**:200, 1978.

Vasilakus, G. J., Nygaard, V. K., and DiPalma, D. M.: Vitamin D resistant rickets: A review and case report of an adolescent boy with a history of dental problems. **J. Oral Med 35**:19, 1980.

Wesley, R. K., Wysocki, G. P., Mimtz, S. M., and Jackson, J.: Dentin dysplasia Type 1. **Oral Surg. 41**:516, 1976.

Witkop, C. J., Brearley, L. J., and Gentry, W. C.: Hypoplastic enamel, onycholysis, and hypohidrosis inherited as an autosomal dominant trait: A review of ectodermal dysplasia syndromes. **Oral Surg. 39**:71, 1975.

Chapter 8

Dental Caries and Pulpal and Periodontal Disease

INTRODUCTION

The panoramic radiograph is not an effective substitute for intraoral films in the detection of dental caries and early periapical and periodontal disease. Panoramic films do not have the image clarity required to adequately examine these diseases. However, the panoramic film does reveal a larger area of the maxilla and mandible than intraoral films at a decreased radiation exposure to the patient. In the detection of dental caries and periapical and periodontal disease, only gross pathologic changes resulting from these diseases will be revealed on the panoramic radiograph. It functions best as a survey film to pinpoint areas of greatest concern and further study.

When the panoramic radiograph is supplemented by posterior bitewings, a radiographic survey with a broadened scope of examination (panoramic radiography) and the image clarity (posterior bitewings) necessary to read interproximal caries and interalveolar bone crest resorption in the posterior regions of the jaws can be obtained. Of course, when using such a survey, single periapical radiographs should be ordered at the discretion of the dentist, depending on the results of the clinical examination and the interpretation of the panoramic radiograph and posterior bitewings. Sometimes the examination indicates the need for a complete radiographic survey; in other cases, only a few single periapical radiographs are needed to complete the diagnosis.

The panoramic radiograph will, in most cases, alert the dentist to chronic periapical disease; however, a periapical radiograph is required for definitive examination of the area. There are many times when the panoramic radiograph will not reveal changes in the interdental alveolar bone as a result of periodontal disease. The clinical examination and history will, in most cases, indicate to the dentist that a periapical radiograph of these regions is needed.

If the patient has periodontal disease or multiple dental problems, a complete intraoral periapical survey with posterior bitewings is the radiographic survey of choice. The periapical films should be taken utilizing the paralleling or right-angle technique to accurately assess the position of the marginal bone in relation to the teeth, dental caries, interproximal restorations, and the true relationships of anatomic structures. A panoramic film may be ordered to supplement the intraoral survey. A larger view of the bone beyond the apices of the teeth is sometimes desired. The intraoral survey will not reveal the entire osseous state of the jaws or those pathologic conditions situated at some distance from the teeth.

RADIOLOGIC INTERPRETATION OF CARIES

Dental caries or tooth decay is a pathologic process of localized destruction of the teeth by microorganisms. For caries to occur, a susceptible host (particularly the saliva and teeth), cariogenic microflora (*Streptococcus mutans* and others), and suitable substrate (diet) must be present for a suitable length of time. Dental caries is considered a chronic disease in man because it develops over a period of months or years.

The intraoral radiographs (the bitewing and the periapical radiograph taken by the paralleling technique) are indispensable in the detection of interproximal caries. Although many carious lesions are easily accessible for examination by the explorer and mirror, a great percentage of them, especially the interproximal lesions, cannot be readily detected by routine procedures.

Several studies have shown that bitewing radiographs are an important aid in the interpretation of interproximal caries (Dunning and Ferguson; Haugejorden and Slack; Hansen). In 1946, Dunning and Ferguson found that the detection of posterior interproximal dental caries increased by 215 per cent when posterior bitewing radiographs were used in addition to the clinical examination. In a recent investigation by Hansen, four times as many posterior interproximal carious lesions were found when posterior bitewings were used as compared with the number of lesions found by clinical methods alone. In the same study, the panoramic radiograph was found to be of little value in the detection of interproximal caries. The bitewing radiograph demonstrated 79.5 per cent of the carious lesions to be diagnosed, whereas the panoramic radiograph disclosed only 33.0 per cent of the carious lesions. Figure 8–1 illustrates why it is important to supplement the panoramic radiograph with bitewings for posterior interproximal caries detection. These findings substantiate a previous study by Hurlburt and Wuehrmann, who found that the panoramic radiograph is ineffective in the detection of interproximal caries.

Since dental caries is essentially a process of decalcification, a certain percentage of calcium and phosphorus must be destroyed before the decreased density can be visualized on the radiograph. It has been estimated that bone has to be decalcified by approximately 50 per cent before a radiolucency will be revealed on the radiograph (Early, Razzak, and Dodee).

The radiographic appearance of caries will be discussed according to its location on the tooth: (1) proximal; (2) occlusal; (3) facial/lingual; (4) root or cemental; and (5) recurrent or secondary (immediate vicinity of preexisting restoration).

PROXIMAL CARIOUS LESIONS

The proximal carious lesion is the most easily recognized lesion on the dental radiograph. This is probably due to the fact that there is less volume of normal tooth structure through which the x-rays must penetrate to reach the carious lesion on the proximal surface than on the other tooth surfaces. Proximal caries usually begins just below the contact point and appears clinically as a chalky white spot that becomes slightly roughened owing to early demineralization. It has a classic V-shaped appearance, with the base of the triangle at the surface of the tooth and, usually, a rounded apex toward the dentino-enamel junction. No possible reason can be given for this configuration except that the carious process tends to follow the course of the enamel rods, which are usually oriented at right angles to the dentino-enamel junction. Since the proximal surface of the teeth is usually convex, the enamel rods then tend to converge at the dentino-enamel junction, which, in turn, produces the classic triangular or V-shaped radiographic appearance. However, there are exceptions to the rule, and many different shapes and sizes of proximal enamel carious lesions may be seen radiographically.

As the carious lesion reaches the dentino-enamel junction, it usually first spreads laterally, and then tends to proceed toward the pulp following the dentinal tubules, forming another triangular radiolucency with its base at the dentino-enamel junction (Fig. 8–3).

There is a need in private practice and teaching clinics for a scoring code to classify the radiographically discernible proximal carious lesions. Several systems have been developed for clinical research of various caries inhibitory agents (Wagg; Zamir and associates; Haugejorden and Slack).

Only by the use of a written description of each stage of caries penetration of the proximal surface can the clinician properly record a baseline from which he can determine whether the lesion has progressed or stabilized from one office visit to the next. Not all radiographically detected early or incipient proximal carious lesions should be restored. The decision to restore a tooth depends on the results of the clinical examination as well as many other factors. The clinician may want to institute preventative caries control measures rather than restorative procedures for the small carious lesion. At any rate, a radiographic caries classification system is shown in Figure 8–4 (as suggested by Haugejorden and Slack). In Figure 8–5, examples of each of the penetration stages of proximal caries are illustrated.

The factors responsible for variation in individual susceptibility to caries are not clearly defined (Mandel). This is demonstrated in a study by Shannon, Gibson, and Terry. In their study of 5,298 Air Force recruits (average age of 20, all with rather homogenous backgrounds and environments), 1 per cent were found to be virtually caries immune, and 5 per cent had rampant caries. The middle range of recruits followed a rather typical distribution curve. The radiographic appearances of several cases of rampant caries are shown in Figure 8–6.

OCCLUSAL CARIES

On the occlusal surface of the teeth, the carious process usually begins in the pits and fissures. Enamel caries that begins in the pits and fissures takes on an appearance opposite that of proximal enamel caries in that the apex of the triangle is toward the outer surface of the tooth and the base of the triangle is at the dentino-enamel junction. The occlusal carious lesion is usually not seen radiographically until it has reached the dentino-enamel junction and spread in all directions. This is due to the great mass of enamel tissue superimposed over the occlusal enamel lesion. Only when the carious lesion has reached the dentin can occlusal caries be seen on the radiograph. Usually, occlusal caries is first seen as a dark radiolucent line or area just under the enamel cap of the occlusal surface (Fig. 8–7). The radiograph is not a reliable diagnostic aid for the detection of occlusal caries. It can only alert the clinician to occlusal surfaces that should be examined more thoroughly. A mirror and a sharp explorer are much better diagnostic aids in the detection of occlusal caries.

FACIAL AND LINGUAL CARIES

Caries on the facial and lingual surfaces of the teeth begins in either the pits and fissures or the cervical region of the tooth. Caries developing in pits on the facial and lingual surfaces appears on the radiograph as round dots on the tooth surface. Cervical caries extends laterally toward the proximal surfaces, forming a typical crescent-shaped cavity. However, the cavity may also be round or oval in shape. It almost always seems to be a wide-open cavity dissimilar to that found in proximal and occlusal

Text continued on page 216

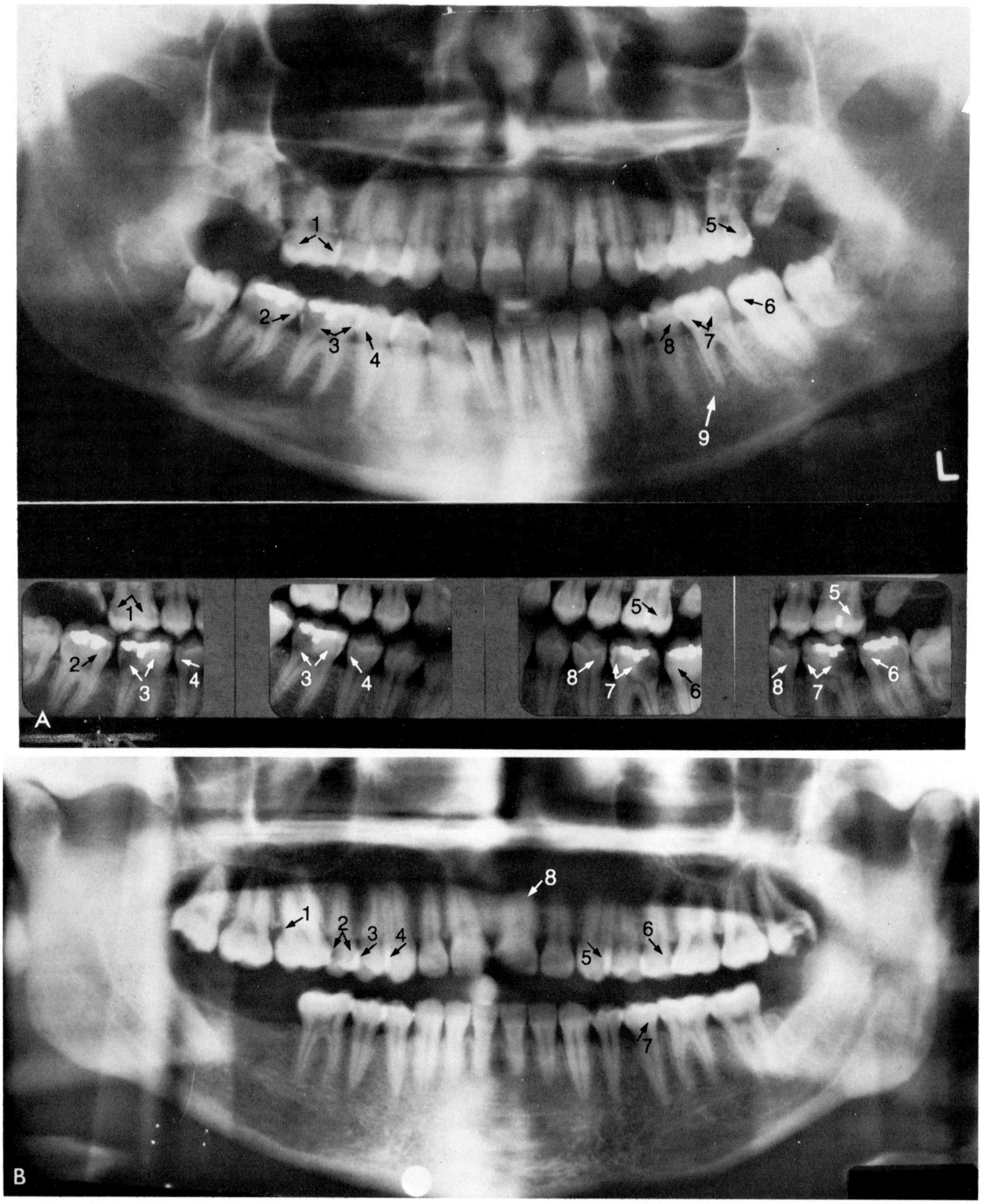

Figure 8–1. Dental caries comparison. **A.** Radiographic appearance of caries on panoramic and bitewing radiographs. Compare the following carious lesions of the same patient in teeth identified as (1), (2), (3), (4), (5), (6), (7), and (8). It is evident from this example that the panoramic radiograph cannot be solely relied upon to reveal interproximal dental caries; the bitewing radiograph is essential in the diagnosis of dental caries. Also, note the thickened periodontal space at (9) (the panoramic radiograph), a sequela of the large carious lesion in the tooth. **B.** Panoramic radiograph of patient with dental caries and periapical pathology of maxillary central incisor (8). (See **C** and **D**).

Illustration continued on opposite page

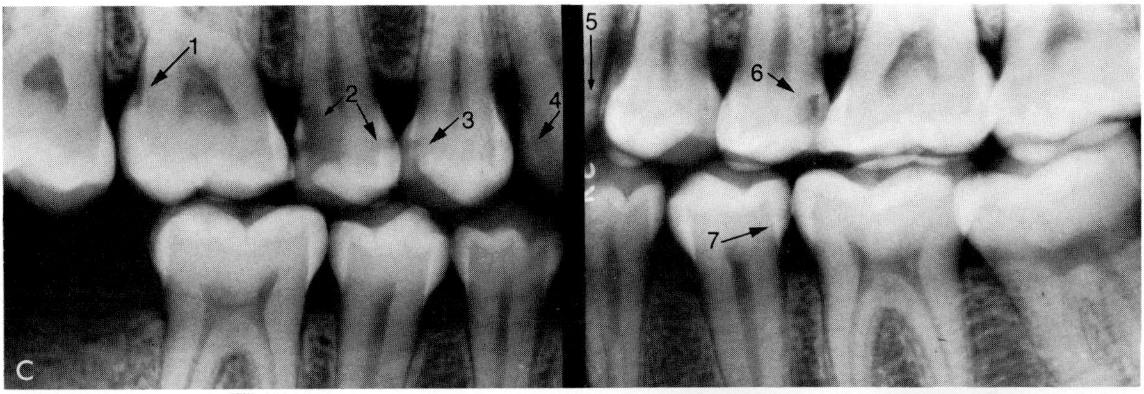

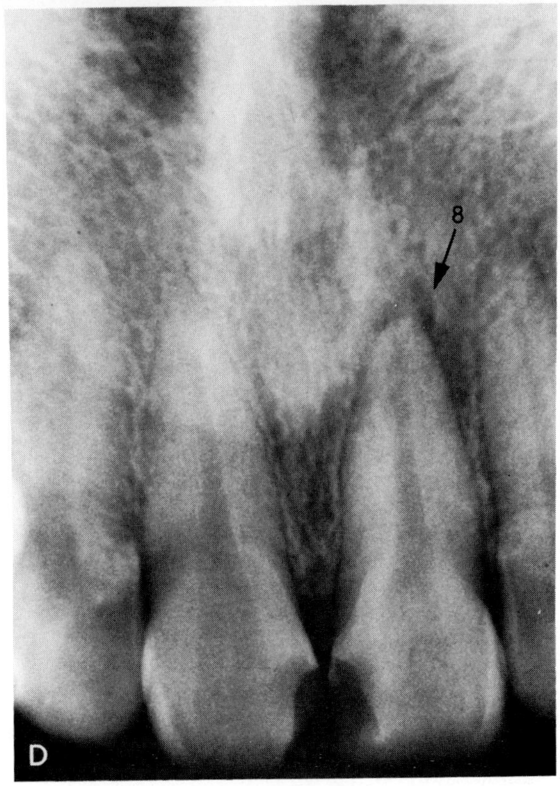

Figure 8–1 *Continued.* **C.** Bitewing radiograph of patient in **B.** Compare the cervical burnout (1) in both radiographs as well as dental caries at (2), (3), (4), (5), (6), and (7). **D.** Periapical radiograph of patient in **B.** Compare periapical lesion at (8) with that in **B. B, C,** and **D** show the need to supplement the panoramic radiograph with bitewing and indicated periapical radiographs.

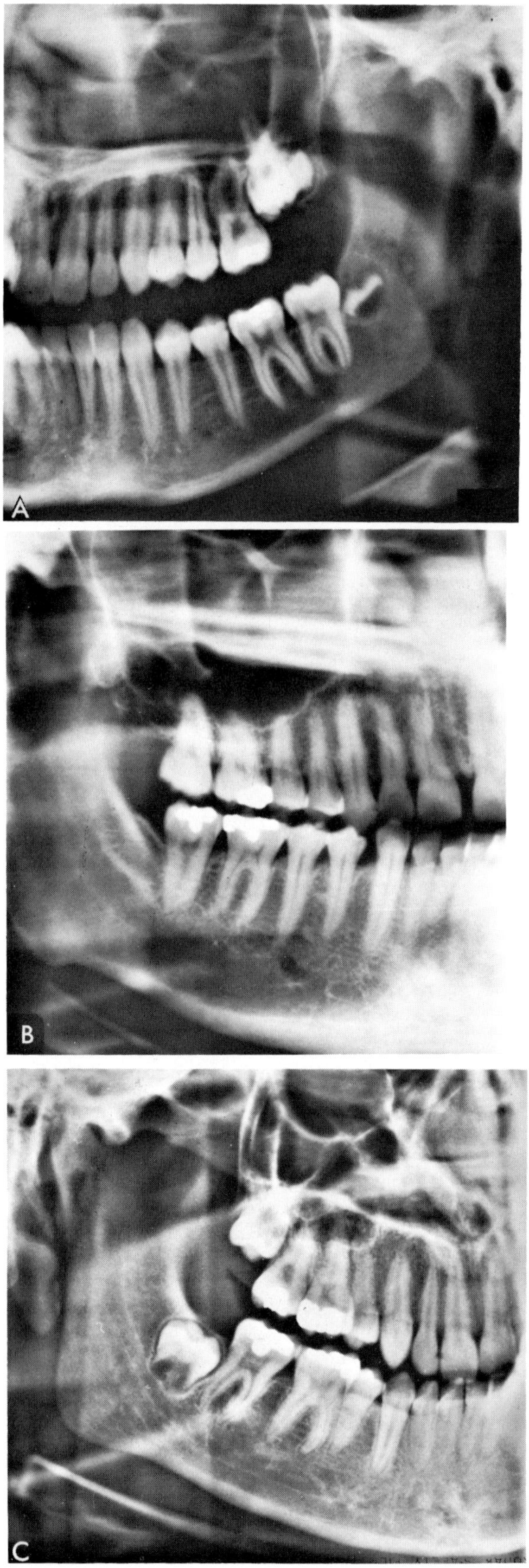

Figure 8–2. **A.** Note triangular or V-shaped caries in distal surfaces of maxillary and mandibular second bicuspids. **B.** Note triangular or V-shaped caries in mesial surface of maxillary cuspid. **C.** Note triangular or V-shaped caries in mesial surface of maxillary lateral incisor.

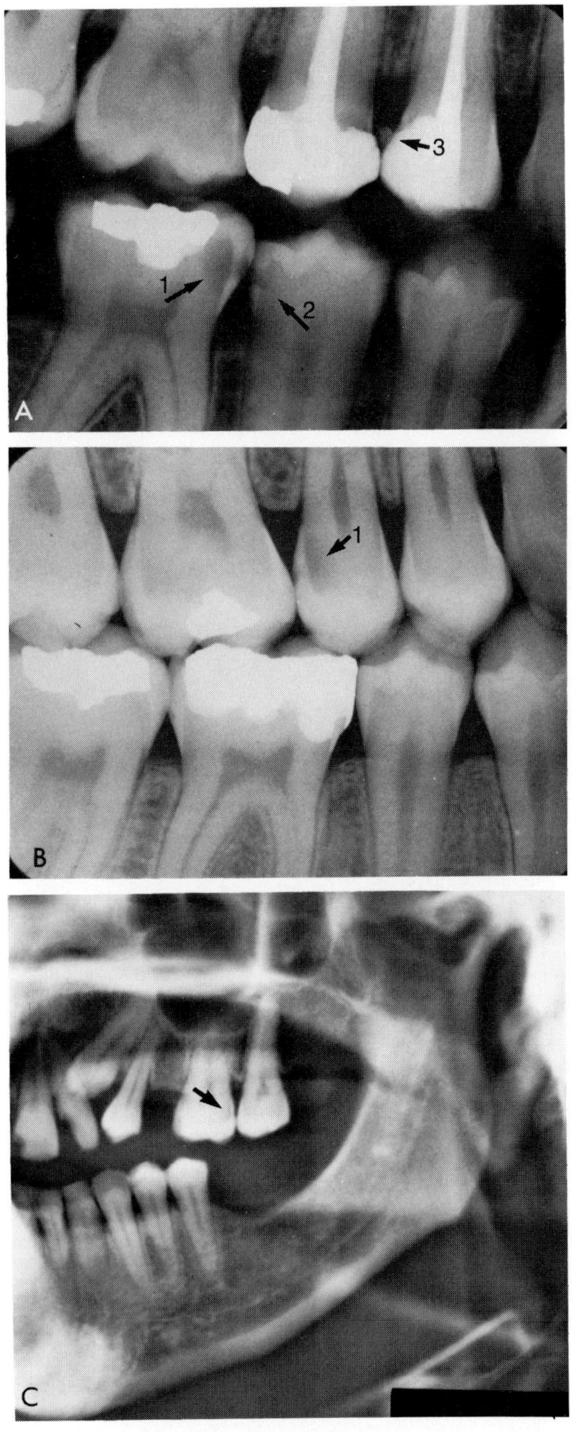

Figure 8–3. **A.** Dentinal caries spreads laterally, first along the dentino-enamel junction, and then tends to follow the dentinal tubules to the pulp. Notice the dentinal caries at (1) and (2). (3) denotes interproximal calculus. **B.** Dentinal caries can be diagnosed when there is a small radiolucency revealed in the enamel presented with seemingly normal enamel and an ill-defined radiolucency in the dentin. This can be explained by the ratio of normal tooth to carious tooth tissue, which varies in different areas of the tooth. In the area where this ratio is high, the x rays become attenuated so that the carious lesion will not be reproduced on the radiograph. This phenomenon is illustrated at (1) in the bitewing radiograph. **C.** Observe the dentinal caries spread at dentino-enamel junction of maxillary first molar (arrow).

Classification of Radiographic Caries

C-1. Enamel caries *less* than 1/2 way through enamel (sometimes called incipient caries). Do not record these lesions if doubtful of their existence.

C-2. Enamel caries penetrating at least 1/2 way through enamel, but *NOT* involving dentino-enamel junction.

C-3. Caries of enamel and dentine definitely at or through the dentino-enamel junction extending less than 1/2 way to pulp cavity.

C-4. Caries of enamel and dentine penetrating more than 1/2 way dentine toward pulp cavity.

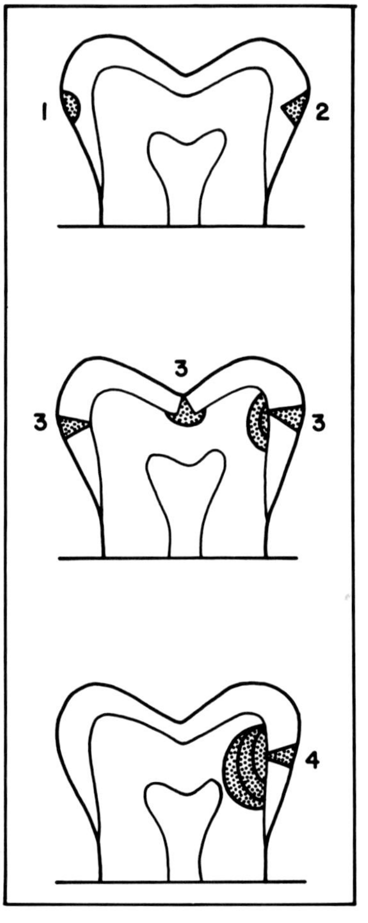

Record the lesser score if there is doubt concerning depth of lesion.

Since occlusal caries is first seen radiographically when the caries penetrates the dentine, a score of C-3 or C-4 is given for occlusal caries.

Enamel caries of C-1 and C-2 cannot be scored if overlapping of interproximal surfaces occurs.

Figure 8–4. A radiographic classification of dental caries according to depth of penetration.

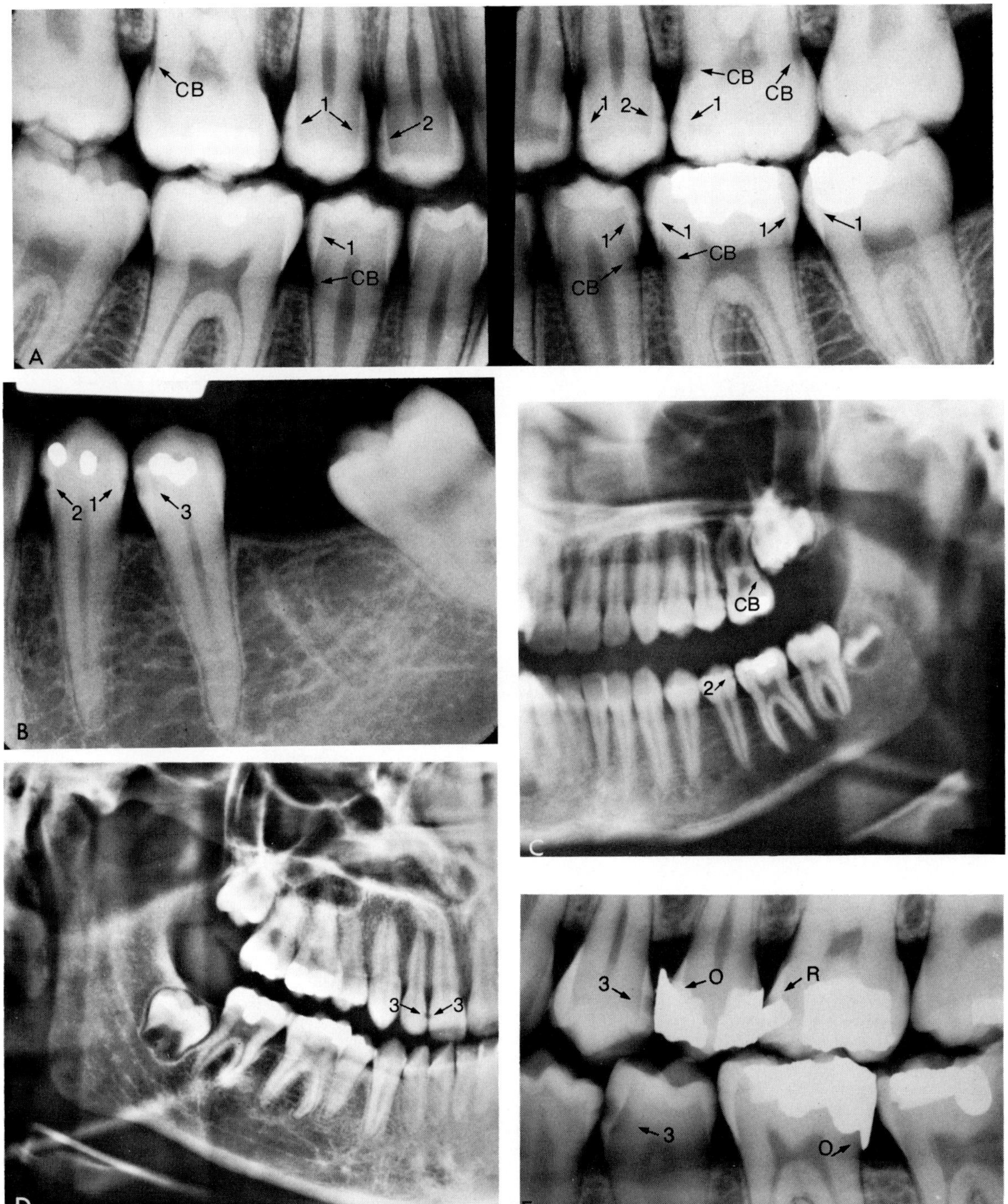

Figure 8–5. Examples of caries penetration. Depth of penetration is indicated by classification number on each radiograph. **A.** Bitewing radiographs (left and right). (CB) = cervical burnout. **B.** Periapical radiograph of mandibular bicuspids. **C.** Panorex radiograph. Possible complex odontoma involving maxillary second molar region. Class 2 caries in mandibular second bicuspid. **D.** Panorex radiograph. Class 3 caries in anterior teeth. This radiograph illustrates the difficulty in determining when caries has reached the dentino-enamel junction. **E.** Posterior bitewings. (R) = recurrent caries. (O) = overhang.

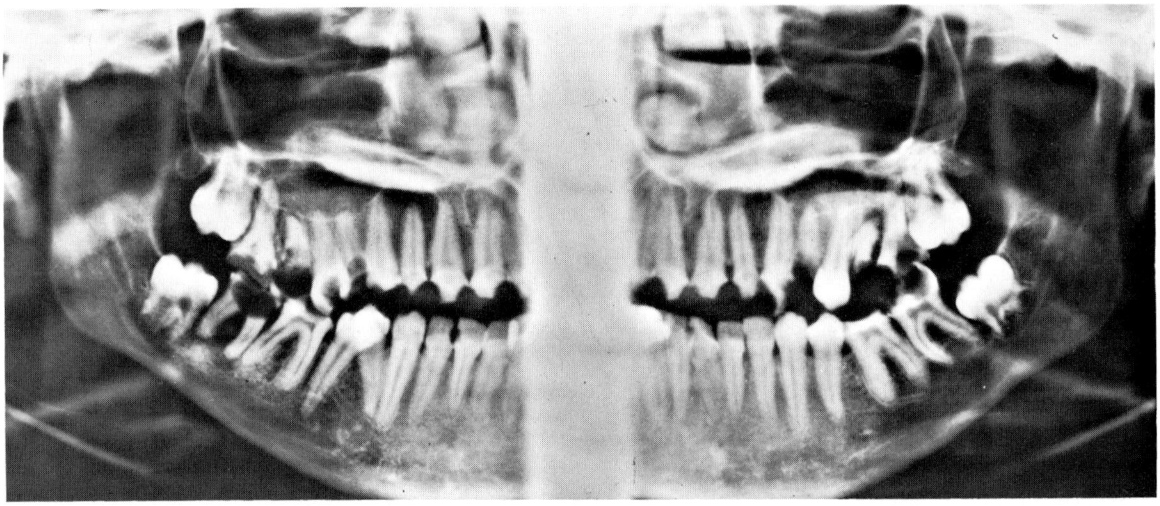

Figure 8–6. Panoramic radiograph of 21-year-old with rampant caries.

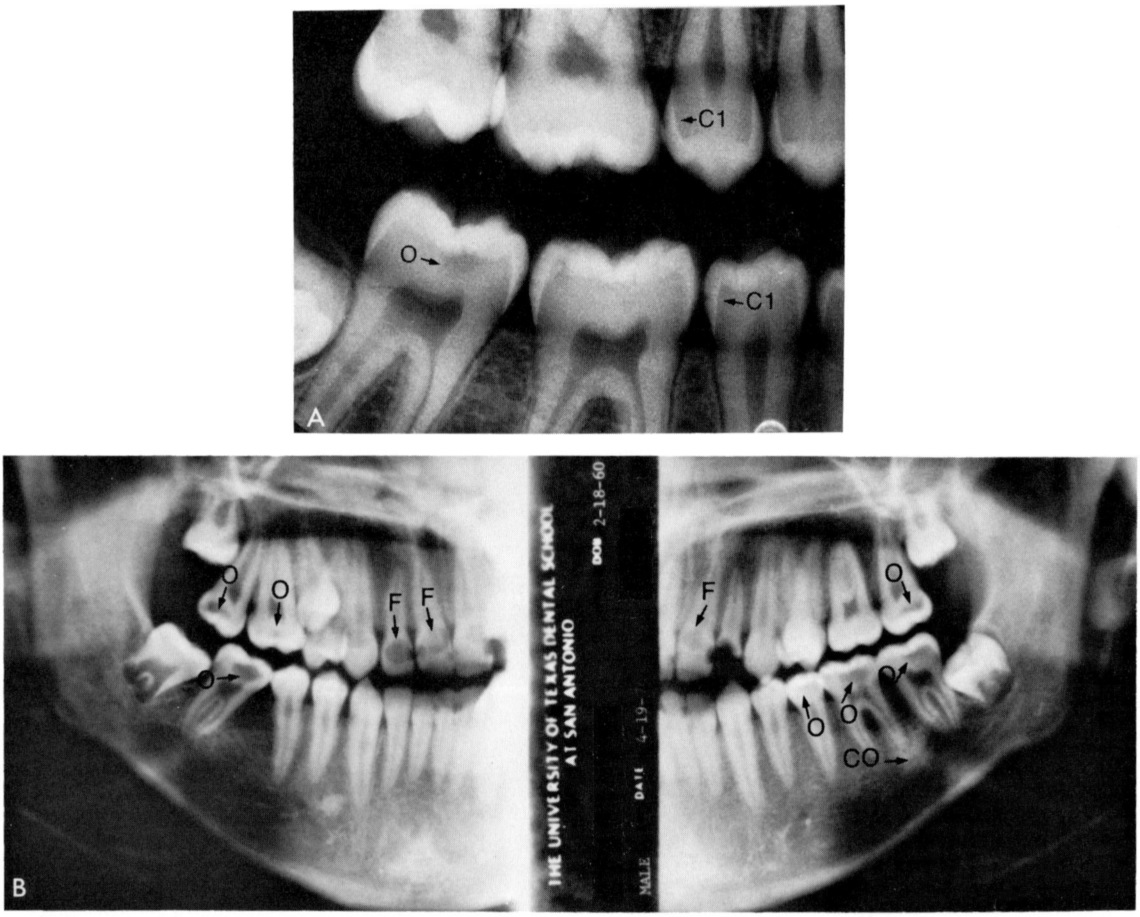

Figure 8–7. Occlusal caries. **A.** Bitewing radiograph. Class 1 caries indicated by (C1). (O) = occlusal caries of mandibular second molar. **B.** Panorex radiograph of 16-year-old. Patient has impacted maxillary second bicuspids. (O) = occlusal caries. (F) = facial caries. (CO) = condensing osteitis.

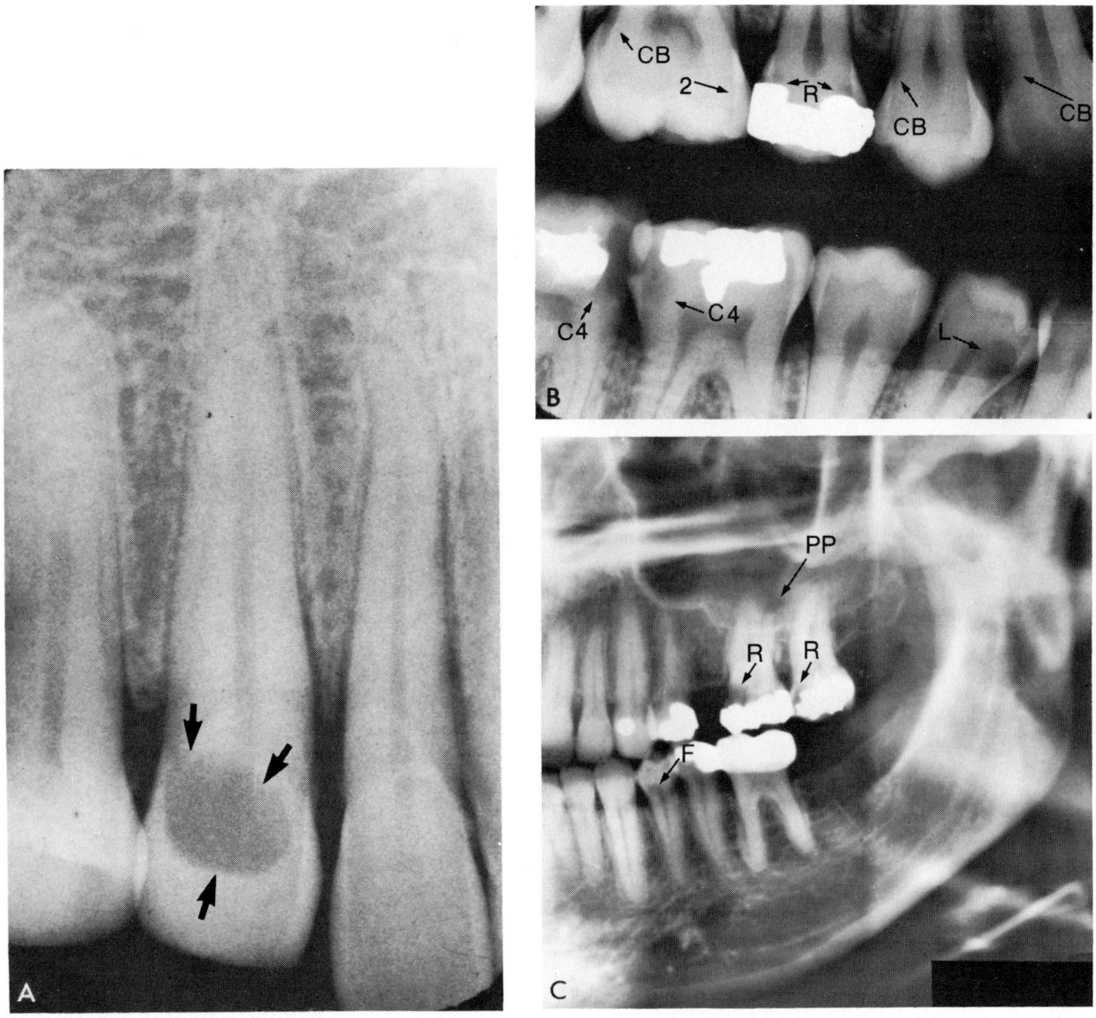

Figure 8–8. **A.** Periapical radiograph. Facial caries of maxillary lateral incisor (arrows). **B.** Bitewing radiograph. Caries classification indicated by number. (L) = lingual or facial caries (clinically it was lingual caries). (CB) = cervical burnout. (R) = recurrent caries. **C.** Panorex radiograph. (F) = crescent-shaped facial caries of mandibular first bicuspid. (R) = recurrent caries. (PP) = periapical pathology.

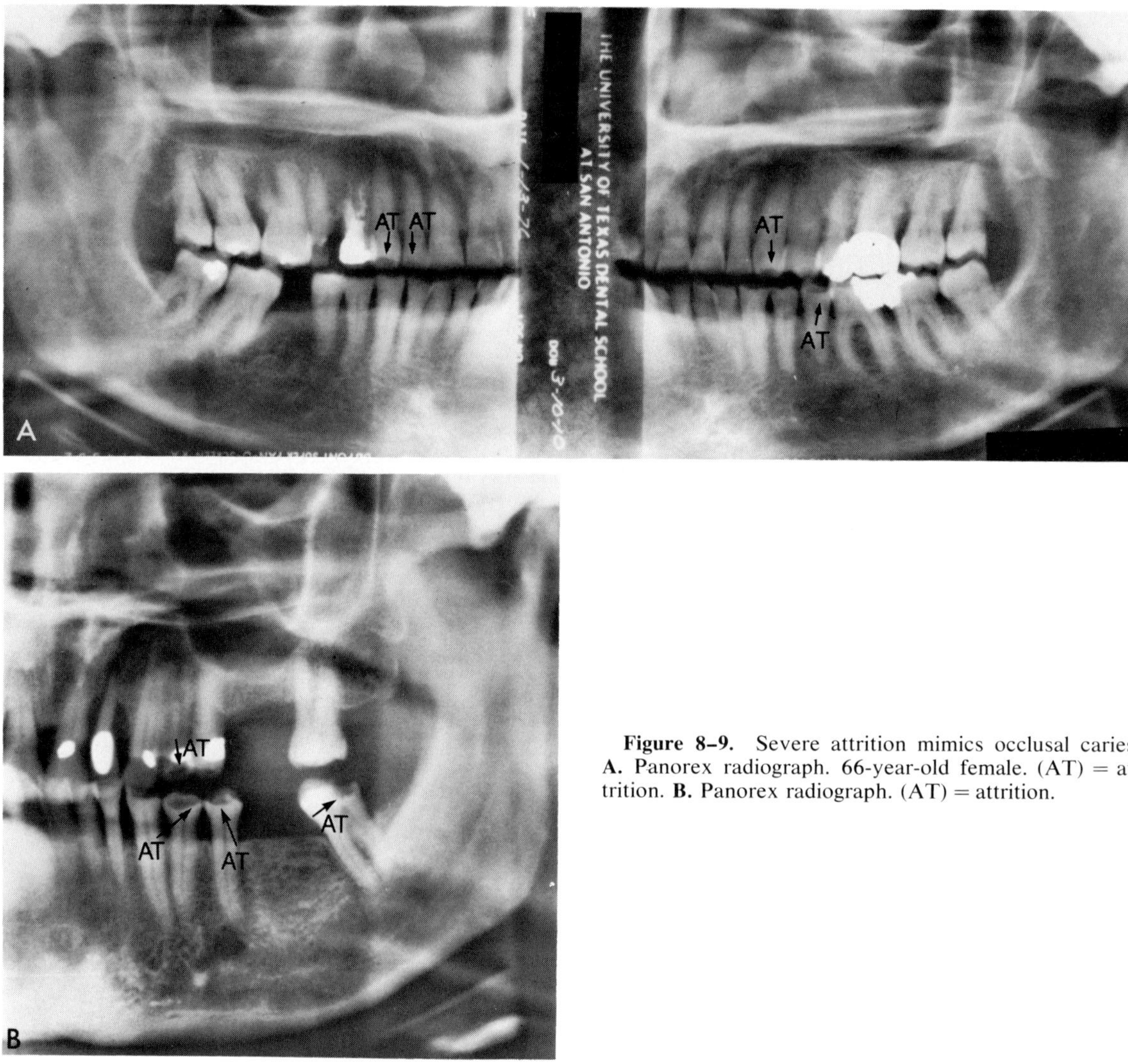

Figure 8–9. Severe attrition mimics occlusal caries. **A.** Panorex radiograph. 66-year-old female. (AT) = attrition. **B.** Panorex radiograph. (AT) = attrition.

caries, which has a narrow area of penetration. Figure 8–8 illustrates examples of facial and lingual caries. The radiographic film serves only to alert the clinician to caries of the facial or lingual surface. It will not routinely detect carious lesions of these surfaces as well as a good clinical examination with a sharp explorer and mirror.

CEMENTAL (ROOT) CARIES

Caries of the roots of the teeth is often referred to as cemental or senile caries. It usually occurs in the elderly who suffer from xerostomia, gingival recession, and food impaction from loose contacts caused by severe attrition. Severe attrition may mimic occlusal caries (Fig. 8–9). Cemental caries is revealed on the radiograph as an ill-defined, cupped-out radiolucent lesion on the surface of the root (Fig. 8–10).

Root caries may at times be misinterpreted as cervical burnout, which is seen normally in the cervical region of the teeth as a radiolucent triangular area on the proximal surfaces of the posterior teeth and as a radiolucent band on the anterior teeth. This can be explained by the tissue density differences of the cervical region, the crown, and the root of the tooth. The cervical area of the tooth is somewhat constricted as compared with the other portions of the tooth and is not covered by enamel or bone. Therefore, the x-radiation penetrates this region more readily than the rest of the tooth, resulting in a greater radiolucency in the cervi-

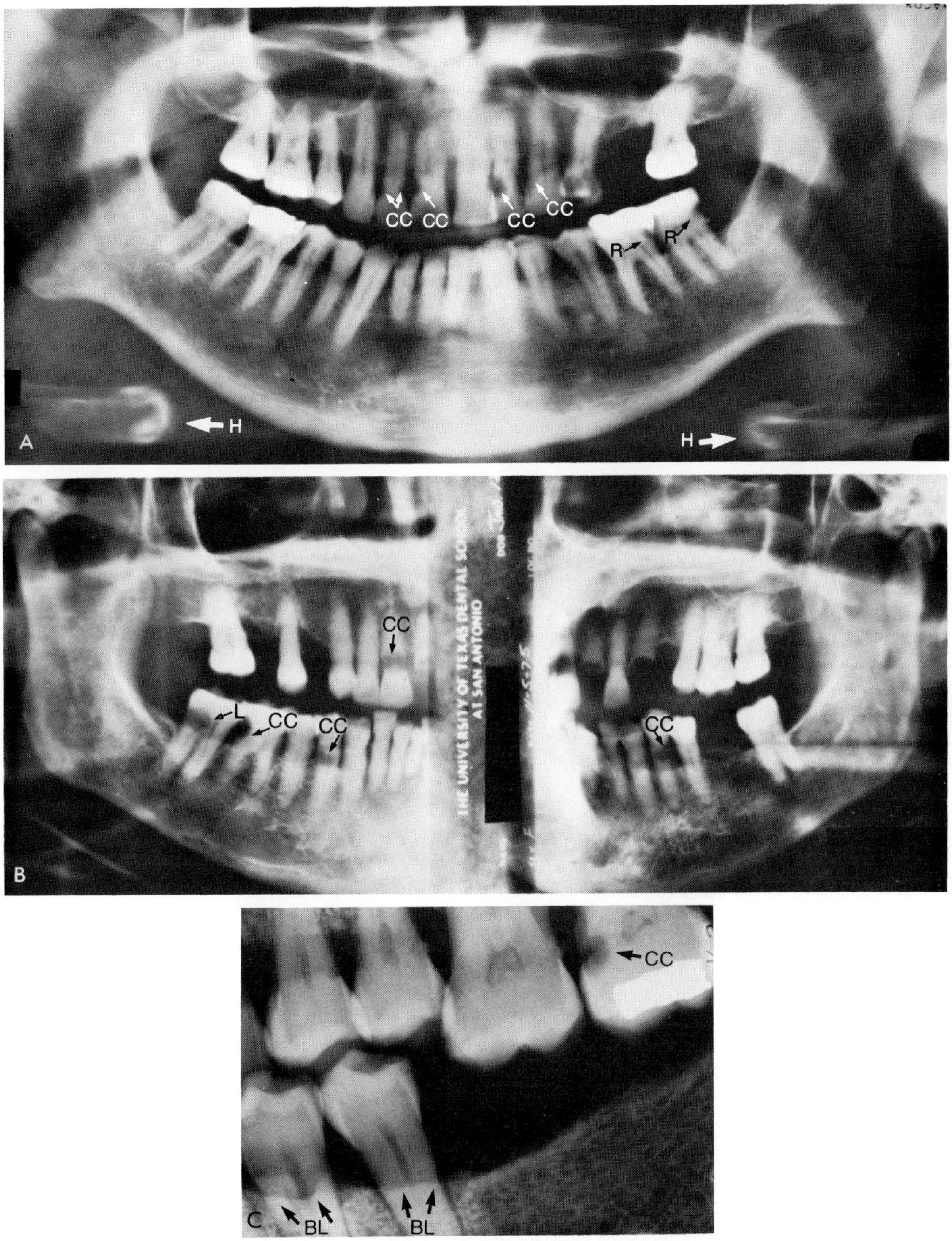

Figure 8–10. Caries of the cementum. This usually occurs in elderly persons who have gingival recession. **A.** Panoral radiograph. Patient with cemental (root) caries (CC). (H) = horseshoe-shaped hyoid bone. (R) = recurrent caries. **B.** Panorex radiograph. (CC) = cemental (root) caries. (L) = lingual caries. **C.** Bitewing radiograph. Cemental caries (CC). Supra-eruption of maxillary second molar exposed root of tooth and caries subsequently developed on the mesial root surface. (BL) = bone level.

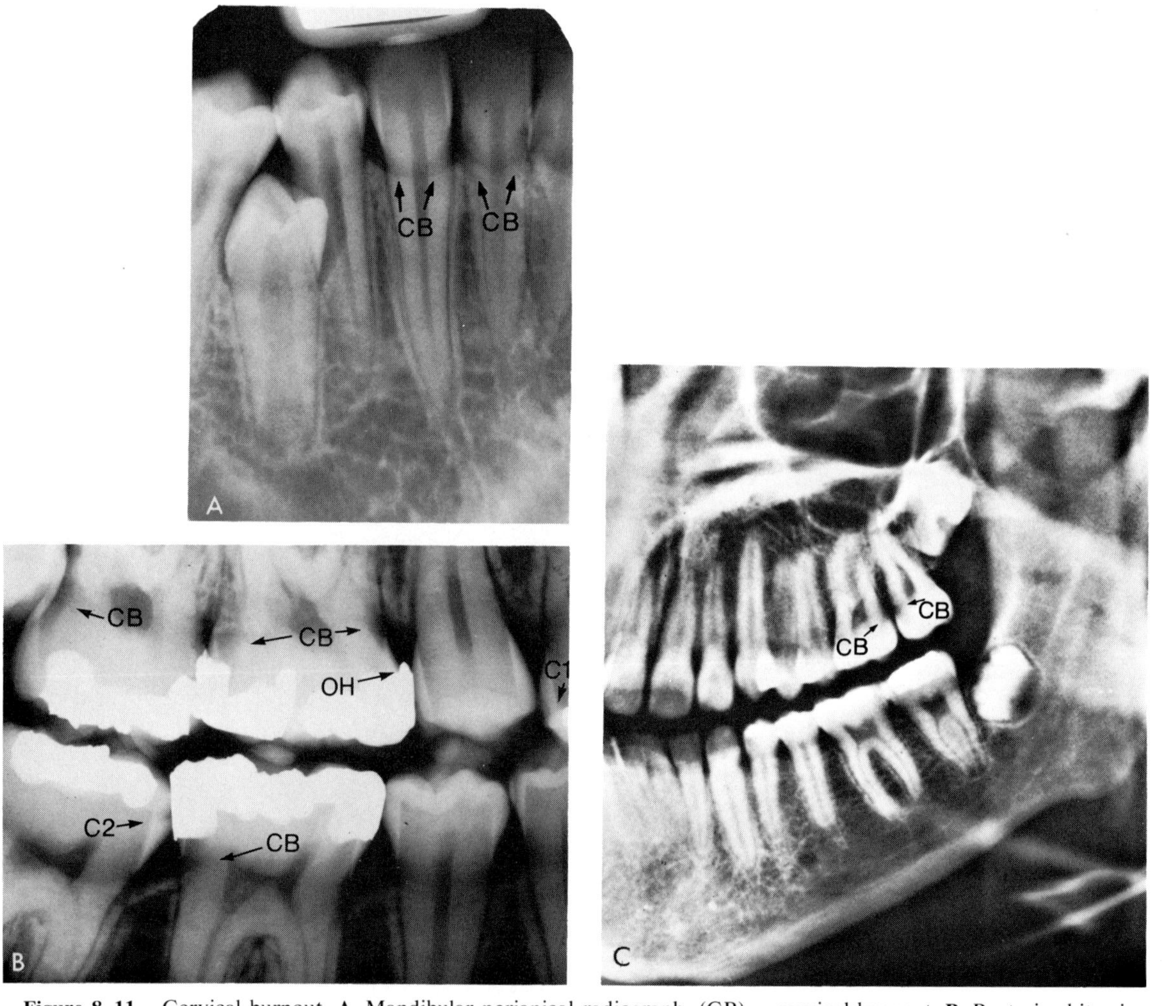

Figure 8–11. Cervical burnout. **A.** Mandibular periapical radiograph. (CB) = cervical burnout. **B.** Posterior bitewing radiograph. Caries classified by number. (CB) = cervical burnout. (OH) = overhang. **C.** Panorex radiograph. (CB) = cervical burnout.

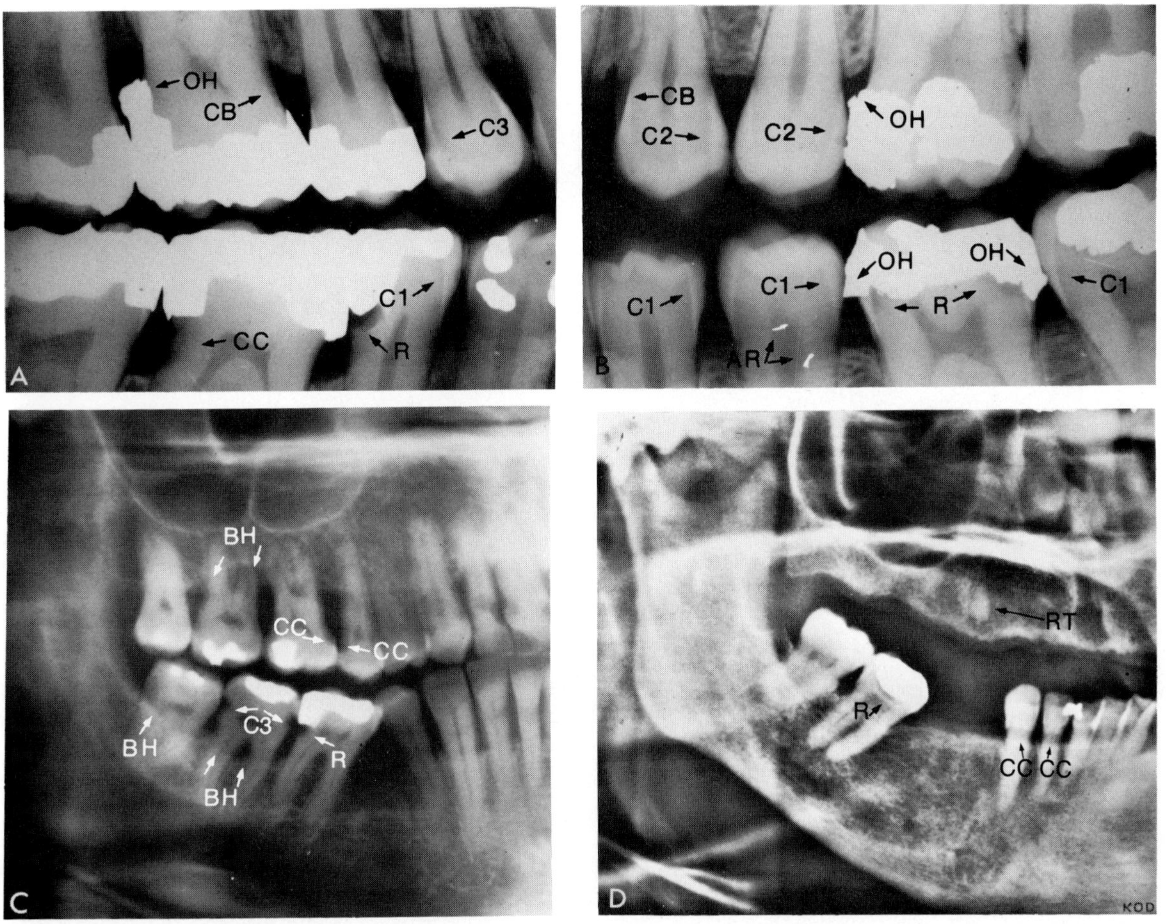

Figure 8–12. Recurrent (secondary) caries. **A.** Posterior bitewing radiograph. Interproximal caries classified by number. (R) = recurrent caries. (OH) = overhang. (CB) = cervical burnout. (CC) = cemental (root) caries. **B.** Posterior bitewing radiograph. Interproximal caries classified by number. (R) = recurrent caries. (AR) = artifacts. (OH) = overhang; (CB) = cervical burnout. **C.** Panoramic radiograph. (R) = recurrent caries. (BH) = bone height; (CC) = cemental (root) caries. **D.** Panorex radiograph. (R) = recurrent caries. (RT) = root tip. (CC) = cemental (root) caries.

cal region. (See Figure 8–11 for examples of cervical burnout.) In many cases, an examination of the area by an explorer is the only method of differentiating between root caries and cervical burnout. Root caries takes on a cupped-out or saucer-shaped dark appearance rather than the wedge-shaped, more diffuse radiolucency seen in cervical burnout.

RECURRENT (SECONDARY) CARIES

Recurrent (secondary) caries originates in the immediate vicinity of a preexisting restoration. In most cases, it occurs because of (1) inadequate extension of the cavity preparation; (2) improper adaptation of the restorative material to the margins of the cavity preparation, resulting in leaky margins; or (3) incomplete removal of all caries prior to placement of the restoration. For an example of recurrent caries see Figure 8–12.

RESTORATIVE MATERIALS

Silicates, resins, and many of the composites are radiolucent and may be misinterpreted as caries. They can be differentiated from carious lesions by the fact that cavity preparations in the anterior teeth have characteristic shapes and, sometimes, opaque cement bases beneath the restorations. Carious lesions of the proximal surfaces of the anterior teeth are usually more radiolucent and triangular in shape (Fig. 8–13).

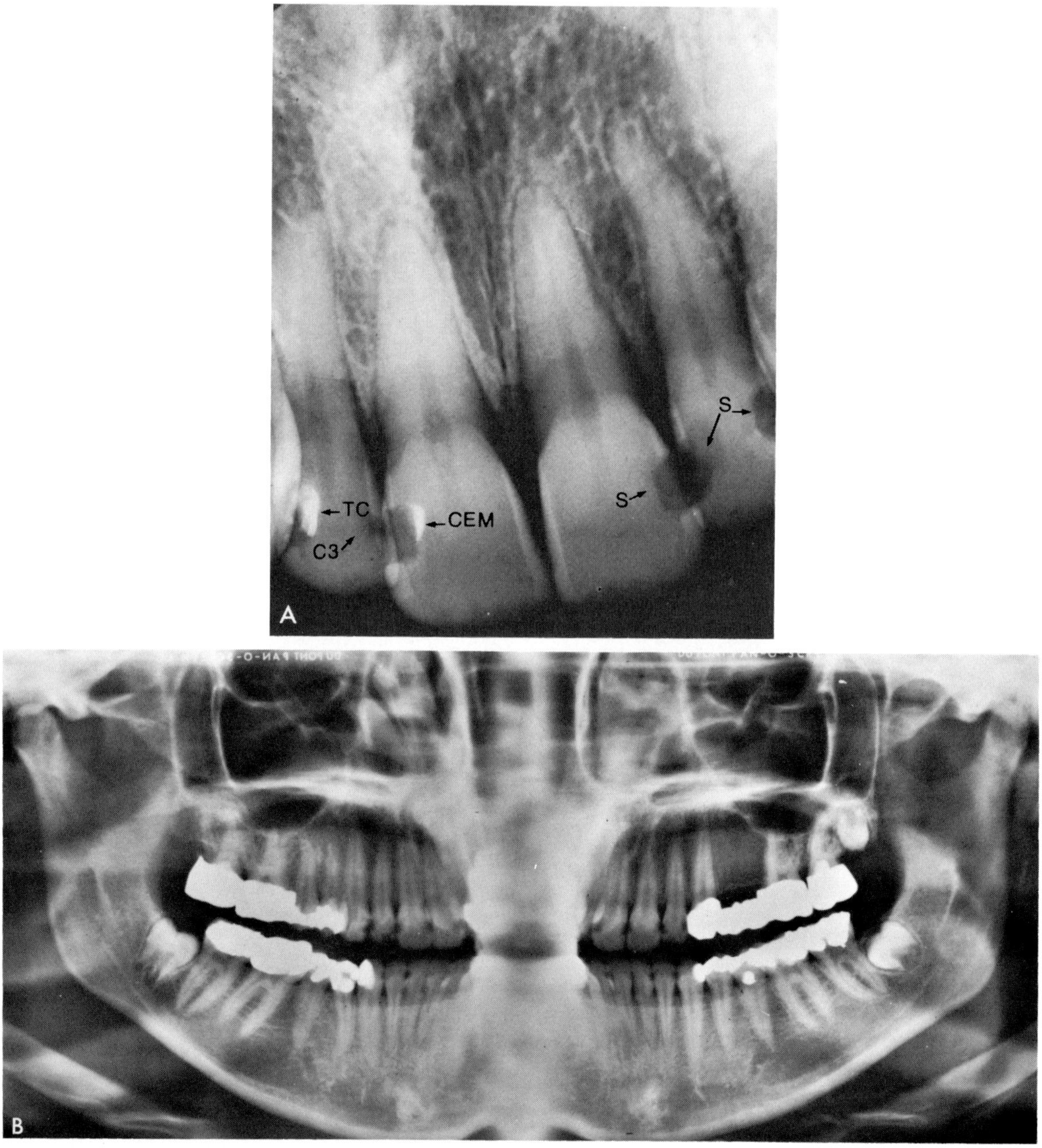

Figure 8–13. Radiolucent restorations. **A.** Periapical radiograph. Silicate restorations. (S) = silicate. (TC) = temporary cement. CEM = cement base. **B.** Panorex radiograph taken by one of the first Panorex x-ray machines produced. The x-radiation was not interrupted during the chair shift in the first Panorex machines, causing a blurring in the middle of the radiograph. This patient has many Class 3 silicates in the maxillary and mandibular incisors.

Illustration continued on opposite page

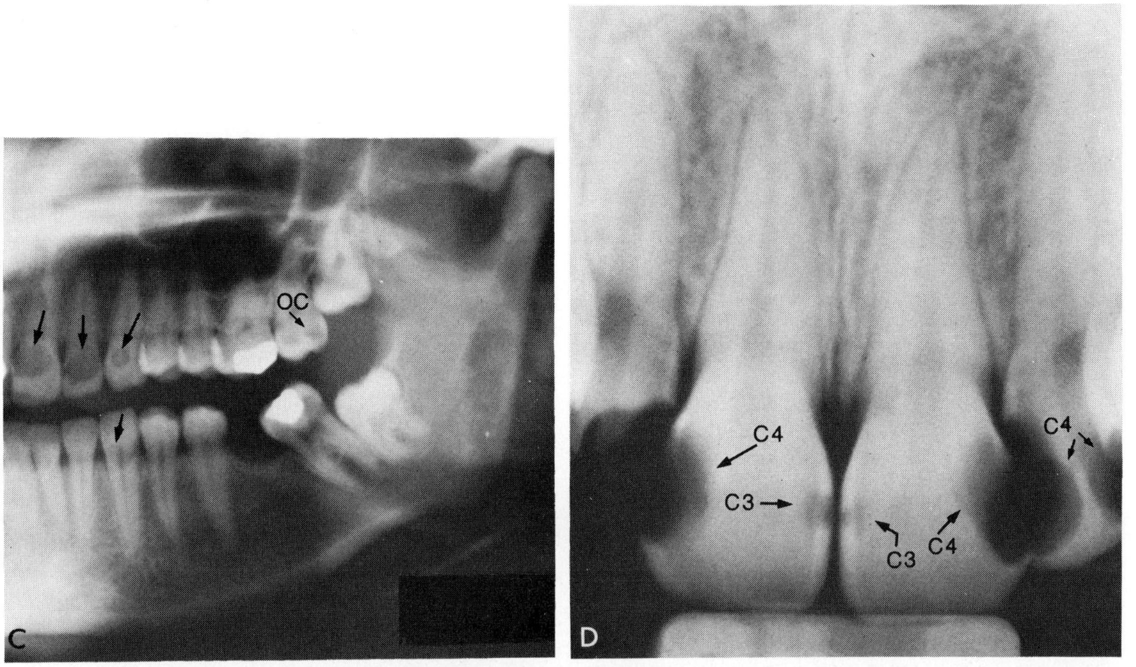

Figure 8–13 *Continued.* **C.** Panorex radiograph. Arrows indicate facial tooth-colored filling material restorations. (OC) = occlusal caries. **D.** Periapical radiograph. Anterior interproximal caries classified according to depth of penetration. Dental caries usually has a different density and configuration than tooth-colored filling material restorations. (**B** courtesy of Jack Faude, Dental Products Div., Pennwalt Corp., Phila., PA.)

PULPAL AND PERIAPICAL DISEASE

SECONDARY DENTIN

The dental pulp becomes smaller with the formation of secondary dentin, which is formed after the primary dentition has been completed. Secondary dentin is formed in two ways as a response to various stimuli.

1. **Physiologically,** dentin formation occurs as a response to the normal aging process (so-called senile dentin). The odontoblasts, which lie adjacent to the dentin, send out fibrils through the dentinal tubules to the dentino-enamel junction and undergo degenerative changes with advancing age. Aging has an adverse effect on the quality and quantity of blood vessels supplying the dental pulp. Blood vessels of the pulp undergo arteriosclerotic changes, resulting in a diminished blood supply to the cells of the pulp, which, in turn, stimulates secondary dentin deposition (Fig. 8–14).

2. The pulp also responds **pathologically** to severe irritants such as dental caries, abrasion, attrition, erosion, cavity preparation, and tooth fracture. Odontoblasts of the pulp are stimulated by these irritants to deposit secondary dentin (sclerotic type) for added protection of the pulp.

PULP CALCIFICATIONS

Calcifications of various forms are found in the pulp with such regularity that it can be questioned whether they are the result of a pathologic state or are within the range of normal biologic variation. Hill reported that, in a group of young persons between 10 and 20 years of age, 66 per cent of all teeth examined had calcifications, and, in a group of persons between 50 and 70 years of age, 90 per cent of all teeth examined had calcifications.

Pulp calcifications are found in two morphologic forms: (1) discrete calcifications (pulp stones and pulp denticles or nodules) and (2) diffuse calcifications. Pulp stones are localized masses of calcified tissue, nodular in shape, that are found more commonly in the pulp chamber than in the root canal. Diffuse calcifications are seen more commonly in the root canal and are usually identified histologically as amorphous, unorganized linear columns lying parallel to the blood vessels of the pulp. Very seldom are they seen radiographically.

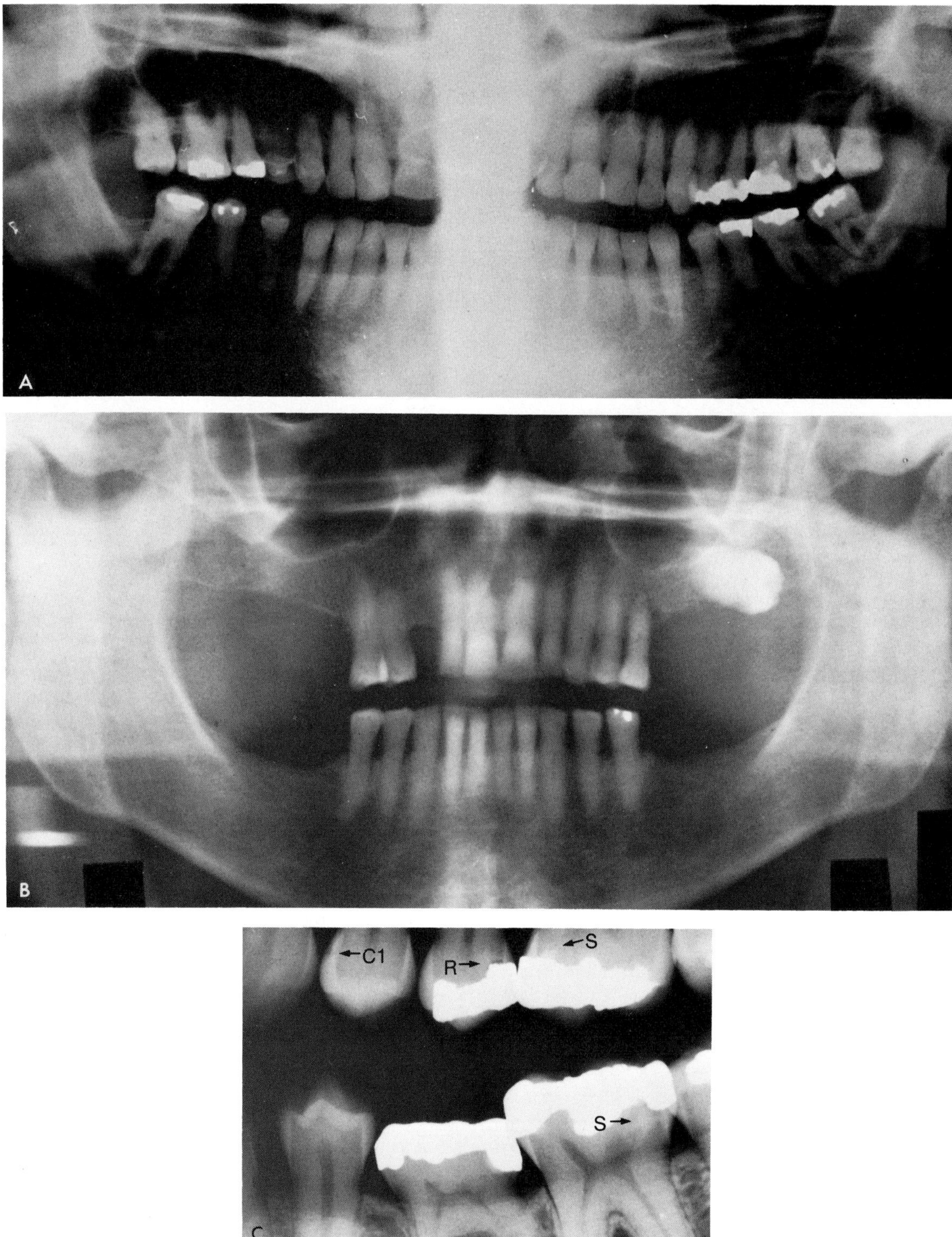

Figure 8–14. Secondary dentin and dentinal sclerosis. **A.** Panorex radiograph. Elderly individual with decrease in size of the pulp chambers and root canals as a result of secondary dentin formation in almost all the teeth. **B.** Panelipse radiograph. Elderly person with generalized secondary dentin formation as a response to stimuli associated with the normal aging process. Note embedded maxillary third molar. **C.** Posterior bitewing of sclerotic dentin. Mineralization of the dentinal tubules as a result of injury to the dentin by caries, abrasion, or cavity preparation. Sclerotic dentin is more highly calcified than normal dentin and, therefore, more radiopaque. Caries classified according to depth. Note submerged retained mandibular second primary molar. (S) = sclerotic dentin. (R) = recurrent caries.

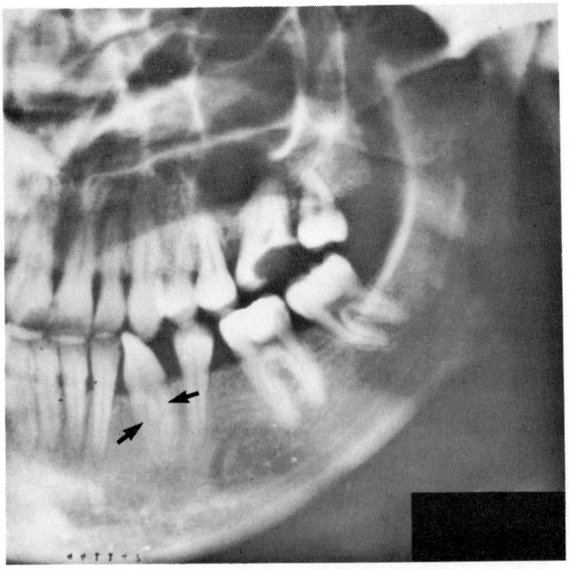

Figure 8–15. Panoramic radiograph. Note the large pulp stone in the mandibular cuspid (arrows).

Pulp stones can be seen quite regularly in the radiograph (Fig. 8–15). In past literature pulp stones have been reported to cause pain (Garretson; White; Stafne and Szabo). However, at present, most investigators believe that seldom, if ever, will pulp stones cause dental pain. In light of our present knowledge, the finding of a pulp stone does not have any clinical significance except that it may cause difficulty in removing the pulp tissue and shaping the canal for reception of root canal filling material.

RESORPTION OF TEETH

The teeth may resorb in many ways other than that associated with the shedding of the primary teeth. There are two types of resorption — internal and external. When the resorption arises from within the tooth it is called **internal resorption**. When the resorption begins at the periphery of the tooth it is called **external resorption**. The chief causes of tooth resorption are as follows (from Shafer, Hine, and Levy):

1. External resorption:
   a. Periapical inflammation
   b. Reimplantation of teeth
   c. Tumors and cysts
   d. Excessive mechanical or occlusal forces
   e. Impaction of teeth
   f. Idiopath
2, Internal resorption:
   a. Idiopath
   b. Chronic hyperplastic pulpitis

For examples of external resorption see Figure 8–16.

Internal resorption begins centrally within the tooth, and its cause is obscure. The stimulus apparently comes from a form of inflammatory hyperplasia of the pulp. Internal resorption is usually seen as a well-defined, round radiolucent defect in the tooth. It rarely affects more than two teeth in the same individual. It is possible that internal resorption does not exist, but that the defect is a result of external resorption of the tooth and subsequent invasion of the pulp. For examples of internal resorption see Figure 8–17.

DISEASES OF THE DENTAL PULP

The dental pulp is composed of delicate connective tissue freely interspersed with minute blood vessels, lymphatics, nerves, and undifferentiated connective tissue cells. It reacts to bacterial infection or other stimuli by an inflammatory reaction very much like that of other connective tissues of the body with some exceptions. The nature of the response is altered because the pulpal tissue is enclosed within calcified walls and fed by means of vessels entering through a small apical foramen, which makes it almost impossible to develop a collateral blood supply to the inflamed area.

Almost all types of pulpitis are caused by dental caries, which allows for the invasion of the pulpal tissue by bacteria. Other causes of pulpitis include the following:

1. **Mechanical irritants**: operative manipulations, cavity preparations, crown preparations, and pin placements.

2. **Thermal irritants:** improper cooling procedures during crown preparations and use of hot modeling compound impressions. Cements used as bases under restorations often induce heat in the pulp (especially if improperly mixed).

3. **Chemical irritants:** silicates and other tooth-colored filling materials need proper insulation if the cavity preparation is large. Also, various dentinal sterilizing agents can produce inflammatory responses in the pulp.

4. **Trauma:** this includes tooth fractures and high tooth restorations. Tooth fractures expose the tooth to fluids and produce a pathway by which microorganisms can enter the pulp. Severe trauma to a tooth can cause irreversible pulpitis, which results in some degree of odontalgia, which is defined as "a spontaneous

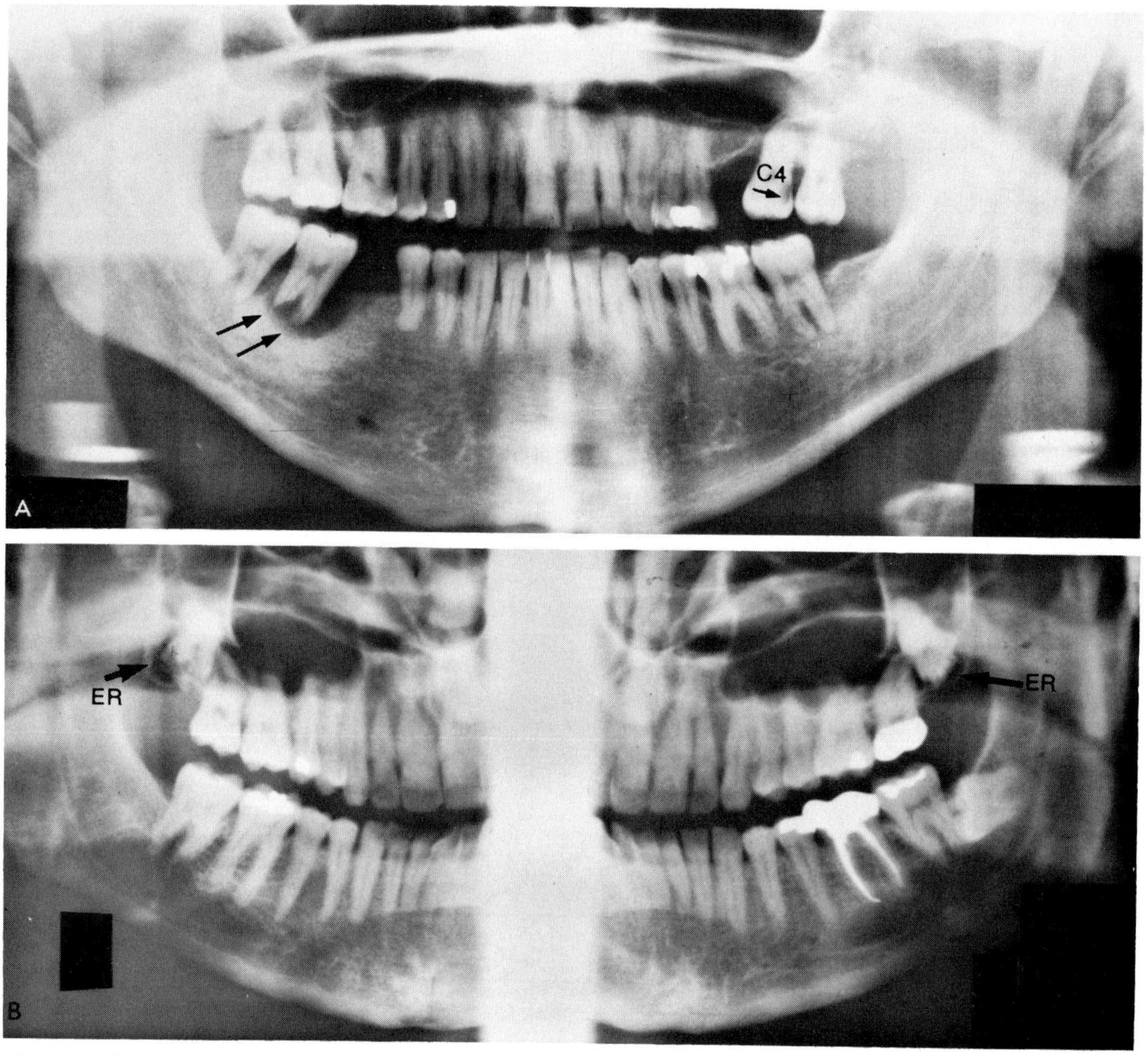

Figure 8–16. External resorption. **A.** Panelipse radiograph. External resorption most likely caused by an inflammatory process associated with the mandibular second molar (arrow). **B.** Panorex radiograph. External resorption (ER) of crowns of impacted maxillary third molars (possible cyst formation).

Illustration continued on opposite page

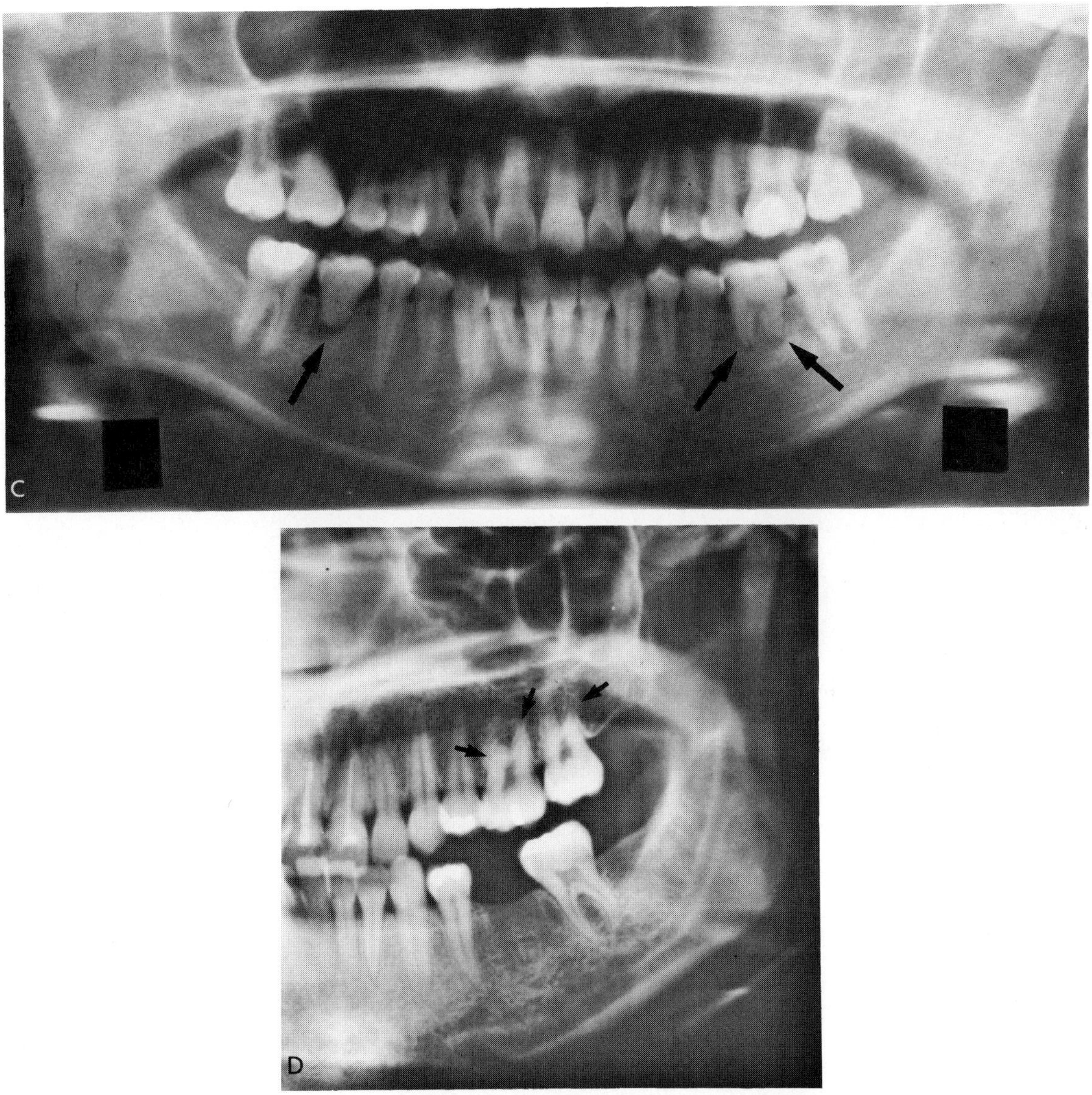

Figure 8–16 *Continued.* **C.** Panelipse radiograph. External resorption of mandibular molars, which were third molar transplants into first molar position (arrows). **D.** Panorex radiograph. External resorption of buccal roots of maxillary first molar from either idiopathic causes or excessive mechanical forces of orthodontic appliances.

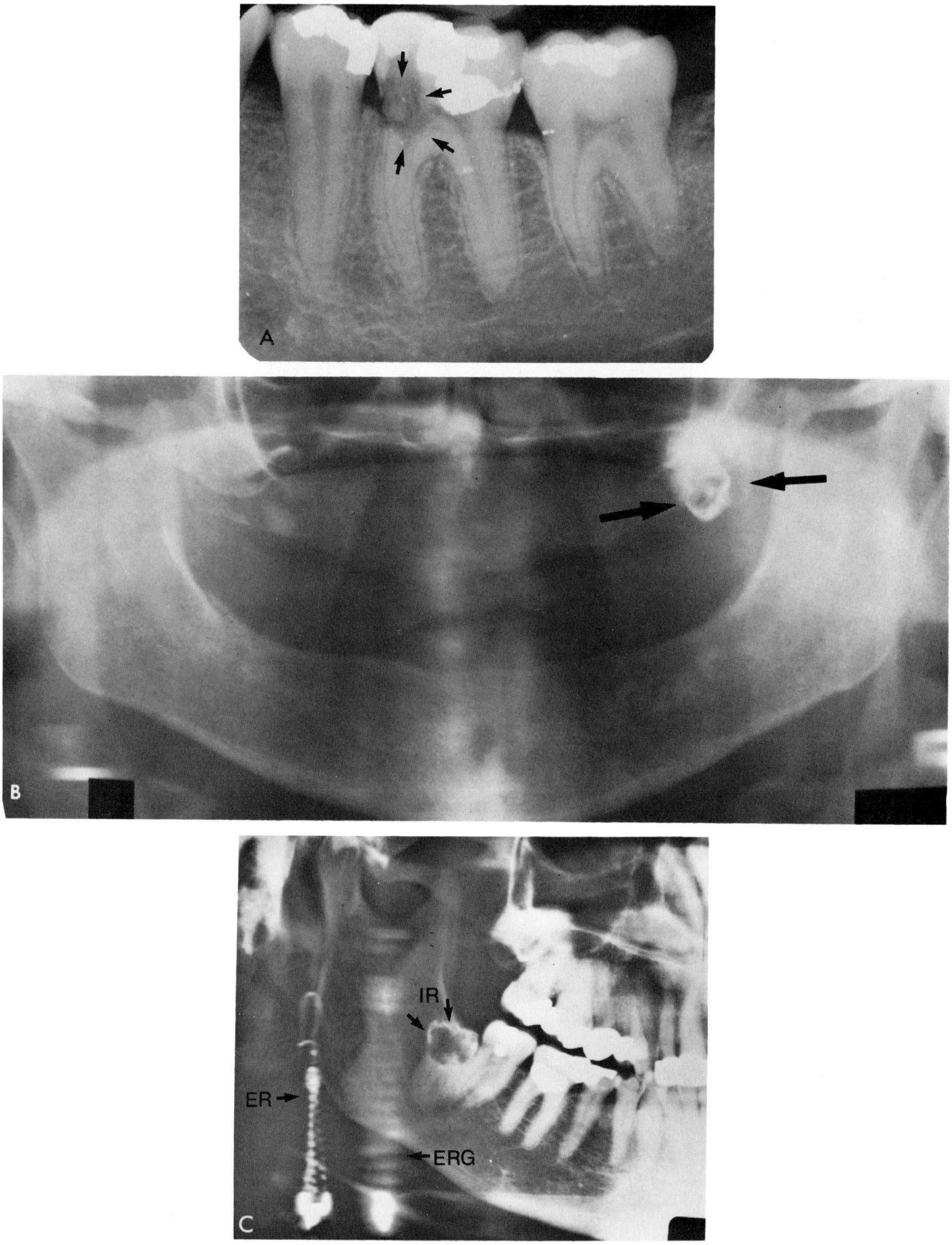

Figure 8–17. Internal resorption. **A.** Periapical radiograph. Internal resorption of mandibular first molar (arrows). **B.** Panelipse radiograph. Internal resorption of impacted maxillary third molar. **C.** Panorex radiograph. Internal resorption (IR) of crown of mandibular third molar (arrows). Note earring (ER) and earring ghost (ERG).

pain in a tooth due to involvement of the pulp or periodontal membrane" (Stedman's Medical Dictionary).

Odontalgia should be differentiated from reversible hyperactive pulpalgia, which is "pulpal sensitivity characterized by short, sharp shooting pains but *not* spontaneous and is precipitated by stimuli such as heat, cold, sweet, and sour" (Maurice).

Reversible hyperactive pulpalgia is, as the name implies, a reversible condition, provided the irritant is removed before the pulp becomes severely injured. Teeth with this condition usually have high restorations, large restorations without bases, restorations with defective margins, or large carious lesions. The pain is usually slight or moderate (can be controlled with aspirin), and percussion and palpation tests are negative. Negative tests are good indications that the pulp can be salvaged.

ODONTALGIA

The acute pain of odontalgia is caused by increased tissue pressure in the pulp or periodontal ligament due to inflammation of these tissues (Beveridge and Brown). In the area of inflammation, localized edema causes pressure on the sensory nerve endings, resulting in pain (Greenbaum).

Ludlow reports five potential pathologic conditions that can produce odontalgia. He also presents the proper treatment of each condition (Fig. 8–18).

1. Acute pulpitis. This is characterized by **vital** but inflamed pulp, usually in the coronal portion of the tooth. Percussion tests and radiographs are negative. The spontaneous, painful symptoms of acute pulpitis are a result of severe intrapulpal pressure. The pain is diffuse and not readily localized by the patient because only pain nerve fibers (no proprioceptive nerve fibers) are found within the pulp. Emergency therapy consists of a pulpotomy (removal of the coronal portion of the pulp) in teeth with multiple canals or pulpectomy in teeth with single canals. A sedative dressing of eugenol or chlorobutanol is sealed in the pulp chamber. After approximately 15 days, routine root canal therapy is completed.

2. Acute pulpitis with apical periodontitis. This condition is characterized by inflammation in the **vital** pulp that has spread to the periapical tissue. Percussion tests are positive. If the percussion test elicits pain, the inflammation has moved into the periodontal ligament. It

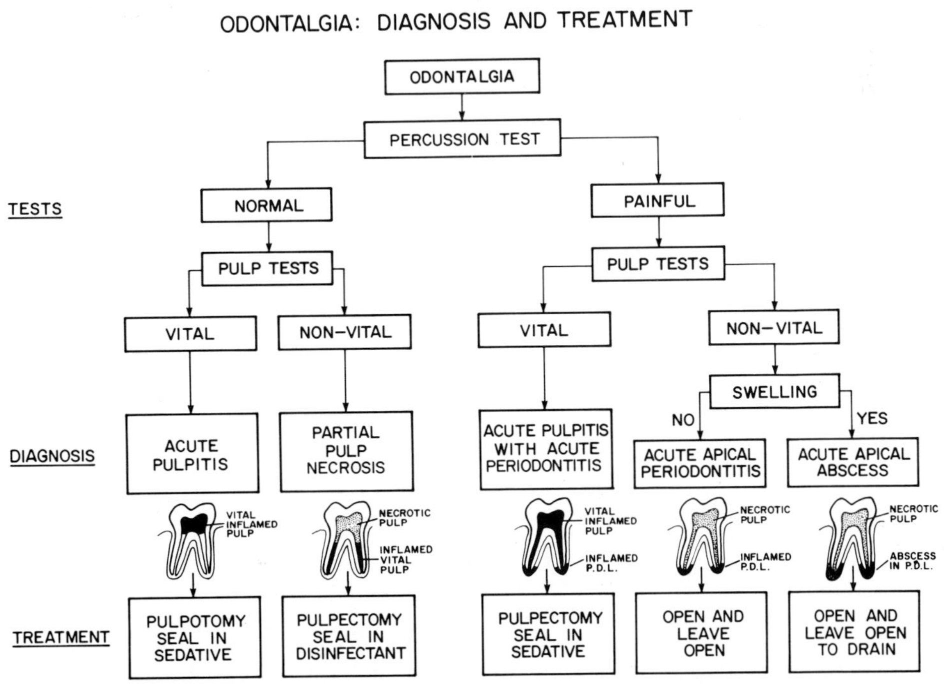

Figure 8–18. Odontalgia chart. (Courtesy of Dr. M. O. Ludlow, Creighton University Dental School, Omaha, NE.)

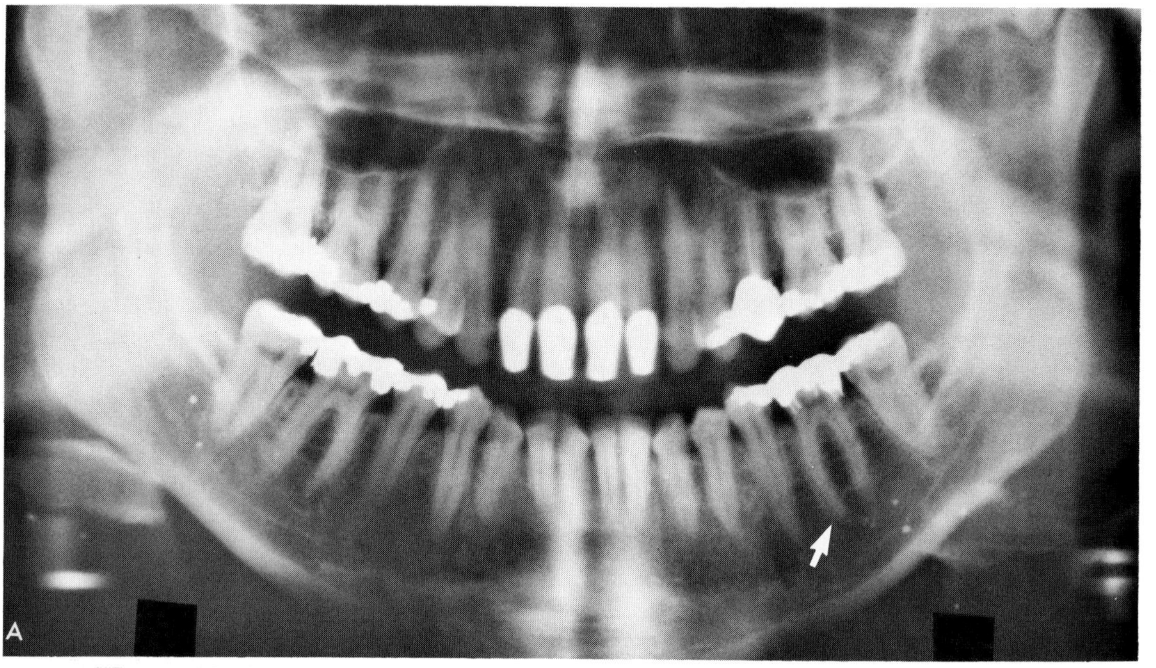

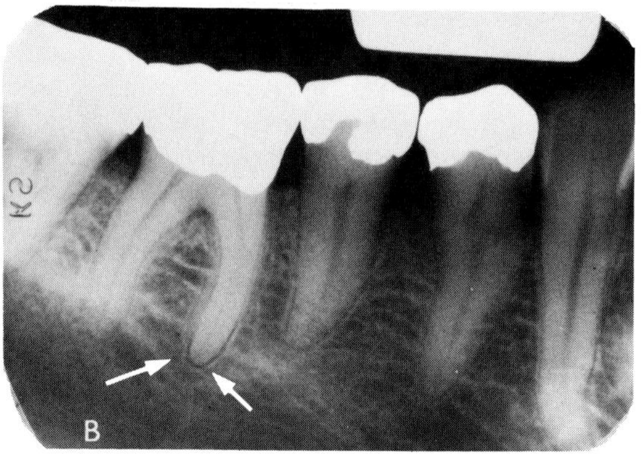

Figure 8–19. Acute pulpitis with apical periodontitis (vital tooth with percussion pain). **A.** Panelipse radiograph. Note apical periodontal ligament space thickening (arrow), diagnosed as acute pulpitis with apical periodontitis. Also note amalgam pins in close association with pulp chamber of tooth. **B.** Periapical radiograph. Mandibular first molar with full gold crown diagnosed as acute pulpitis and apical periodontitis. Note slightly thickened periodontal ligament space (arrows).

must be remembered that periodontal disease and maxillary sinusitis will also elicit positive percussion signs. Three out of four patients with acute maxillary sinusitis will respond positively to percussion tests. Sometimes in acute pulpitis with apical periodontitis a slightly thickened periodontal ligament space can be seen at the apex of a tooth on the radiograph (Fig. 8–19). In the early stages of this condition there is slight tenderness of the tooth, and as pressure increases, the periodontal ligament fibers stretch and elevate the tooth slightly. The tooth will become increasingly tender so that even the slightest pressure will induce mild pain. A **positive radiograph** is seen in acute apical inflammation when there has been a 30 to 60 per cent loss of mineral content in the bone. Consequently, resorption is rarely sufficient to be detected radiographically until 10 days or so after the initial onset of the acute apical inflammation. Emergency treatment consists of pulpectomy, especially removal of the inflamed apical pulpal tissue, because it is the source of the pressure and pain. To obtain anesthesia, a local anesthetic may have to be injected directly into the pulp under pressure. After the canals have been debrided, a sedative dressing of eugenol or chlorobutanol is placed in the pulp chamber.

3. Partial pulp necrosis (chronic pulpitis). This condition is characterized by necrosis of the coronal pulpal tissue; however, **vital** inflamed tissue remains in the root portion of the tooth. The periapical tissue is not inflamed as yet. The tooth is essentially **nonvital;** however, it may give high readings on the electric pulp tester. The percussion tests and radiographs are **negative.** Pain may be absent; if present, it will be a dull vague pain, which can usually be kept under control with aspirin. The patient will often report the pain begins late in the day, usually when the patient is tired or when he lies down. The pain of chronic pulpitis refers vague pains throughout a region, making it difficult, at times, to locate the offending tooth. Emergency treatment consists of total debridement of all root canals, followed by rinsing with a disinfectant solution such as sodium hypochlorite and sealing the pulp chamber with another disinfectant drug, usually camphorated monochlorophenol (CMCP), for approximately 15 days.

4. Acute apical periodontitis. In this condition, the pulp is necrotic and the periapical tissues are inflamed with a serous exudate, causing pressure in the periodontal membrane. The pulp is **nonvital,** and percussion tests are positive. There is no swelling or tenderness on palpation of the soft tissue over the apex of the offending tooth. This indicates that the inflammation is confined to the apical region of the tooth. The radiograph may reveal a slight thickening of the periodontal ligament space at the apex of the tooth (Fig. 8–20). Pain will range from a slight tenderness experienced in the initial stages to an intense, constant throbbing easily localized by the patient. There is an additional feeling of fullness in the area. Emergency treatment consists of complete canal debridement to remove necrotic irritants from the root canal or canals. The canals should be disinfected with sodium hypochlorite irrigation and the tooth left open, leaving only a small pellet of dry cotton in the pulp chamber to keep oral debris out of the pulp canals. The pulp is left open to provide an outlet for any remaining edema. After approximately 15 days, the root canals are cleaned and shaped and left open for another 24 hours. At the third appointment the tooth is irrigated, dried, and sealed with a cotton pellet saturated with disinfectant placed in the pulp chamber. Often the canal can be closed at the fourth appointment.

5. Acute apical abscess. This is characterized by a necrotic pulp and liquefaction necrosis of the periapical tissues, which results in edema and abscess formation in the apical periodontal ligament. The tooth is **nonvital** and painful on percussion. Often there is swelling in the soft tissues above the offending tooth, and sometimes facial cellulitis is present. The pain is intense, constant, and sometimes throbbing. It increases as pus formation adds to the periapical pressure. As the pain becomes more intense, the patient experiences a feeling of fullness in the area. The vestibular region above the root end of the tooth may be painful and fluctuant on palpation. The radiograph will usually show a thickening of the periodontal ligament space of the tooth eliciting the pain (Fig. 8–21). Emergency treatment requires opening a pathway through the tooth for draining the suppurative exudates. If anesthesia is required, a nerve block should be used, because injection should not be made through an area of swelling or edema. After the tooth is open and drained, the root canals should be debrided and irrigated to remove necrotic irritants and to

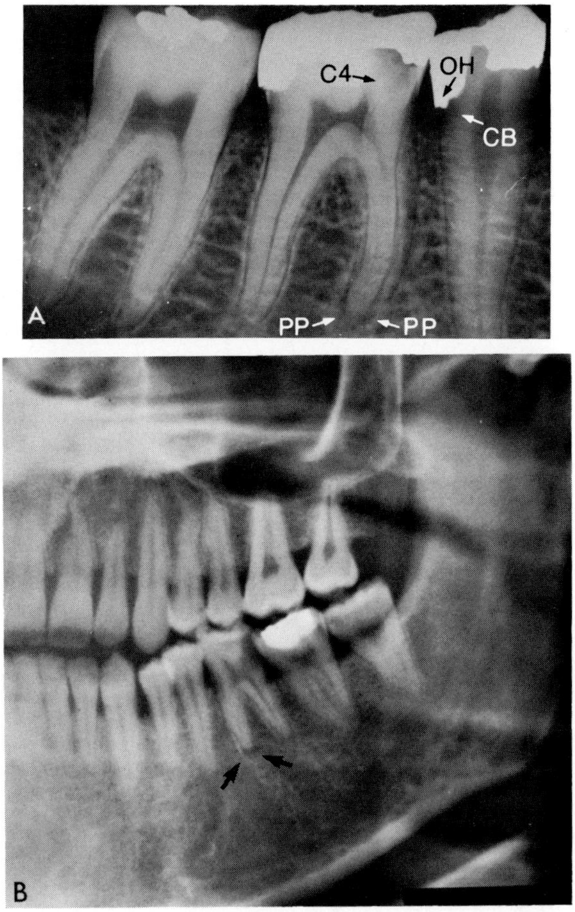

Figure 8–20. Acute apical periodontitis (nonvital tooth with positive percussion test, no swelling, and no tenderness to palpation). **A.** Periapical radiograph. Mandibular first molar diagnosed as acute apical periodontitis. Note the large secondary carious lesion under restoration and the thickened periodontal ligament space of mesial root. (PP) = periapical pathology. (C4) = dentinal caries encroaching upon pulp of tooth. (OH) = overhang. (CB) = cervical burnout. **B.** Panorex radiograph. Mandibular first molar with large carious lesion diagnosed as acute periodontitis (nonvital tooth with positive percussion test and no swelling at apices of tooth). Note the thickened periodontal ligament space at mesial root apex of mandibular first molar (arrows).

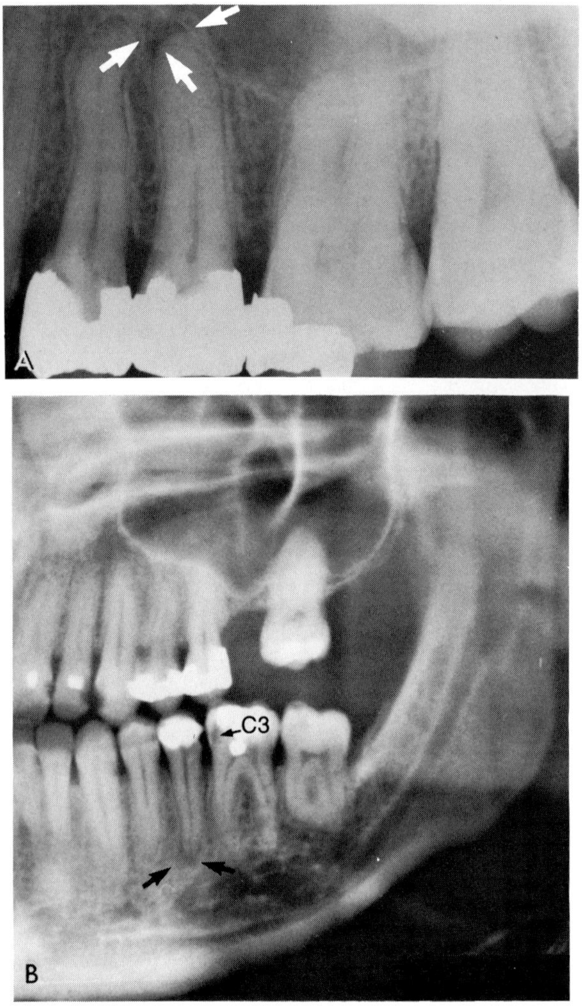

Figure 8–21. Acute apical abscess (nonvital tooth, painful percussion, swelling, and tender palpation). **A.** Periapical radiograph. Maxillary second bicuspid diagnosed as acute apical abscess. Note thickened periodontal ligament space (arrows). **B.** Panoramic radiograph. Mandibular second bicuspid diagnosed as acute apical abscess. Note radiolucency at apex of tooth (arrows).

provide a pathway for drainage. The tooth should be left open, and a small dry pellet of cotton should be placed in the chamber to prevent oral debris from lodging in the pulp chamber. Sometimes the abscess may have to be incised and drained through the soft tissue, especially if the soft tissue is fluctuant. Depending on the clinical signs and symptoms, patients with acute apical abscesses may be given systemic antibiotics and hourly warm saline rinses (Natkin).

The same procedure for closing should be followed as that for acute apical periodontitis. According to Weine, Healey, and Theiss, teeth that have been left open should not be closed at the same appointment they are instrumented because acute symptoms sometimes reappear if the teeth are closed too quickly.

The clinician should be cautioned not to use the panoramic film exclusively to interpret periapical pathology. Besides not supplying the needed definition, superimposed anatomic structures in the radiographic film may, at times, be misinterpreted as periapical lesions. One of these possible misinterpretations is the superimposition of the nasal cavities over the apices of the anterior teeth (Fig. 8–22).

CHRONIC PERIAPICAL DISEASE

There are a number of chronic reactions of the periapical tissue to the toxic irritants from an infected pulp. The type of reaction depends on the number and virulence of the invading organisms and the tissue resistance of the host. Pain is minimized or absent in chronic conditions because the intraperiapical pressure from the exudate is lessened and balanced.

Chronic periapical diseases are inflammatory defense responses of the periapical connective tissue to pulpal irritants. The response is usually a growth of granulation tissue in which the microorganisms have been destroyed. The teeth are nonvital and asymptomatic. The radiograph reveals a radiolucent apical lesion of varying size, shape, and appearance. The clinician cannot make a definitive diagnosis of the chronic periapical lesion from the radiograph alone. A definitive diagnosis can be made only after microscopically examining the lesion after its removal. However, the clinician can make a provisional diagnosis from the radiograph, which provides sufficient accuracy of interpretation so that appropriate treatment can be planned for the type of lesion revealed. The following four chronic periapical diseases will be discussed (Fig. 8–23).

1. **Chronic apical abscess** (suppurative apical periodontitis, chronic alveolar abscess).
2. **Apical granuloma** (chronic apical periodontitis, dental granuloma).
3. **Apical cyst** (apical periodontal cyst, radicular cyst).
4. **Condensing osteitis** (sclerosing osteitis, chronic focal sclerosing osteomyelitis).

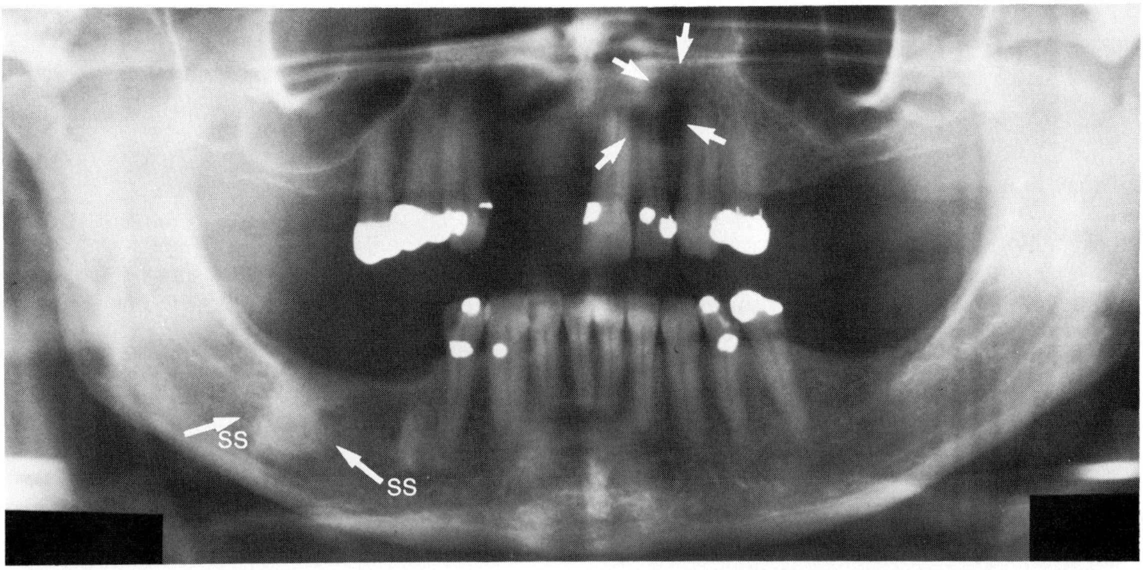

Figure 8–22. Superimposed anatomic structures simulating pathology. Panelipse radiograph. Radiolucencies of nasal cavities superimposed over periapical regions of teeth will simulate periapical pathology (arrows). (SS) = socket sclerosis.

CHRONIC APICAL ABSCESS

This is a low-grade suppurative process of the periapical region. There are two types, one without a fistula and one with a fistula. The process without a fistula develops directly from an acute apical abscess. The acute symptoms of pain, tenderness, and swelling have subsided. However, the transition from an untreated acute apical abscess to an apical granuloma is usually quite rapid, leaving very little time for the development of a chronic apical abscess.

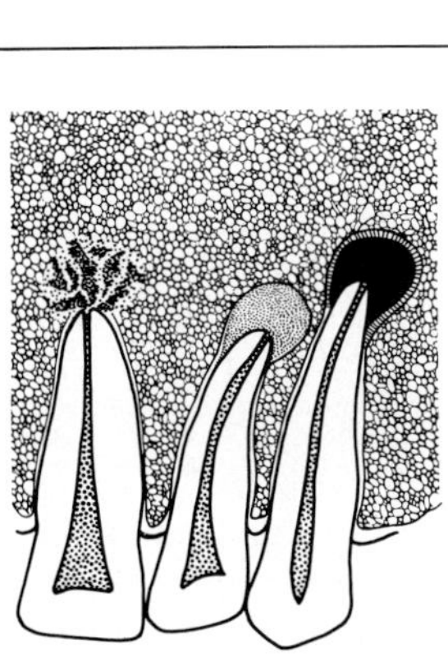

Figure 8–23. Chronic apical conditions.

Most acute apical abscesses are treated by either extraction or pulp therapy because of the pain associated with them. Of course, the acute symptoms of pain, swelling, and tenderness will vary, depending on the number and virulence of the invading organisms and the resistance of the patient.

Most chronic apical abscesses seen are those with fistulas. These abscesses are characterized by active pus formation draining from a fistulous opening. A chronic apical abscess can develop from an acute apical abscess if pus is allowed to drain freely by means of a sinus tract. However, if the fistulous tract becomes blocked, it will give rise to the acute symptoms of pain, tenderness, and swelling of the acute apical abscess again.

More commonly, the chronic apical abscess develops from an apical granuloma. Sometimes the apical granuloma becomes overwhelmed by masses of pulpal irritants; the granulation tissue breaks down, forming an abscess cavity filled with pus, accompanied by all the clinical symptoms of an acute apical abscess.

As soon as drainage is established through the mucoperiosteal tissue by excision or by a fistulous tract, the acute symptoms terminate, and the lesion becomes a chronic apical abscess, which has milder symptoms.

The classic radiographic appearance of a chronic apical abscess is a radiolucent diffuse area at the apex of the tooth, which may extend for a considerable distance along the side of the root surface. If a fistulous tract is present, a radiolucent canal may sometimes be seen leading toward the mucoperiosteal surface of the bone. The borders of the radiolucency are indefinite and irregular and fade indistinctly into normal bone (Fig. 8–24). To localize the fistulous tract, a gutta-percha point may be inserted into the orifice of the fistulous tract prior to radiographing the area. In many cases this will establish which tooth or root is involved.

To successfully treat a chronic apical abscess, it is necessary to first establish proper drainage, followed by removal of necrotic pulp and the application of an adequate apical seal. Usually the chronic apical abscess heals without special treatment of the sinus tract. Some clinicians like to operate on the large lesions to assist healing and repair. Actually, this interferes with healing and repair in most cases because it removes the granulation tissue that is already organized for this very purpose.

APICAL GRANULOMA (CHRONIC APICAL PERIODONTITIS)

One of the most common chronic apical conditions resulting from pulpitis is the apical granuloma. It is essentially a growth of apical granulation tissue in response to pulpal infection. It has a continuous collagenous fiber capsule separating the granulation tissue from the bone. The term granuloma is a misnomer —

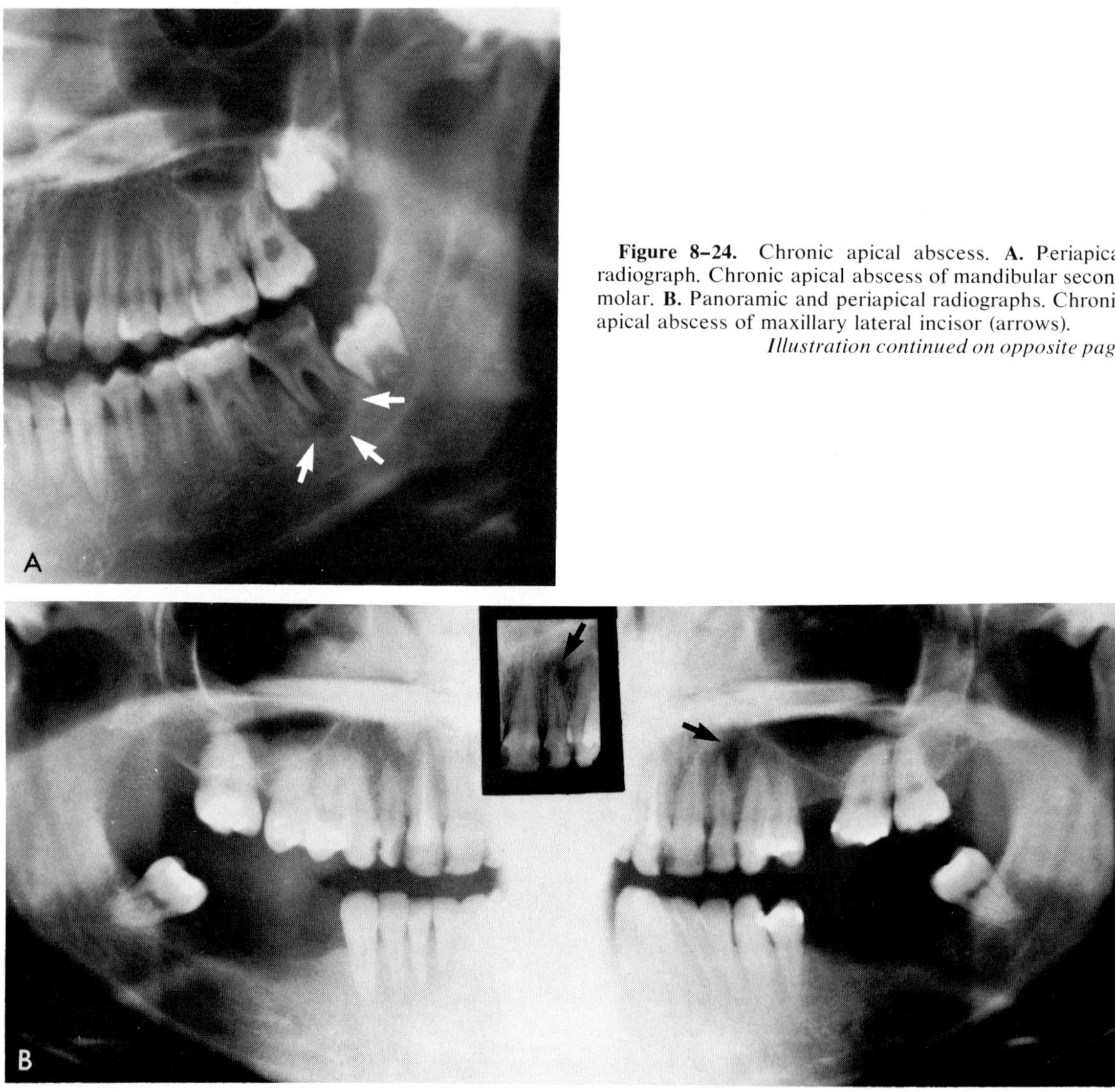

Figure 8–24. Chronic apical abscess. **A.** Periapical radiograph. Chronic apical abscess of mandibular second molar. **B.** Panoramic and periapical radiographs. Chronic apical abscess of maxillary lateral incisor (arrows).

Illustration continued on opposite page

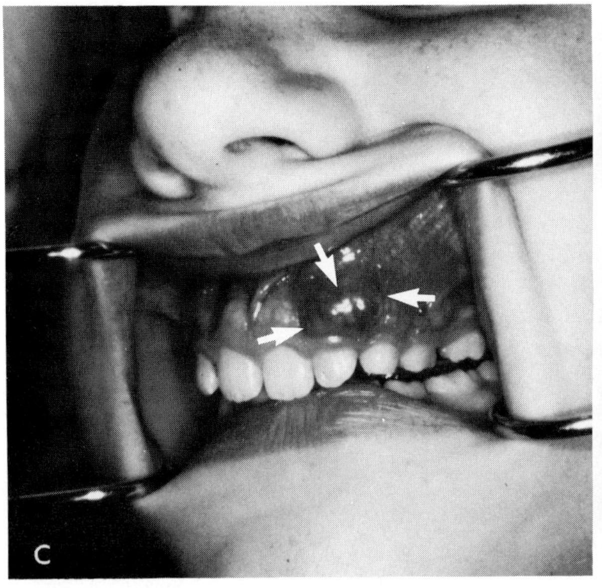

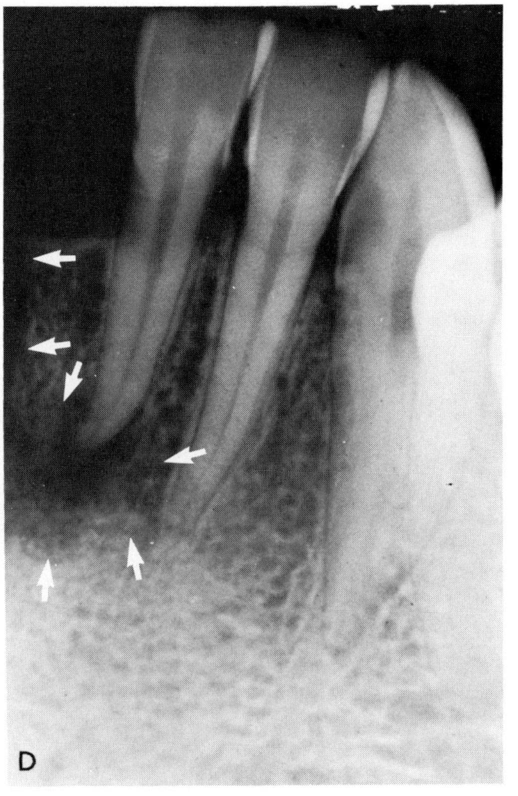

Figure 8–24 *Continued.* **C.** Chronic apical abscess with parulis (gum boil) above maxillary lateral of young child (arrows). **D.** Chronic apical abscess with fistulous tract through alveolar bone from mandibular central incisor to oral cavity (arrows).

it implies a tumor, but actually the apical granuloma is a mass of granulation tissue that has developed in response to irritation. However, the term dental granuloma is so ingrained in the dental literature that it is difficult to change the terminology. The apical granuloma is composed of chronic inflammatory tissue. It is not a place in which bacteria grow, but a place in which they are destroyed. The tooth is nonvital and asymptomatic.

Radiographically, the apical granuloma is a definitely limited or circumscribed area of radiolucency. It maintains a somewhat rounded, rather defined, outline. The periphery of the apical granuloma may appear as a thin wall of compact cancellated bone, and the apex of the tooth may project into the bone cavity. The radiolucency is not as dark as the radicular cyst, and trabeculations of bone, which are actually superimposed over the lesion, may be seen within the apical granuloma (Fig. 8–25).

Treatment depends on the effective removal of the necrotic material from the root canal, followed by sufficient sealing of the apical portion of the tooth. Once the pulpal irritants are removed, the granulation tissue of the apical granuloma heals and repairs the destroyed bone tissue.

APICAL CYST (RADICULAR CYST)

The apical cyst may develop from the apical granuloma, but this is not an inevitable occurrence. The apical cyst is a true cyst in that it consists of a pathologic cavity lined by epithelium that is usually filled with a sterile fluid, but it may be an infected, purulent fluid. It is thought that the epithelial lining of the cyst is derived from the epithelial rests of Malassez, which are found in the periodontal ligament. These epithelial cell rests are stimulated to proliferate by periapical inflammation. They multiply to such an extent that the central cells grow away from their source of nutrition. Therefore, they die and liquefy, forming a cyst.

The radiographic appearance of the apical cyst is an area of radiolucency at the apex of a tooth, usually bounded by an unbroken line of sclerotic bone. The radiolucent area is generally rounded in outline, except where it approximates the adjacent teeth, at which point it is flattened in outline, presenting a more or less oval pattern. The apical cyst has little sign of internal bone trabeculation, and the radiolucency is very dark (Fig. 8–26).

Treatment is based on removal of the necrotic products of the canals and adequate apical

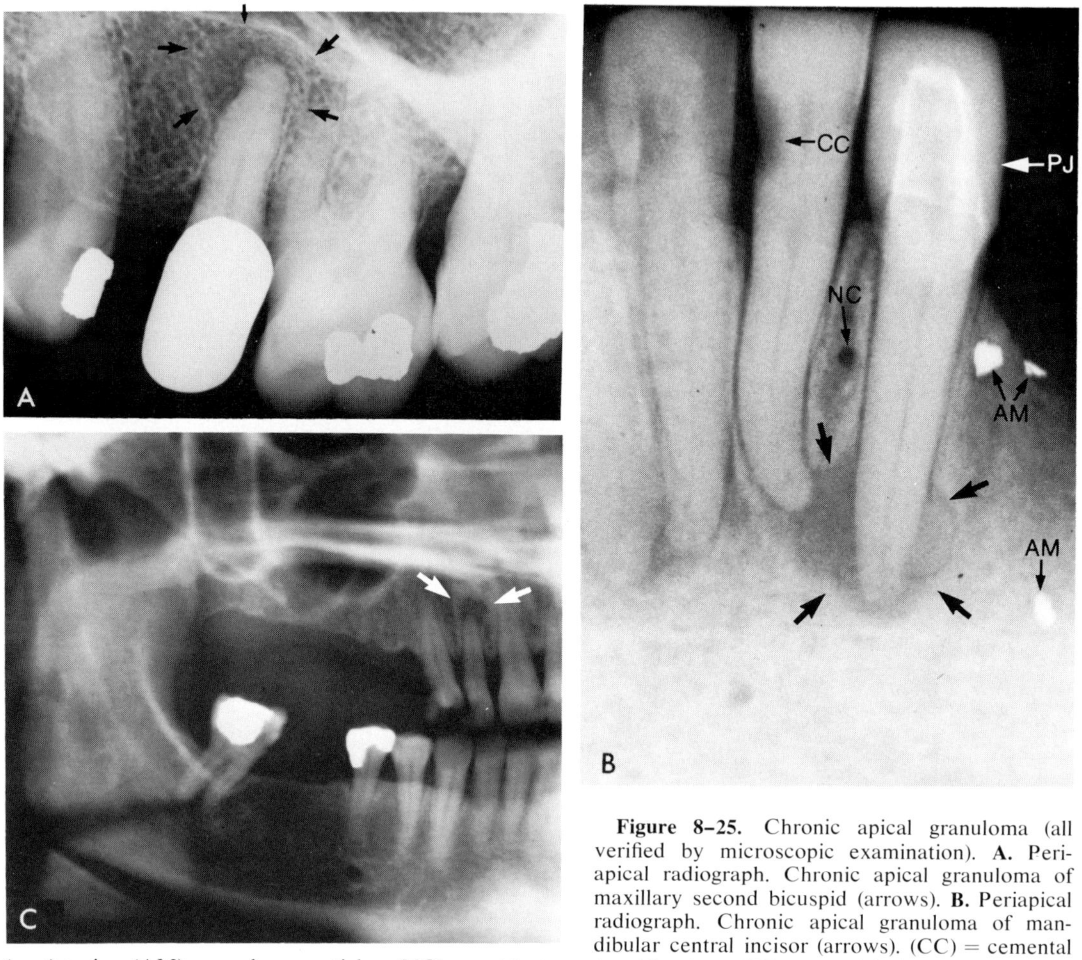

Figure 8–25. Chronic apical granuloma (all verified by microscopic examination). **A.** Periapical radiograph. Chronic apical granuloma of maxillary second bicuspid (arrows). **B.** Periapical radiograph. Chronic apical granuloma of mandibular central incisor (arrows). (CC) = cemental (root) caries. (AM) = amalgam particles. (NC) = nutrient canal and foramen. (PJ) = porcelain jacket. **C.** Panorex radiograph. Chronic apical granuloma of maxillary lateral incisor (arrows).

sealing. In many cases, apical cysts will heal without surgical enucleation after proper endodontic therapy. If left untreated, the apical cyst will increase in size at the expense of the surrounding tissue (Fig. 8–27). If the tooth is removed and the epithelial lining of the apical cyst is not adequately destroyed or removed, a residual cyst will develop.

CONDENSING OSTEITIS (CHRONIC FOCAL SCLEROSING OSTEOMYELITIS)

This is an unusual apical bone reaction to infection seen in people with extremely high tissue resistance or in those with low-grade infections. It is a form of osteomyelitis and occurs almost exclusively in young persons under the age of 20. The mandibular first molar is the tooth most commonly involved. Usually a large carious lesion is present. The tooth is **nonvital** and asymptomatic.

Radiographically, a small radiolucent area is seen around the apex of the tooth surrounded by a larger area of denser bone. The entire root outline is, in most cases, visible, which differentiates condensing osteitis from a benign cementoblastoma. Condensing osteitis is an osteogenic reaction of the bone to the toxic products of the pulp rather than the usual osteolysis. These toxic products act as stimuli rather than irritants (Fig. 8–28). The sclerotic bone is not attached to the tooth and remains after the tooth is extracted. This dense area of bone is usually not remolded and may be recognized in the radiograph years later as osteosclerosis.

If the tooth is worth saving, treatment consists of removal of necrotic material in the root canals and effective sealing of the apex of the roots. The dental radiograph can be used to monitor endodontic therapy to determine whether treatment has been successful (Fig. 8–29).

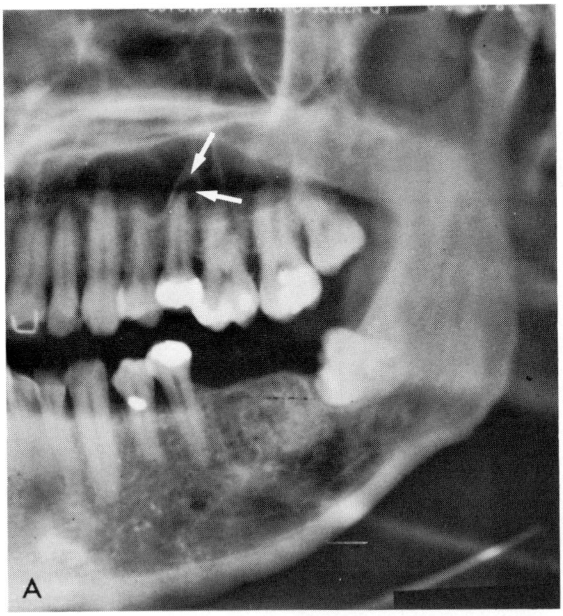

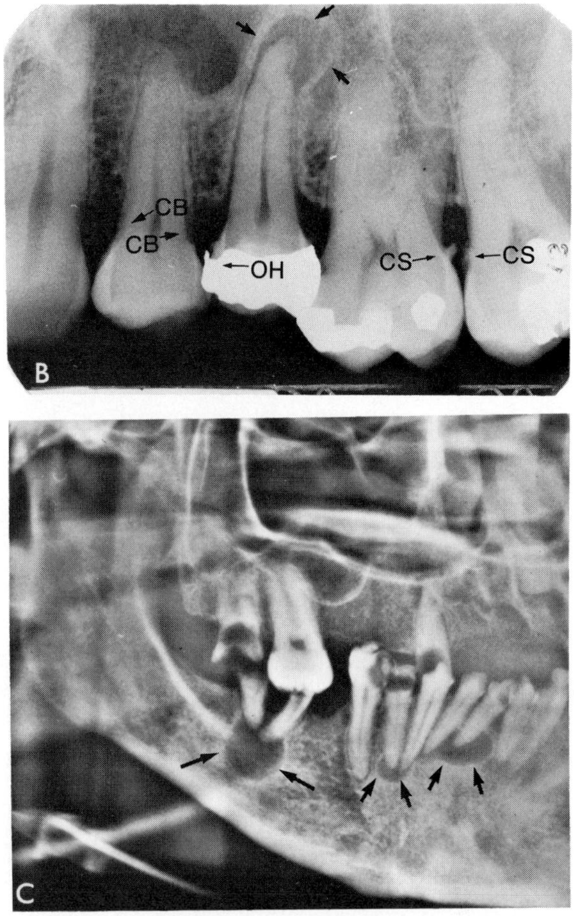

Figure 8–26. Apical cyst (later verified by microscopic study). **A.** Panoramic radiograph. Apical cyst of maxillary second bicuspid (arrows). **B.** Periapical radiograph. Same patient as in **A.** (CS) = calculus spur. (CB) = cervical burnout. (OH) = overhang. **C.** Panoramic radiograph. Multiple apical cysts (arrows).

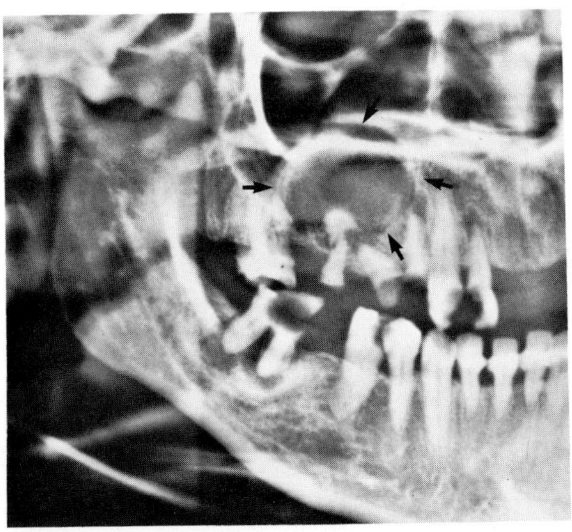

Figure 8–27. Panoramic radiograph. Large apical cyst in maxillary molar region (arrows).

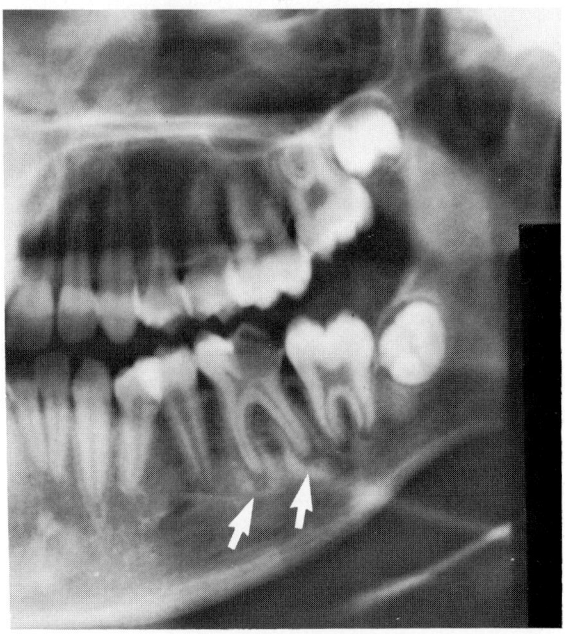

Figure 8–28. Panoramic radiograph. Condensing osteitis in a teenager. This large carious lesion is in the mandibular first molar, which is nonvital.

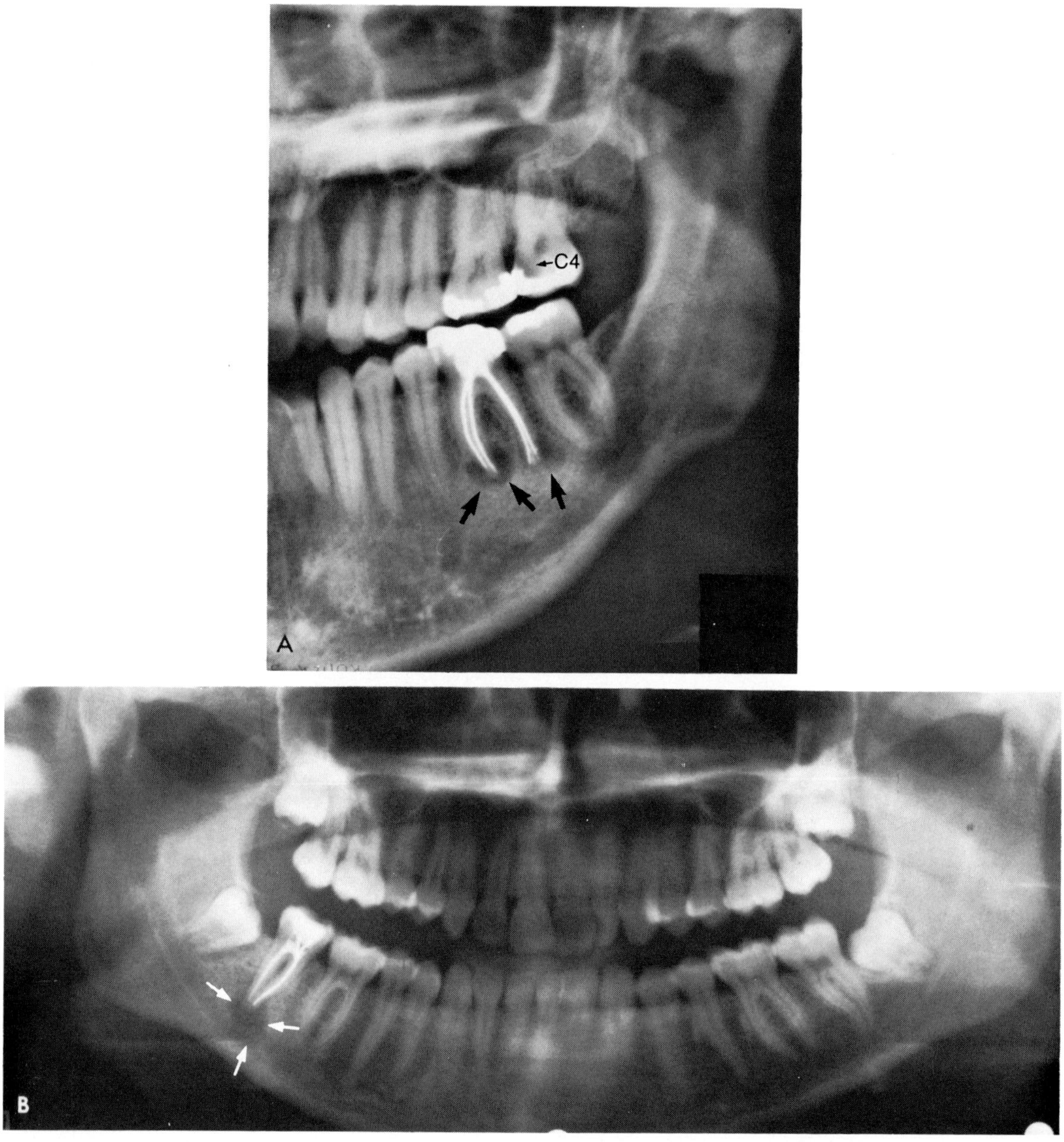

Figure 8–29. Possible unsuccessful endodontic therapy. Radiographic indication of unsuccessful endodontic therapy is when a periapical radiolucency develops on a tooth that preoperatively had normal periapical tissue or when a previous periapical radiolucency does not reduce in size and may, in fact, grow larger. **A.** Panorex radiograph. Endodontic therapy completed one year previous to when radiograph was taken. The periapical radiolucencies associated with the roots of the mandibular first molar have grown in size (arrows). The failure is probably due to an incompletely sealed apex. (C4) = Class 4 secondary caries in maxillary second molar. **B.** Panoral radiograph. Periapical radiolucency of mandibular second molar (arrows) has grown larger since endodontic treatment. Tooth was retreated.

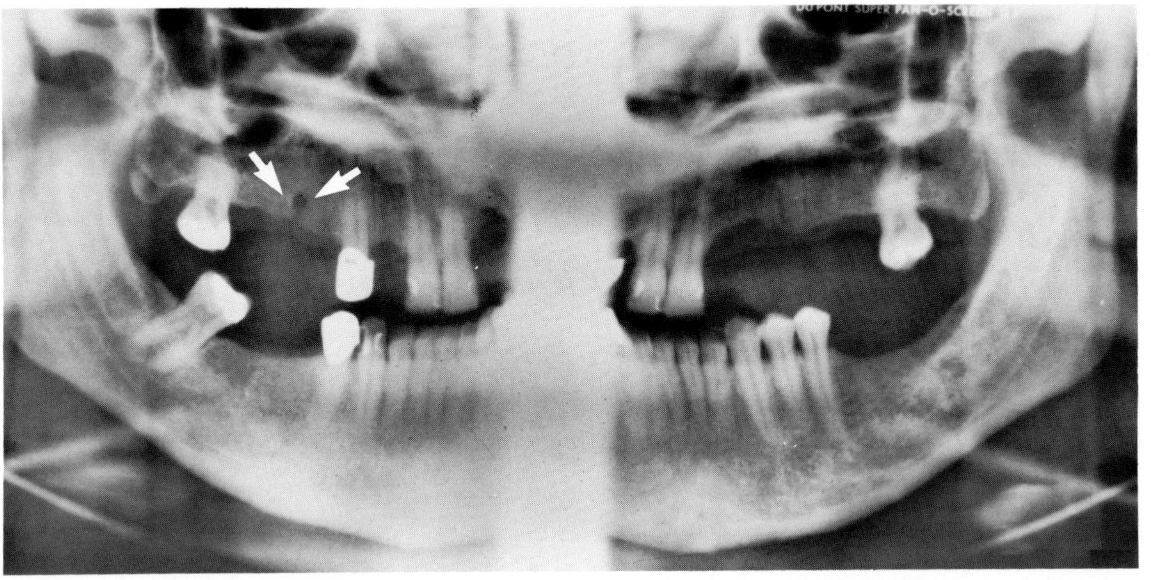

Figure 8–30. Fibrous healing defect. Panorex radiograph with round radiolucency in area of maxillary second bicuspid. This proved to be a fibrous healing defect in which large areas of facial and lingual cortical bone, along with periosteum and marrow, were removed during a previous surgical procedure, leaving a deformity in the bone with a cystlike appearance (arrows).

There are times when a solitary radiolucent lesion will be seen in the alveolar bone. If there has been a history of previous surgery in the area, it is possible that the radiolucency is a fibrous healing defect. Fibrous healing defects usually occur when the facial and lingual cortical plates are destroyed during a surgical procedure or as a result of trauma (Fig. 8–30).

RADIOLOGIC INTERPRETATION OF PERIODONTAL DISEASE

The panoramic radiograph is limited in its ability to depict periodontal disease because of the lack of definition and the routine overlapping of the teeth. However, the panoramic radiograph does provide the clinician with a single, continuous view of the bone of both jaws, which does have some value in the diagnosis of periodontal disease. Therefore, the panoramic radiograph is often used as a supplement to the intraoral radiographic exam in periodontal diagnosis.

The intraoral radiograph that has been properly projected, preferably by the paralleling or right-angle technique, and exposed by a high kilovoltage, long-scale contrast technique will provide information essential to the overall diagnosis of periodontal disease. The accurate radiograph serves primarily to detect the resorption of calcified tissues especially in the interproximal alveolar bone region, because the facial and lingual alveolar bones are obscured by the radiopaque tooth. By the time periodontal bone destruction is seen on the radiograph, it has usually progressed beyond its earliest stages (Bender and Seltzer; Ramaden and Mitchell).

The periodontal pocket, which is a gingival sulcus pathologically deepened (beyond 3 mm in depth) by periodontal disease, will not be recorded on the radiograph because it is composed of soft tissue. In some instances, the pocket depth can be recorded on the radiograph by the use of radiopaque points inserted into the pocket prior to x-ray exposure.

The earliest radiographic signs of periodontal disease are a fuzziness and a break in the continuity of the cortical bone at the crest of the septal bone. This break results from the extension of inflammation from the gingiva into the bone, which, in turn, widens the vessel channels and results in a reduction of calcified tissue per unit of bone at the septal crest (Fig. 8–31). By extension of the inflammation and subsequent resorption of the bone, the height of the septal bone is reduced. Sometimes, on severely inclined teeth, pseudo-infrabony pockets and pseudohyperostosis can be seen in the radiographs (Fig. 8–32).

The properly exposed intraoral radiographic

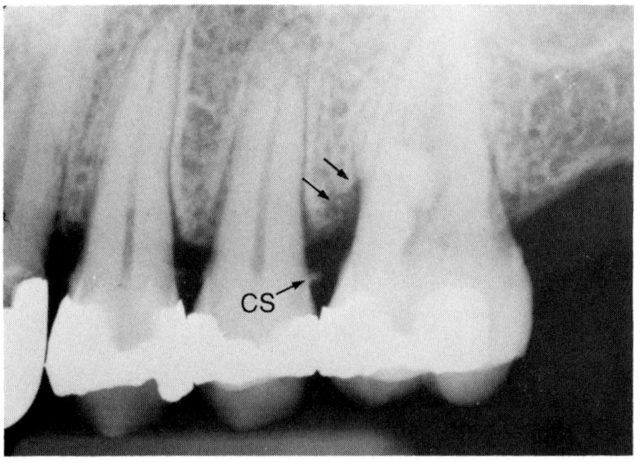

Figure 8–31. Periapical radiograph. Earliest sign of periodontal disease. Fuzziness and a break in continuity of the crest of septal bone (arrows). (CS) = calculus spur.

survey assists the clinician in the periodontal examination in several ways as follows:

1. Estimating the amount of septal bone loss or destruction.
2. Locating the area of bone destruction.
3. Monitoring the clinical examination, confirming and suggesting areas for additional examination.
4. Determining the clinical crown–to–clinical root ratio as well as the shape and size of the roots.

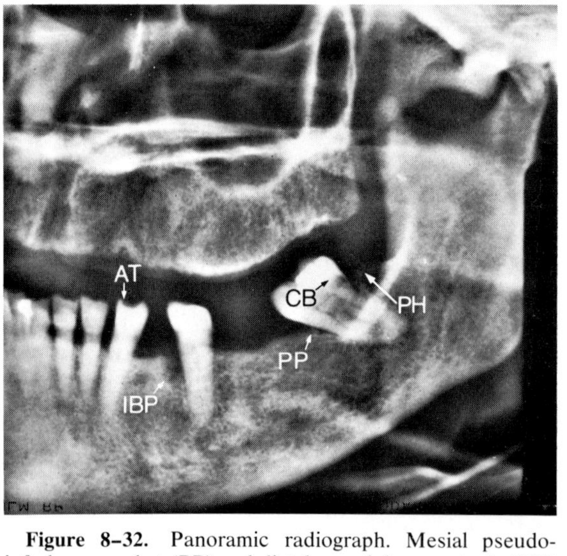

Figure 8–32. Panoramic radiograph. Mesial pseudo-infrabony pocket (PP) and distal pseudohyperostosis (PH) resulting from severely inclined tooth. (IBP) = actual infrabony pocket (mandibular second bicuspid): base of pocket is apical to crest of alveolar ridge (this is probably a one-wall variety with only the mesial wall left standing). (AT) = attrition simulating incisal caries. (CB) = cervical burnout.

5. Determining the pattern or direction of the bone destruction.
6. Determining the distribution of bone destruction or bone loss.
7. Estimating the activity of the destructive process.
8. Detecting local irritating factors such as calculus, overhanging restorations, loose contacts, and trauma.

ESTIMATING THE AMOUNT OF BONE LOSS OR DESTRUCTION

The radiograph may be used indirectly to determine the amount of bone loss in periodontal disease. Actually, the radiograph indicates the amount of bone remaining rather than the amount of bone lost. The amount of bone loss is the difference between the remaining coronal bone height and the assumed normal bone level for the patient. In a normal individual, the alveolar bone level is located 1 to 1.5 mm apical to the cementoenamel junction.

Although bone loss occurs on all surfaces of the root, the density of the tooth obscures the radiographic image of the bone level on the facial and lingual surfaces. However, at times it is possible to read facial and lingual bone levels by using two different procedures:

1. Follow the line of the lamina dura coronally until it loses its opacity. This is the true height of the bone. The bone above this level has been cast coronally by excessive angulation.
2. Examine the tubular pattern of the bone, starting at the apex of the tooth and viewing toward the crown. The appearance of the trabecular pattern of the bone will terminate at the true height of the facial and lingual bone levels. It will give the appearance of a line running across the tooth (Fig. 8–33).

Invasions of the furca areas in the teeth are difficult to identify. They will not be seen until the bone resorption extends apically beyond the furca. The mandibular furca involvement is much more sharply defined than that in the maxillary molar furca because it does not have a palatal root superimposed over the furca, as does the maxillary molar (Fig. 8–34).

The radiograph also acts as a monitor for the clinical examination, confirming or suggesting areas for additional examination. For instance, pericoronal infection around the crown of an unerupted or partially erupted mandibular third molar may be pinpointed by the radiograph. In these cases, there is usually a deep pocket distal

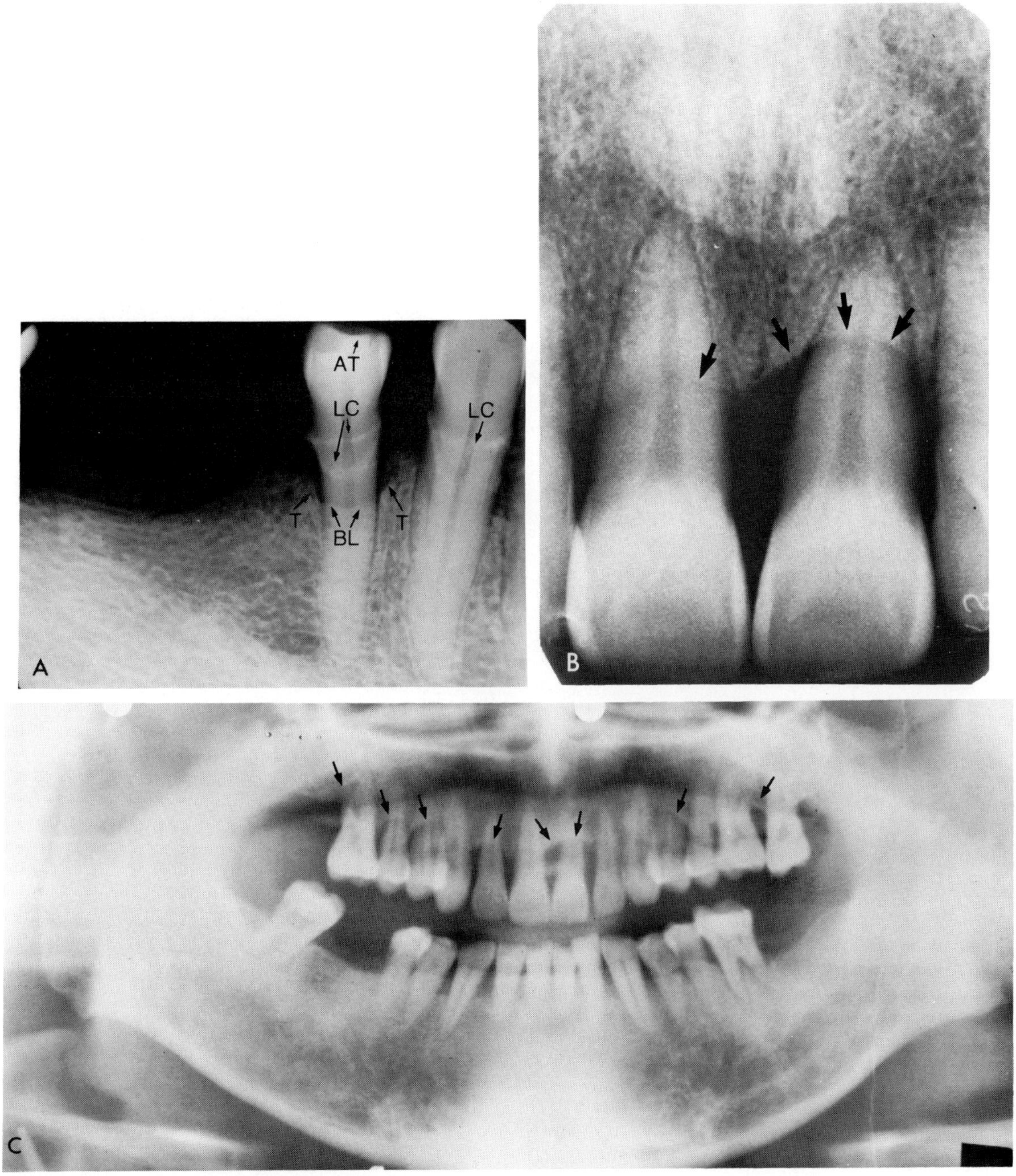

Figure 8–33. Radiographic appearance of height of bone on facial and lingual surfaces of teeth. **A.** Periapical radiograph. (BL) = facial/lingual bone level. (T) = triangulation: widening of periodontal space at crest of ridge (sign of bone degeneration). (LC) = line calculus on facial and lingual surfaces. (AT) = attrition. **B** and **C.** Periapical radiograph. Facial/lingual bone level outlined by arrows.

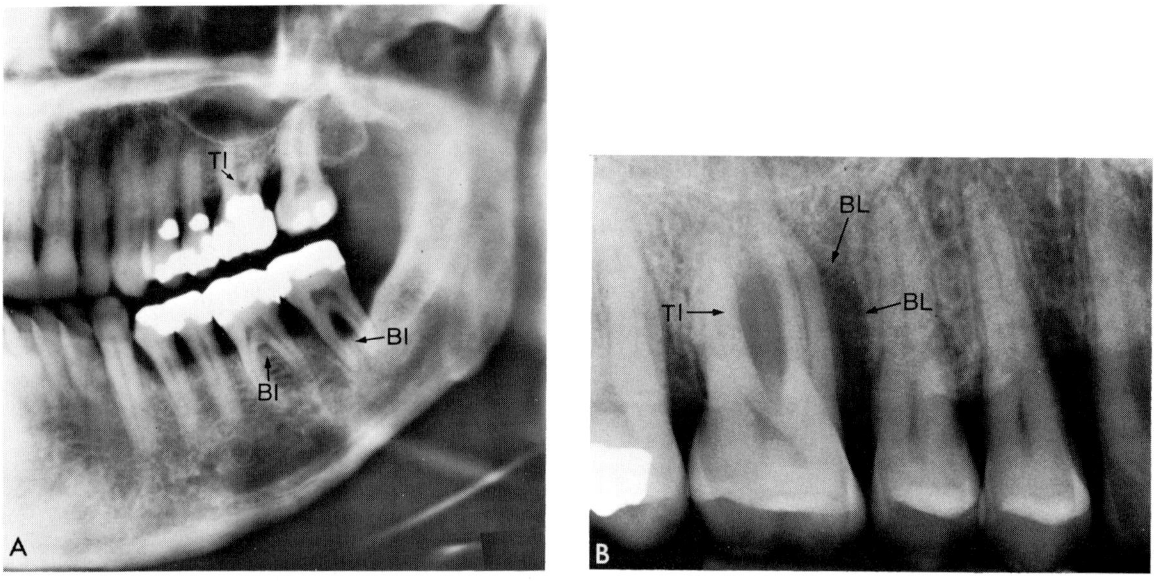

Figure 8–34. Furca invasions. They are visible radiographically only after bone resorption extends apically past the furca of the tooth. **A.** Panoramic radiograph. The radiodensity of trifurcation involvement (TI) of the maxillary molar teeth is *not* as radiolucent as that of bifurcation involvement (BI) of the mandibular molars because of the superimposition of the radiopaque lingual root of the maxillary molars. The thickened periodontal ligament space of the mandibular first molar should be investigated clinically, especially because of the bone loss on the adjacent roots. **B.** Periapical radiograph. Furca invasion of the maxillary molar may invade from the buccal, distal, or mesial aspect. The most common invasion site is the mesial surface. Bone resorption is probably from both the buccal and mesial aspects in this patient. Whenever there is severe bone loss associated with a single molar tooth (as shown here), the furcation is almost always involved. (BL) = bone loss. (TL) = trifurcation involvement.

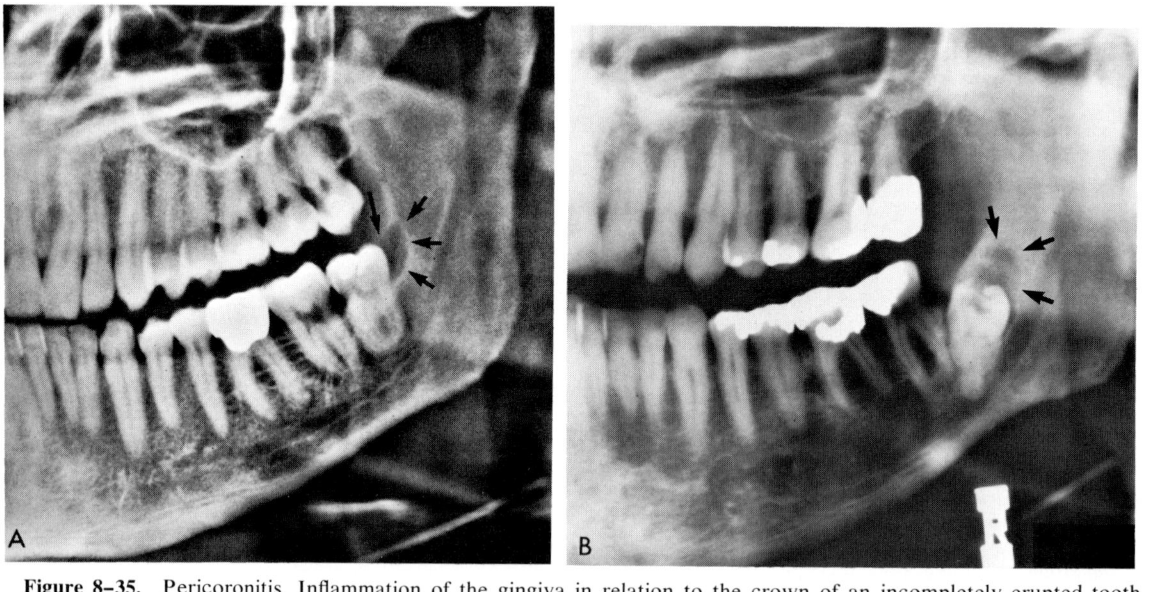

Figure 8–35. Pericoronitis. Inflammation of the gingiva in relation to the crown of an incompletely erupted tooth. This occurs most frequently in the mandibular third molar region. **A.** Panoramic radiograph. Pericoronitis of the mandibular third molar (arrows). Note the typical flame-shaped radiolucency distal to the crown of the third molar. **B.** Panoramic radiograph. Pericoronitis of impacted mandibular third molar. Patient had a severe localized form of pericoronal abscess, which spread posteriorly into the throat and medially into the floor of the mouth, making it difficult to swallow. There was submandibular and cervical lymph node involvement.

to the crown, which makes an ideal incubating area for bacteria.

In the acute phase of pericoronal infection there may be no apparent radiographic change, but in those acute cases preceded by a chronic phase, a radiolucency of bone may be seen. The typical symptoms of acute inflammation are present — redness, swelling, and usually some trismus (Fig. 8–35).

The amount of bone loss should not be the sole determining factor in periodontal diagnosis as to whether a tooth should be sacrificed or

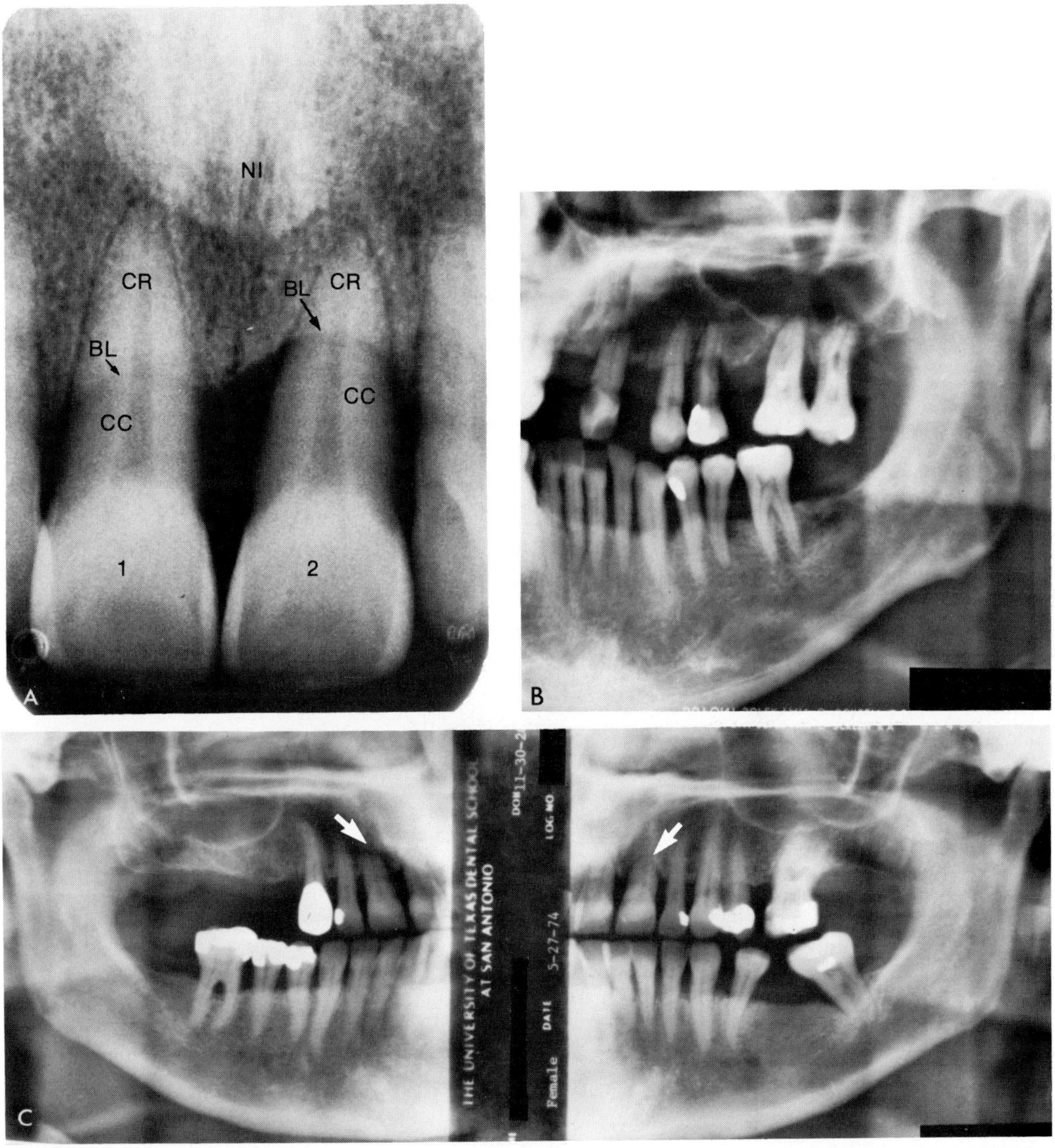

Figure 8–36. Clinical crown–to–clinical root ratio. The clinical crown is the amount of tooth not retained in bone, and the clinical root is the portion of tooth retained in bone. The more the clinical crown lengthens, the less the periodontium will be able to withstand the occlusal forces put upon it. **A.** Periapical radiograph. Central incisor #1 has a more favorable clinical crown–to–clinical root ratio than central incisor #2. (BL) = bone level. (CR) = clinical root. (CC) = clinical crown. (NI) = nose image. **B.** Panoramic radiograph. Clinical crown–to–clinical root ratio is unfavorable. However, the long roots of this patient preserved a favorable clinical crown–to–clinical root ratio for more years than is usual. **C.** Panoramic radiograph. Unfavorable clinical crown–to–clinical root ratio of maxillary centrals due to a combination of short roots and alveolar bone loss (arrows).

treated. Therapy should be determined using the radiograph as a diagnostic aid only. The final decision to perform periodontal therapy should be based on all the diagnostic information collected.

DETERMINING THE CLINICAL CROWN-TO-CLINICAL ROOT RATIO

The clinical crown-to-clinical root ratio is determined by comparing the portion of the tooth outside the bone with the length and contour of the root that is invested in the bone. This ratio is one of the criteria used to determine whether splinting or a fixed prosthesis is indicated in certain cases (Fig. 8–36).

The radiograph records the shape and length of the roots of the teeth, which are important in establishing a prognosis. Teeth that are short and spiked-shaped have a guarded prognosis if periodontically involved (Fig. 8–37).

DETERMINING THE PATTERN OR DIRECTION OF BONE DESTRUCTION

The direction of the bone loss is determined using the cementoenamel junction as the plane of reference. When the bone loss occurs on a plane that is parallel to a line drawn from the cementoenamel junction of one tooth to that of an adjacent tooth, it is called horizontal bone loss (Fig. 8–38). When there is greater bone destruction on the proximal aspect of one tooth than on the adjacent tooth, the bone level is angular or not parallel to a line joining the cementoenamel junctions. This type of bone loss is called vertical bone loss (Fig. 8–39).

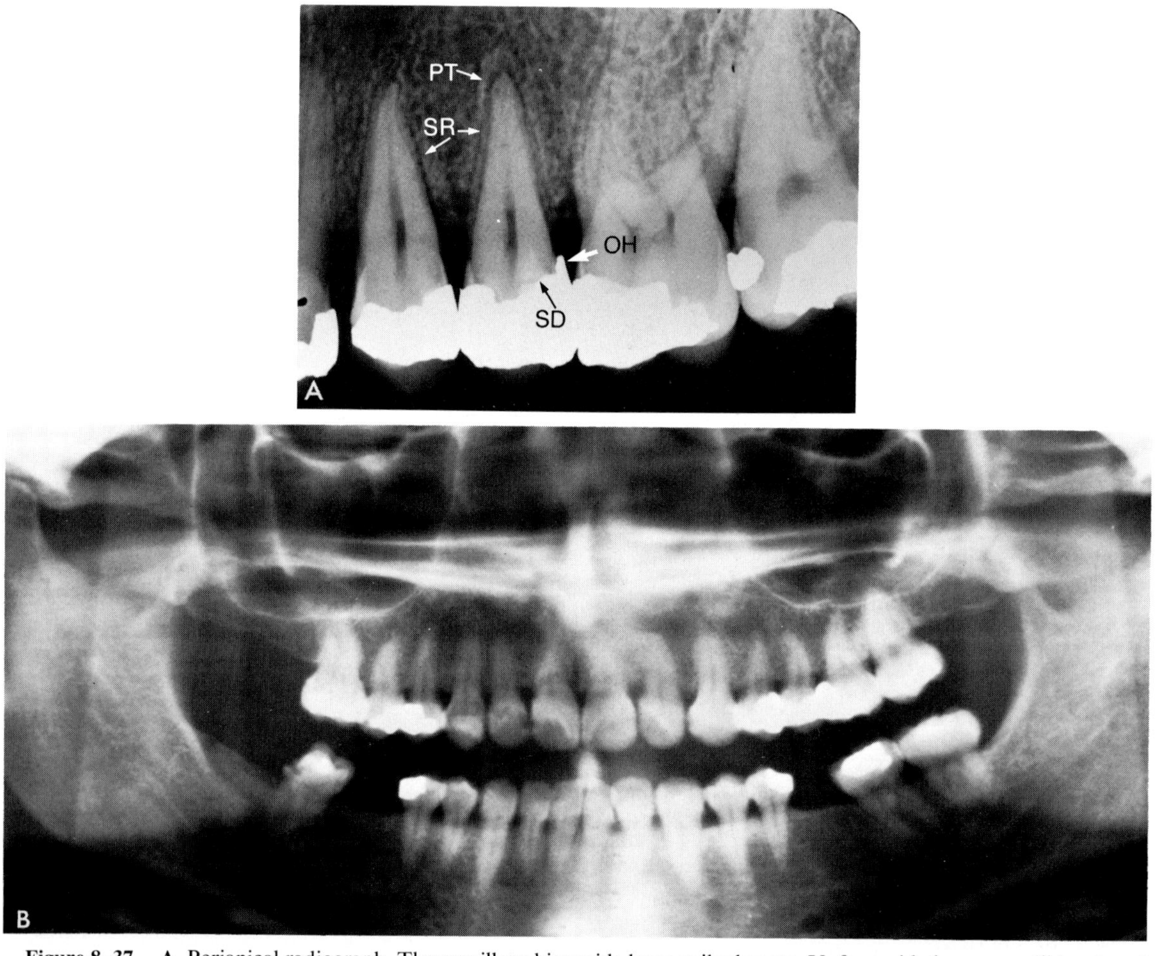

Figure 8–37. **A.** Periapical radiograph. The maxillary bicuspids have spiked roots. Unfavorable leverage will be placed upon the periodontium of these teeth if there is any amount of alveolar bone loss. There is a slight amount of periodontal ligament space thickening (PT) at the apex of the maxillary second bicuspid. (OH) = overhang. (SR) = spiked roots. (SD) = sclerotic dentin. **B.** Panoramic radiograph of patient with short, spike-shaped roots.

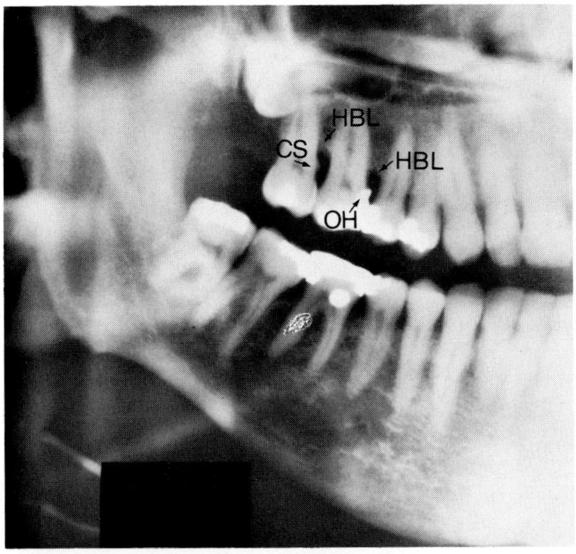

Figure 8–38. Panorex radiograph. With a horizontal bone loss (HBL) or defect, the interseptal bone is reduced in height, with the alveolar crest horizontal and perpendicular to the long axis of the adjacent teeth. The sole source of this type of bone destruction is thought to be inflammation in response to local irritants. (OH) = overhang. (CS) = calculus spur.

Horizontal bone loss is consistent with the uniform resorption of bone in response to the inflammation caused by local factors. Angular or vertical bone loss was at one time thought to be associated with a more complex etiology such as, possibly, of systemic origin. Proof of this has not been demonstrated, and, therefore, vertical and horizontal bone losses have not been as critical in the clinical diagnosis as was formerly believed. Even so, vertical bone loss is still thought by many to be derived from a more complex etiology than horizontal bone loss (most likely, a combination of traumatic occlusion and local irritation factors).

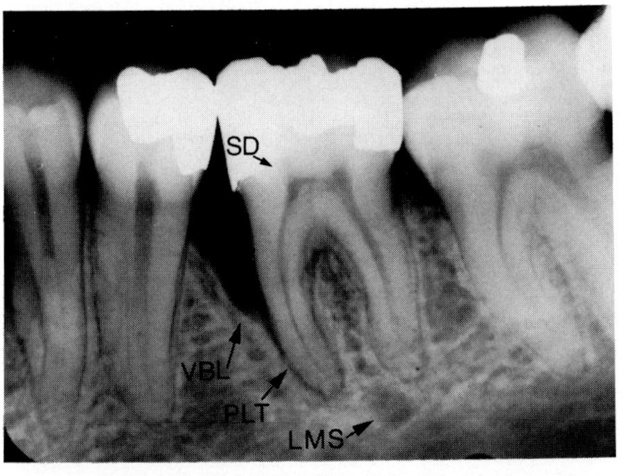

Figure 8–39. Periapical radiograph. An angular pattern of bone destruction or vertical bone loss is thought to be due to a combination of inflammation and trauma from occlusion. (LMS) = large medullary space. (SD) = sclerotic dentin. (VBL) = vertical bone loss. (PLT) = periodontal ligament thickening.

DETERMINING THE DISTRIBUTION OF BONE DESTRUCTION OR LOSS

Bone destruction or bone loss may be localized in one area of the dental arches or it may be generalized throughout the mouth. It is an important diagnostic sign. The overall prognosis is bad if there are not enough good teeth to support a satisfactory prosthesis (Fig. 8–40).

In the terminal stages of chronic destructive periodontal disease, the teeth may be exfoliated because of complete lack of periodonal ligament attachment and bony support of the teeth. In the radiograph, the teeth seem to be hanging in air (Fig. 8–41). Inflammation may spread from the gingiva into the alveolar bone and periodontal ligament and may reach the pulp through the root apices or accessory pulp canals near the apex or the furcation. In these cases, survival of the tooth depends on combined periodontal-endodontic treatment (Fig. 8–42).

ESTIMATING THE ACTIVITY OF THE DESTRUCTIVE PROCESS

The activity of the destructive process of the bone is best evaluated by a series of radiographs taken over a period of time. When the bone is reduced in height with an irregular and roughened crest and without bone condensation, it is most likely that an active destructive process is at work (Fig. 8–43). The process is most likely static or slowly destructive if, in the presence of bone loss, the crestal region of the bone is smooth, with bone condensation (Fig. 8–44).

DETECTING LOCAL IRRITATING FACTORS

Several local irritating factors may be detected by the radiograph. They are calculus, faulty restorations, food-packing areas, and occlusal overstress. The radiograph plays no role in determining the etiology of these conditions

Text continued on page 252

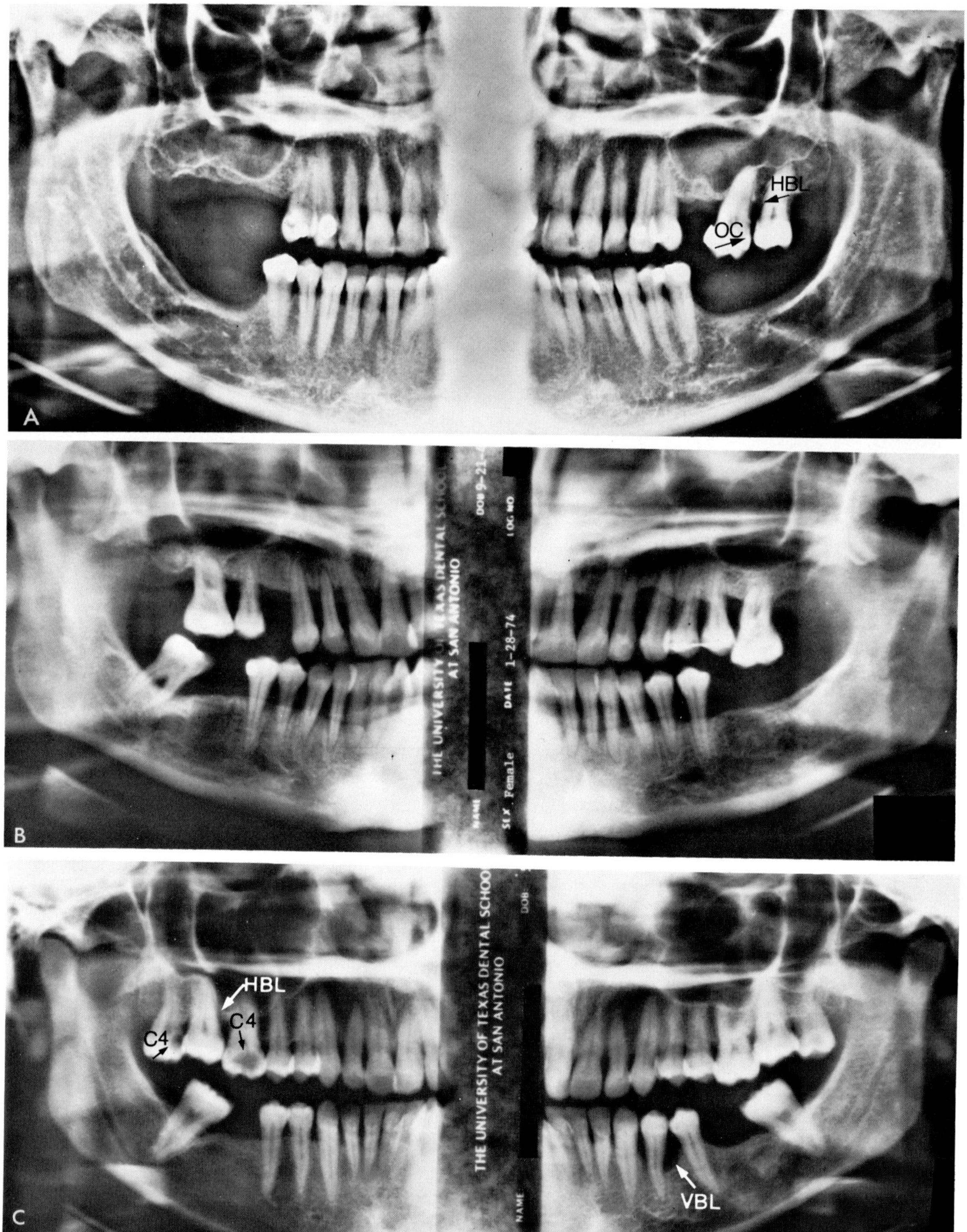

Figure 8–40. Localized and generalized bone loss. **A.** Panorex radiograph. The distribution of the bone destruction is an important diagnostic sign. If the bone loss is severe and generalized, the prognosis is poor. (HBL) = localized horizontal bone loss between maxillary molars. (OC) = open contact. **B.** Panoramic radiograph. Generalized horizontal bone loss in female patient with chronic destructive periodontitis. **C.** Panorex radiograph. Localized vertical (VBL) or angular bone loss of mandibular first bicuspid. In the early stages of periodontal disease, the loss of alveolar bone is usually localized and tends to be generalized as the disease progresses. (HBL) = horizontal bone loss. (C4) = dentinal caries encroaching upon pulp.

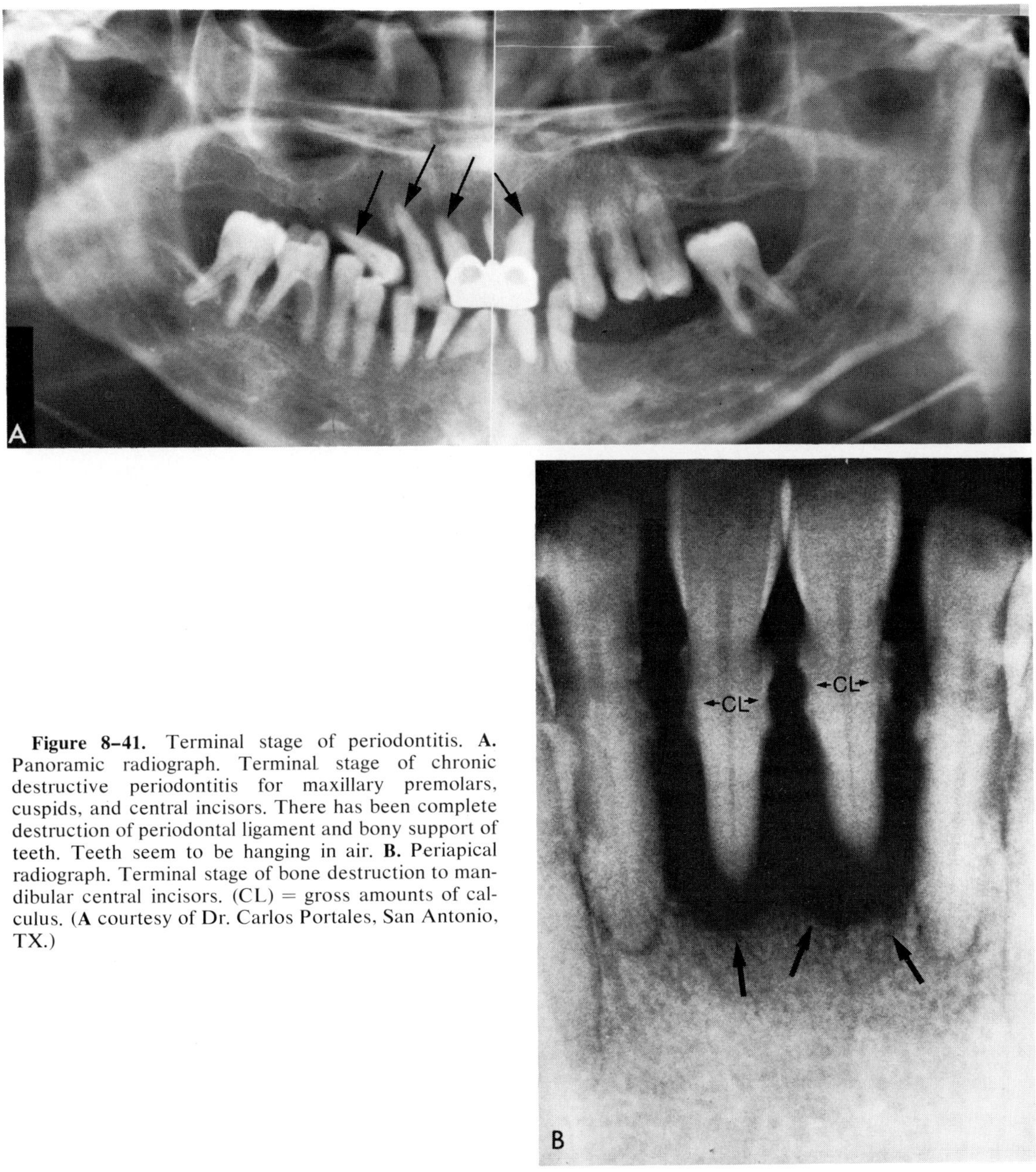

Figure 8–41. Terminal stage of periodontitis. **A.** Panoramic radiograph. Terminal stage of chronic destructive periodontitis for maxillary premolars, cuspids, and central incisors. There has been complete destruction of periodontal ligament and bony support of teeth. Teeth seem to be hanging in air. **B.** Periapical radiograph. Terminal stage of bone destruction to mandibular central incisors. (CL) = gross amounts of calculus. (**A** courtesy of Dr. Carlos Portales, San Antonio, TX.)

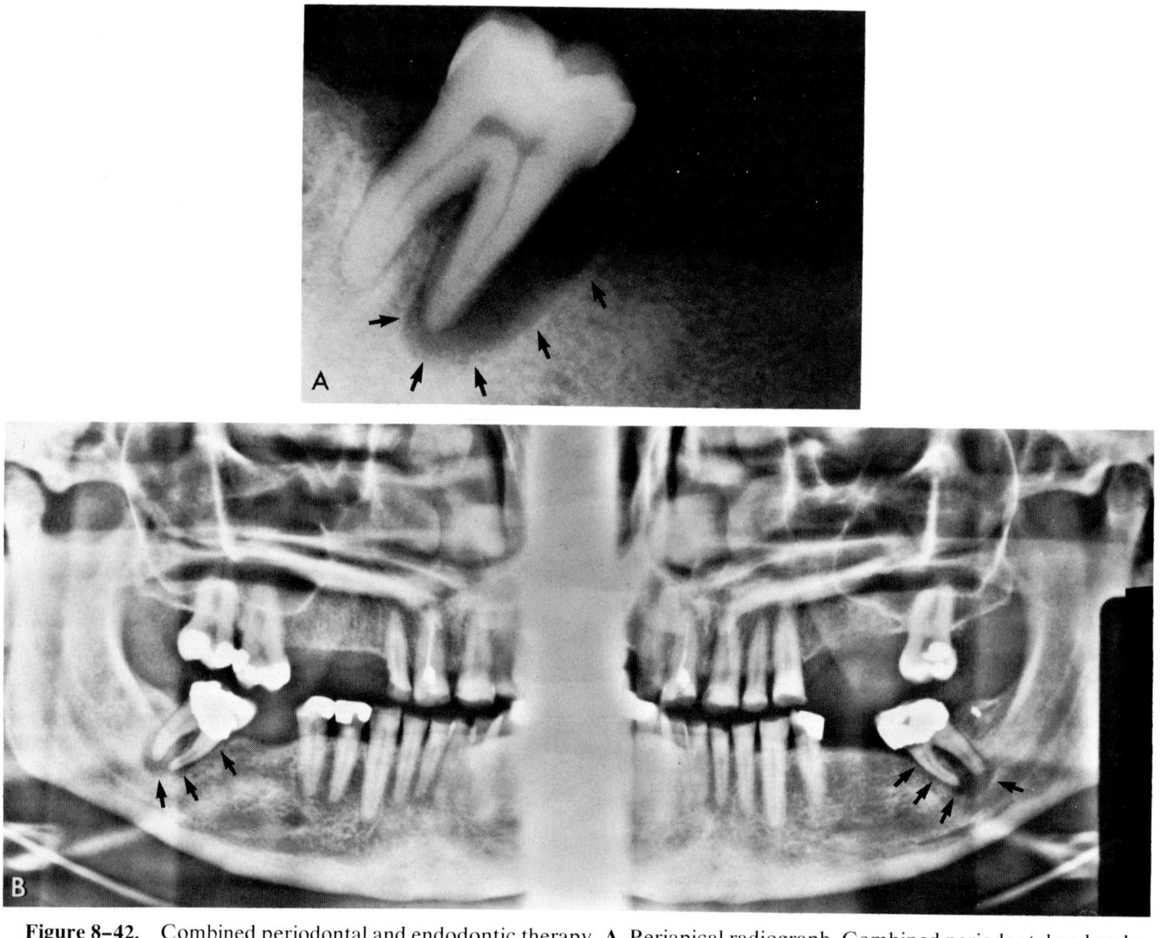

Figure 8–42. Combined periodontal and endodontic therapy. **A.** Periapical radiograph. Combined periodontal and endodontic therapy. There was a continuous tract from the gingival crest to the apex of the tooth. This was determined by probing. The mesial root of the tooth was nonvital. The prognosis of this type of therapy is best when the teeth are firm and the destruction is confined to one root surface of single-rooted teeth and one root surface of multirooted teeth. **B.** Panorex radiograph. Possible combined periodontal-endodontic therapy was contemplated for both mandibular molars. The periodontal destruction is continuous from the gingival crest to the apices of both teeth. Both teeth are nonvital. Trauma from occlusal disharmony was one of the causative factors in this case.

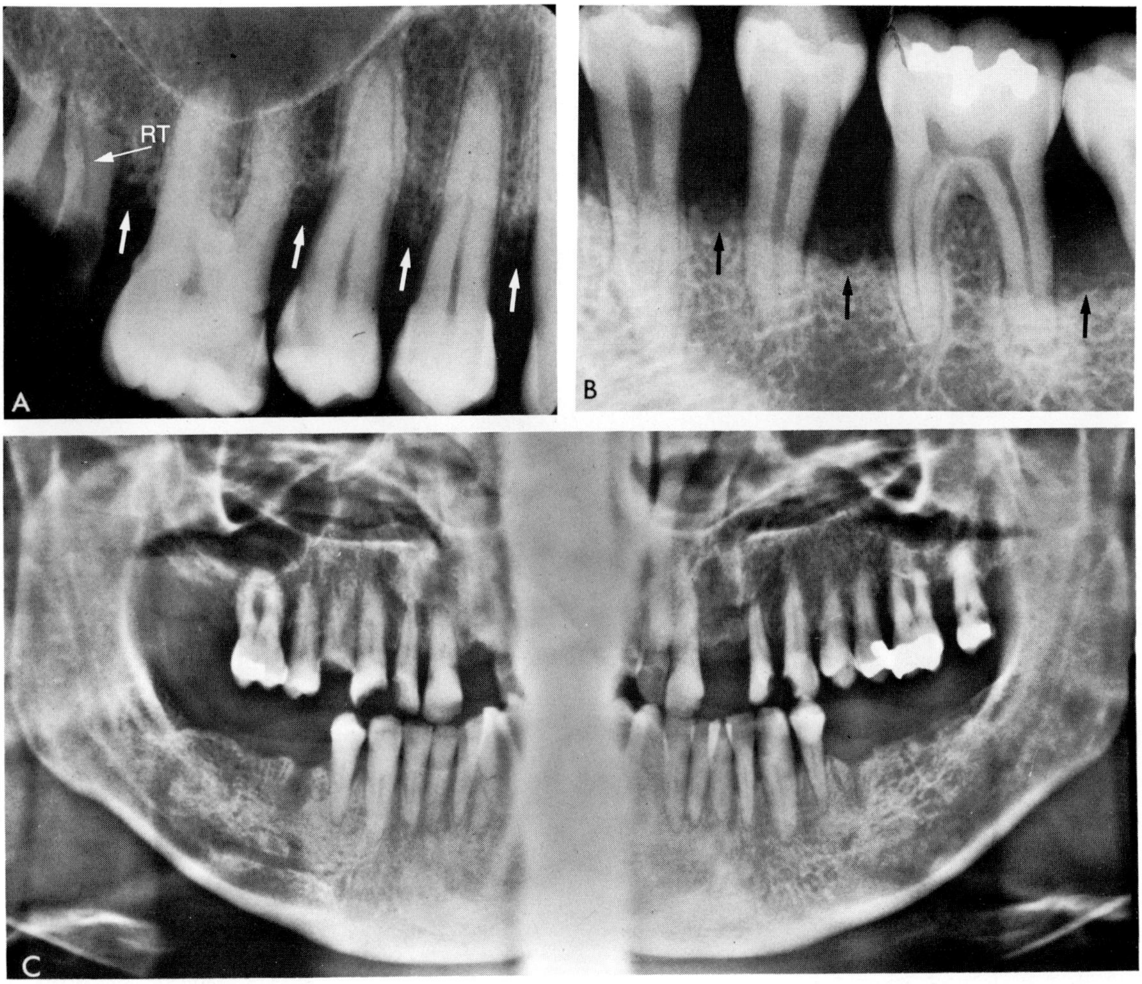

Figure 8–43. Active bone destruction. **A.** Periapical radiograph. Active destruction of maxillary alveolar bone in posterior region from periodontal disease. The height of the bone is reduced and the crest of the interseptal bone is roughened and irregular (arrows). The maxillary first molar is supraerupted. (RT) = root tips. **B.** Periapical radiograph. Active bone destruction from periodontal disease in mandibular posterior arch (arrows). **C.** Panorex radiograph. Active bone destruction of maxillary arch by periodontal disease. Note the osteoporotic appearance of the bone and the reduced height of the irregular bone crests between the teeth.

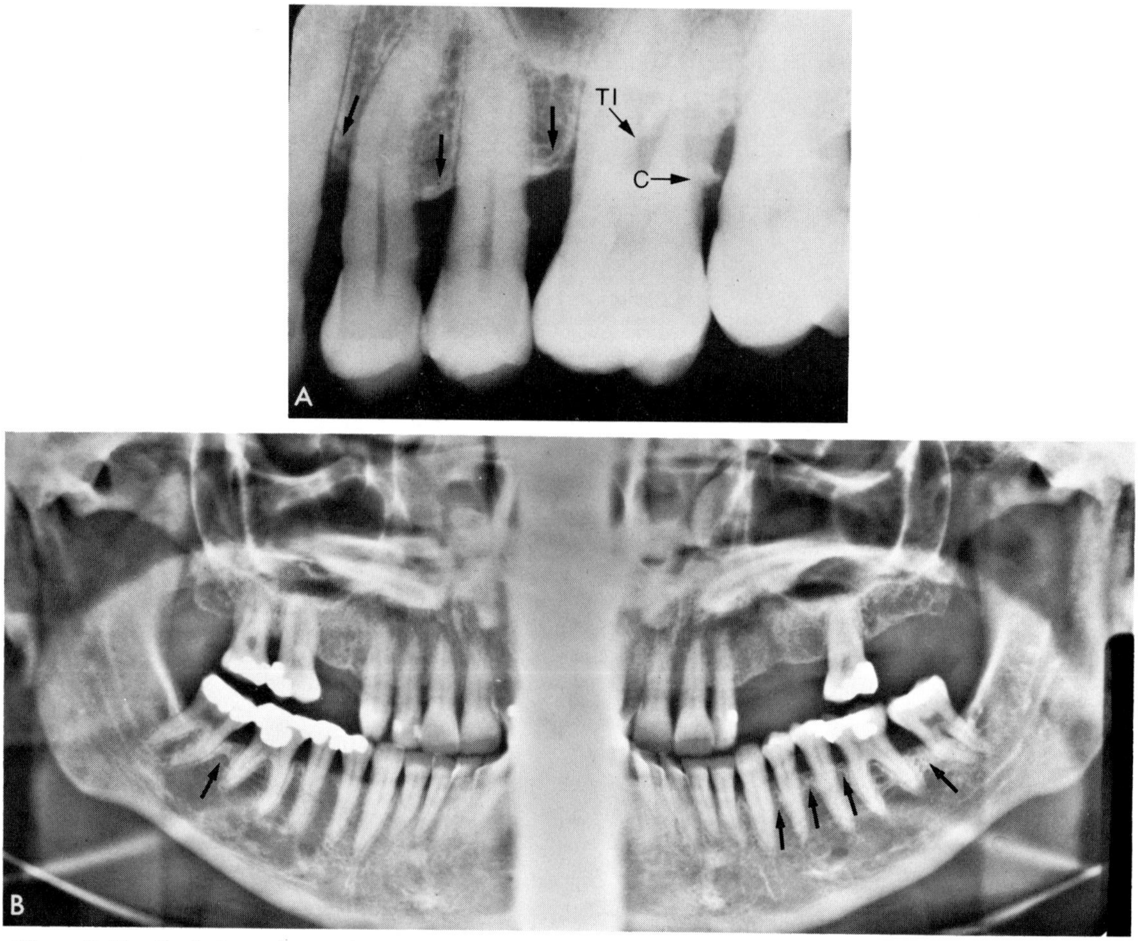

Figure 8–44. Static bone destruction. **A.** Periapical radiograph. Static or slowly destructive process. Bone height is reduced, but the crest of septal bone is smooth with condensed bone (arrows). (C) = calculus. (TI) = trifurcation involvement. **B.** Panorex radiograph. Static or slowly destructive activity. Bone height of interseptal bone is reduced, but it is smooth in contour.

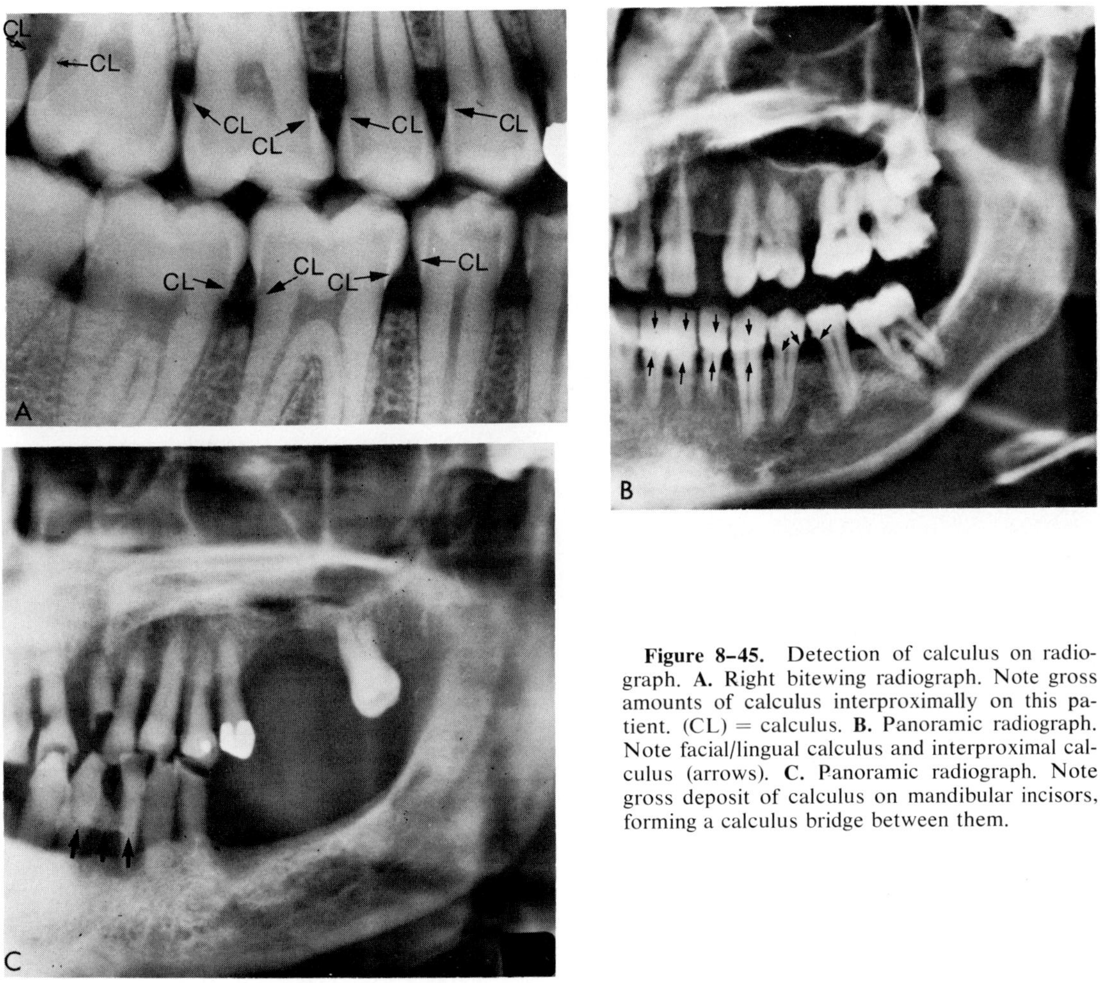

Figure 8-45. Detection of calculus on radiograph. **A.** Right bitewing radiograph. Note gross amounts of calculus interproximally on this patient. (CL) = calculus. **B.** Panoramic radiograph. Note facial/lingual calculus and interproximal calculus (arrows). **C.** Panoramic radiograph. Note gross deposit of calculus on mandibular incisors, forming a calculus bridge between them.

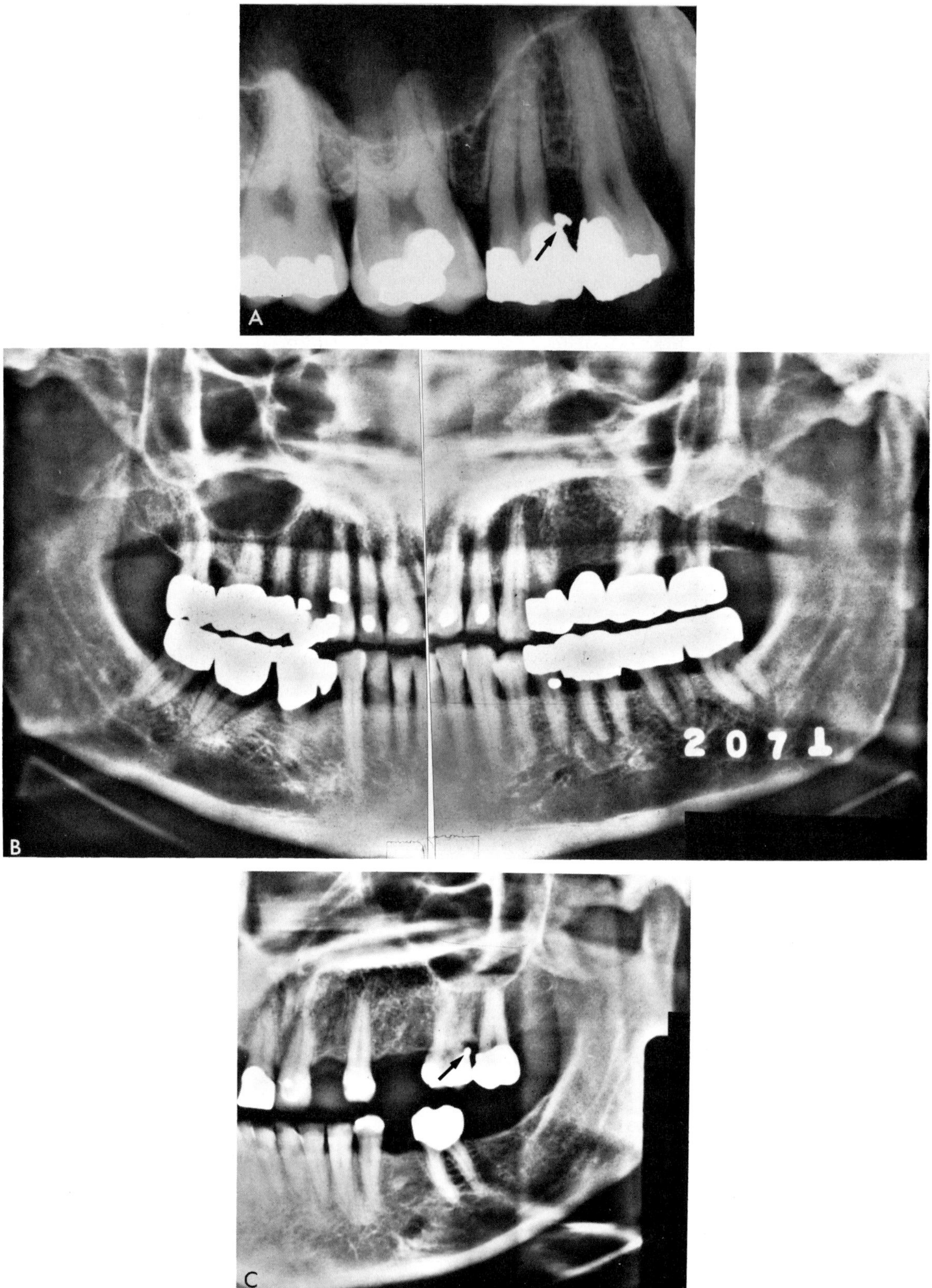

Figure 8–46. Faulty restorations (overhangs). **A.** Periapical radiograph. Overhang interproximal restoration shaped like a hook. **B.** Panoramic radiograph. Oversized crowns throughout both arches. **C.** Panoramic radiograph. Overhang distal to maxillary first molar (arrow).

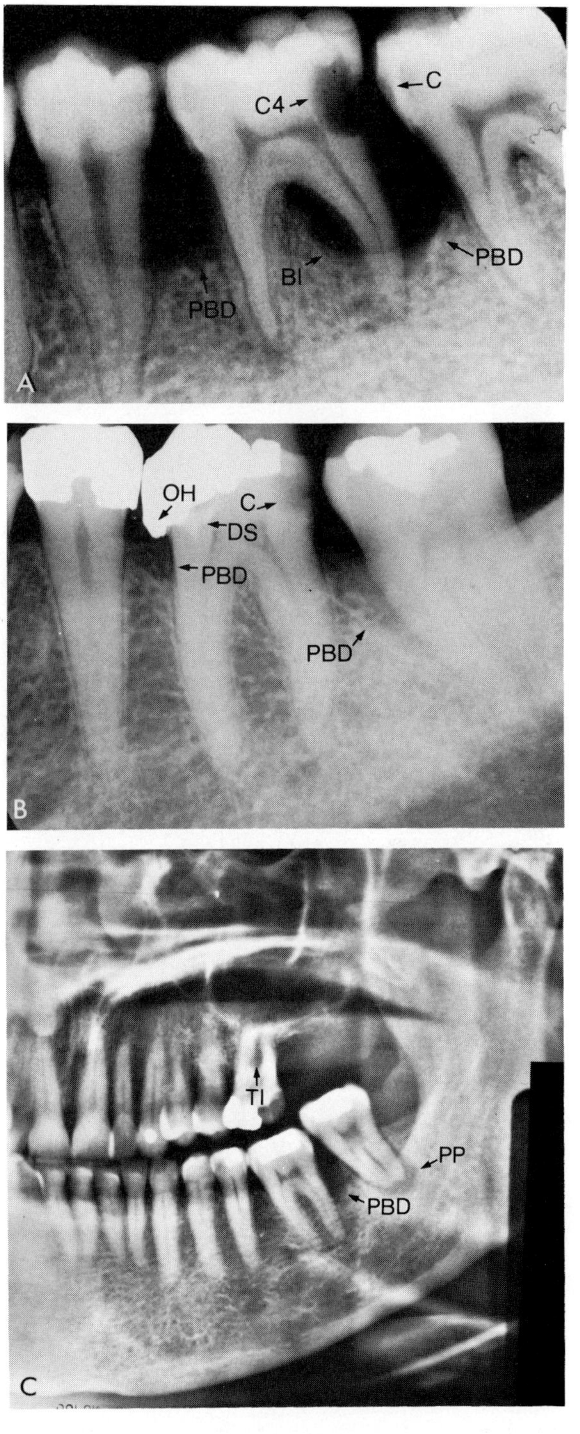

Figure 8–47. Loose contacts. **A.** Periapical radiograph. Loose contact between first and second molars resulting in caries (C), periodontal bone destruction (PDB), and bifurcation involvement (BI). **B.** Periapical radiograph. Loose contact from interproximal caries (C) on the distal aspect of first molar, resulting in food packing area and periodontal bone destruction (PBD). Note overhang (OH) on mesio-occlusal restoration in same tooth and beginnings of bone destruction. (DS) = dentinal sclerosis. **C.** Panoramic radiograph. Loose contact resulting from supraerupting mandibular second molar. Note periodontal bone destruction (PBD) between mandibular first and second molars, periapical pathology (PP) at apex of mandibular second molar, and trifurcation involvement (TI) of maxillary first molar.

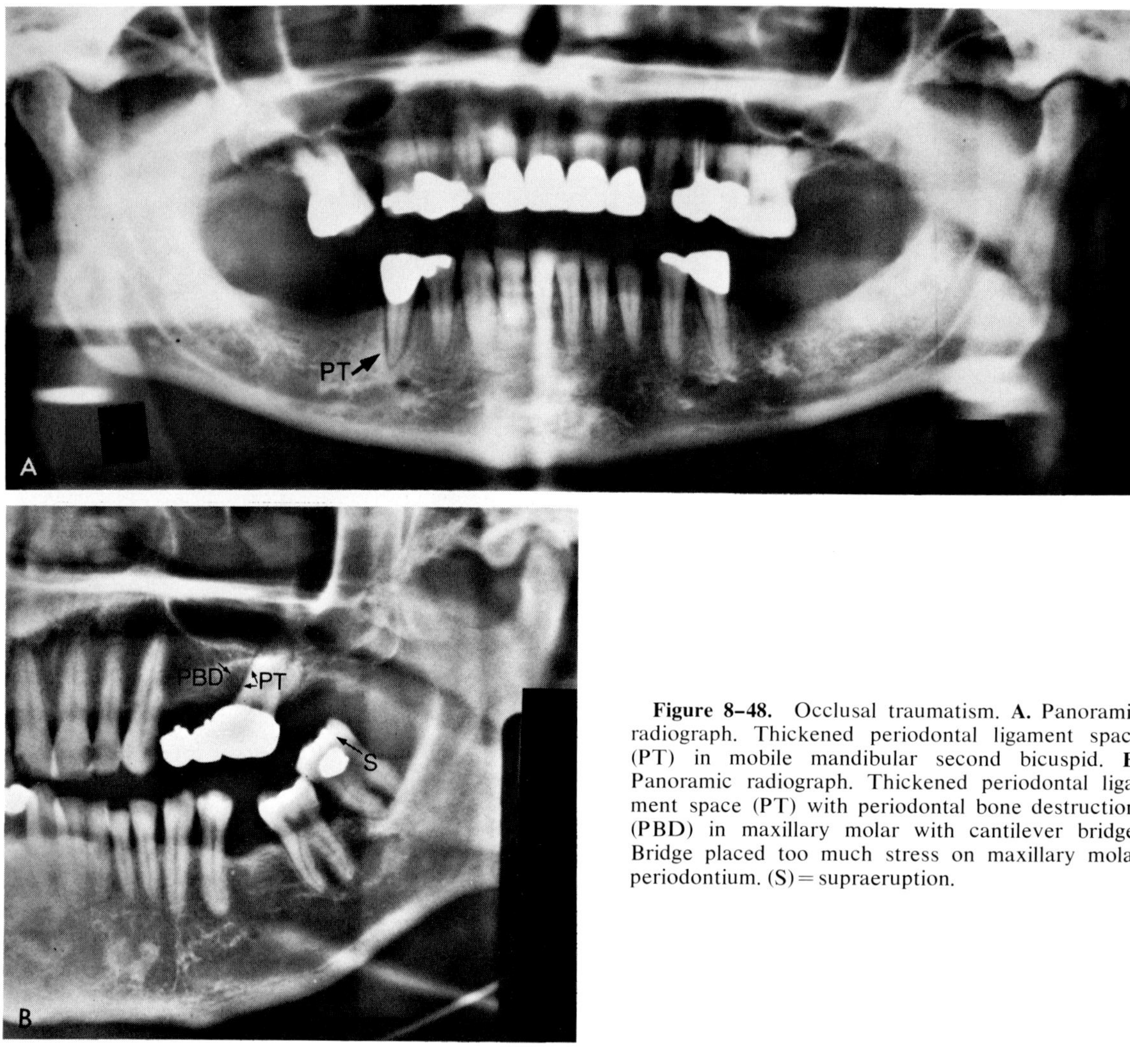

Figure 8–48. Occlusal traumatism. **A.** Panoramic radiograph. Thickened periodontal ligament space (PT) in mobile mandibular second bicuspid. **B.** Panoramic radiograph. Thickened periodontal ligament space (PT) with periodontal bone destruction (PBD) in maxillary molar with cantilever bridge. Bridge placed too much stress on maxillary molar periodontium. (S) = supraeruption.

other than detecting the presence of certain types of irritations.

The radiograph will detect gross deposits of calculus interproximately and sometimes on the facial and lingual surfaces (Fig. 8–45). The bone level has to be reduced sufficiently to reveal facial/lingual calculus formation. The radiograph cannot be relied upon for the detection of all calculus. The use of a sharp explorer is the only sure way to examine the teeth for calculus.

Some of the local irritating factors caused by faulty restorations are overhangs, imperfectly formed embrasures, and ill-shaped facial/lingual contours (Fig. 8–46). Loose contacts provide areas for food impaction, another source of local irritation to the periodontal tissues (Fig. 8–47).

The supporting periodontal structures can be injured when restorations are placed that do not conform to the occlusal wear patterns of the teeth. Radiographic signs of traumatic occlusion include: (1) widening of the periodontal ligament space; (2) thickening of the lamina dura; (3) vertical septal bone destruction; and (4) root resorption (Fig. 8–48).

REFERENCES

Barr, J. H., and Stephens, R. B.: **Dental Radiology**. Philadelphia: W. B. Saunders, 1980, pp. 297–326.

Bender, I. B., and Seltzer, S.: Roentgenographic and direct observation of experimental lesions in bone: I. **J.A.D.A. 62**:152, 1961a.

Bender, I. B., and Seltzer, S.: Roentgenographic and direct observations of experimental lesions in bone: II. **J.A.D.A. 62**:708, 1961.

Beveridge, E. E., and Brown, A. C.: The measurement of human dental intrapulpal pressures and its response to clinical variables. **Oral Surg., 19**:655, 1965.

Dunning, J. M., and Ferguson, G. W.: Effect of bitewing roentgenograms on Navy dental examination findings. **U.S. Naval Med. Bull. 46**:83, 1946.

Early, P. J., Razzak, M. A., and Dodee, D. B.: **Textbook of Nuclear Medicine Technology**. 3rd Edition. St. Louis: C. V. Mosby, 1979, p. 379.

Garretson, J. E.: Neuralgia dependent on granules of osteodentine. **Dent. Cosmos 14**:25, 1872.

Glickman, I.: **Clinical Periodontology,** 4th Edition. Philadelphia: W. B. Saunders, 1972, pp. 336–337, 483, 499–516.

Greenbaum, L. M.: Inflammation and the role of endogenous pain-producing substances. **Dent. Clin. North Am. 22**:47, 1978.

Hansen, B. F.: Clinical and roentgenologic caries detection. **Dent. Max.-Fac. Radiol. 9**:34, 1980.

Haugejorden, O.: A study of the methods of radiologic diagnosis of dental caries in epidemiological investigations. **Acta Odontol. Scand. (Suppl. 65),** 1974.

Haugejorden, O., and Slack, G. L.: A study of intra-examiner caries at different diagnostic levels. **Acta Odontol. Scand. 33**:169, 1975.

Haugejorden, O., and Slack, G. L.: The construction and use of diagnostic standards for radiographic caries incidence scores. **Acta Odontol. Scand. 35**:95, 1977.

Hill, T. J.: Pathology of the dental pulp. **J.A.D.A. 21**:820, 1934.

Hurlburt, C. E., and Wuehrmann, A. H.: Comparison of interproximal carious lesion detection in panoramic and standard intraoral radiography. **J.A.D.A. 93**:1154, 1976.

Ludlow, M. O.: Endodontic first aid for the patient with odontalgia. **Dent. Surv. 42**:25, 1979.

Mandel, I. D.: Dental caries. **Am. Sci. 67**:661, 1979.

Maurice, C. G.: **An Annotated Glossary of Terms Used in Endodontics.** 3rd Edition. Atlanta: Am. Assoc. of Endodontics, 1973.

Natkin, E.: Treatment of endodontic emergencies. **Dent. Clin. North Am. 18**:243, 1974.

Nebrun, E.: **Cariology.** Baltimore: Williams & Wilkins, 1979, pp. 15–43.

Orban, B.: **Oral Histology and Embryology.** St. Louis: C. V. Mosby, 1944, p. 55.

Pindborg, J. J.: **Pathology of the Dental Hard Tissues.** Philadelphia: W. B. Saunders, 1970, pp. 256–275, 326–338.

Prichard, J. F.: **Advanced Periodontal Disease,** 2nd Edition. Philadelphia: W. B. Saunders, 1972, pp. 103–107, 142–196, 381.

Ramaden, A. B. E., and Mitchell, D. F.: A roentgenographic study of experimental bone destruction. **Oral Surg. 15**:934, 1962.

Shafer, W. G., Hine, M. K., and Levy, B. M.: **A Textbook of Oral Pathology,** 3rd Edition. Philadelphia: W. B. Saunders, 1974, pp. 295, 366–432, 704–753.

Shannon, I. L., Gibson, W. A., and Terry, J. M.: Caries experience in the U.S. Air Force. **J. Public Health Dent. 26**:206, 1960.

Spouge, J. D.: **Oral Pathology.** St. Louis: C. V. Mosby, 1973, pp. 3–40, 83–124.

Stafne, E. C., and Szabo, S. E.: The significance of pulp nodules. **Dental Cosmos 75**:160, 1933.

Stedman's Medical Dictionary, 23rd Edition. Baltimore: Williams & Wilkins, 1976, p. 1459.

Updegrave, W. J.: Accurate radiography for diagnosis of periodontal disease. *In* Ward, H. (ed.): **A Periodontal Point of View.** Springfield, Ill.: Charles C Thomas, 1973, pp. 389–419.

Wagg, B. J.: ECSI — A new index for evaluating caries progression. **Community Dent. Oral Epidemiol. 2**:219, 1974.

Weine, F. S.: **Endodontic Therapy.** St. Louis: C. V. Mosby, 1973, pp. 40–50, 95–119.

Weine, F. S., Healey, H. J., and Theiss, E. P.: Endodontic emergency dilemma: Leave open or keep closed. **Oral Surg. 40**:531, 1975.

White, T. C.: Secondary dentine nodules. **Br. J. Dent. Sci., 14**:80, 1871.

Wuehrmann, A. H., and Manson-Hing, L. R.: **Dental Radiology,** 4th Edition. St. Louis: C. V. Mosby, 1977, pp. 297–334.

Zamir, T., Fischer, D., Fishel, D., and Sharav, Y.: A longitudinal radiographic study of the rate and spread of human approximal dental caries. **Arch. Oral Biol. 21**: 523, 1976.

Chapter 9

Pericoronal Radiolucencies

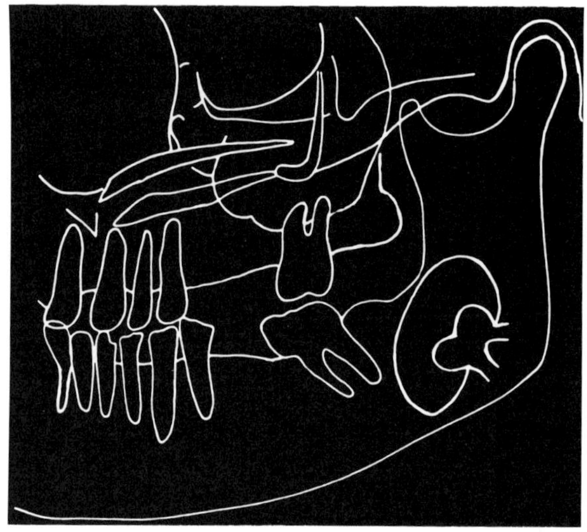

PERICORONAL RADIOLUCENCIES THAT DO NOT TEND TO CONTAIN RADIOPAQUE FLECKS

NORMAL FOLLICULAR SPACE (Follicular Sac)

BRIEF OVERVIEW

This pericoronal radiolucency is usually seen about the crowns of normally **erupting** teeth. It is important to recognize the features of the follicular space because radiographs are extremely valuable in distinguishing this entity from the follicular cyst.

RADIOGRAPHIC FEATURES (Figs. 9–1 to 9–3)

A normal follicular space generally measures up to 3 mm on panoramic films and 2.5 mm on intraoral films. There is usually some magnification associated with panoramic films, although the amount varies from one machine to another. Exceptions to this measurement occur in the permanent cuspids, especially those in the maxilla, which may normally have a **larger** follicular space. Unerupted teeth in middle-aged or older patients may have **little or no** follicular space. In marginal cases involving younger patients, it is important to evaluate the degree of root formation. If the follicular space appears enlarged and root formation is complete as indicated by the closure of the apex, then the eruptive potential of the tooth is greatly diminished and cystic transformation of the follicular sac has probably occurred. In such cases, further observation is of little value and treatment should be initiated.

If a small radiopacity is associated with the follicular space of a nearly erupted tooth, an eruption sequestrum, which is of no consequence, should be suspected (see Fig. 9–3). It is usually of the same density as bone, and the patient may complain of mild discomfort or

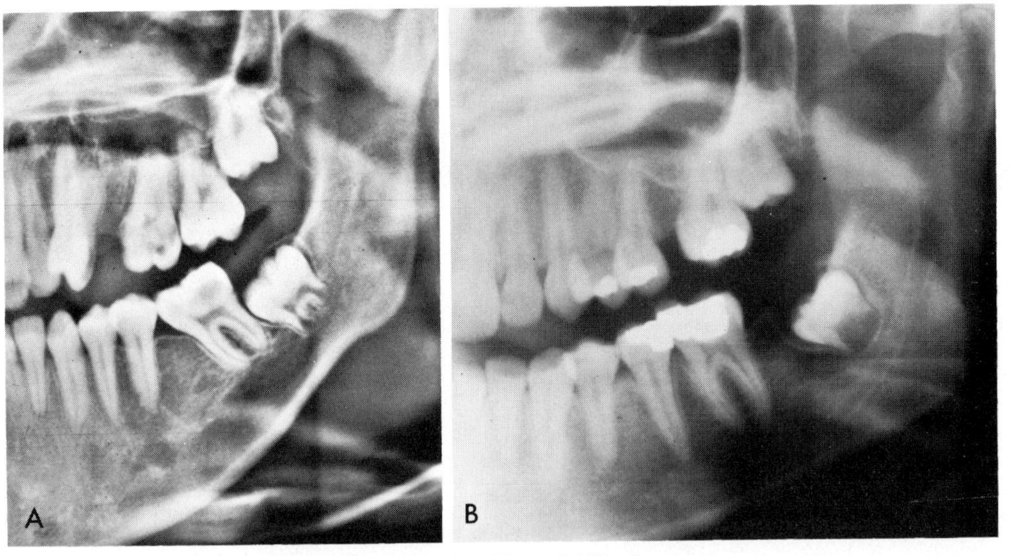

Figure 9–1. **A** and **B**. Normal follicular space.

pain. If, however, the radiopacity is denser than bone, a developing odontoma or other radiopaque lesion should be suspected and may be of considerable consequence. In this instance, the patient may be asymptomatic, and further evaluation and follow-up is indicated.

PERICORONITIS (Operculitis, Every's Syndrome)

BRIEF OVERVIEW

Pericoronitis is an inflammation of the soft tissue surrounding the crown of a partly erupted or impacted tooth. The condition is often painful, and there may be trismus and an associated cellulitis. Pericoronitis often involves a lower third molar. The inflamed and swollen operculum is sometimes traumatized by the maxillary third molar, usually the palatal cusp tip. A variant of this condition, known as Every's syndrome, involves a buccally erupting maxillary third molar. There is temporomandibular joint pain and trismus, and the internal pterygoid muscle may be tender on palpation. Generally, the patient reports a vague previous history of pain involving an upper molar and a rapid onset of acute symptoms, usually first discovered upon awakening in the morning. It is important to distinguish this condition from

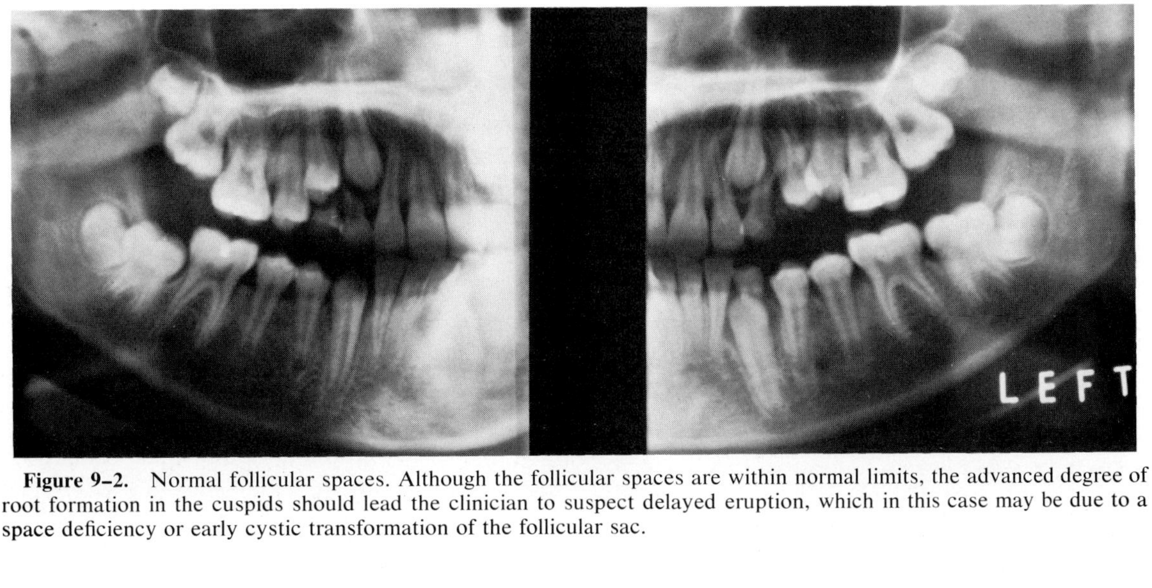

Figure 9–2. Normal follicular spaces. Although the follicular spaces are within normal limits, the advanced degree of root formation in the cuspids should lead the clinician to suspect delayed eruption, which in this case may be due to a space deficiency or early cystic transformation of the follicular sac.

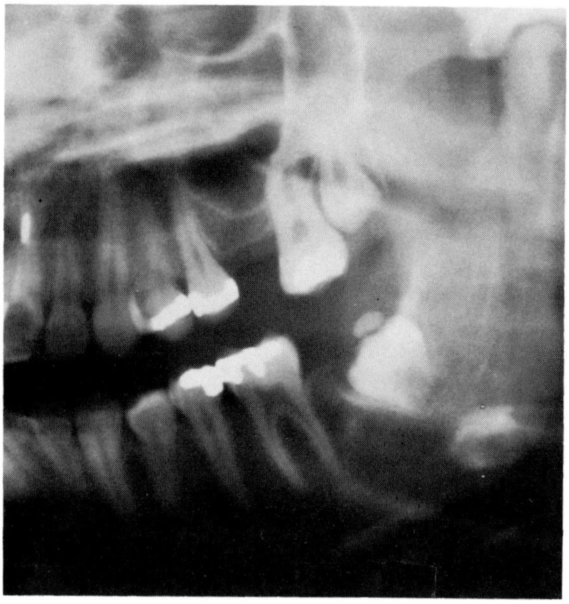

Figure 9–3. Eruption sequestrum.

the temporomandibular joint pain associated with myofascial pain-dysfunction syndrome or the referred temporomandibular joint pain associated with a pulpally involved tooth. These conditions are further discussed in Chapter 16.

Initial treatment in both cases usually consists of either reducing the offending cusp tip, flushing out the infected area, and administering antibiotics; or removing the maxillary third molar. This may be followed by removal of the remaining third molars.

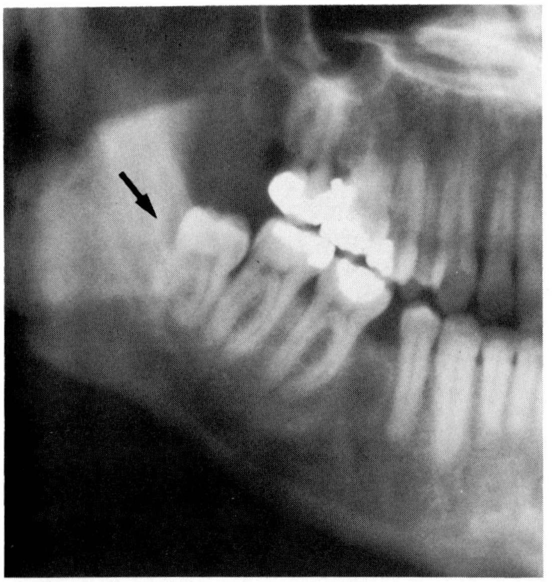

Figure 9–4. Pericoronitis. Note the absence of a cortical outline and the complete root formation in the third molars.

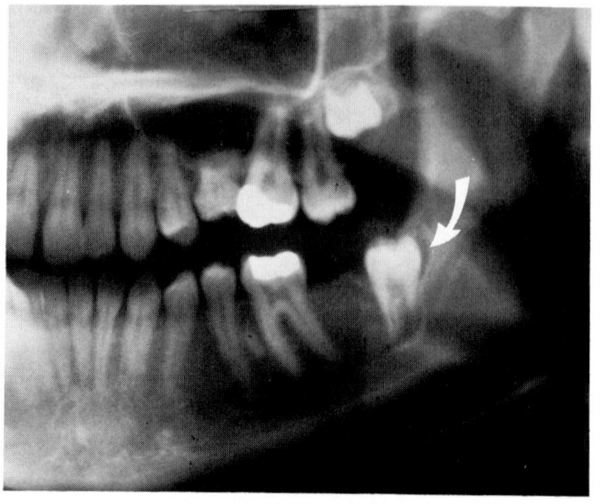

Figure 9–5. Normal follicular space. Note the cortical outline and the incomplete root formation.

The panoramic radiograph is particularly helpful in evaluating this condition, as intraoral films may be impossible to obtain owing to the trismus.

RADIOGRAPHIC FEATURES (Figs. 9–4 to 9–6)

The radiographic features of pericoronitis may not be seen when only the soft tissue is involved. However, in many instances there is an underlying osteitis, usually of the bone surrounding the distal portion of an impacted lower third molar. In this situation, a small, characteristic flame-shaped radiolucency may be seen. There is generally no cortical outline, thus distinguishing this condition from the follicular space of an erupting tooth that has just broken through into the soft tissue. In Every's syndrome, a buccally erupting third molar is noted, along with normal findings, on the temporomandibular joint films, which can also be taken with most panoramic machines.

DENTIGEROUS CYST (Follicular Cyst, Eruption Cyst)

BRIEF OVERVIEW

This is the most common pathologic pericoronal radiolucency. It arises from the reduced enamel epithelium about the crown of an unerupted or impacted tooth, often a third

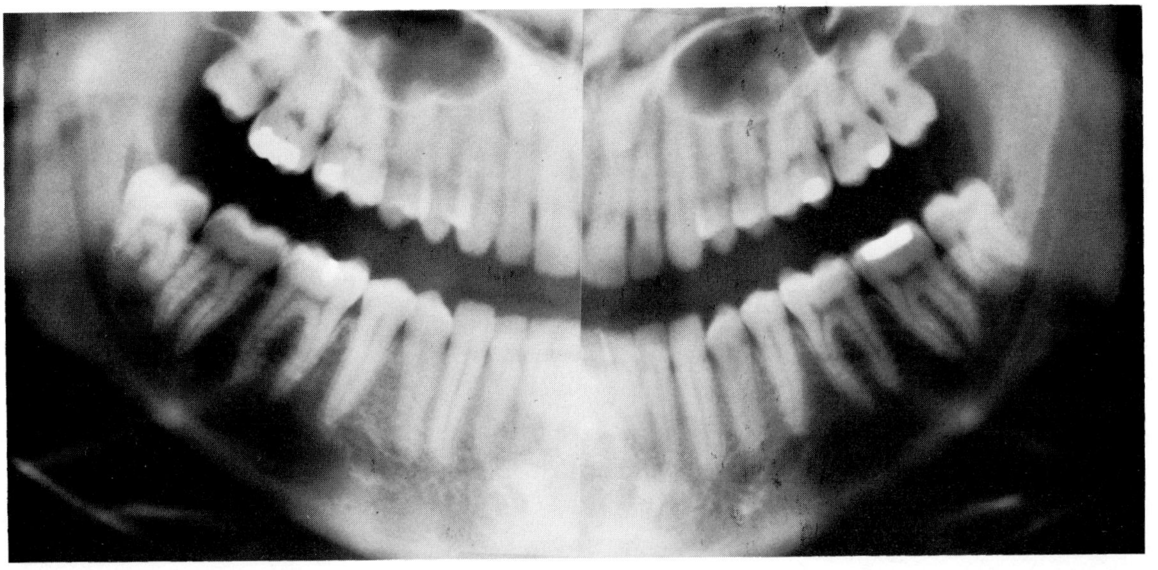

Figure 9–6. Bilateral pericoronitis.

molar or cuspid. The **eruption cyst** is considered by most to be a variant of the follicular cyst, which is close to the surface. Clinically, a bluish, domelike bump on the gingiva may be seen, and this represents the crestal portion of the follicular cyst, which has eroded through the alveolar ridge and is expanding into the soft tissue. The bluish color may be due to the refractory properties of the cystic fluid as seen through the soft tissue or it may represent blood due to trauma from the opposing tooth.

Although the radiograph is extremely helpful in distinguishing the follicular cyst from a normal follicular space, all suspected follicular cysts should be submitted for histopathologic examination for the following clinically significant reasons: the epithelial lining may be an odontogenic keratocyst; the epithelial lining may give rise to an ameloblastoma; and, on occasion, the lining may also give rise to a central epidermoid carcinoma or a central mucoepidermoid carcinoma. The presence of these

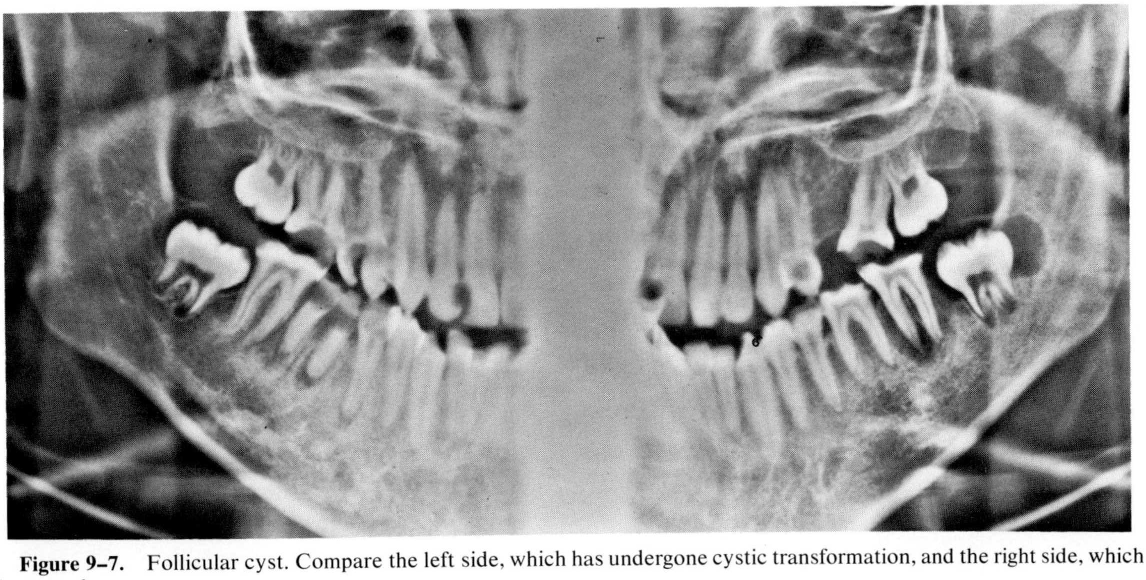

Figure 9–7. Follicular cyst. Compare the left side, which has undergone cystic transformation, and the right side, which is normal.

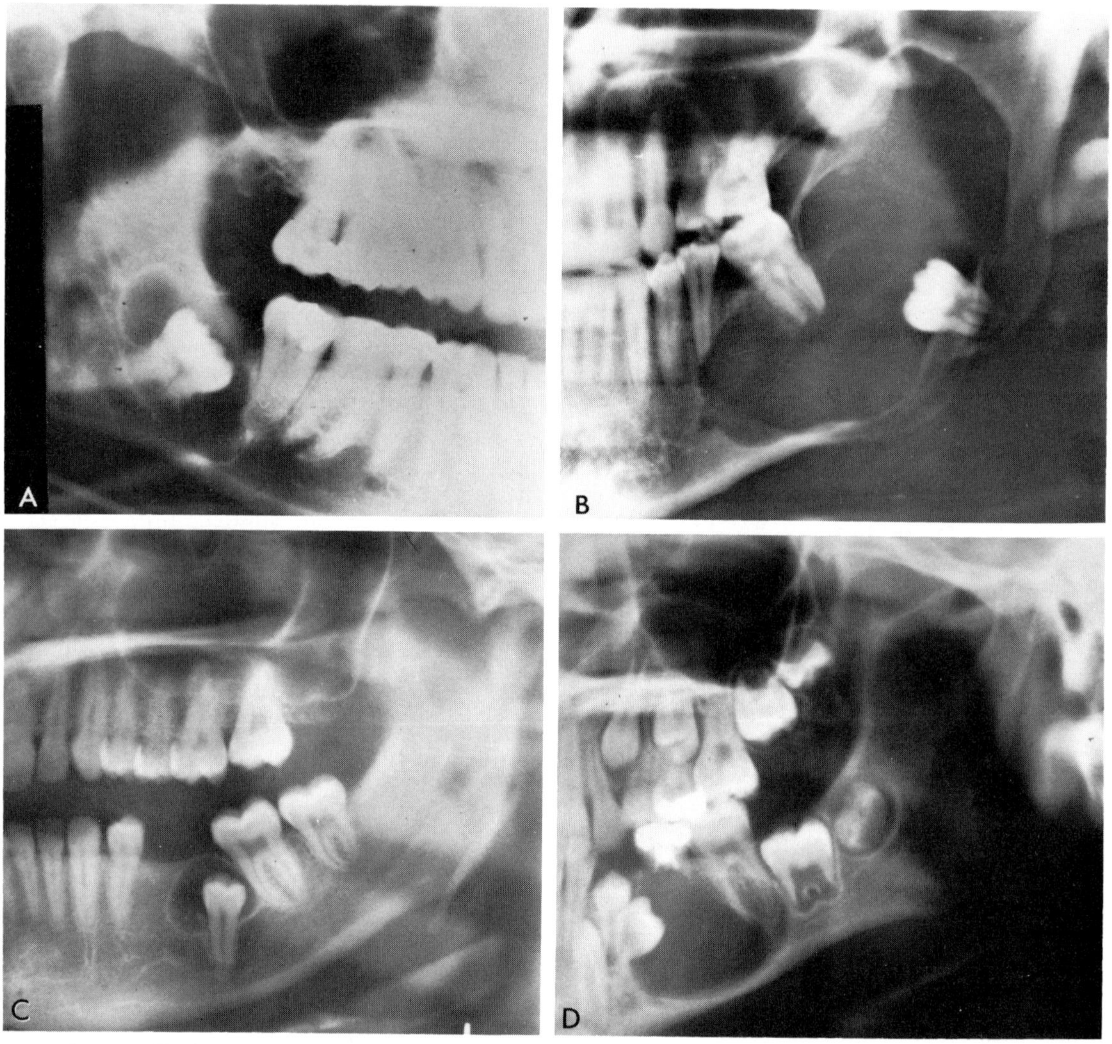

Figure 9–8. Follicular cyst. **A.** Courtesy of Drs. Frank Sammis Jr. and Carlos Portales, San Antonio, TX. **B.** Courtesy of Dr. Chris Nortjé, University of Stellenbosch, Tygerberg, South Africa. **C.** Courtesy of Dr. Steven Bricker, San Antonio, TX. **D.** In children the differential diagnosis for this particular lesion would include odontogenic keratocyst, odontogenic fibroma, and ameloblastic fibroma.

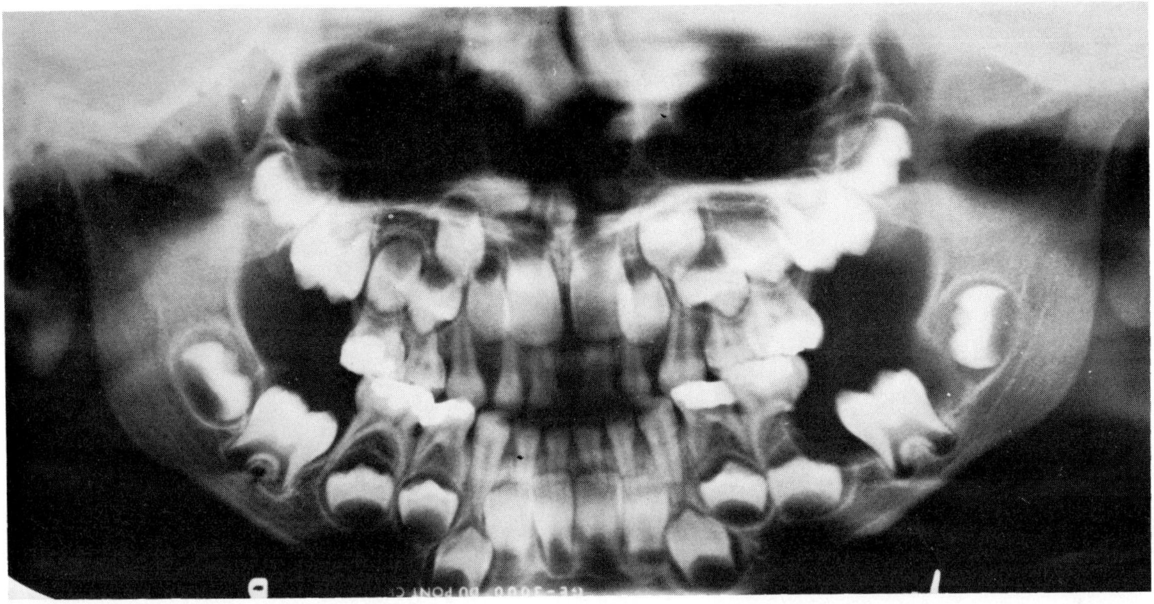

Figure 9–9. Eruption cyst. (Courtesy of Dr. Chris Nortjé, University of Stellenbosch, Tygerberg, South Africa.)

conditions affects the diagnosis, treatment, prognosis, and follow-up of the case. Treatment generally consists of enucleation of the cyst and removal or orthodontic traction of the involved tooth.

RADIOGRAPHIC FEATURES (Figs. 9–7 to 9–10)

This cyst classically consists of a well-corticated pericoronal radiolucency, which exceeds 3 mm when measured from the edge of the crown to the periphery of the lesion. It is usually distributed symmetrically about the crown of the involved tooth but may occur to one side or the other, in which case it is referred to as a lateral dentigerous cyst. In the eruption cyst variant, the superior portion of the cortical outline may be lost, and a gingival soft tissue swelling may be noted (see Fig. 9–9).

The follicular cyst may be expansile and may achieve very large proportions. It may be multilocular on occasion. It may be associated with displaced, unerupted, or impacted teeth. Additionally, when these variants appear radiographically, keratinizing metaplasia or the other transformations previously discussed should be suspected. When the follicular cyst gives rise to any of these conditions, it may acquire the characteristic radiographic appearance of the new lesion.

A further variation in the radiographic appearance of the follicular cyst occurs when radiopaque foci are seen within the lumen of the lesion. In this instance, the radiopaque material may represent an odontoma, a supernumerary tooth, or a paramolar. These entities may also give rise to follicular cysts.

Histopathologic examinations may reveal a completely different diagnosis when radiopaque foci are present, such as a Pindborg tumor, a Gorlin cyst, or an adenomatoid odontogenic tumor. The odontogenic keratocyst (see Fig. 9–10), a follicular cyst sub-type, will be discussed separately in Chapter 11.

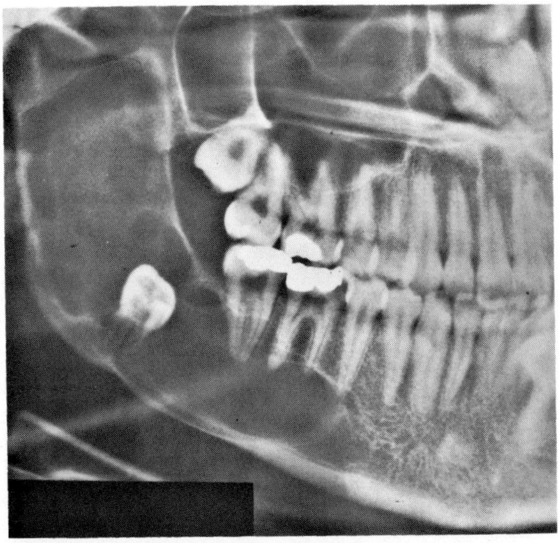

Figure 9–10. Odontogenic keratocyst; follicular cyst type. This type of cyst is discussed further in Chapter 11.

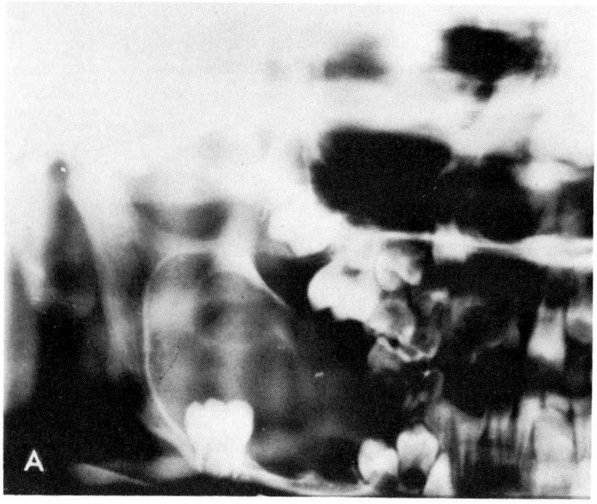

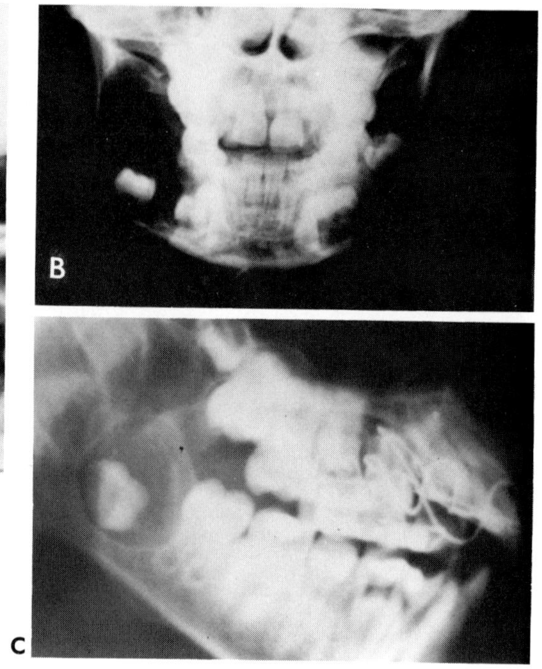

Figure 9–11. Ameloblastic fibroma. A. Panoramic view. B. PA view in an 8-year-old girl. C. Note the cyst-like pericoronal radiolucency and displacement of the developing mandibular third molar in this 10-year-old boy. (A and B courtesy of Dr. de V. Joubert, Tygerberg, South Africa.)

AMELOBLASTIC FIBROMA

BRIEF OVERVIEW

The ameloblastic fibroma is an uncommon lesion. It is classified as a true mixed odontogenic tumor because it contains strands and nests of ameloblastlike epithelium and primitive dental papillalike connective tissue. It occurs most frequently in the mandibular molar region in teenage males and is usually discovered on routine radiographic examination. The lesion is not aggressive like an ameloblastoma and rarely recurs when treated by simple curettage.

RADIOGRAPHIC FEATURES (Figs. 9–11 and 9–12)

The ameloblastic fibroma may be associated with an impacted or unerupted tooth in the mandibular molar region and may greatly resemble a follicular cyst. However, it also may be located between the teeth and may resemble a lateral periodontal cyst. Occasionally the lesion may be multilocular, and slight expansion may be present. This lesion is usually well demarcated with a smooth, corticated, peripheral outline. There may be displacement of the involved tooth.

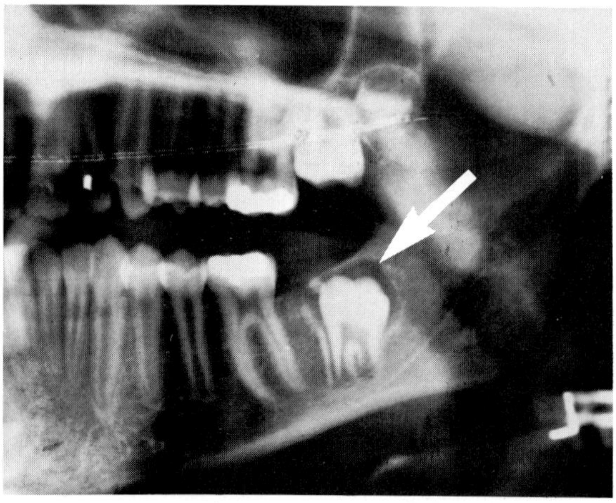

Figure 9–12. Ameloblastic fibro-odontoma. (Courtesy of Dr. Doug Stoneman, Toronto, Canada.)

PERICORONAL RADIOLUCENCIES THAT MAY CONTAIN RADIOPAQUE FLECKS

AMELOBLASTIC FIBRO-ODONTOMA

BRIEF OVERVIEW

This lesion is mentioned here to distinguish it from the ameloblastic odontoma and the ameloblastic fibroma. Basically, the ameloblastic fibro-odontoma behaves like the ameloblastic fibroma. It occurs predominantly in teenage males under the age of 15 years and, like the odontoma component, may be located in either jaw.

In a recent series of seven cases reported by Miller and associates, the chief presenting complaints were noneruption of one or several permanent teeth, facial swelling, and facial asymmetry. The lesion is not considered aggressive and may be treated by simple enucleation.

RADIOGRAPHIC FEATURES (Fig. 9–12)

The most striking feature of the 26 cases reported by Hooker and those reported by Miller and associates is that all cases were associated with an impacted or unerupted tooth. The pericoronal radiolucency may vary from very small to large, sometimes expanding into the ramus, but maintains a smooth, well-defined, cortical outline. The central radiopaque area may resemble a composite or complex odontoma, or it may consist of nonspecific radiopaque flecks distributed throughout the lesion. A reliable and accurate histopathologic diagnosis is essential to distinguish this lesion from the ameloblastic odontoma, as the two conditions behave very differently in terms of aggressiveness and recurrence.

ADENOMATOID ODONTOGENIC TUMOR (Odontogenic Adenomatoid Tumor, Adenoameloblastoma)

BRIEF OVERVIEW

The adenomatoid odontogenic tumor is uncommon but typical in its presentation. It most often affects an unerupted or impacted maxillary cuspid, occurring more frequently in females between the ages of 11 and 20. In the series reported by Courtney and Kerr, 60 per cent of the cases occurred in the maxilla and 90 per cent of all cases involved a cuspid or an area anterior to the cuspid. The most common presenting complaint was painless swelling. The pathogenesis is not fully understood, but clinically and radiographically the adenomatoid odontogenic tumor neither resembles nor behaves like an ameloblastoma, as had been previously implied by the old name. The lesion is surrounded by a thick connective tissue capsule and is removed by simple enucleation. Recurrence is exceedingly rare.

RADIOGRAPHIC FEATURES (Fig. 9–13)

The lesion often consists of a well-corticated radiolucency, and in the series of Courtney and Kerr, 40 per cent involved an unerupted or impacted tooth, usually the maxillary cuspid of a teenage female. It may become quite large and expansile and may eventually surround the whole tooth and displace the adjacent teeth. It is not always associated with an impacted tooth. Radiopaque foci of calcification are sometimes seen in association with this benign neoplasm. In the absence of radiopaque foci, this lesion may resemble a globulomaxillary cyst, an incisive canal cyst, a median mandibular cyst, or a lateral periodontal cyst as well as a number of other benign cysts and neoplasms.

CALCIFYING EPITHELIAL ODONTOGENIC TUMOR (Pindborg Tumor)

BRIEF OVERVIEW

The Pindborg tumor is like the ameloblastoma in most respects, except that it is much more rare in occurrence. The features of this neoplasm have been recently reviewed by Franklin and Pindborg. This odontogenic tumor of epithelial origin occurs twice as frequently in the mandible as in the maxilla (in the molar-ramus area). There is no sex predilection, and the mean age of patients with this tumor is 40 years for both sexes. This lesion is locally aggressive, tends to recur, and should be treated by excision for smaller lesions and by bloc resection for larger tumors.

Postoperative radiographic follow-up is recommended, and the lesion may recur many years later. A peripheral variant of this lesion occurs on the anterior gingiva as an epulislike growth. The mean age of patients with this lesion is 31 years, and it is rare in occurrence.

RADIOGRAPHIC FEATURES (Fig. 9–14)

There does not seem to be any real agreement as to the radiographic features of the typical lesion. There are, however, two features that are commonly seen: about one half of all lesions are associated with an unerupted or impacted tooth that would normally not tend to be impacted, most commonly a first or second molar; secondly, there may be flecks of radiopaque material present in varying quantities, which are sometimes said to resemble driven snow. These radiopaque flecks correspond to calcified amyloid, a degenerative product of the neoplastic epithelial cells. The calcification occurs in an annular fashion in the form of Liesegang's rings

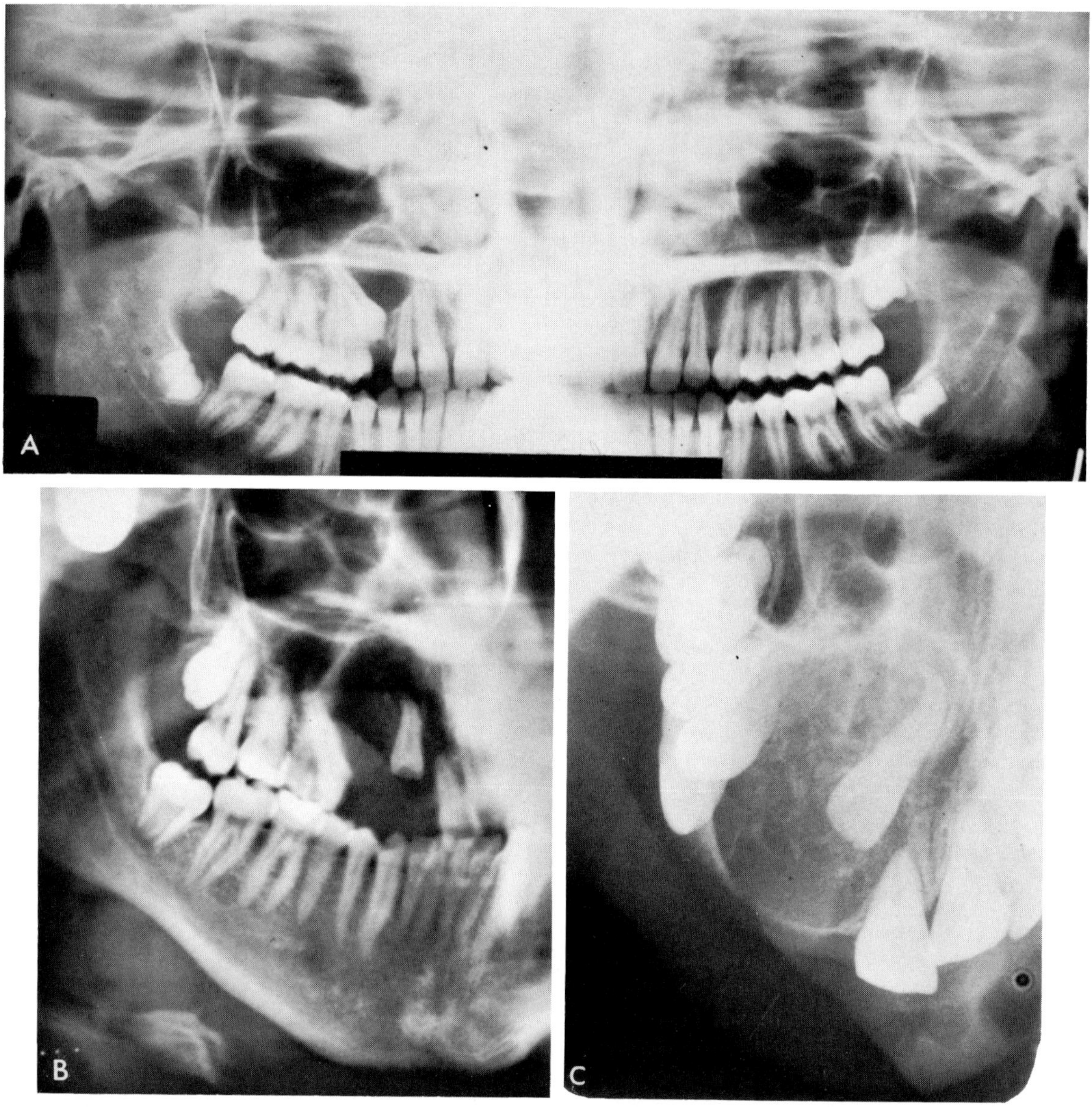

Figure 9–13. Adenomatoid odontogenic tumor. **B** and **C**. Both radiographs are of the same patient. (Figure 9–13 courtesy of Dr. Gus Pappas, Columbus, OH.)

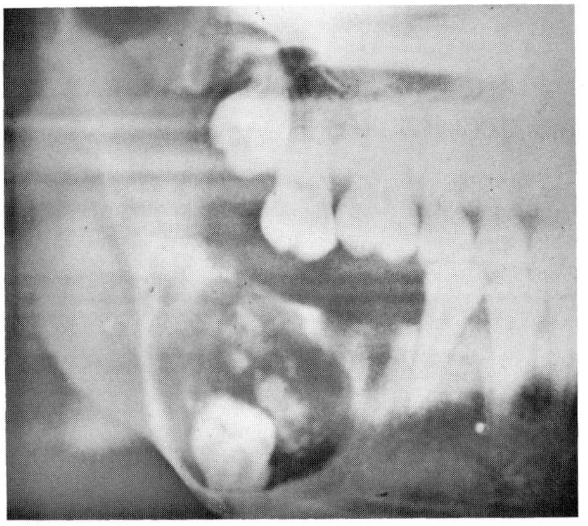

Figure 9–14. Calcifying epithelial odontogenic tumor of Pindborg. (Courtesy of Dr. Steven Kaltman, Pittsburgh, PA.)

and histologically is a characteristic feature of the Pindborg tumor. Other radiographic patterns include a predominantly unilocular radiolucency with or without fine trabecular septae; a multilocular radiolucency; or a fairly dense, mottled radiopacity. Expansion, root resorption, tooth displacement, and poorly defined, noncorticated borders are also features. Lesions in the maxilla may expand into the antrum.

KERATINIZING AND CALCIFYING ODONTOGENIC CYST (Gorlin Cyst, Calcifying Odontogenic Cyst, Calcifying Odontogenic Tumor)

BRIEF OVERVIEW

The Gorlin cyst is a true epithelium-lined cyst that contains the characteristic ghost cells, which may be keratinized or calcified. This cyst occurs primarily in the mandibular molar-ramus area, with no age or sex predilection. Most lesions occur centrally in bone, but a rare peripheral variant occurs as an epulislike growth on the mandibular gingiva.

According to Farman and associates, the Gorlin cyst often contains components characteristic of, or mimicking, other odontogenic tumors such as ameloblastoma, complex odontomas, adenomatoid odontogenic tumor, ameloblastic odontoma, and ameloblastic fibro-odontoma. Their case of a Gorlin cyst with areas resembling ameloblastic fibro-odontoma is illustrated in Fig. 9–16**A** and **B**. The Gorlin cyst may recur, and treatment is by thorough excision.

RADIOGRAPHIC FEATURES (Figs. 9–15 and 9–16)

Since this cyst is rare in occurrence, it is difficult to ascribe typical radiographic features

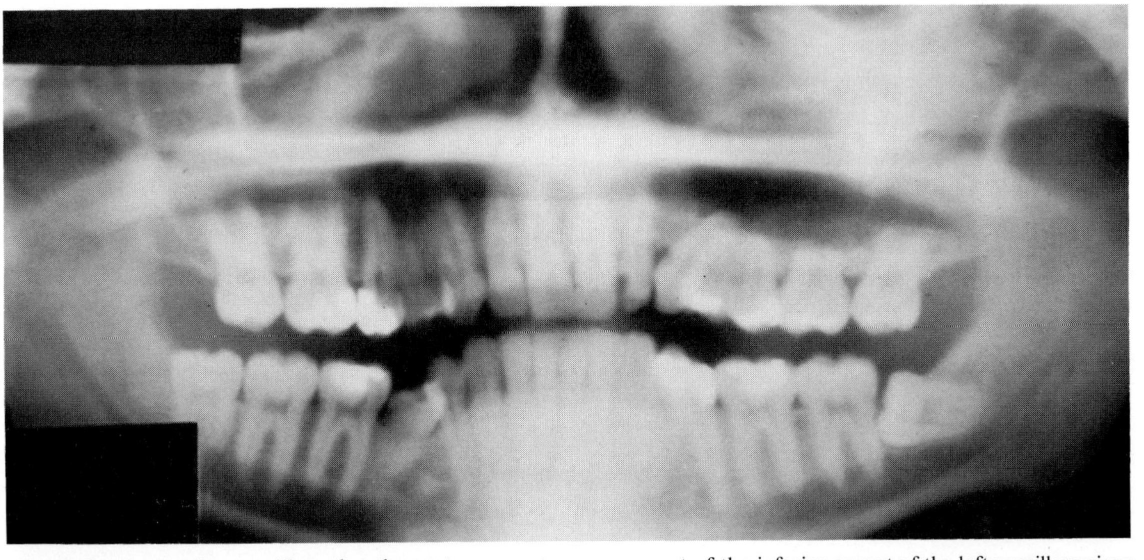

Figure 9–15. Gorlin cyst. Note that the cyst appears to occupy most of the inferior aspect of the left maxillary sinus. Part of the superior outline is corticated. The sinus is expanded anteriorly to the lateral incisor area. There is root resorption of the apices of the associated teeth. (Courtesy of Dr. Edward Rossi, Cleveland, OH.)

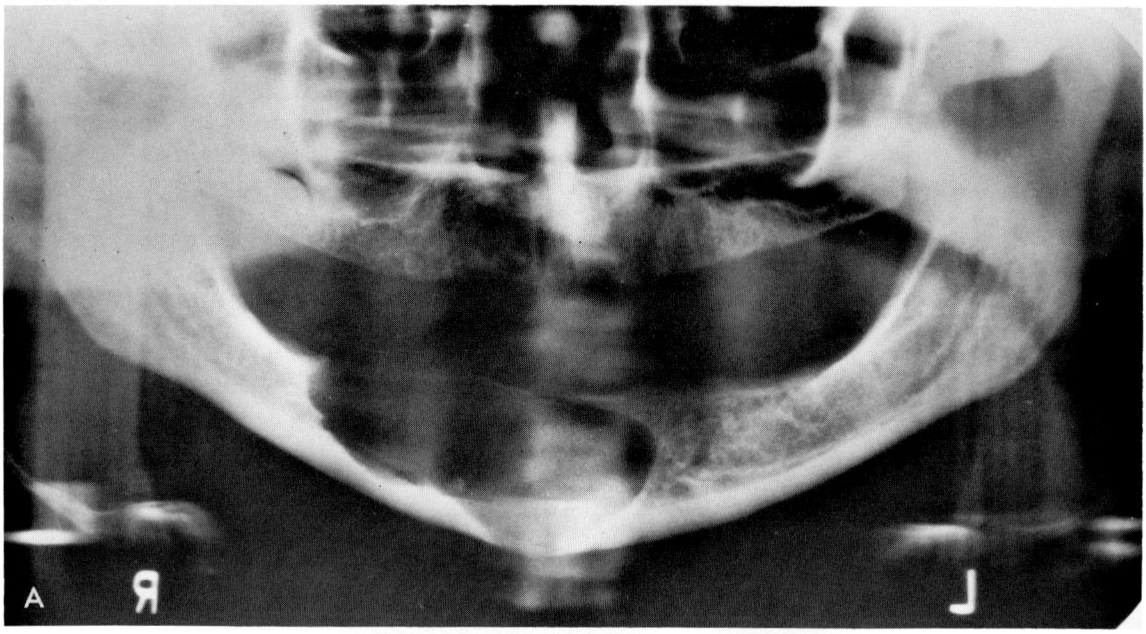

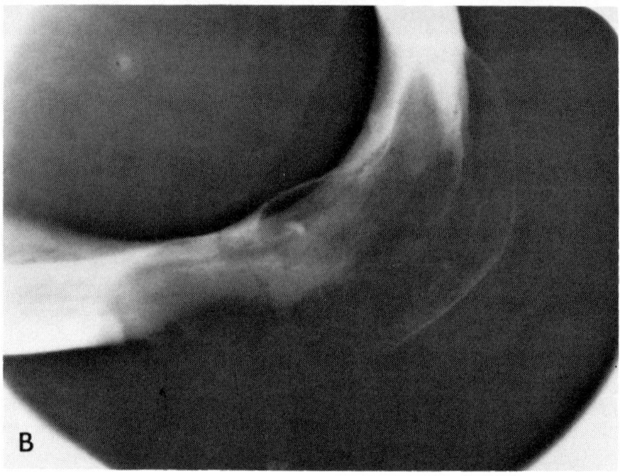

Figure 9–16. **A** and **B.** Gorlin cyst. The patient is a 46-year-old female. (Courtesy of Dr. Chris Nortjé, University of Stellenbosch, Tygerberg, South Africa.)

to it. The central lesion is associated with an impacted or unerupted tooth in 20 per cent of cases. The lesion is probably most commonly unilocular, with radiopaque flecks or a central radiopaque mass with a peripheral radiolucent outline. Displacement of the adjacent teeth has been reported by Sellinger and Reyneke. Expansion also occurs. The borders are usually well defined and corticated. In Figure 9–15, note that the lesion that occupies most of the maxillary sinus appears to be causing resorption of the apices, but the resorbed apices do not appear to be protruding into the lesion. This is a radiographic finding suggestive of a cystic lesion rather than a neoplastic one.

REFERENCES

Reference Texts

Eversole, L. R.: **Clinical Outline of Oral Pathology.** Philadelphia: Lea & Febiger, 1978, pp. 199–204.

Shafer, W. G., Hine, M. K., and Levy, B. M.: **A Textbook of Oral Pathology,** 3rd Edition. Philadelphia: W. B. Saunders, 1974, pp. 237–242, 258–261.

Wood, N. K., and Goaz, P. W.: **Differential Diagnosis of Oral Lesions.** St. Louis: C. V. Mosby, 1975, pp. 303–314.

Worth, H. M.: **Principles and Practice of Oral Radiologic Lesions.** Chicago: Year Book Medical Publishers, 1963, pp. 458, 466–472.

Selected References

Courtney, R. M., and Kerr, D. A.: The odontogenic adenomatoid tumor. **Oral Surg.** 39:424, 1975.

Farman, A. G., Smith, S. N., Nortje, C. J., and Grotepass,

F. W.: Calcifying odontogenic cyst with ameloblastic fibro-odontoma: One lesion or two? **J. Oral Path.** 7:19, 1978.

Franklin, C. D., and Pindborg, J. J.: The calcifying epithelial odontogenic tumor: A review and analysis of 113 cases. **Oral Surg.** 42:753, 1976.

Fredrickson, C., and Cherrick, H. M.: Central mucoepidermoid carcinoma of the jaws. **J. Oral Med.** 33:80, 1978.

Hager, R. C., Taylor, C. G., and Allen, P. M.: Ameloblastic fibroma: Report of a case. **J. Oral Surg.** 36:66, 1978.

Hooker, S. P.: Ameloblastic odontoma: An analysis of twenty-six cases. **Oral Surg.** 24:375, 1967.

Miller, A. S., Lopez, C. F., Pullon, P. A., and Elzay, R. P.: Ameloblastic fibro-odontoma: Report of seven cases. **Oral Surg.** 41:354, 1976.

Seelinger, J. E., and Reyneke, J. P.: The calcifying odontogenic cyst: Report of a case. **J. Oral Surg.** 36:469, 1978.

Sheteyer, A., Lustmann, J., and Lewin-Epstein, J.: The mural ameloblastoma: A review of the literature. **J. Oral Surg.** 36:866, 1978.

Smith, R. A., Roman, R. S., Hansen, L. S., Lundell, W. J., and Riley, R. W.: The calcifying epithelial odontogenic tumor. **J. Oral Surg.** 35:160, 1977.

Tsakamis, P. J., Carpenter, W. M., and Shade, N. L.: Odontogenic adenomatoid tumor: Report of case and review of the literature. **J. Oral Surg.** 35:146, 1977.

Chapter 10

Solitary, Single, or Multiple Radiolucencies with Distinct Borders

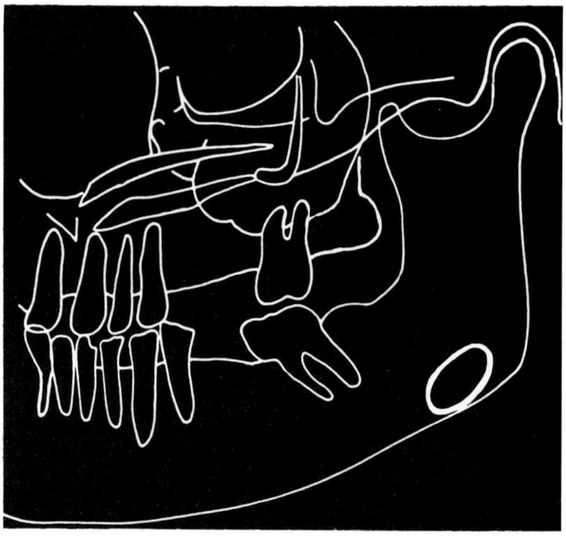

VARIATIONS IN TRABECULAR PATTERNS AND MARROW SPACES

BRIEF OVERVIEW

These variations do occur and are particularly evident on the panoramic radiograph. If such a variation is suspected, a normal intraoral or extraoral film should be taken. Often the pattern cannot be duplicated on standard films. If the clinician is still uncertain after the standard films are taken, the area should be biopsied or followed by periodic radiographic examination.

RADIOGRAPHIC FEATURES (Fig. 10–1)

These variations may mimic cystlike radiolucent lesions. However, there may be some aspect of the area that does not seem to fit any particular pattern; a normal variation may be suspected in this situation, especially in the absence of symptoms or clinical findings. These variations are often seen in the mandibular anterior area on panoramic films.

EARLY STAGE TOOTH CRYPTS

BRIEF OVERVIEW

If early stage tooth crypts are not recognized, the clinician may perceive the lesion as mimicking a pathologic condition. Early stage tooth crypts may be seen from birth to late adolescence.

RADIOGRAPHIC FEATURES (Figs. 10–2 and 10–3)

The uncalcified crypt usually consists of a bilateral, well-corticated, solitary radiolucency

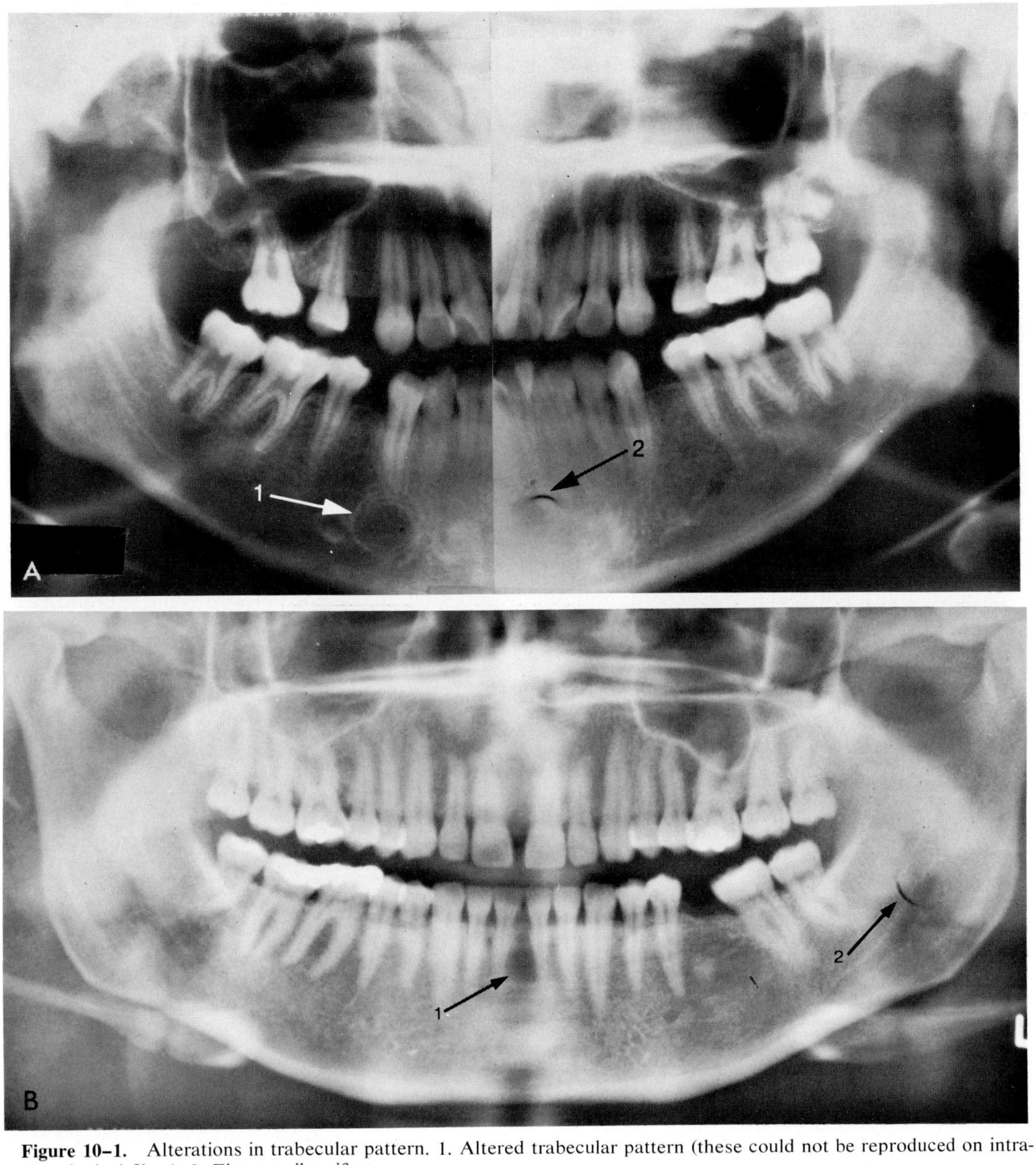

Figure 10–1. Alterations in trabecular pattern. 1. Altered trabecular pattern (these could not be reproduced on intraoral periapical films). 2. Finger nail artifact.

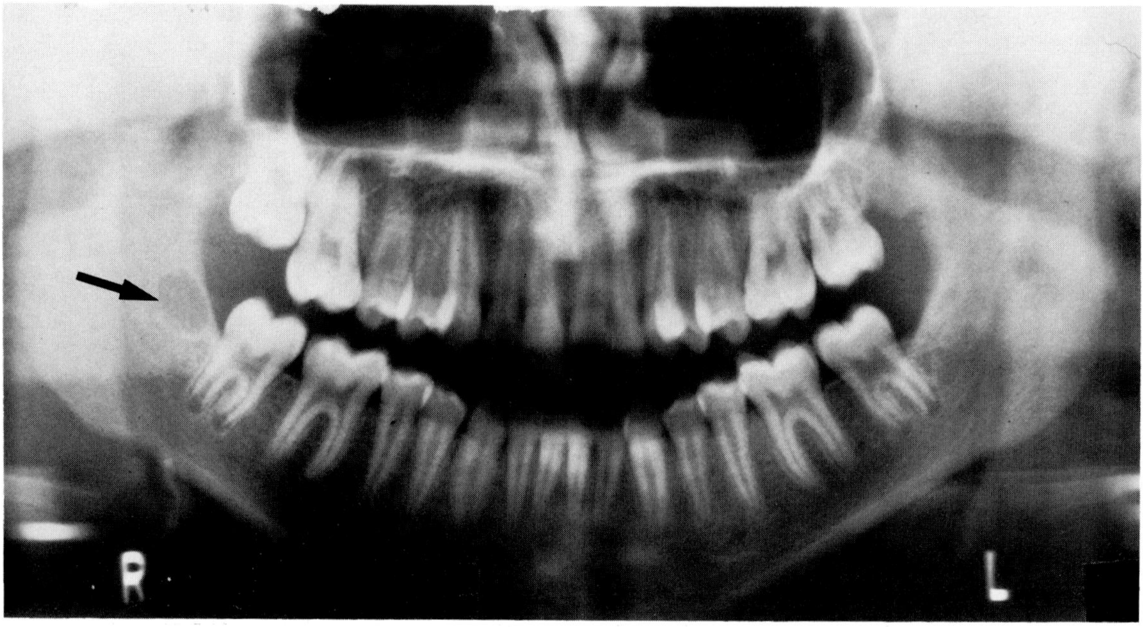

Figure 10–2. Tooth crypt.

of the approximate diameter of the crown of the developing tooth. In the permanent teeth, especially the bicuspids, the uncalcified crypt may resemble a small central lesion or radiolucency of pulpal origin, particularly when the radiolucency occurs at the bifurcation of a primary molar. Bifurcation radiolucencies of pulpal origin are common findings in primary teeth and contribute to the development of Turner's enamel hypoplasia involving the occlusal portions of the affected bicuspids.

In the permanent molars, the uncalcified crypts are located just under the crest of the ridge and may strongly resemble primordial cysts or large marrow spaces. As the cusp tips begin to calcify, circumflex or inverted V-shaped radiopacities appear, mimicking solitary radiolucent lesions, which may have flecks or islands of calcification such as the adenomatoid odontogenic tumor, Gorlin cyst, Pindborg tumor, or the central cemento-ossifying fibroma.

POSTEXTRACTION SOCKET

BRIEF OVERVIEW

Generally, postextraction sockets are easily identified radiolucencies. They are usually apparent on the radiograph for 6 to 12 months,

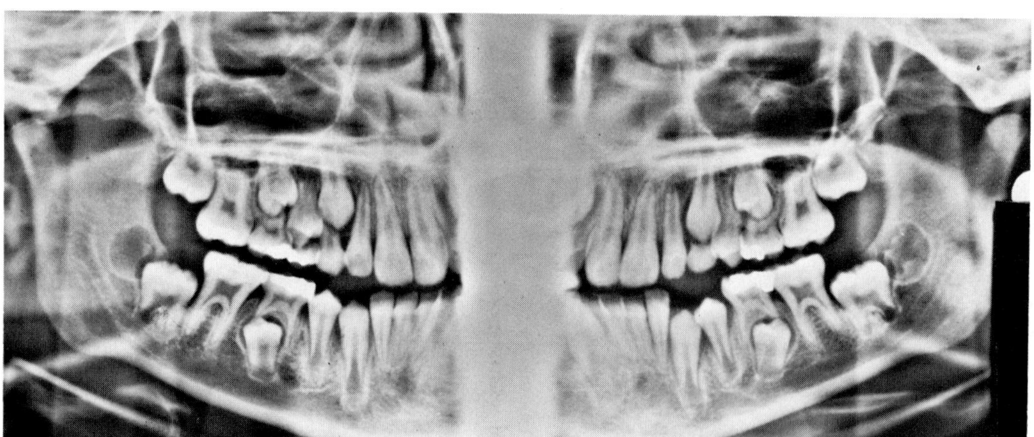

Figure 10–3. Early stage tooth crypts. Note the circumflex calcification pattern of the cusp tips.

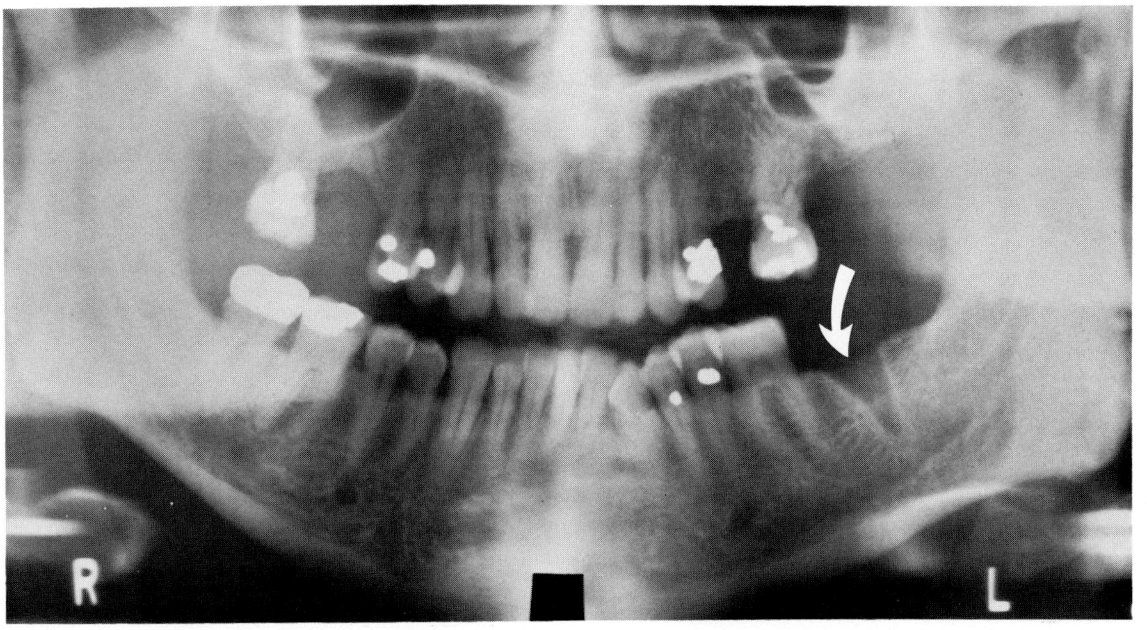

Figure 10–4. Postextraction socket.

after which time they become indistinguishable from the surrounding alveolar bone. A variation of this condition occurs when bone fails to deposit at the extraction site. Instead, normal red or yellow bone marrow fills the area. This asymptomatic lesion has been termed by Standish and Shafer the **focal osteoporotic bone marrow defect of the jaws.** This condition is more common in middle-aged females and occurs predominantly in the mandible. This lesion should be enucleated, as diagnosis can only be made by histopathologic examination.

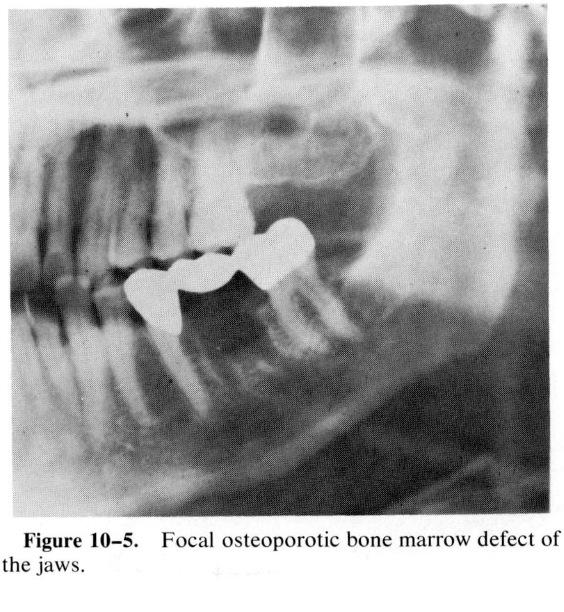

Figure 10–5. Focal osteoporotic bone marrow defect of the jaws.

RADIOGRAPHIC FEATURES (Figs. 10–4 and 10–5)

As healing of the socket occurs, the cortical outline of the roots disappears. The area fills with bone trabeculae and marrow spaces and becomes indistinguishable from the surrounding bone. When an exuberant repair process occurs, socket sclerosis may develop. This condition is discussed in Chapter 14.

The **focal osteoporotic bone marrow defect** generally does not have a well-corticated outline. The crest of the ridge is usually intact, and the area is basically radiolucent, with some fine trabeculations. Usually there is a history of previous tooth extraction.

FIBROUS HEALING DEFECT (Surgical Defect, Apical Scar, Fibrous Union)

BRIEF OVERVIEW

Healing of any alveolar bone wound will proceed normally if the cortical plates are intact and if they are covered by healthy periosteum. If the cortical plate and periosteum are destroyed by a pathologic condition such as a neoplasm, inflammation, or an extensive surgical procedure, the periosteal source of new osteoblasts is lost, and the probability of developing a fibrous healing defect is increased. Although the exact mechanism is not known, fibrous healing defects may develop in any of

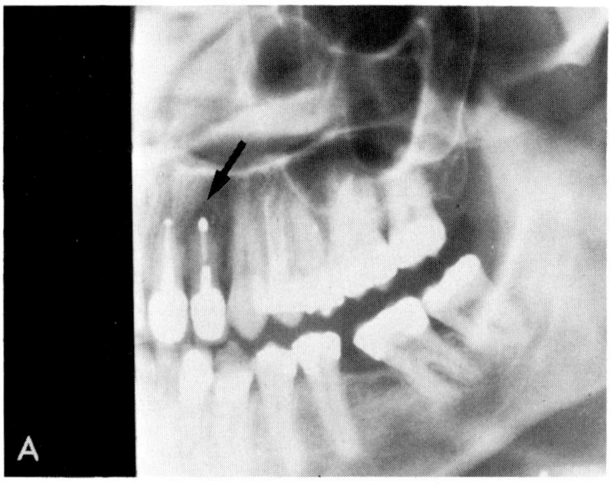

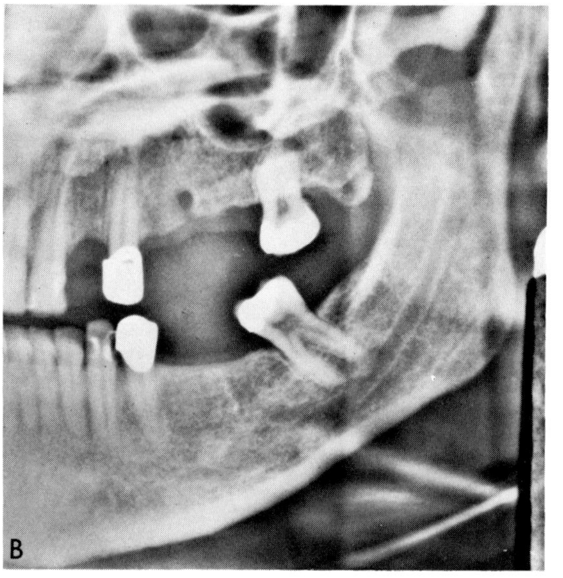

Figure 10–6. Fibrous healing defect.

the following situations: following apicoectomy; following excision of large lesions; at extraction sites, particularly those of difficult extractions; at fracture sites; or at the sites of orthognathic surgical margins. Movement of the approximated bony margins plays a role in the development of fibrous healing defects in the latter two situations.

An apical scar is a residual periapical radiolucency resembling a widely thickened apical periodontal membrane space. This fibrous healing defect develops as a sequela of inflammation and successful routine endodontic therapy. In the absence of symptoms or further radiographic change, these cases should not be retreated. Generally, all types of fibrous healing defects are quite stable once they develop. They are asymptomatic and do not tend to change in size or appearance over many years of follow-up. Conversely, a recurrent radiolucent lesion at the site of previous surgery tends to increase in size and may be symptomatic.

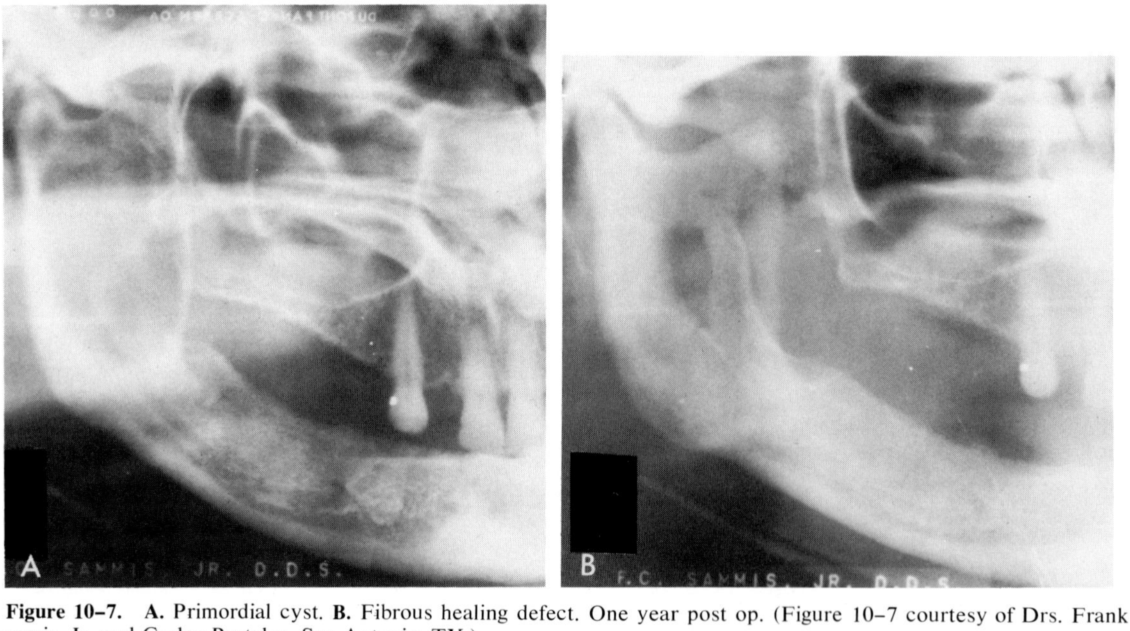

Figure 10–7. **A.** Primordial cyst. **B.** Fibrous healing defect. One year post op. (Figure 10–7 courtesy of Drs. Frank Sammis, Jr. and Carlos Portales, San Antonio, TX.)

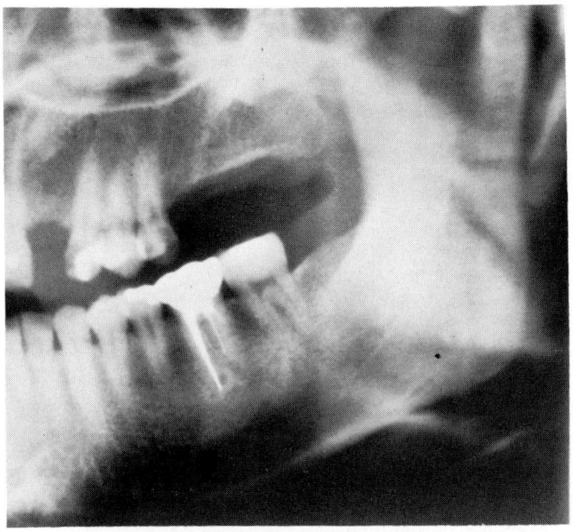

Figure 10–8. Apical scar.

RADIOGRAPHIC FEATURES (Figs. 10–6 to 10–8)

Fibrous healing defects occur at the sites of previous injury. They may or may not be well corticated but are usually well demarcated from the surrounding bone. Because of the lack of cortical bone covering these areas, they have a distinct radiolucent punched-out or see-through appearance, which is usually characteristic. It is interesting to note that some fibrous healing defects seen in edentulous areas initially resemble small residual cysts, but, as the ridge resorbs they take on a cupped-out appearance at the crest of the ridge and eventually disappear with further resorption.

DEVELOPMENTAL LINGUAL MANDIBULAR SALIVARY GLAND DEPRESSION (Developmental Bone Defect of the Mandible, Stafne's Cyst, Static Bone Cyst, Latent Bone Cyst)

BRIEF OVERVIEW

This developmental condition has a predilection for adult males. The defect has also been reported in children in rare instances. It is asymptomatic and is usually found on routine radiographic examination. This depression occurs in two locations; the most common site is on the lingual aspect of the mandible below the mandibular canal in the second molar-ramus area. This posterior variant consists of a concavity on the lingual cortical plate of the bone, which has been resorbed from the outside, causing a depression with a rough inner surface. On several occasions, surgical exploration and sialography have revealed salivary gland tissue in close proximity to the defect. More often, an empty cavity is found.

The second, less common variant is the an-

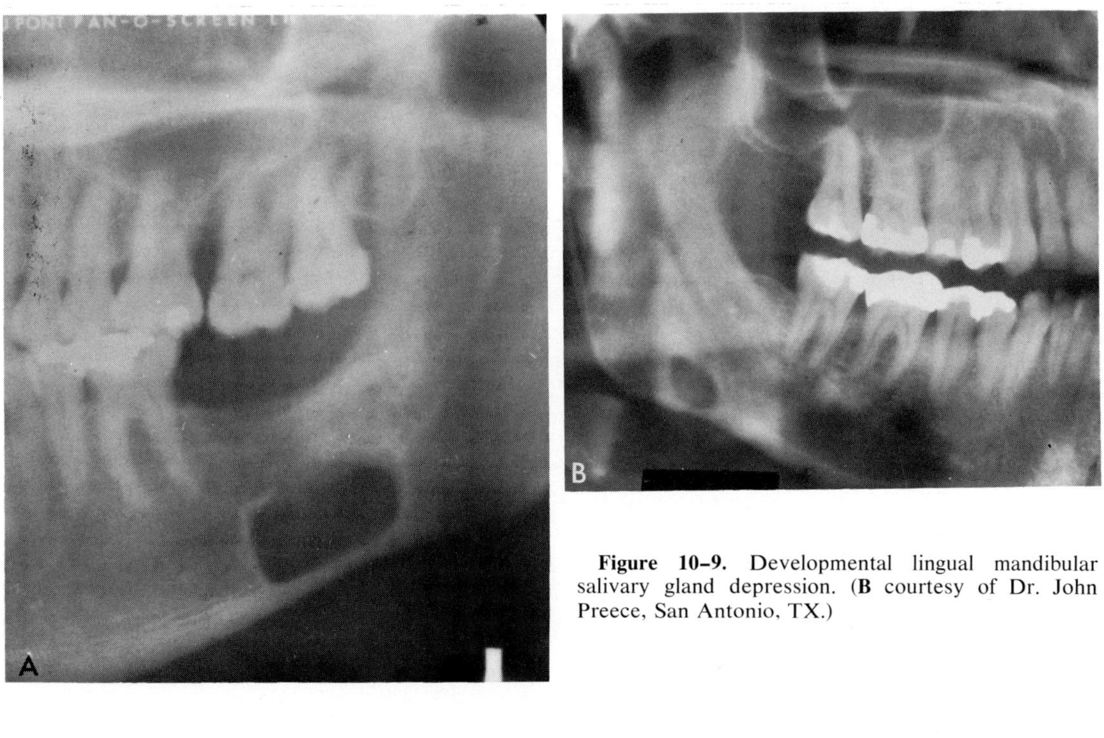

Figure 10–9. Developmental lingual mandibular salivary gland depression. (**B** courtesy of Dr. John Preece, San Antonio, TX.)

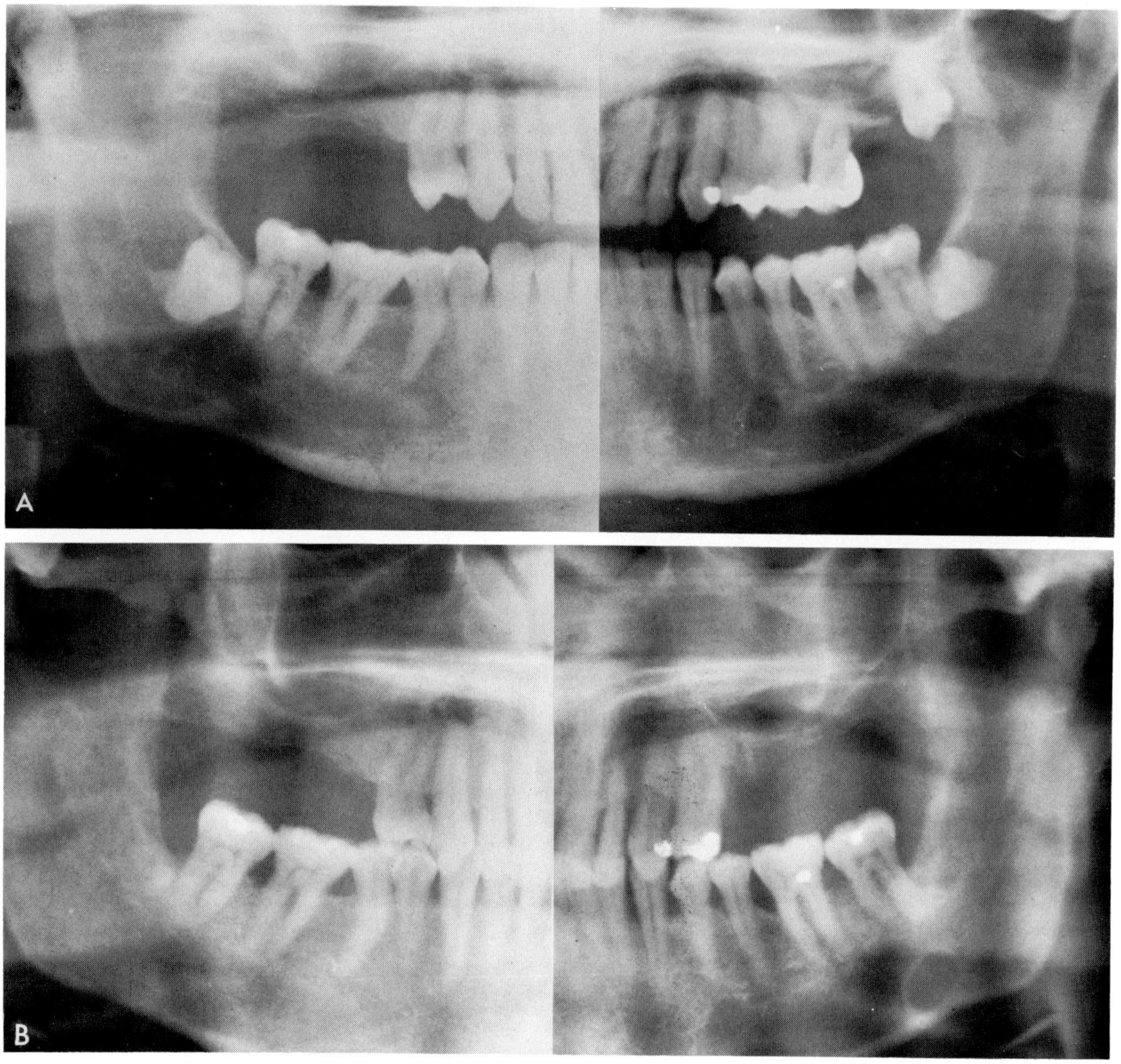

Figure 10–10. Developmental lingual mandibular salivary gland depression. (Note: **B** is the same patient three years later.) (Figure 10–10 courtesy of Drs. Frank Sammis, Jr. and Carlos Portales, San Antonio, TX.)

terior depression, which is thought by the authors to consist of a smooth concavity of bone on the lingual aspect of the mandible in the cuspid–lateral incisor area, with no evidence of resorption of the lingual cortical plate but rather a smooth thinning of the depressed lingual cortex. Although salivary gland tissue has been reported to be present in this defect, many surgical reports have failed to identify salivary gland tissue or the exact nature of the depression.

Because of the characteristic radiographic features of the posterior variant, the depression should simply be recognized; no further treatment is recommended. The anterior depression is not as characteristic radiographically as the posterior depression and should probably be explored surgically to rule out other conditions.

RADIOGRAPHIC FEATURES (Figs. 10–9 and 10–10)

The posterior defect is characteristic and consists of a 1- to 2-cm round, oval, or triangular, well-corticated radiolucency located below the mandibular canal in the second molar-ramus area of the mandible. This depression may be intimately associated with the inferior border of the mandible, in which case the inferior cortical plate will have a cupped-out appearance. The condition may be bilateral.

The anterior depression is less well corticated but, nevertheless, well defined. It is usually located about one-third to one-half way up on the root of a vital mandibular cuspid and/or lateral incisor, or it may be located at, or slightly below, the apices of these vital teeth. It is usually round or oval in shape. Relatively fewer cases of the anterior variant have been reported than of the posterior variant, and it would appear that it does not achieve as large proportions as the posterior depression. In no instances have anterior and posterior variants been reported in the same individual.

PRIMORDIAL CYST

BRIEF OVERVIEW

The primordial cyst arises from a developing tooth that undergoes cystic degeneration prior to calcification. It develops with equal frequency in males and females. Although they are often present by early adulthood, primordial cysts are often not discovered until many years later. The most common locations are in the mandibular third molar-ramus area and at the sites of supernumerary teeth, such as the mandibular bicuspid and maxillary central incisor. Primordial cysts occur in two histologic types, nonkeratinizing and keratinizing, the latter being by far the most frequent histologic type. Keratocysts tend to recur, usually within three to five years postoperatively.

RADIOGRAPHIC FEATURES (Fig. 10–11)

In the early lesion or in the younger patient, the primordial cyst is usually a round or oval, well-corticated radiolucency. It is often asymptomatic and is discovered on routine radiographic examination.

In older patients or if the cyst is of the keratocyst type at any age, it may be very large, expansile, and scalloped or multilocular. It may have a cloudy lumen, may displace impacted or unerupted teeth, and may show evidence of cortex perforation. These features are true of most keratocysts. Keratocysts will be discussed and illustrated separately in Chapter 11.

LATERAL PERIODONTAL CYST

BRIEF OVERVIEW

There is some controversy as to the origin of the lateral periodontal cyst. The older school of thought ascribes two theories of origin: (1) the cyst grows out of the epithelial rests in the periodontal ligament; or (2) it is a follicular cyst of a tooth that eventually erupted. The modern school considers it to be a primordial cyst of a supernumerary tooth. Since the lateral periodontal cyst may be of either the nonkeratinizing or keratinizing type and since it tends to occur in the mandibular premolar area where supernumerary teeth are commonly found, the mod-

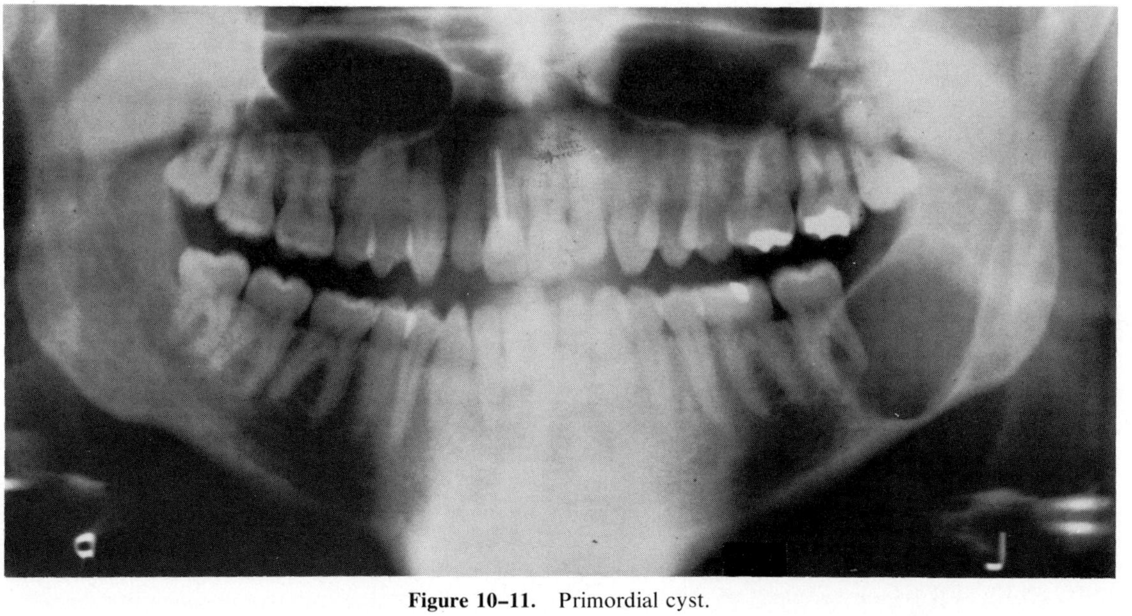

Figure 10–11. Primordial cyst.

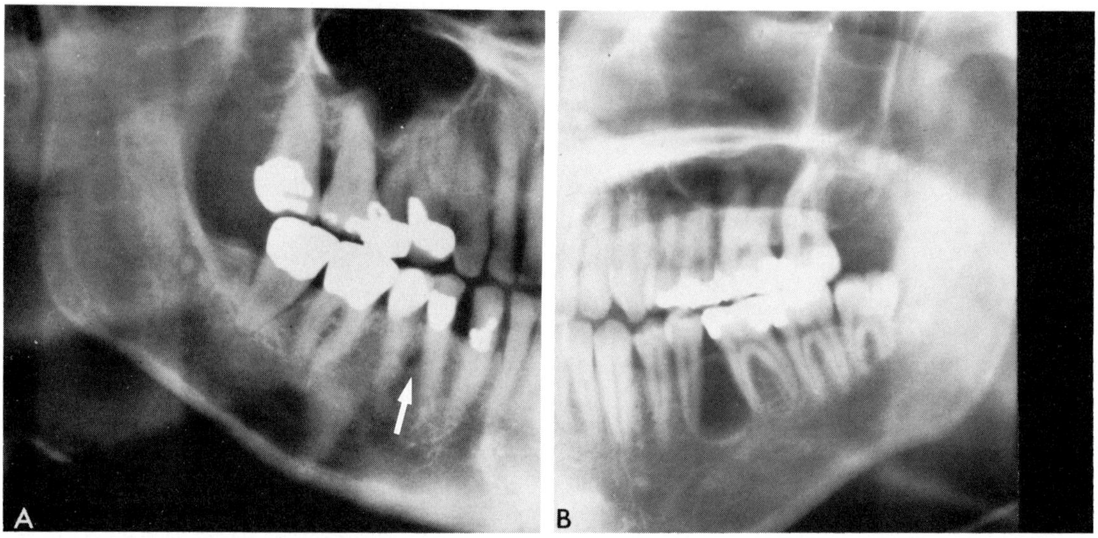

Figure 10–12. Lateral periodontal cyst.

ern school is perhaps the more credible. Once diagnosed, the keratocyst type should be closely followed radiographically on a yearly basis after removal, as recurrence is high.

RADIOGRAPHIC FEATURES (Fig. 10–12)

The lateral periodontal cyst is often a small, round, well-corticated radiolucency. It is usually intimately associated with the root of a vital mandibular bicuspid, often about half way up on the root. These cysts may sometimes enlarge and cause divergence of the involved roots and expansion of the cortical plates.

Although this cyst is usually found in adults, it may closely resemble the ameloblastic fibroma, the botryoid odontogenic cyst, a developing ameloblastoma, and a variety of other lesions, especially when the lateral periodontal cyst achieves larger proportions or when it is located in an area other than the mandibular bicuspid region.

INCISIVE CANAL CYST (Median Anterior Maxillary Cyst, Nasopalatine Duct Cyst)

BRIEF OVERVIEW

The incisive canal cyst is the most common of the developmental cysts. It develops from epithelial remnants of the nasopalatine duct, which remains patent for a short time during embryogenesis. This cyst occurs mainly in adults, and a soft tissue swelling in the area of the incisive papilla may sometimes be noted clinically. The cyst should be enucleated and followed up radiographically.

RADIOGRAPHIC FEATURES (Fig. 10–13)

The incisive canal cyst is classically described as a heart-shaped, well-corticated radiolucency located between the roots of vital maxillary central incisors. It may also be round or oval in shape and may be located to one side of the midline, especially in smaller lesions. This cyst can become very extensive.

When in the midline, the incisive canal cyst is radiographically indistinguishable from a primordial cyst of a mesiodens or a **median palatal cyst,** which is said to arise from embryonic epithelium entrapped at the midline of the hard palate. Owing to the focal trough, the median palatal cyst may be difficult to detect on panoramic radiographs.

When it occurs on one side of the midline, the incisive canal cyst may resemble a lateral periodontal cyst, an apical periodontal cyst, or even the superior foramen of the incisive canal.

GLOBULOMAXILLARY CYST

BRIEF OVERVIEW

As is the case for many fissural cysts, there is dispute as to the origin of the globulomaxillary cyst. Classically, it is thought to arise from embryonic epithelium somehow entrapped be-

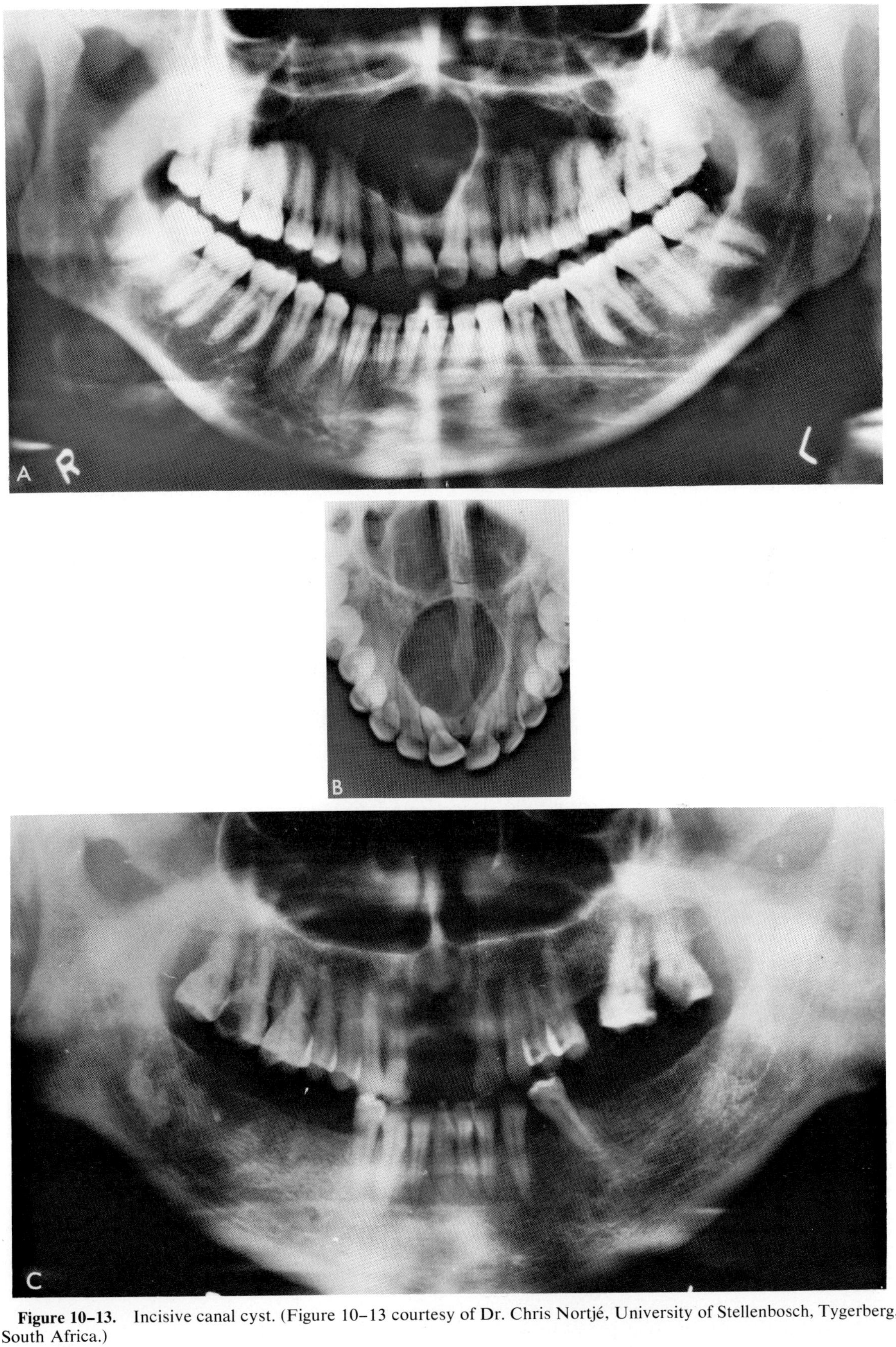

Figure 10–13. Incisive canal cyst. (Figure 10–13 courtesy of Dr. Chris Nortjé, University of Stellenbosch, Tygerberg, South Africa.)

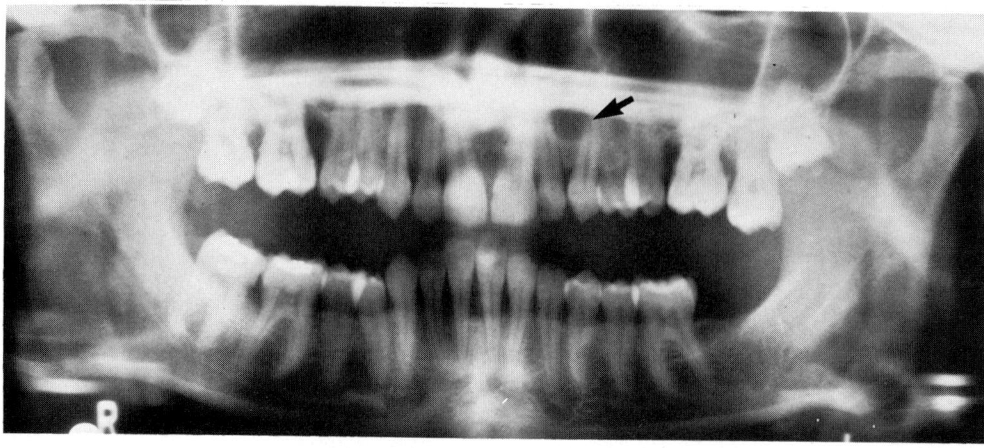

Figure 10–14. Globulomaxillary cyst.

tween the globular portion of the median nasal process and the maxillary process. Others believe it to be an odontogenic cyst such as a primordial cyst of a supernumerary tooth, whereas some have shown that upon reexamination, many so-called globulomaxillary cysts are simply apical periodontal cysts of a nonvital lateral incisor or cuspid. The treatment of choice is surgical enucleation. Globulomaxillary cysts do not tend to recur.

RADIOGRAPHIC FEATURES (Figs. 10–14 and 10–15)

The globulomaxillary cyst is classically described as a pear-shaped, well-corticated radiolucency, located between and causing divergence of the roots of vital maxillary lateral incisors and cuspids. Particularly in this area, it is important to consider a radiolucent lateral fossa, an apical periodontal cyst, and an adenomatoid odontogenic tumor in the differential diagnosis. The **nasoalveolar** or **nasolabial cyst** occurs in this area, is located exclusively in soft tissue, and is not visible radiographically unless injected with radiopaque material (see Fig. 10–15**A** and **B**).

MEDIAN MANDIBULAR CYST

BRIEF OVERVIEW

The median mandibular cyst is a rare fissural cyst whose origin remains unclear. According to most recent reviews, including that of Soskolne and Shteyer, there are probably less than 24 reported cases. Classically, it has been said to arise from embryonic epithelium trapped between the two halves of the mandible in the region of the symphysis. It has also been called a primordial cyst of a supernumerary tooth and a lateral periodontal cyst. This cyst should be removed by enucleation and followed up radiographically.

RADIOGRAPHIC FEATURES (Fig. 10–16)

Because of the rarity of this cyst, there is probably no classic description. It is basically a well-corticated radiolucency that is variable in size. It is located between vital mandibular central incisors, and the smaller lesion may resemble a small lateral periodontal cyst. The larger cyst may be slightly expansile and may cause divergence of the roots of the central and lateral incisors.

RESIDUAL CYST

BRIEF OVERVIEW

Residual cyst is a broad term referring to an odontogenic cyst that remains after the associated tooth has been extracted. It therefore refers to radicular (periapical cysts, apical periodontal cysts), lateral periodontal, or follicular (dentigerous) cysts. Additionally, the latter two may be of either the nonkeratinizing or, more importantly, the keratinizing type. All residual cysts should be enucleated and submitted for histopathologic diagnosis. They may resemble or give rise to other conditions, and an accurate diagnosis is important for future follow-up procedures. Martinelli, Melhado,

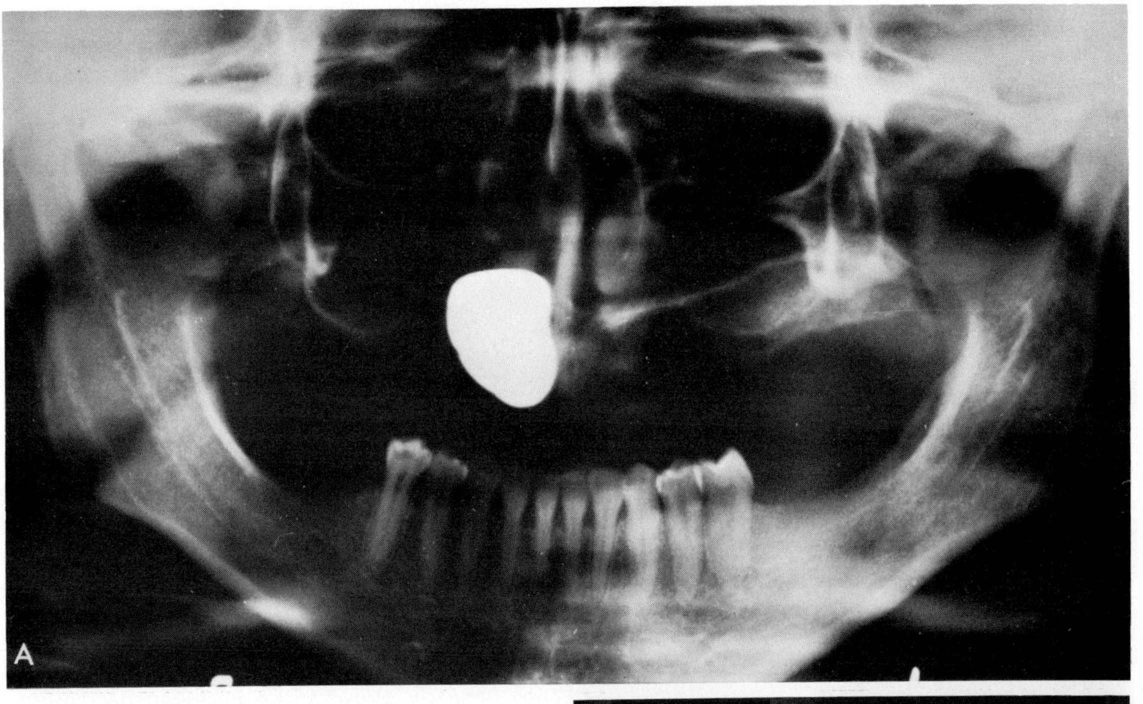

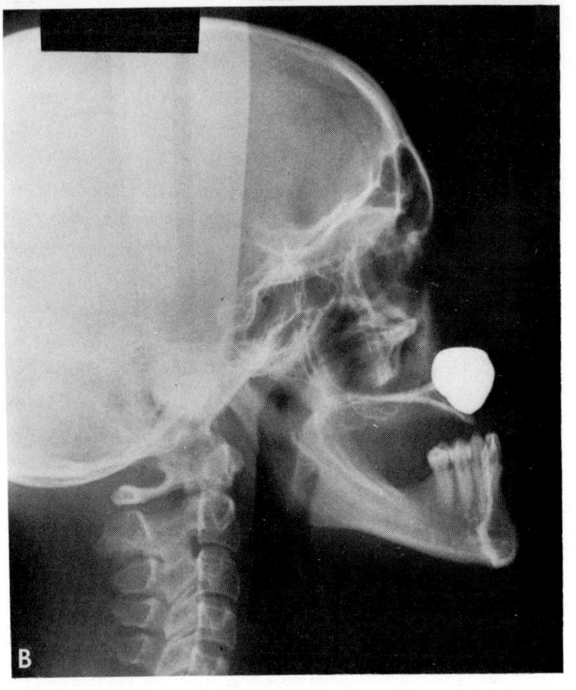

Figure 10–15. Nasolabial cyst. This is a soft tissue cyst and must be injected with radiopaque medium to be visualized radiographically. (Figure 10–15 courtesy of Dr. Chris Nortjé, University of Stellenbosch, Tygerberg, South Africa.)

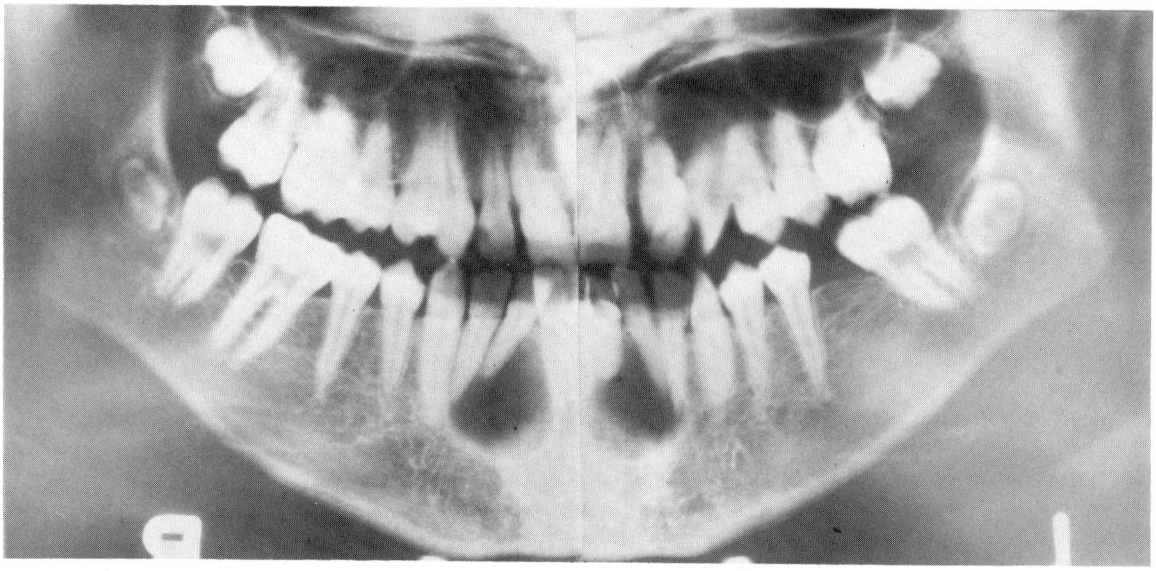

Figure 10–16. Median mandibular cyst. This was a single midline lesion on a split-image radiograph, which was subsequently trimmed for this photo. (Courtesy of J. Brugeman, St. Louis, MO.)

and Callestini have reported a case of squamous cell carcinoma in a residual cyst.

RADIOGRAPHIC FEATURES (Figs. 10–17 and 10–18)

Residual cysts are usually well-corticated, round radiolucencies, most often about 1 cm in diameter. They are frequently located in edentulous areas previously occupied by teeth. They may, however, be very large and may exhibit all the characteristics of a keratocyst. Residual cysts are often confused with the focal osteoporotic bone marrow defect or mistaken radiographically for primordial cysts or other de novo or recurrent central solitary odontogenic or nonodontogenic neoplasms.

TRAUMATIC CYST (Solitary Bone Cyst, Hemorrhagic Bone Cyst, Extravasation Cyst, Simple Bone Cyst, Unicameral Cyst)

BRIEF OVERVIEW

The traumatic cyst is one of several pseudocysts, as it contains no epithelial lining. The other pseudocysts are the aneurysmal bone cyst and Stafne's cyst (salivary gland depression).

In a recent review of the literature, Kuroi reports that the traumatic cyst occurs most frequently in adolescents and young adults and has a slight predilection for males. The cause of this condition is unknown, and a history of trauma is elicited in about half the cases. Kuroi reports that although most cases were asymptomatic, fully 18 per cent presented with pain or swelling.

Although the radiographs may be highly suggestive of a traumatic cyst, a definitive diagnosis is made by entering the area surgically. An empty cavity is usually found, but it may, on occasion, contain serosanguineous fluid. It may or may not be lined by a thin connective tissue membrane. In any case, gentle curettage of the walls of the cavity to stimulate bleeding and subsequent closure will usually bring about resolution within approximately one year.

RADIOGRAPHIC FEATURES (Fig. 10–19)

Classically, the traumatic cyst is described as an asymptomatic radiolucency that occurs most frequently in the mandible in the bicuspid-molar region. As reported by Kuroi, the ratio of mandibular to maxillary lesions is 6.5 to 1, and in the maxilla there is a marked predilection for the anterior area. Traumatic cysts are usually located in the peripapical area above the mandibular canal, and the superior margin appears scalloped as it spreads up in between the roots of the associated teeth. The periphery of the lesion may or may not be corticated. The cyst does not tend to resorb teeth, cause divergence of the roots, or destroy the lamina dura. The smaller traumatic cyst may resemble a small periapical radiolucency of pulpal origin, whereas larger lesions may be expansile, may

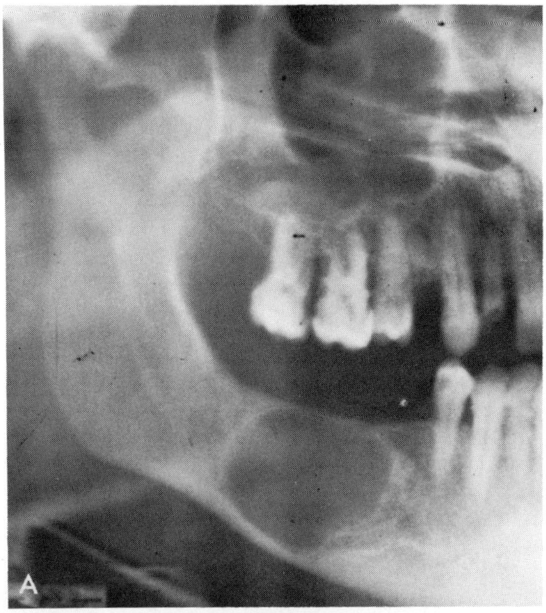

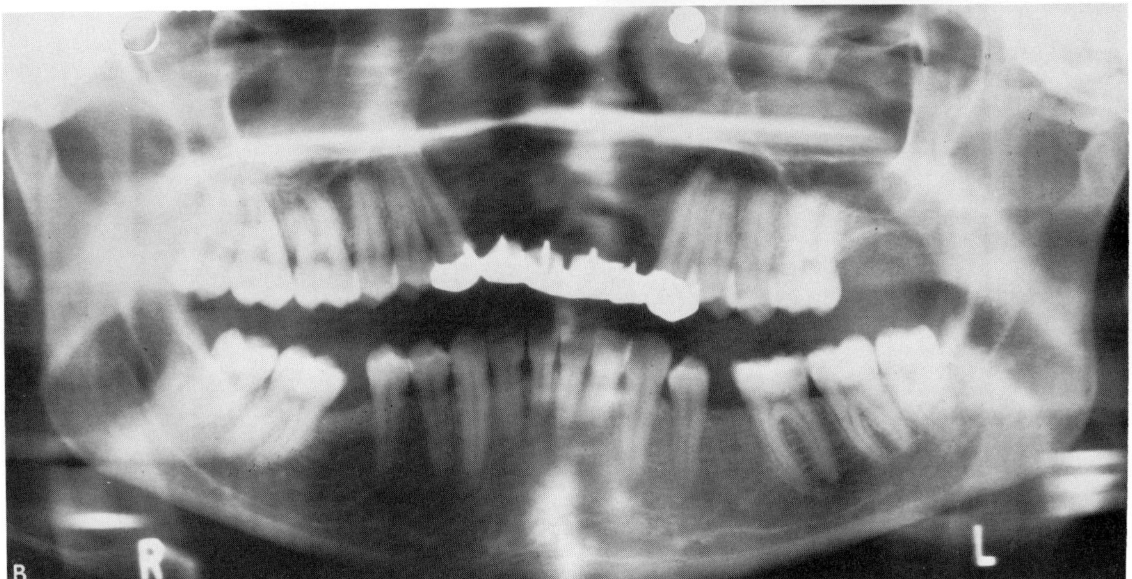

Figure 10–17. **A.** Residual cyst. **B.** The 28-year-old female patient was completely unaware of the presence of this cyst. (**B** courtesy of Dr. Steven Bricker, San Antonio, TX.)

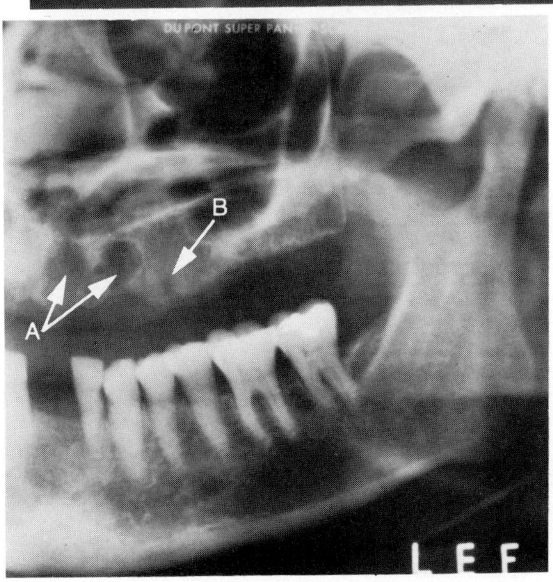

Figure 10–18. **A.** Residual cysts. **B.** Fibrous healing defect.

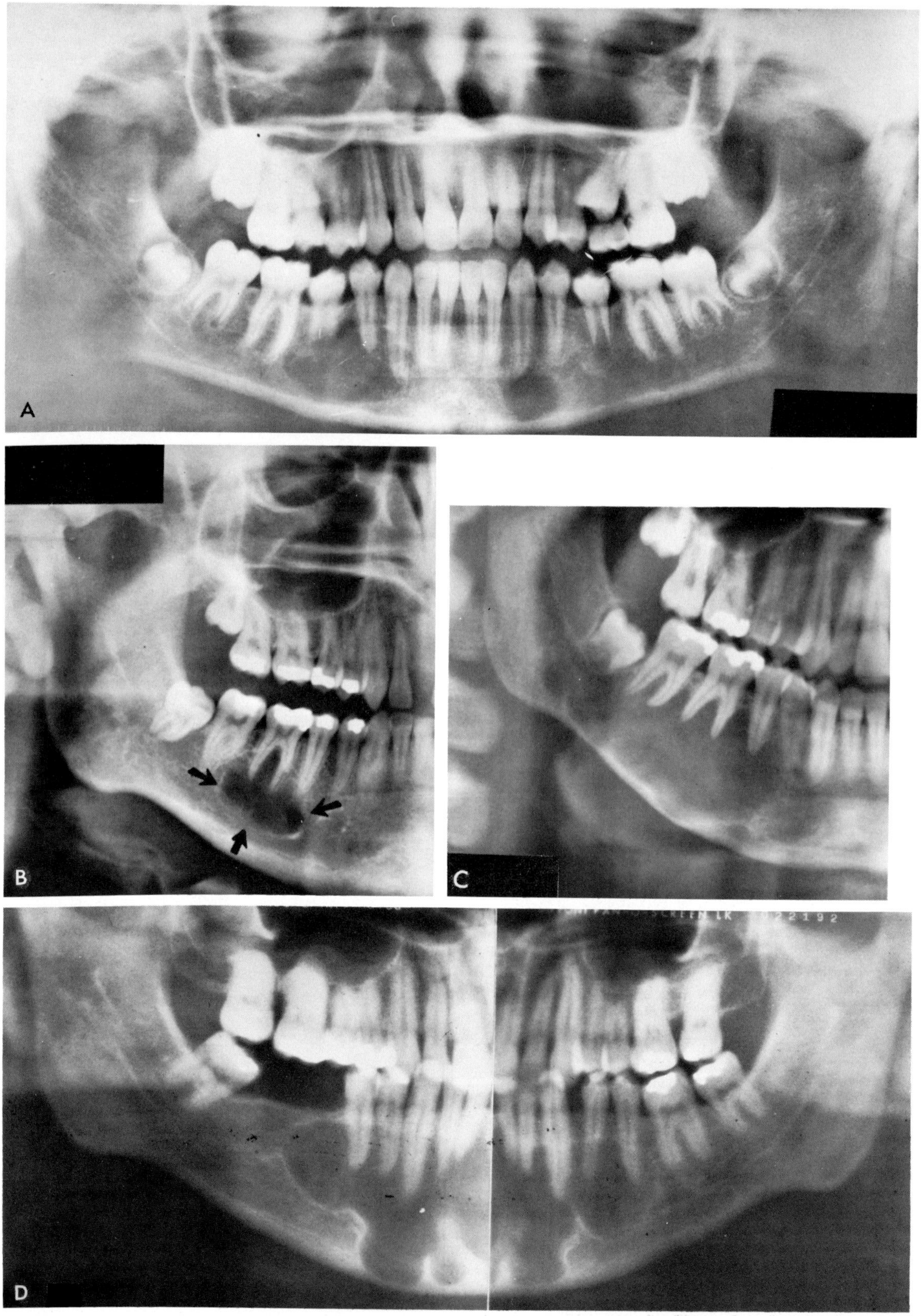

Figure 10–19. Traumatic cyst. **A.** This lesion was bilateral, crossing the midline, although it did not appear to do so in this radiograph. (**A, B,** and **C** courtesy of Dr. Gus Pappas, Columbus, OH.)

cause resorption of the inferior cortex of the mandible, and may occupy the entire body and ramus of the mandible. In this instance, the traumatic cyst may appear multilocular and may have a cloudy lumen if spontaneous or surgically stimulated resolution is in progress, thus greatly resembling an odontogenic keratocyst. Additionally, the traumatic cyst may be located in and cross the midline and, in rare instances, may be bilateral. Owing to the asymptomatic nature of this condition, the panoramic radiograph is an invaluable aid in discovering the presence of these lesions.

NEUROMA, NEUROFIBROMA, NEURILEMOMA

BRIEF OVERVIEW

Central tumors of neural origin are rare in the jaws. Neuromas usually develop as a sequela to trauma such as fracture, orthognathic surgery, or removal of a tumor or a tooth. The neuromas of the neuropolyendocrine syndrome do not usually occur centrally in bone, as they are generally confined to the mucosa.

Central neurofibromas may occur as a separate finding or may present in association with the skin and mucosal neurofibromas of von Recklinghausen's disease.

Central neurilemomas may occur as a single finding or may present in association with other neurilemomas involving the skin or mucosa. Multiple lesions are not associated with any particular disease or syndrome.

Central neural lesions are often discovered because of the symptoms of expansion, pain, and paresthesia. The patient usually complains of burning, tingling, or aching sensations. Since these lesions are treated by surgical excision, residual sensations such as anesthesia or paresthesia may persist.

RADIOGRAPHIC FEATURES (Fig. 10–20)

The most common radiographic finding for central neural lesions is a symmetric widening of the mandibular canal, which may become extensive. Usually the cortical outline of the canal remains intact. Larger lesions may have scalloped borders with a tendency towards multilocularity and may displace both erupted and unerupted teeth. Evidence of involvement of the mandibular canal may or may not be present. In some instances the borders may not be well corticated but nevertheless remain fairly well defined. Peripheral or parosteal neurofibromas of the gingiva or alveolar mucosa may produce a cupping-out of the crest of the alveolar ridge, thus producing a saucerlike defect in the area. In one case reported by Ellis, Abrams, and Melrose, the radiolucency contained a central radiopaque mass, which was histologically identified as dystrophic calcification.

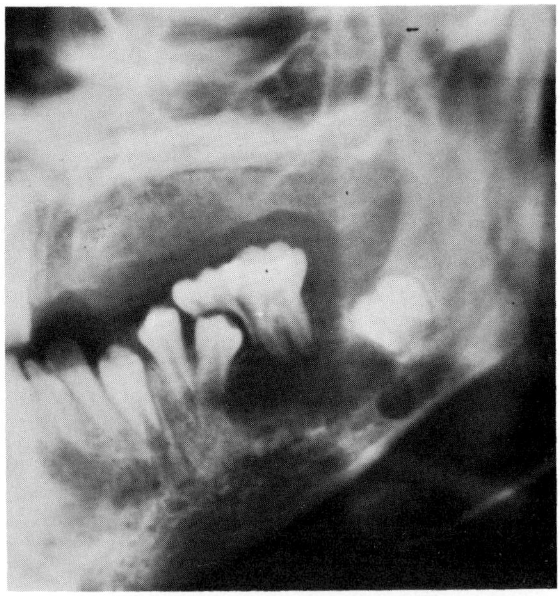

Figure 10–20. Central neurofibroma. This was a case of neurofibromatosis (von Recklinghausen's disease). (Courtesy of Dr. Philip Boyne, Loma Linda, CA.)

REFERENCES

Reference Texts

Eversole, L. R.: **Clinical Outline of Oral Pathology,** Philadelphia: Lea & Febiger, 1978, pp. 185–190.

Shafer, W. G., Hine, M. K., and Levy, B. M.: **A Textbook of Oral Pathology,** 3rd Edition. Philadelphia: W. B. Saunders, 1974, pp. 33–34, 67–71, 189–196, 237, 243–245, 451, 494–496, 550–555.

Wood, N. K., and Goaz, P. W.: **Differential Diagnosis of Oral Lesions.** St. Louis: C. V. Mosby, 1975, pp. 319–326, 333–335, 338–347.

Selected References

Christ, T. F.: The globulomaxillary cyst: An embryologic misconception. **Oral Surg. 30**:515, 1970.

Correll, R. W., Jensen, J. L., and Rhyne, R. R.: Lingual cortical mandibular defects: A radiographic incidence study. **Oral Surg. 50**:287, 1980.

Crawford, B. E., and Weathers, D. R.: Osteoporotic marrow defects of the jaws. **J. Oral Surg. 28**:600, 1970.

Ellis, G. L., Abrams, A. M., and Melrose, R. J.: Intraosseous benign neural sheath neoplasms of the jaws: Report of seven new cases and review of the literature. **Oral Surg. 44**:731, 1977.

Fantasia, J. E.: Lateral periodontal cyst: An analysis of forty-six cases. **Oral Surg. 48**:237, 1979.

Gallo, W. J., Moss, M., Shapiro, D. N., and Gaul, J. V.:

Neurilemoma: Review of the literature and report of five cases. **J. Oral Surg. 35**:235, 1977.

Hall, A. M.: The solitary bone cyst: Report of two cases. **Oral Surg. 42**:164, 1976.

Hansen, L. S., Saporre, J., and Sproat, R. C.: Traumatic bone cysts of jaws: Report of sixty-six cases. **Oral Surg. 37**:899, 1974.

Hansson, L-G.: Development of a lingual mandibular bone cavity in an 11-year-old boy. **Oral Surg. 49**:376, 1980.

Kuroi, M.: Simple bone cyst of the jaw: Review of the literature and report of a case. **J. Oral Surg. 38**:456, 1980.

Langlais, R. P., Cottone, J. A., and Kasle, M.: Anterior and posterior lingual depressions of the mandible. **J. Oral Surg. 34**:502, 1976.

Lorsan, E. L., DeLong, P. E., Osborn, D. B., and Dolaw, K. D.: Neurofibromatosis with central neurofibroma of the mandible: Review of the literature and report of a case. **J. Oral Surg. 35**:733, 1977.

Martinelli, C., Melhado, R. M., and Callestini, E. A.: Squamous cell carcinoma in a residual mandibular cyst. **Oral Surg. 44**:274, 1977.

Morris, C. R., Steed, D. L., and Jacoby, J. J.: Traumatic bone cysts. **J. Oral Surg. 28**:188, 1970.

Nanavati, S. D., and Ghandi, P. R.: Median mandibular cyst. **J. Oral Surg. 37**:422, 1979.

Nortje, C. J., and Farman, A. G.: Nasopalatine duct cyst: An aggressive condition in adolescent negroes from South Africa? **Int. J. Oral Surg. 7**:65, 1978.

Oikariven, V. J., Wolf, J., and Julku, M.: A stereosialographic study of developmental mandibular bone defects. **Int. J. Oral Surg. 4**:51, 1975.

Pagrel, M. A.: Bilateral solitary bone cysts: Report of a case. **J. Oral Surg. 36**:55, 1978.

Ruprecht, A., and Reid, J. A.: Radiologic appearances of oral and perioral cysts. **Ont. Dent. 52**:9, 1975.

Saporre, J., and Hansen, L.: Traumatic bone cysts of the jaws: Diagnosis, treatment and prognosis. **Oral Surg. 38**:127, 1974.

Soskolne, W. A., and Shteyer, A.: Median mandibular cyst. **Oral Surg. 44**:84, 1977.

Van Gemert, R. J., Yamashita, D. D. R., and Goodsell, J. F.: Multiple neurofibromatosis (von Recklinghausen's disease) with concurrent micrognathia: Review of the literature and report of a case. **Oral Surg. 43**:165, 1977.

Weathers, D. R., and Waldron, C. A.: Unusual multilocular cysts of the jaw (botryoid odontogenic cysts). **Oral Surg. 36**:235, 1973.

Chapter 11
Multilocular Radiolucencies

MULTILOCULAR CYST
ODONTOGENIC KERATOCYST
AMELOBLASTOMA
CENTRAL GIANT CELL GRANULOMA
CHERUBISM
ODONTOGENIC MYXOMA
ANEURYSMAL BONE CYST
CENTRAL HEMANGIOMA OF BONE AND VASCULAR LESIONS
CHONDROMYXOID FIBROMA OF THE MANDIBLE

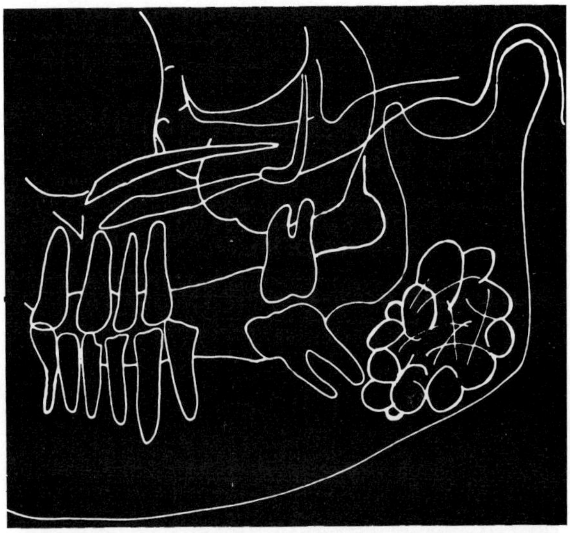

MULTILOCULAR CYST — ODONTOGENIC, NONKERATOCYST TYPE (Botyroid Odontogenic Cyst)

BRIEF OVERVIEW AND RADIOGRAPHIC FEATURES (Figs. 11–1 and 11–2)

The multilocular cyst as a separate entity is probably rare and may in most cases consist of several separate unilocular cysts that have grown to within close proximity of one another. Many of the older reports of multilocular cysts may have in fact been odontogenic keratocysts, which are often multilocular. Certainly, if a histopathologic diagnosis of odontogenic cyst is given, an effort should be made to determine if it is a keratocyst, as this is highly possible. The identification of cysts specifically as keratocysts is of clinical significance.

An extremely rare type of multilocular cyst is the **botryoid odontogenic cyst**, so named by Weathers and Waldron because of its grapelike gross appearance and probable odontogenic origin. The multilocularity was a histologic as well as a radiographic finding in one of the two reported cases. Both cases were located in the mandibular cuspid-bicuspid area, and expansion was present.

ODONTOGENIC KERATOCYST

BRIEF OVERVIEW

It is of clinical importance to identify an odontogenic cyst as either nonkeratinizing or keratinizing. Histologically, the keratocyst's lumen is lined with keratinizing odontogenic epithelium. Large amounts of keratin are sometimes seen filling the entire lumen. Odontogenic

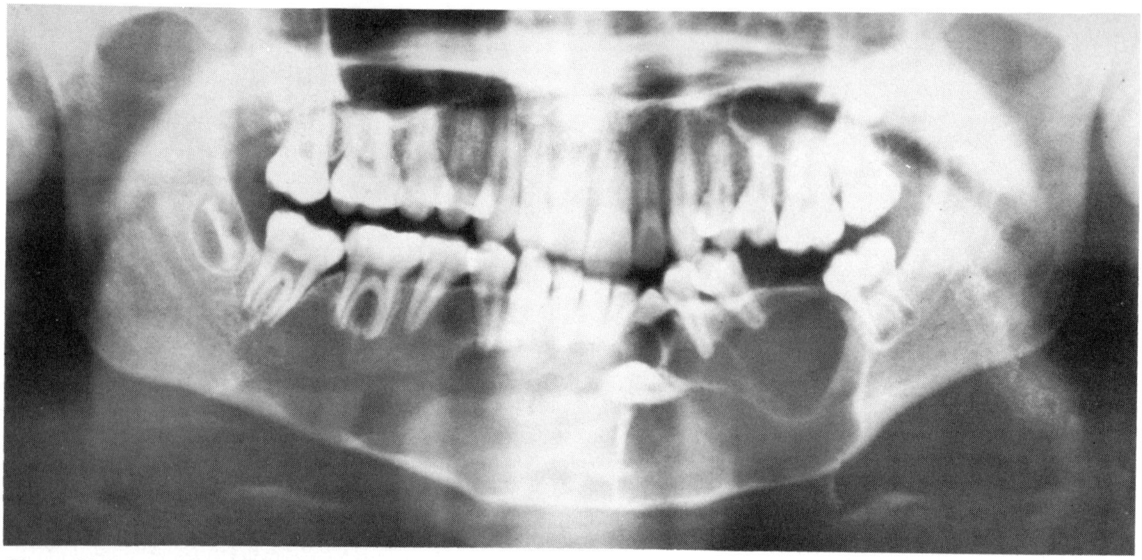

Figure 11–1. Multilocular follicular cyst. Histologic type unknown. (Courtesy of Dr. Gus Pappas, Columbus, OH.)

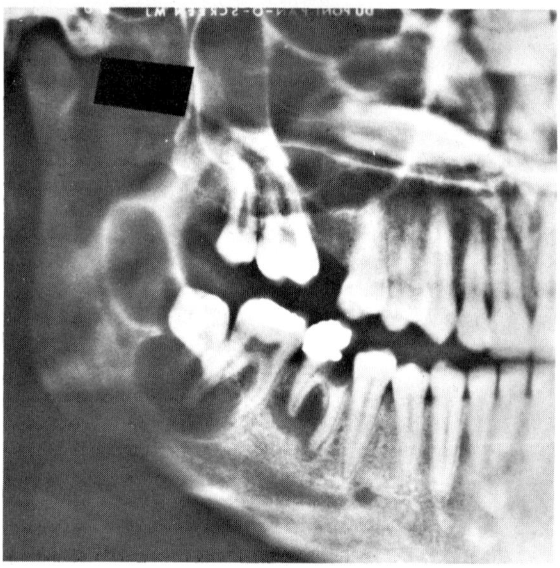

Figure 11–2. Follicular cyst. This was a nonkeratinizing type in near collision with several radiolucencies of pulpal origin.

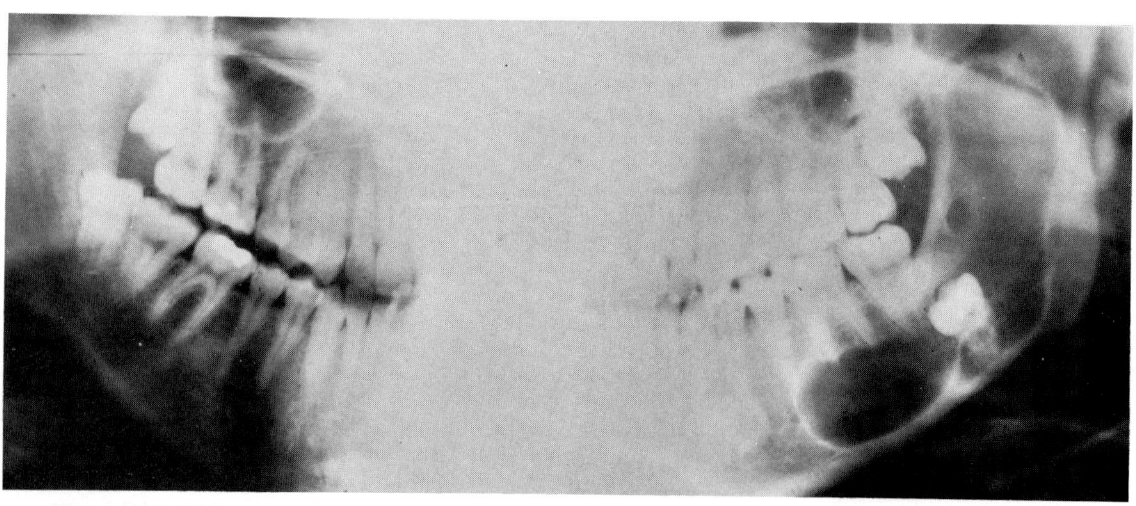

Figure 11–3. Odontogenic keratocyst, follicular sub-type. Note the large size and perforation of the cortex.

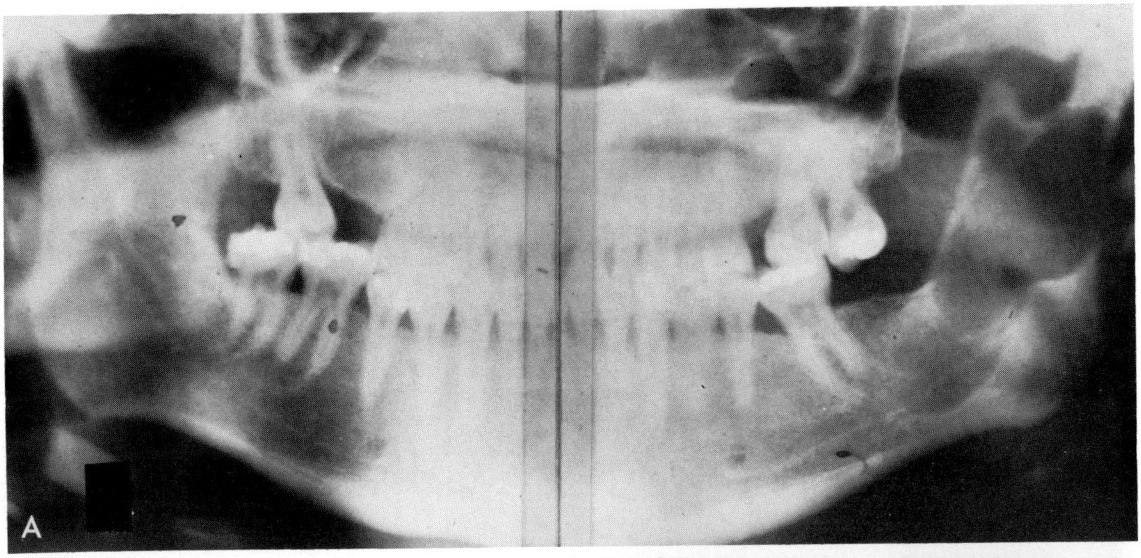

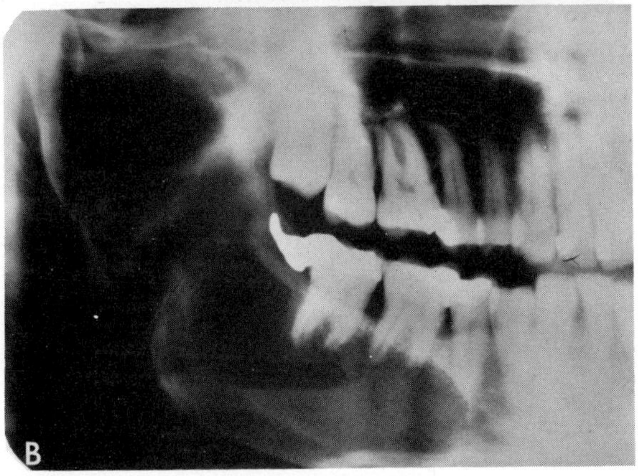

Figure 11–4. Odontogenic keratocyst, primordial sub-type. **A.** Note the large size; scalloped, well-corticated border; and perforation of the posterior cortex of the ramus. **B.** Note the large size, expansion, and multilocular appearance.

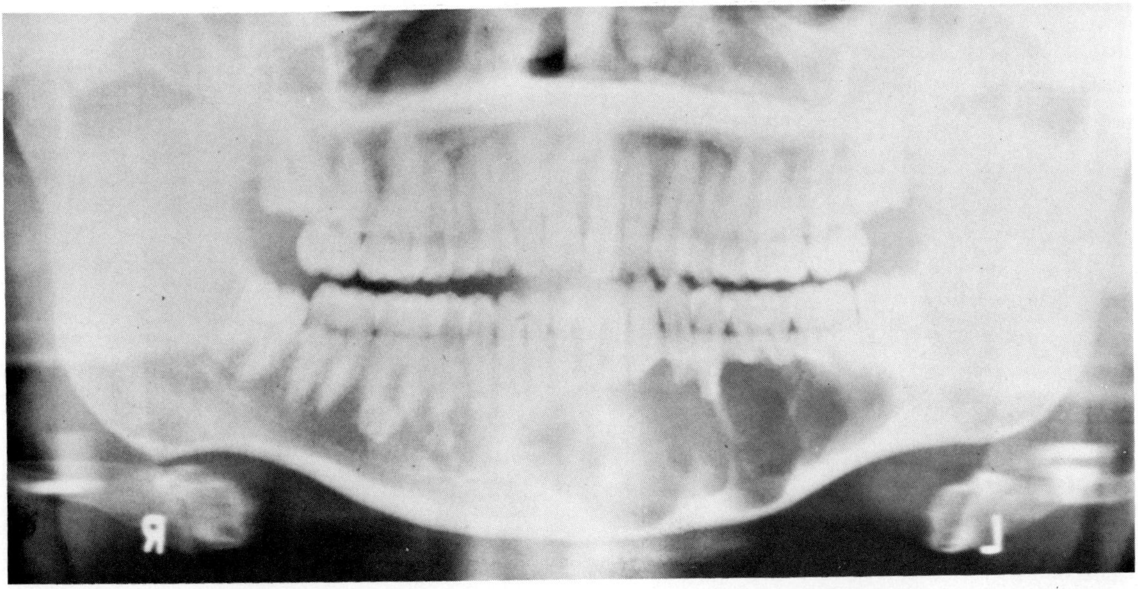

Figure 11–5. Odontogenic keratocyst, idiopathic sub-type. Note the large size, multilocularity, thinning of the inferior cortex, root resorption, and scalloped border. (Courtesy of Dr. Jim Cottone, San Antonio, TX.)

keratocysts have a tendency to recur. Additionally, the odontogenic keratocyst may be more rapidly growing than nonkeratinizing odontogenic and other cysts of the jaws. Therefore, the all important postsurgical radiographic follow-up should be carried out at six months initially and on a yearly basis for the remainder of the patient's life.

Odontogenic keratocysts have been subclassified according to their clinical presentation:

1. Follicular (dentigerous)
2. Primordial
3. Lateral periodontal
4. Jaw cysts of the basal cell nevus, bifid rib syndrome (Gorlin-Goltz syndrome)
5. Idiopathic
6. Residual or recurrent
7. Apical periodontal (radicular)

Keratocysts may resemble ordinary odontogenic nonkeratinizing cysts and other nonodontogenic cysts of the jaws. This is one of the important reasons why all suspected cysts should be biopsied and sent for histopathologic examination to an oral pathologist.

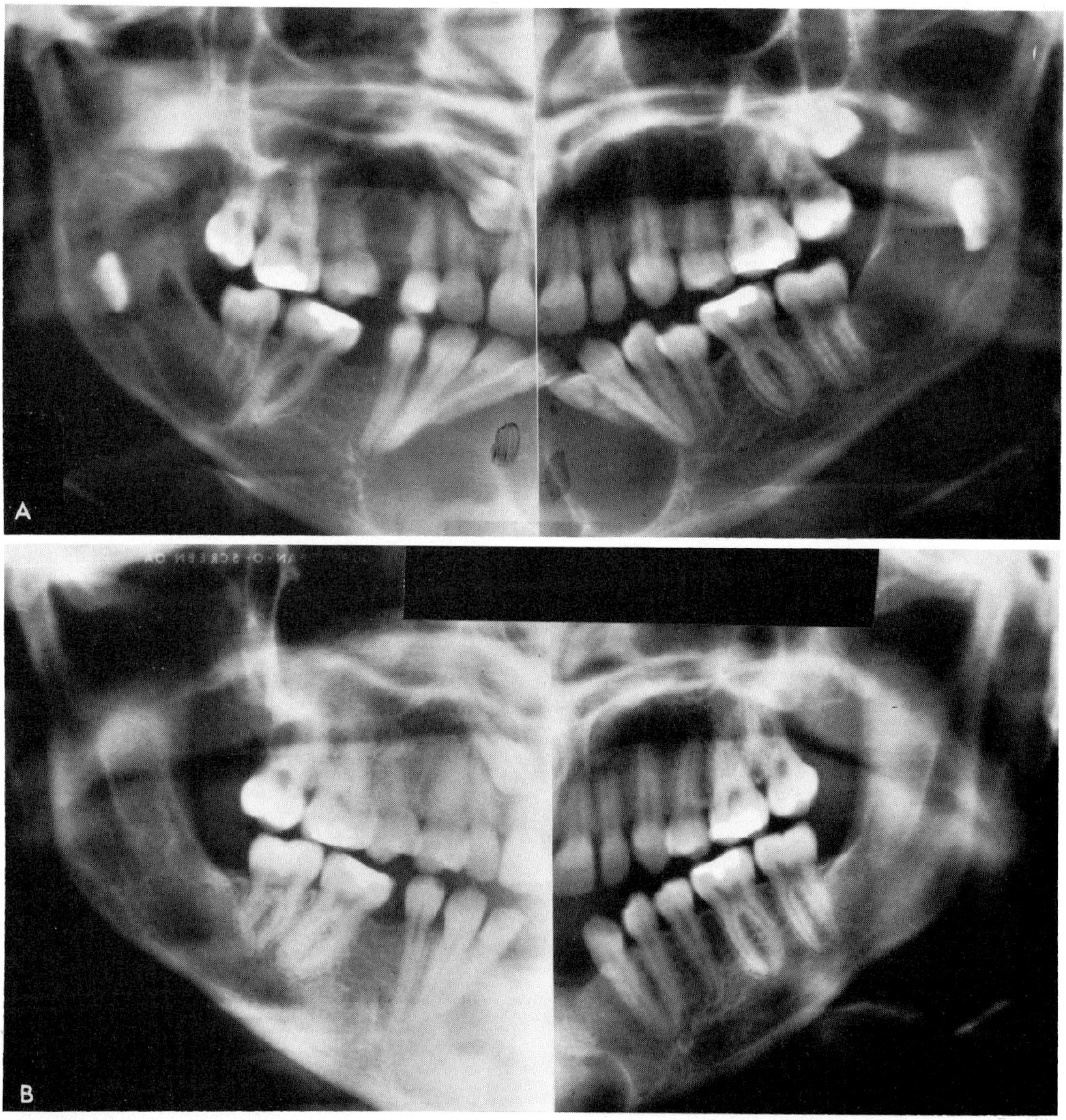

Figure 11–6. Odontogenic keratocyst, Gorlin-Goltz syndrome sub-type. **A.** Age 13, preoperative film. **B.** Six-month postoperative film.

Illustration continued on opposite page

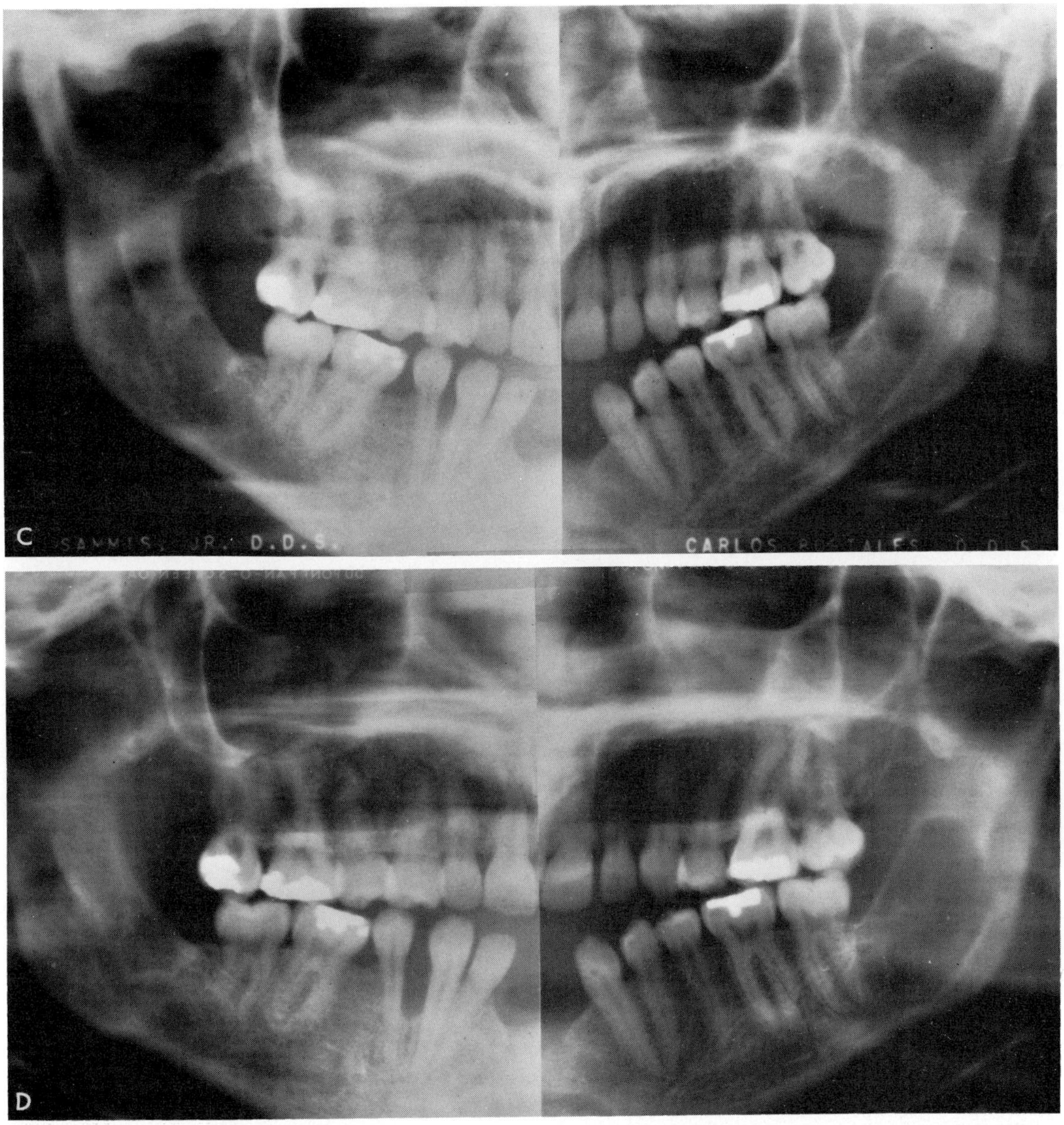

Figure 11–6 *Continued.* **C.** Age 16. **D.** Age 17½. (Figure 11–6 courtesy of Drs. Frank Sammis, Jr. and Carlos Portales, San Antonio, TX.)

RADIOGRAPHIC FEATURES (Figs. 11–3 to 11–7)

When small, odontogenic keratocysts have no particular radiographic features other than a mimicking of other nonkeratinizing cysts of the jaws.

When large, as is often the case, odontogenic keratocysts may exhibit any of the following features:

1. Scalloped and usually well-corticated radiopaque border, greatly contributing to its multilocular appearance;
2. Expansile tendency;
3. Large size;
4. Displacement of unerupted and/or developing teeth;
5. Cloudy or Milky-Way appearance of the lumen;
6. Occasional presence of multiple lesions;

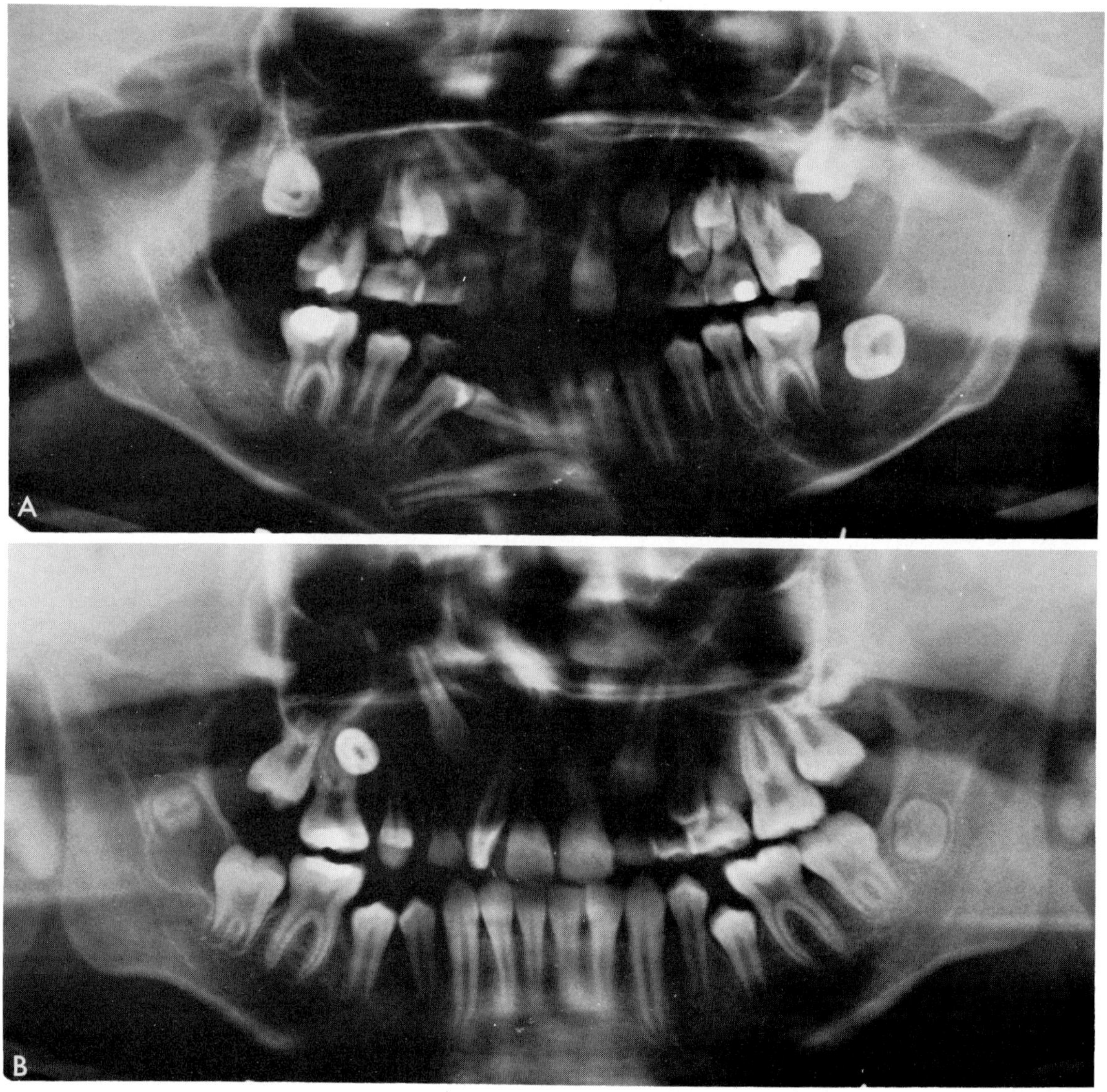

Figure 11–7. Odontogenic keratocyst, Gorlin-Goltz syndrome sub type. **A.** Age 11. **B.** Sibling, age 13. (Figure 11–7 courtesy of Dr. Chris Nortjé, University of Stellenbosch, Tygerberg, South Africa.)

7. A tendency to sometimes break through or perforate the cortical plate, causing a discontinuity or loss of this structure.

AMELOBLASTOMA

BRIEF OVERVIEW

The ameloblastoma occurs in mature adults, the average age being the mid-30s. However, this lesion is seen with some frequency in children. After odontomas of all types, the ameloblastoma was the second most common odontogenic tumor to be diagnosed by biopsy in the series reported by Regezi, Kerr, and Courtney. Whereas odontomas of all types comprised 67 per cent of the series, ameloblastomas occurred with a frequency of 11 per cent.

There are five main histologic types of ameloblastoma: follicular, plexiform, basal cell, acanthomatous, and granular cell. The plexiform type occurs more frequently in the maxilla. The granular cell type, although histologically benign, is said to be the most frequent type to metastasize, usually to the lungs, and therefore to behave as a malignancy. Metastasis is, however, an extremely rare sequela for any ameloblastoma. Although ameloblastomas have a high propensity for recurrence, many can probably be treated by curettage. This is especially true for unilocular and smaller multilocular lesions. Bloc resection may be preferable for more extensive lesions.

Although most ameloblastomas occur in the mandibular molar-ramus area, ameloblastomas do occur in the maxilla, most often involving the maxillary sinus. Because of the aggressive nature of this lesion and the proximity of vital structures, an early diagnosis is essential. Surgery is more complex and potentially more mutilating in the maxilla.

RADIOGRAPHIC FEATURES (Figs. 11–8 and 11–9)

The ameloblastoma classically is a multilocular, expansile radiolucency that occurs most frequently in the mandible, especially the molar-ramus area. In a review of 109 ameloblastomas, Adekeye found that 90 per cent consisted of a multilocular pattern, whereas the remainder were unilocular. This tumor may be associated with an unerupted or impacted tooth or an odontoma and may cause resorption and displacement of the adjacent teeth. All suspected dentigerous cysts should be sent for histopathologic examination, as mural ameloblastomas may arise from the epithelial lining of such cysts with no radiographic evidence of this clinically significant variation. Mural ameloblastomas comprise about 5 per cent of all ameloblastomas. Additionally, when ameloblastomas are unilocular, they may radiographically resemble cysts; thus, histopathologic diagnosis is essential for all such lesions. When ameloblastomas arise in the maxilla,

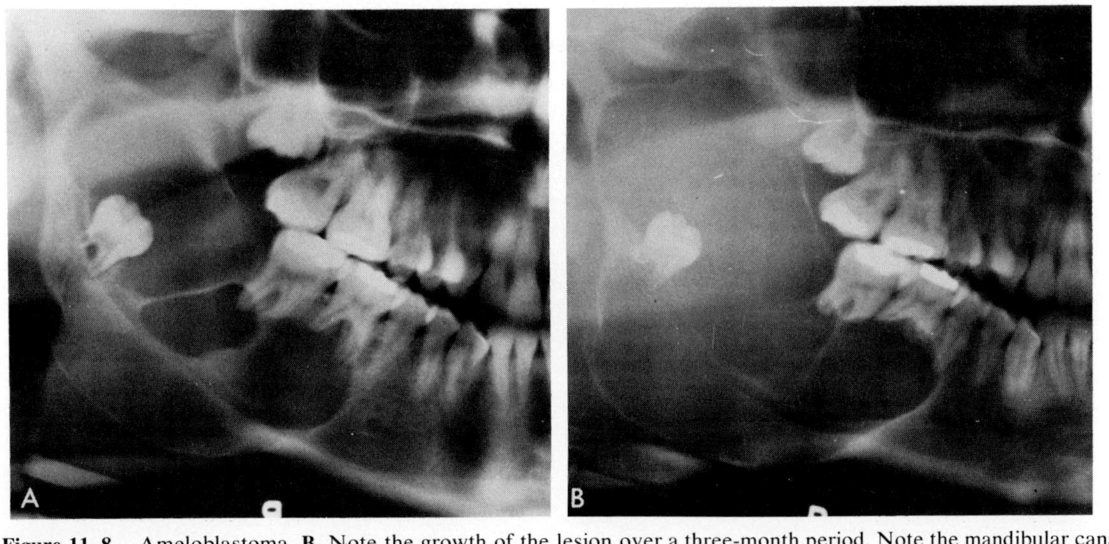

Figure 11–8. Ameloblastoma. **B.** Note the growth of the lesion over a three-month period. Note the mandibular canal within the lesion. **G.** A 78-year-old female. (**A, B, C, E,** and **G** courtesy of Dr. Chris Nortjé, University of Stellenbosch, Tygerberg, South Africa.)

Illustration continued on following page

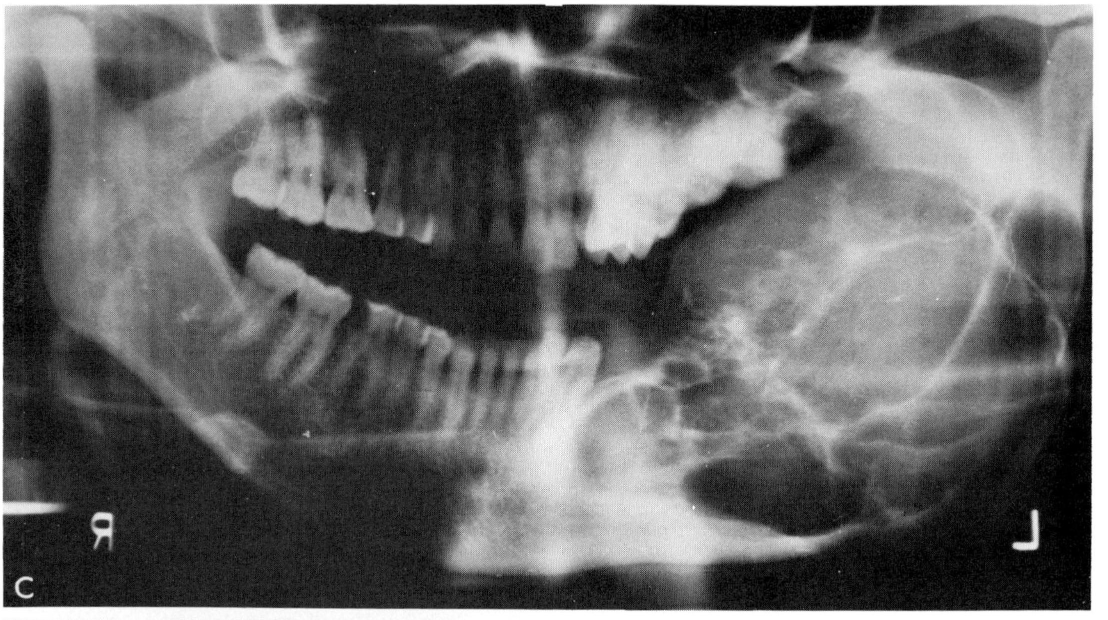

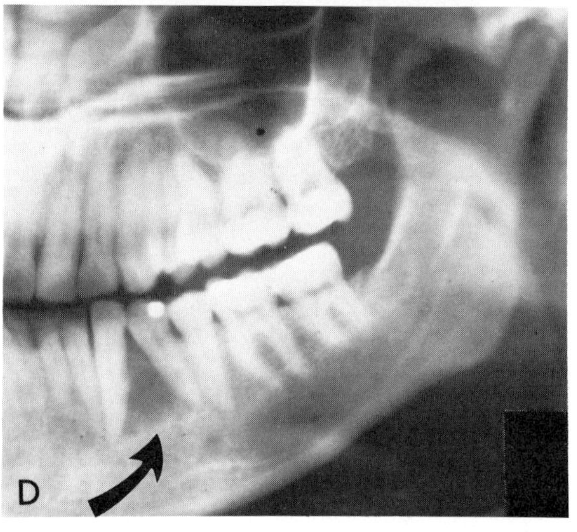

Figure 11–8 *Continued.*
Illustration continued on opposite page

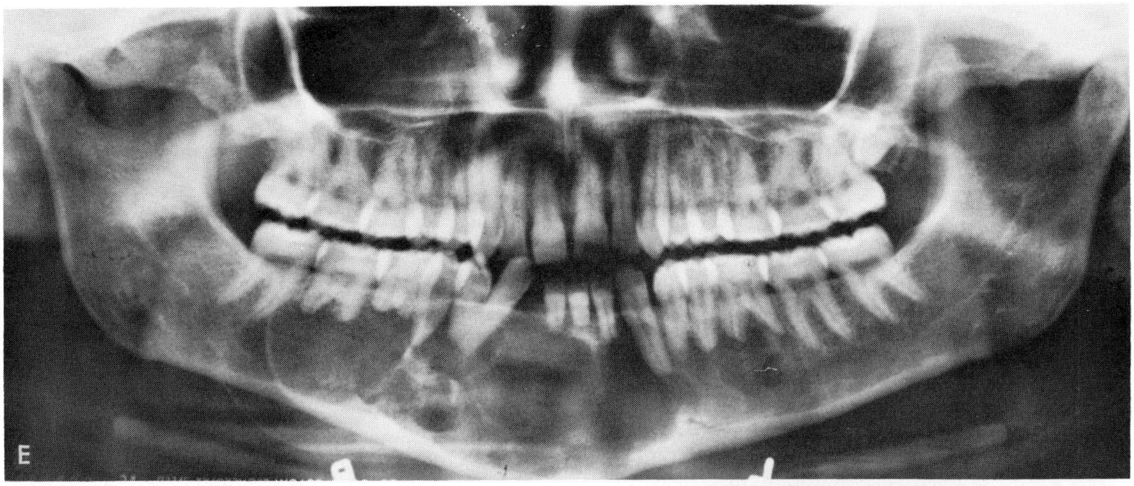

Figure 11-8 *Continued.*

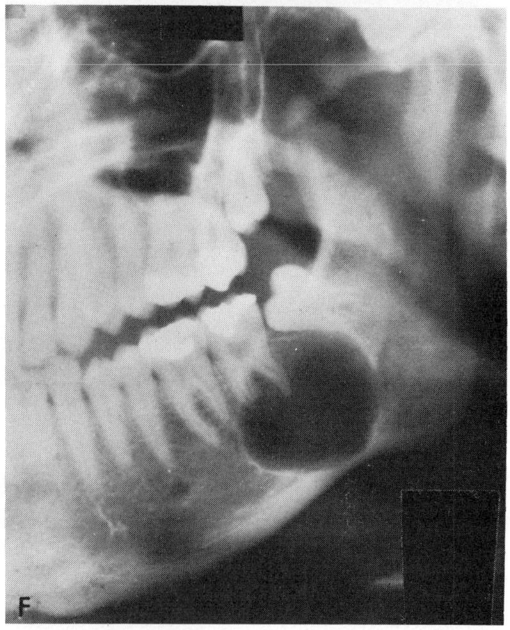

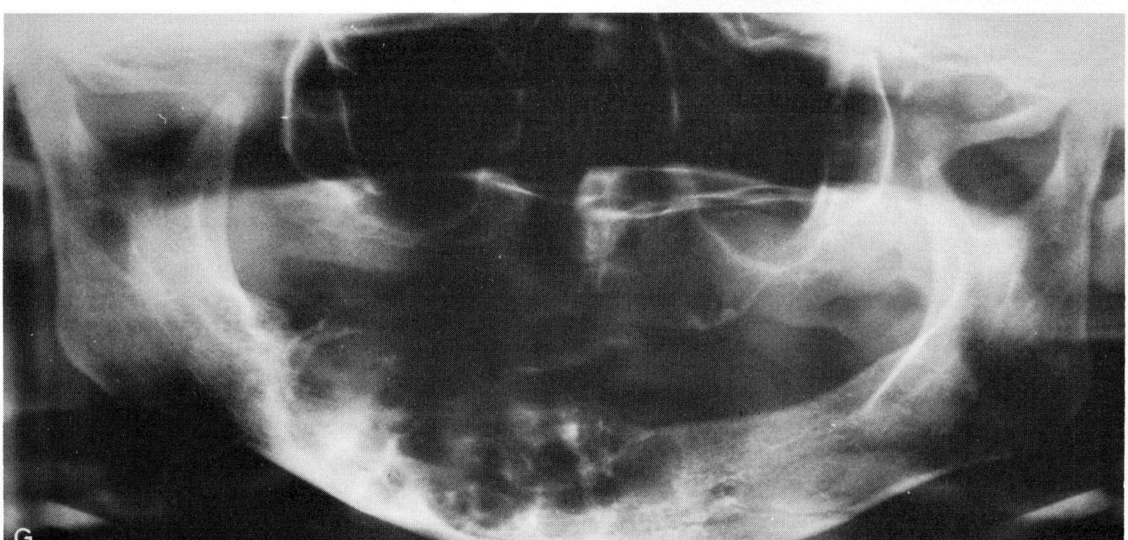

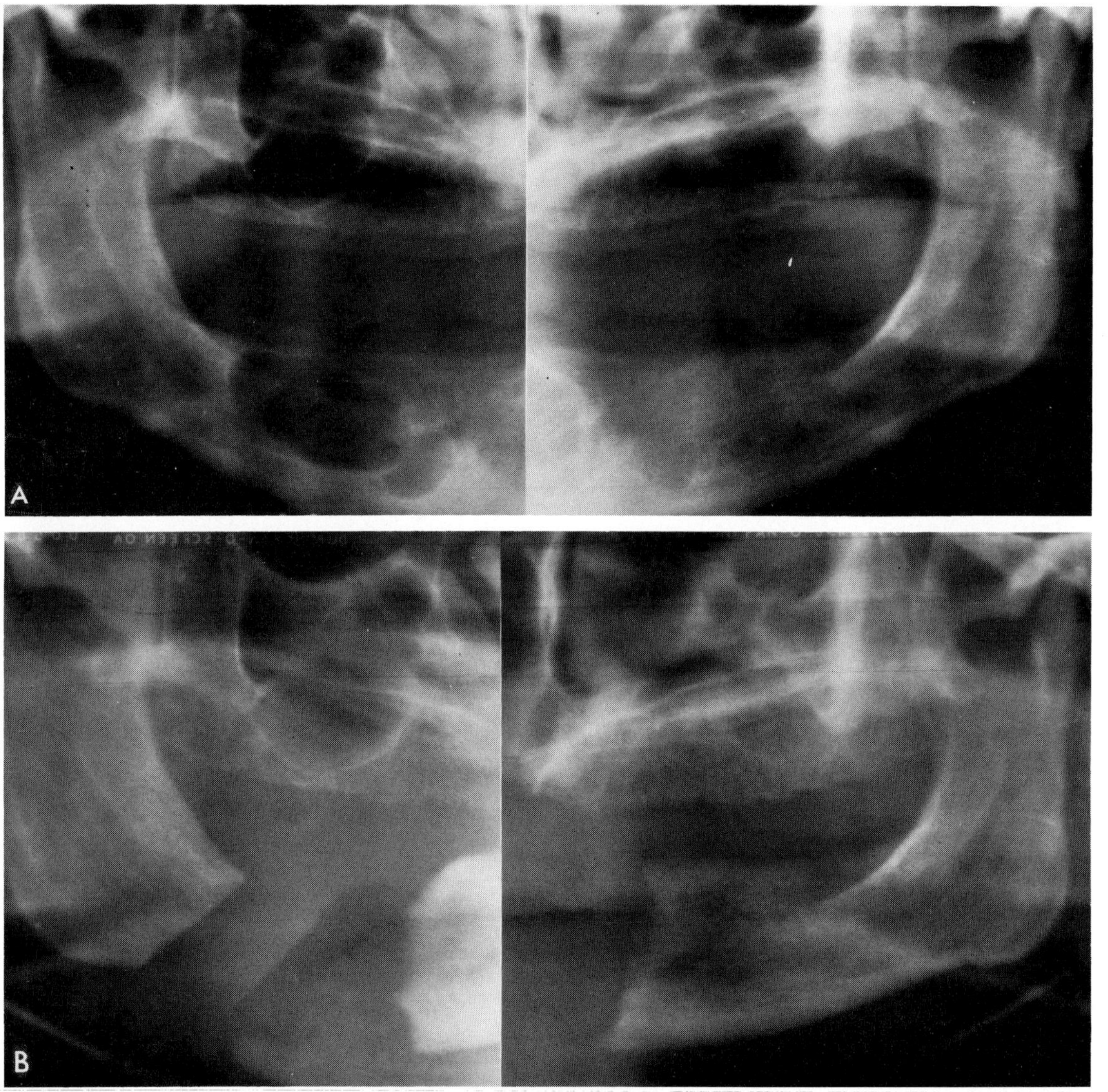

Figure 11–9. Recurrent ameloblastoma. **A.** Preoperative lesion. **B.** One-month postoperative surgical defect.

Illustration continued on opposite page

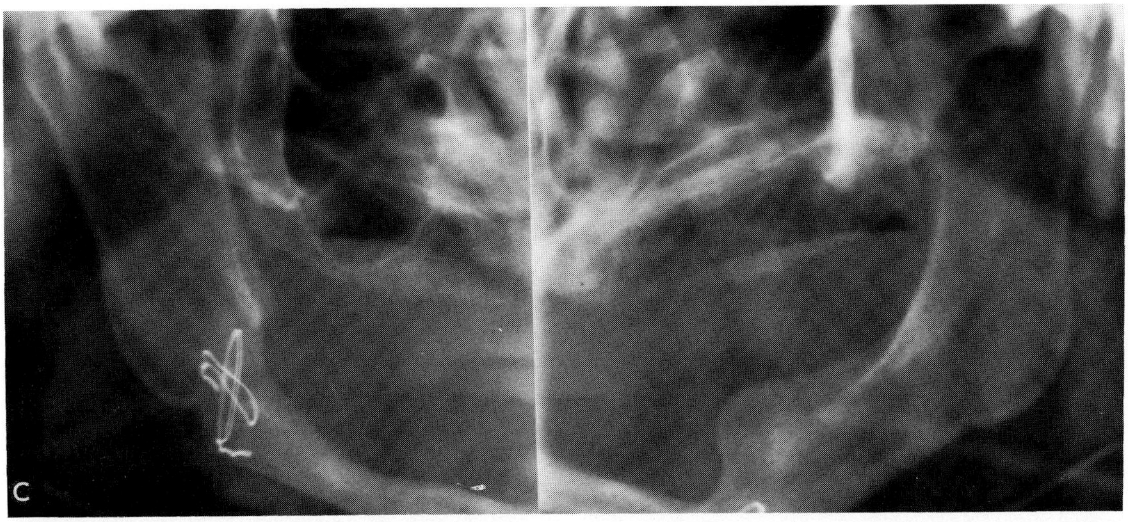

Figure 11–9 *Continued.* **C.** Five years postoperatively, with healed rib graft in place. (Figure 11–9 courtesy of Drs. Frank Sammis, Jr. and Carlos Portales, San Antonio, TX.)

they are most frequently seen in the posterior area and almost invariably involve the maxillary sinus. When the maxillary sinus is involved it would appear, from the limited number of cases available, that the pattern remains essentially multilocular within the sinus.

CENTRAL GIANT CELL GRANULOMA (Central Giant Cell Reparative Granuloma)

BRIEF OVERVIEW

This lesion occurs more frequently in young females, often under the age of 20 years. It occurs most frequently in the mandible, usually anterior to the permanent molars. It may cross the midline and rarely occurs in nontooth-bearing areas of the jaws. The lesion should be treated by curettage. It should be followed up by periodic radiographic examination, as it may recur. It is important to remember that this lesion is histologically indistinguishable from the giant cell (brown) tumor of hyperparathyroidism. Hyperparathyroidism, both primary and secondary, should be ruled out when a histologic diagnosis of central giant cell granuloma is received.

RADIOGRAPHIC FEATURES (Figs. 11–10 to 11–12)

The central giant cell granuloma is classically described as an expansile, painless, multilocular lesion occurring in the anterior mandible of young females. It often displaces, and sometimes resorbs, adjacent teeth and may be associated with an impacted or unerupted tooth. This lesion clinically and radiographically resembles a rare condition known as the **central odontogenic fibroma.** A peripheral giant cell granuloma occurs as an epulislike growth on the gingiva that histologically resembles the central lesion but does not create a central radiolucency. The peripheral giant cell granuloma is said to often exhibit a pathognomonic peripheral cuff of bone when it occurs on edentulous areas of the alveolar ridge (see Fig. 11–12).

CHERUBISM (Familial Fibrous Dysplasia, Familial Intraosseous Swelling of the Jaws)

BRIEF OVERVIEW

Cherubism is a hereditary fibro-osseous condition separate and distinct from fibrous dysplasia. It is transmitted as an autosomal dominant trait and begins to manifest early in childhood, eventually stabilizing during adolescence. Owing to the bilateral bony expansion, these patients exhibit a cherubic-looking facies; when only the mandible is involved, the condition also resembles bilateral masseter hypertrophy. Some individuals exhibit café au lait spots on the skin, and premature shedding of primary teeth is an early feature. If the condition does not stabilize or regress on its own, young adults may be admitted for cosmetic recontouring, although this procedure is usually of little benefit.

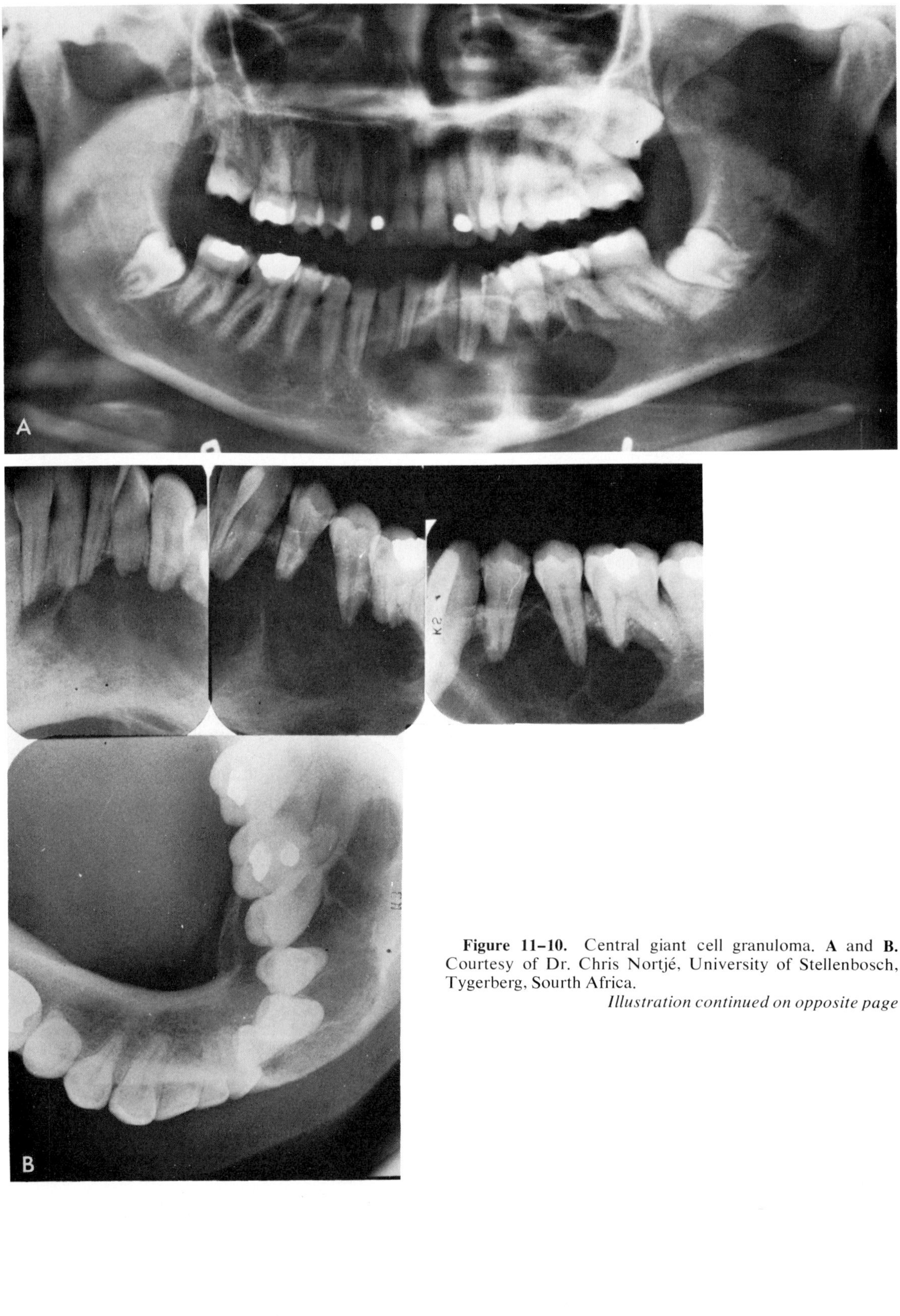

Figure 11–10. Central giant cell granuloma. **A** and **B.** Courtesy of Dr. Chris Nortjé, University of Stellenbosch, Tygerberg, Sourth Africa.

Illustration continued on opposite page

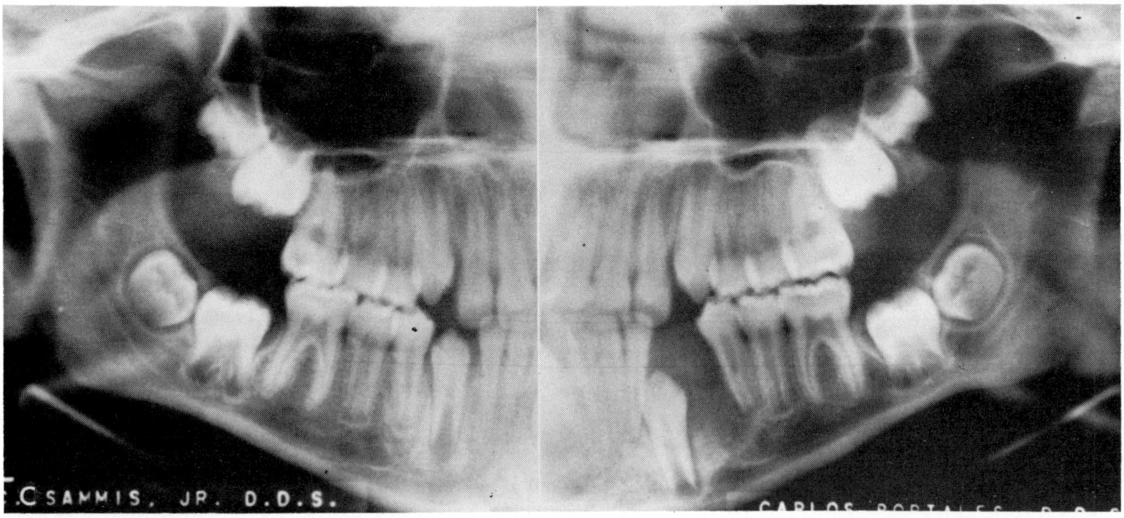

Figure 11–10 *Continued.* C. Courtesy of Dr. Frank Sammis, Jr. and Carlos Portales, San Antonio, TX.)

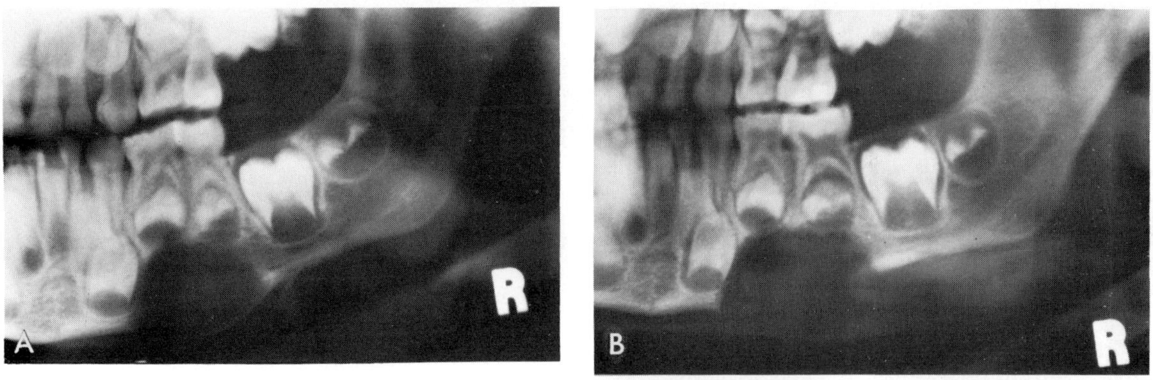

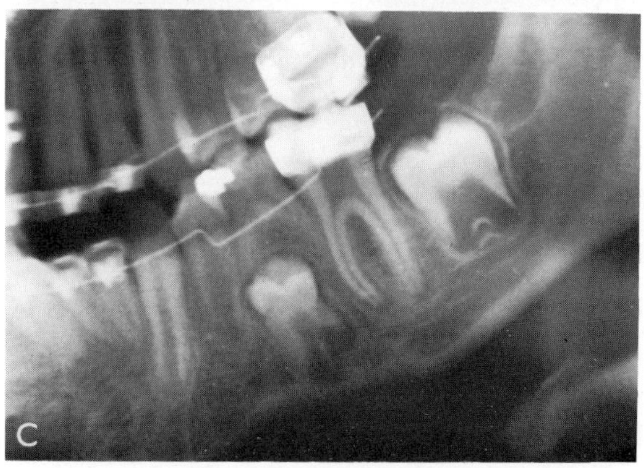

Figure 11–11. Central giant cell granuloma. **A.** Preoperative view. **B.** Postoperative view. **C.** Healed surgical site, one year postoperatively. (Figure 11–11 courtesy of Dr. Stanley Lovestedt, Rochester, MN.)

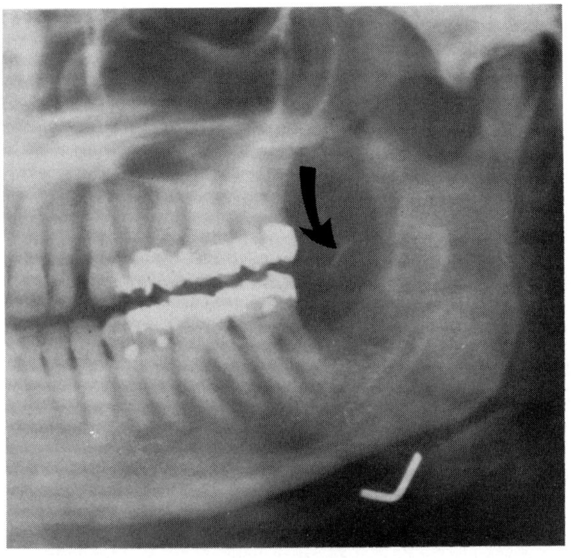

Figure 11–12. Central giant cell granuloma. Note the peripheral cuff of bone, highly suggestive of this lesion in edentulous areas. (Courtesy of Dr. Gus Pappas, Columbus, OH.)

RADIOGRAPHIC FEATURES (Fig. 11–13)

This lesion is classically described as a bilateral, multilocular, cystlike, expansile lesion, usually affecting the mandible and sometimes the maxilla or both jaws of children. There is premature exfoliation of the primary teeth, and there are many missing, malformed, and unerupted permanent teeth present. Although some lesions appear highly destructive, including the loss of cortical bone, pathologic fracture of the jaw is **not** a feature.

Sometimes this lesion strongly resembles the odontogenic keratocyst when the internal loculations become indistinct, leaving only a scalloped peripheral outline. These especially resemble the keratocyst of the jaw cyst, basal cell nevus, and bifid rib syndrome, as these are often bilateral, large, and associated with displaced unerupted teeth.

When all of the classic radiographic features of this disease are present, cherubism is considered radiographically pathognomonic.

ODONTOGENIC MYXOMA (Myxoma, Myxofibroma)

BRIEF OVERVIEW

This lesion is said to occur almost exclusively in the jaws, especially in the mandible of young and middle-aged adults. Maxillary lesions may erode into the maxillary sinus. This lesion has a significant recurrence rate and may be treated by curettage in less extensive cases. Bloc resection may be preferable for more extensive cases. Farman and associates have reported their results of an exhaustive literature review of this lesion.

RADIOGRAPHIC FEATURES (Fig. 11–14)

The odontogenic myxoma is classically described as a multilocular, expansile radiolucency, with a slight predilection for the mandible. The multilocular appearance of this neoplasm is usually caused by radiopaque striae, which may be seen within the area and are characteristically fine and lacy. Displacement of adjacent teeth is a common feature, and the tumor is almost always associated with a clinically missing or unerupted, displaced tooth.

If the dental papilla of a developing tooth is sent for histologic examination, it may be misdiagnosed as an odontogenic myxoma. This may occur easily with third molars, and an accurate history, radiographs, and clinical diagnosis are helpful to the pathologist.

ANEURYSMAL BONE CYST

BRIEF OVERVIEW

This is not a true cyst but a vascular lesion probably caused by a local change in hemodynamics. The cause is not definitely known but may result from trauma and attempted repair. In many cases it is associated with other primary lesions of bone. It shares some similarity with the central giant cell granuloma and, like that lesion, occurs mainly in young persons under the age of 20, with a slight female predilection.

Preoperatively, blood may be aspirated from this lesion. The syringe, however, will not fill as easily or as rapidly as with an arteriovenous malformation or some hemangiomas. Since the aneurysmal bone cyst and the central hemangioma resemble each other radiographically, angiograms are helpful to further distinguish these two lesions. Treatment is by surgical enucleation, and recurrence is rare.

RADIOGRAPHIC FEATURES (Fig. 11–15)

This lesion is classically described as a relatively destructive, slow-growing, multilocular,

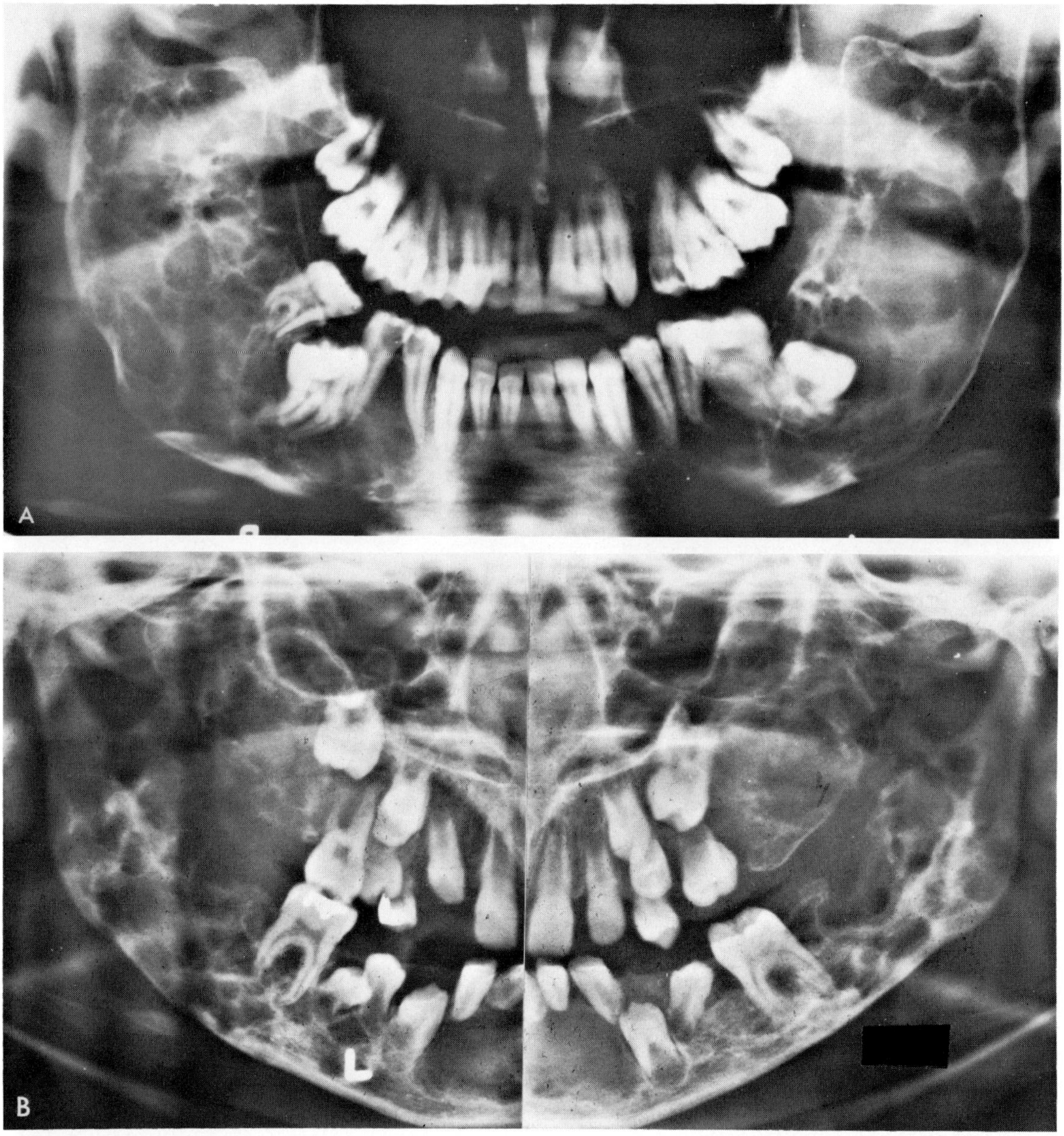

Figure 11–13. Cherubism. **A.** Courtesy of Dr. Chris Nortjé, University of Stellenbosch, Tygerberg, South Africa. **B.** Courtesy of Dr. Edward A. Scott, St. Louis, MO.

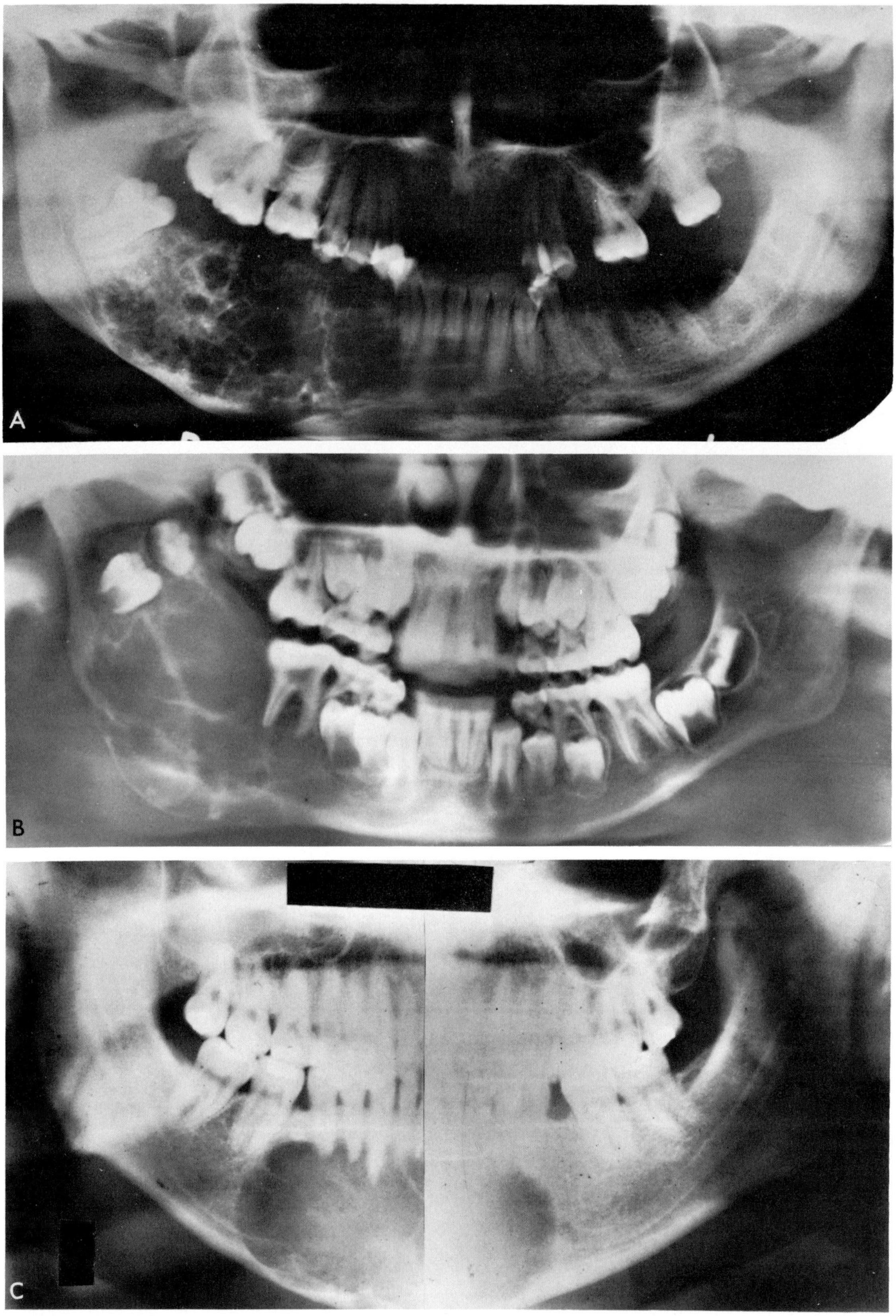

Figure 11–14. Odontogenic myxoma. **A.** A typical soap-bubble pattern, with thin, lacy striae. **B.** A typical multilocular, expansile pattern in a child. **C.** Note the thin, lacy, radiopaque striae. (**A** and **B** courtesy of Dr. Chris Nortjé, University of Stellenbosch, Tygerberg, South Africa.)

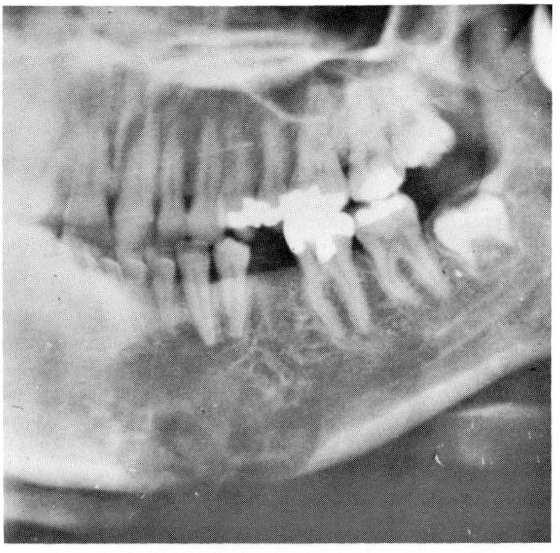

Figure 11–15. Aneurysmal bone cyst. (Courtesy of Dr. Gus Pappas, Columbus, OH.)

expansile radiolucency occurring more frequently in the mandible of young persons under the age of 20. The cortex may be greatly expanded, and teeth may be displaced. Destruction of the cortex is rare, although it may occur.

This lesion does **not** tend to resorb adjacent teeth, as sometimes occurs with the central giant cell granuloma. Also, this neoplasm lacks the multiple foraminae that are sometimes seen in central hemangiomas and arteriovenous (A-V) malformations.

CENTRAL HEMANGIOMA OF BONE AND VASCULAR LESIONS (A-V Malformation, A-V Shunt, A-V Aneurysm, A-V Fistula)

BRIEF OVERVIEW

Although quite common in soft tissue, the hemangioma occurs much less frequently as a central lesion of bone. However, because it is extremely important to suspect this and other vascular lesions clinically before initiating treatment, they will be covered in some detail here. When the jaws are involved, the central hemangioma of bone occurs most frequently in the mandible of young females between the ages of 10 and 20. Expansion and paresthesia may be present. An important clinical feature is the finding of blood oozing from the gingival sulcus of a tooth that may be loose. Additionally, the tooth may exhibit a pumping movement when pressure is applied to it and released. This finding is inconsistent with the presence of either periodontal disease or the normal exfoliation of primary teeth. The mucosa overlying the area may be warm or may display increased surface vascularity or redness. The patient may or may not have other peripheral hemangiomas. The central hemangioma of bone is one of two basic types involving proliferation of small or large blood vessels.

The central hemangioma of bone may be clinically and radiographically indistinguishable from another vascular condition known as the central arteriovenous (A-V) fistula, shunt, or aneurysm. In this situation there is a direct connection between the arteries and veins without the intervening capillaries. Sometimes a distinct bruit may be detected with the stethoscope at the carotid artery in the neck or at the facial artery on the lateral aspect of the mandible. There may be a history of trauma.

Central hemangiomas will readily yield blood upon aspiration, and the pressure of the central arteriovenous shunt may force the plunger right out of the syringe. The clinician should be prepared to cope with possible difficult hemostasis at the puncture site. Such lesions should not be biopsied indiscriminately. Arteriography is helpful in confirming the diagnosis and blood supply of a suspected vascular lesion. Often, ligation of the major vessels that supply and drain the area is a major contingency of the treatment plan.

Although arteriography is usually helpful in delineating the extent of vascular involvement, the arteriogram may not show all of the vascular connections to the lesion. The arteriogram should be studied through the venous phase to evaluate not only the afferent supply but also the efferent drainage from the lesion. In the case reported by Kelly, Terry, and Small, the external carotid artery as well as the inferior alveolar and mental neurovascular bundles were tied off, yet venous-type bleeding persisted at the surgical site. Their explanation is illustrated in Figure 11–19.

The presence of venous blood after arterial ligation is explained by a backflow of venous blood into the area once forward arterial pressure has been cut off. This secondary source of bleeding is an important consideration. It may often be encountered and may also be life threatening.

It is important to remember that there are at least a dozen reported fatalities associated with the surgical removal of central vascular lesions of the jawbones and, undoubtedly, many more unreported cases. Embolization with Gelfoam has been and is being used with some success with larger lesions.

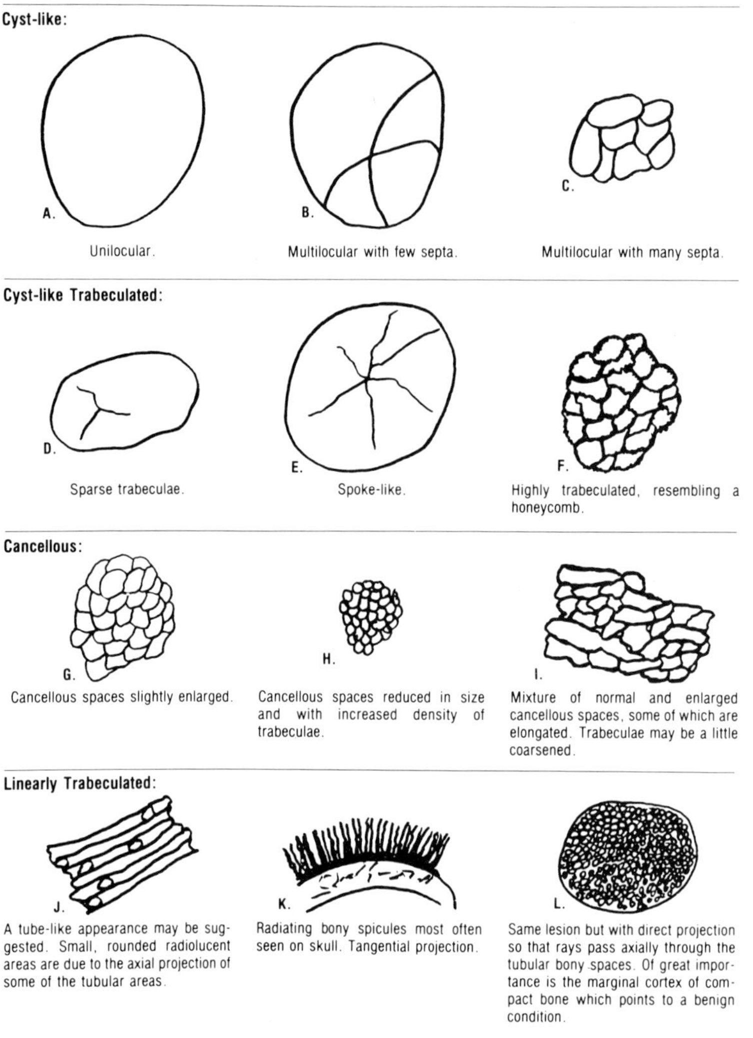

Figure 11–16. Sketches of bone patterns associated with vascular lesions. (Courtesy of Dr. H. M. Worth, Vancouver, Canada; Dr. Doug Stoneman, Toronto, Canada; Eastman Kodak Co., Rochester, NY.)

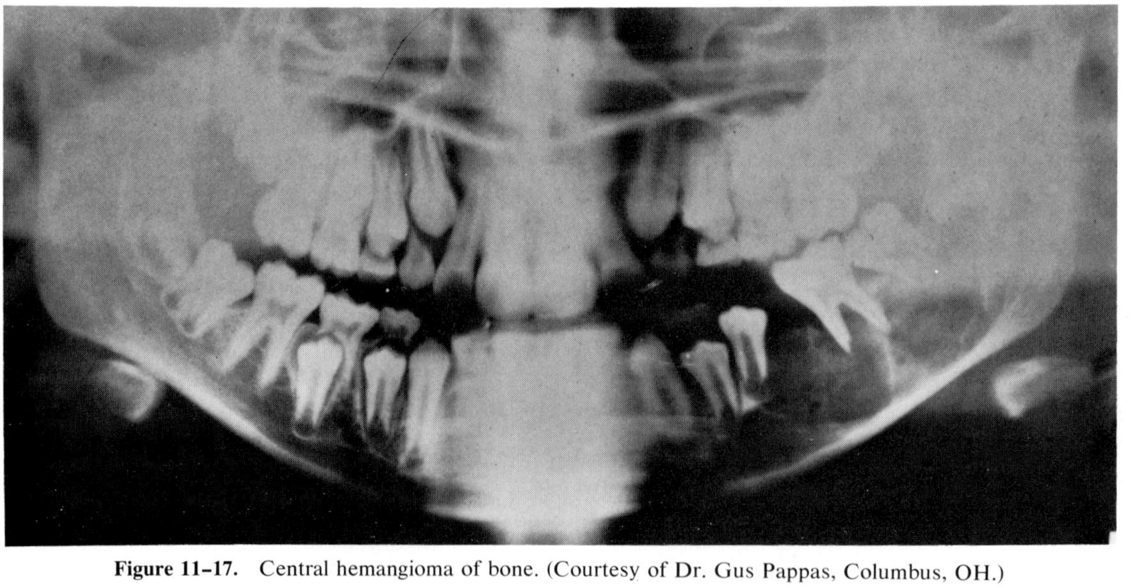

Figure 11–17. Central hemangioma of bone. (Courtesy of Dr. Gus Pappas, Columbus, OH.)

RADIOGRAPHIC FEATURES (Figs. 11–16 to 11–19)

Classically, central vascular lesions usually consist of a multilocular, expansile lesion, which may be associated with displacement and resorption of unerupted and erupted teeth. The cortex usually remains intact. There are, however, a great number of variations and combinations of changes that may lead the clinician to suspect a vascular lesion. These are outlined in Figure 11–16. In forming the basic multilocular

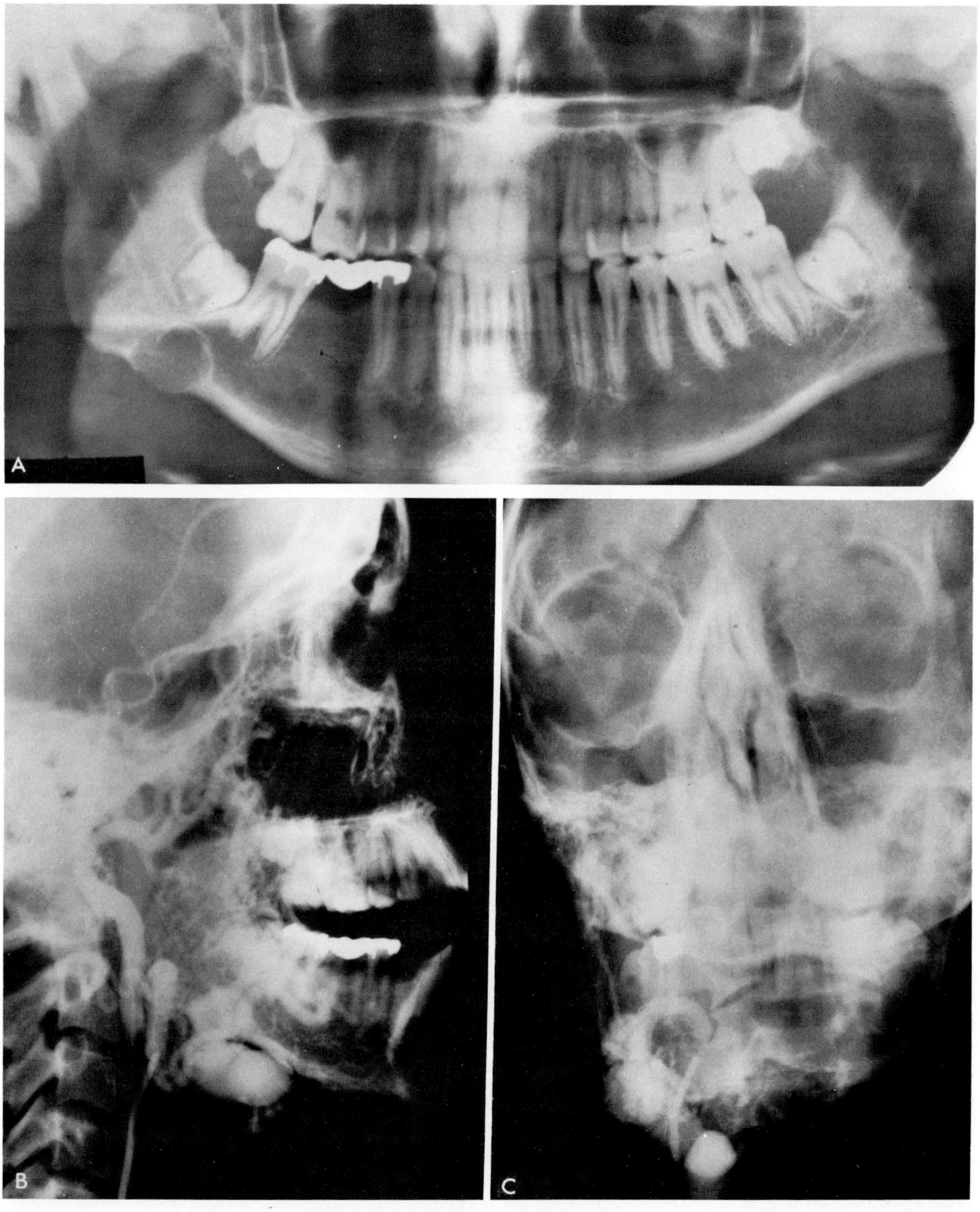

Figure 11–18. A-V aneurysm. **A.** Panoramic view of the lesion. **B** and **C.** Arteriograms of the lesion. (Figure 11–18 courtesy of Dr. Doug Stoneman, Toronto, Canada.)

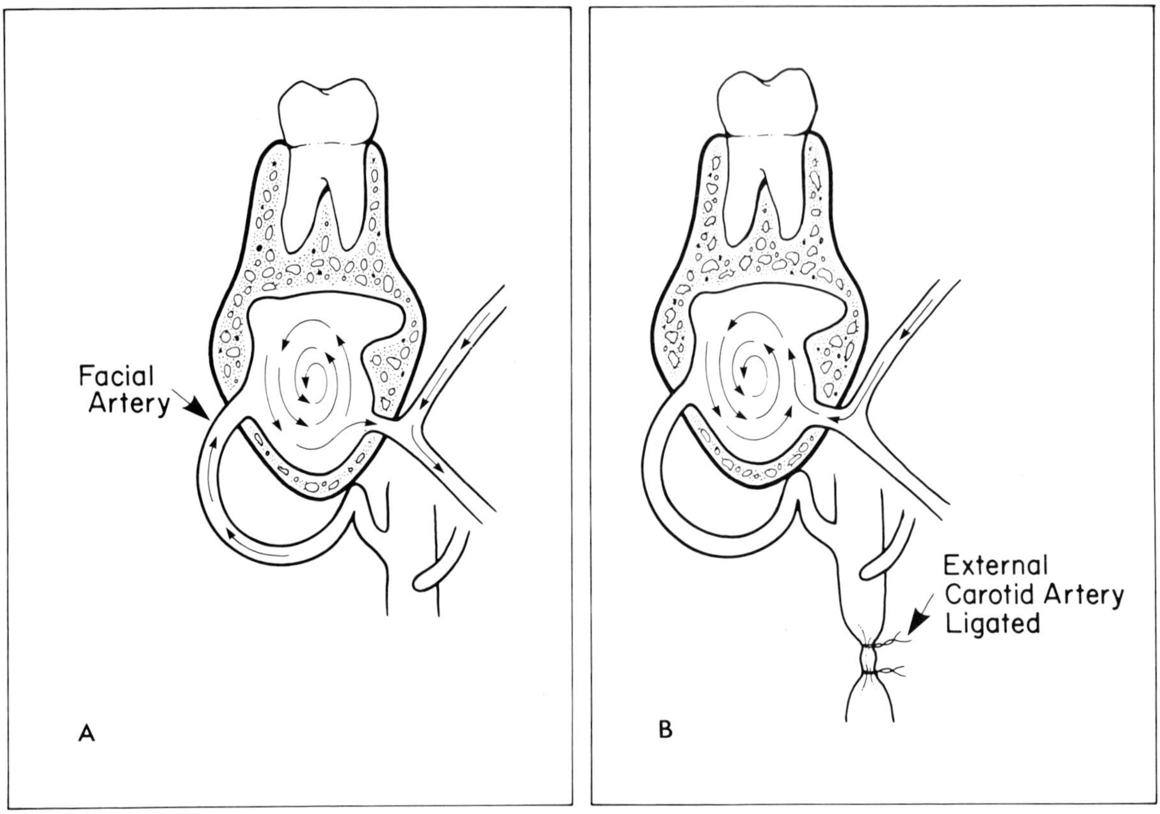

Figure 11–19. Venous backflow into an A-V malformation after ligation of the external carotid artery. (Adapted from Kelly, D. E., Terry, B. C., and Small, E. W.: Arteriovenous malformation of the mandible: Report of a case. *J. Oral Surg.*, *35*:392, 1977.)

pattern, the delicate radiopaque striations may form a few or many loculations and may be arranged in a hub, spokelike, or honeycomb pattern. According to Worth and Stoneman, the slightest hint of a hub is strongly suspect. These findings may be accompanied by the presence of several noncorticated foraminae, which may be single here and there throughout the lesion or may occur in groups of two or three. Additionally, these foramina may be associated with a parallel or tubelike arrangement of radiopaque striae. No other lesion presents this latter pattern. Another variation occurs when the striae are arranged in a sunburst or sunray pattern, resembling an osteogenic sarcoma, a chondrosarcoma, or a complex odontoma. The radiographic findings may be limited to a central, unilocular, well-corticated cystlike radiolucency, or there may be no apparent bony lesion at all with only an altered trabecular pattern and a change in size of the cancellous spaces in the affected area. The presence of phleboliths or a wavy donut-shaped radiopacity representing a large calcified blood vessel wall is helpful. A difference in vertical depth of the mandible from one side to the other is suggestive but may be seen in lymphangioma and neurofibroma. Peripheral vascular lesions may cause smooth, punched-out or cupped-out erosions of the underlying bone.

CHONDROMYXOID FIBROMA OF THE MANDIBLE

BRIEF OVERVIEW

This condition was originally described as a separate entity by Jaffe and Lichtenstein in 1948. Since then, several hundred cases have been reported affecting various bones of the skeleton. According to Grotepass, Farman, and Nortjé, jaw involvement is extremely rare, with only six reported cases in the world literature, all in the mandible. Generally, there is a slight predilection for males, and the condition is rare before the age of 5 and after the age of 60. In most skeletal locations this benign neoplasm is reported to have a recurrence rate of about 25 per cent; therefore, treatment should involve

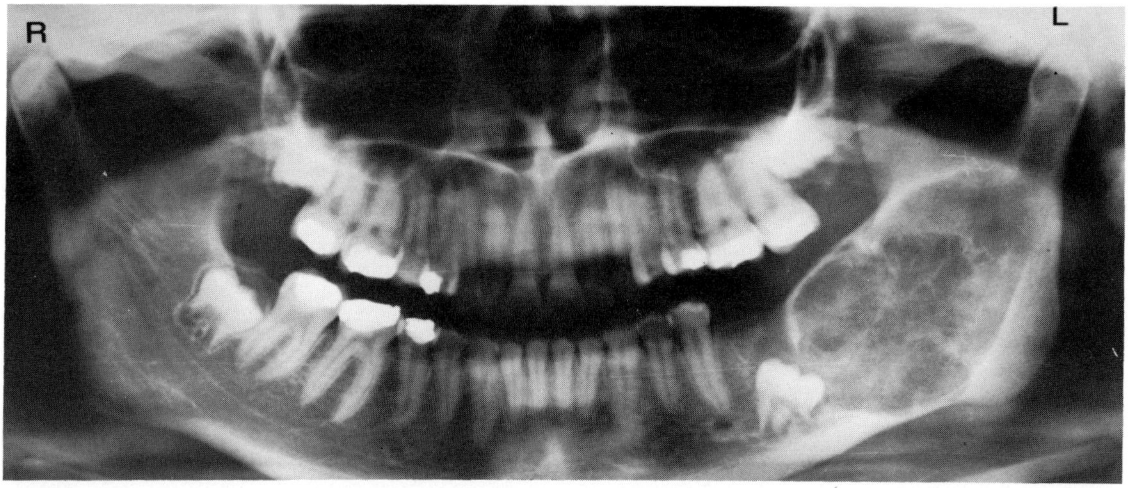

Figure 11–20. Chondromyxoid fibroma of the mandible. (Courtesy of Dr. Chris Nortjé, University of Stellenbosch, Tygerberg, South Africa.) Postscript: This case recurred; the recurrent lesion was a chondrosarcoma.

thorough excision and careful postoperative radiographic follow-up.

RADIOGRAPHIC FEATURES (Fig. 11–20)

Owing to the paucity of mandibular cases, no characteristic features can be attributed to this neoplasm. According to Grotepass, Farman, and Nortjé, the long bone lesion consists of a well-circumscribed, eccentrically located, round or oval metaphyseal defect. This radiolucency usually contains a trabecular pattern and a well-demarcated sclerotic margin.

REFERENCES

Reference Texts

Eversole, L. R.: **Clinical Outline of Oral Pathology.** Philadelphia: Lea & Febiger, 1978, pp. 205–212.

Shafer, W. G., Hine, M. K., and Levy, B. M.: **A Textbook of Oral Pathology.** 3rd Edition. Philadelphia: W. B. Saunders, 1974, pp. 138–140, 142, 145, 247–249, 251–258, 265–266, 646–648.

Stafne, E. C., and Gibilisco, J. A.: **Oral Radiographic Diagnosis,** 4th Edition. Philadelphia: W. B. Saunders, 1975, pp. 169–172, 181–183.

Wood, N. K., and Goaz, P. W.: **Differential Diagnosis of Oral Lesions.** St. Louis: C. V. Mosby, 1975, pp. 354–369.

Selected References

Adekeye, E. O.: Ameloblastoma of the jaws: A survey of 109 Nigerian patients. **J. Oral Surg. 38**:36, 1980.

Brannon, R. B.: The odontogenic keratocyst: A clinico-pathologic study of 312 cases. Part I: Clinical features. **Oral Surg. 42**:54, 1976.

Brannon, R. B.: The odontogenic keratocyst: A clinico-pathologic study of 312 cases. Part II: Histologic features. **Oral Surg. 43**:233, 1977.

Buff, S. J., Chen, J: T., Ravin, C. C., and Moore, J. O.: Pulmonary metastasis from ameloblastoma of the mandible: Report of a case and review of the literature. **J. Oral Surg. 38**:374, 1980.

Donatsky, O., Hjorting-Hansen, E., Philipsen, H. P., and Fejerskov, O.: Clinical, radiologic and histopathologic aspects of 13 cases of nevoid basal cell carcinoma syndrome. **Int. J. Oral Surg. 5**:19, 1976.

Farman, A. G., Nortjé, C. J., Grotepass, F. W., Farman, F. J., and Van Zyl, J. A.: Myxofibroma of the jaws. **Br. J. Oral Surg. 15**:3, 1977–78.

Grotepass, F. W., Farman, A. G., and Nortjé, C. J.: Chondromyxoid fibroma of the mandible. **J. Oral Surg. 34**:958, 1976.

Kelly, D. E., Terry, B. C., and Small, E. W.: Arteriovenous malformation of the mandible: Report of a case. **J. Oral Surg. 35**:387, 1977.

Lamberg, M. A., Tasanen, A., and Jaaskelainen, J.: Fatality from central hemangioma of the mandible. **J. Oral Surg. 37**:578, 1979.

Orbach, S.: Congenital arteriovenous malformations of the face. **Oral Surg. 42**:2, 1976.

Reaume, C., Wesley, R. K., Jung, B., and Grammer, F. C.: Ameloblastoma of the maxillary sinus. **J. Oral Surg. 38**:520, 1980.

Regezi, J., Kerr, D. A., and Courtney, R. M.: Odontogenic tumors: Analysis of 706 cases. **J. Oral Surg. 36**:771, 1978.

Schindel, J., Matz, S., Edlaw, A., and Abraham, A.: Central cavernous hemangioma of the jaws. **J. Oral Surg. 36**:803, 1978.

Shteyer, A., Lustmann, J., and Lewin-Epstein, J.: The mural ameloblastoma: A review of the literature. **J. Oral Surg. 36**:866, 1978.

Singh, J., Sidhu, B. S., and Kanta, S.: Hemangioendothelioma of the mandible: Report of a case. **J. Oral Surg. 35**:673, 1977.

Stewart, S. S., Baum, S. M., Arlen, M., and Elguezabal, A.: Myxoma of the lower jaw. **Oral Surg. 36**:800, 1973.

Tsakmis, P. J., and Nelson, J. F.: The maxillary ameloblastoma: An analysis of 24 cases. **J. Oral Surg. 38**:336, 1980.

Weathers, D. R., and Waldron, C. A.: Unusual multilocular cysts of the jaws (botyroid odontogenic cysts). **Oral Surg. 36**:235, 1973.

Worth, H. M., and Stoneman, D. W.: Radiology of vascular abnormalities in and about the jaws. **Dent. Radiogr. Photog. 52**:1, 1979.

Chapter 12

Solitary, Single, or Multiple Radiolucencies with Indistinct or Ragged Borders

OSTEOMYELITIS
OSTEORADIONECROSIS
PRIMARY INTRA-ALVEOLAR EPIDERMOID CARCINOMA
METASTATIC CARCINOMA
HISTIOCYTOSIS-X GROUP
- Letterer-Siwe Disease
- Hand-Schüller-Christian Disease
- Eosinophilic Granuloma

MULTIPLE MYELOMA
LYMPHOSARCOMA
FIBROSARCOMA
BURKITT'S LYMPHOMA
HISTIOCYTIC LYMPHOMA
EWING'S SARCOMA

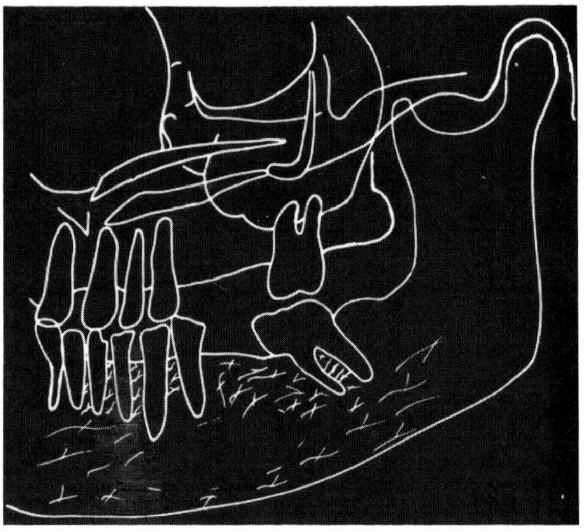

OSTEOMYELITIS

BRIEF OVERVIEW

Osteomyelitis can be acute or chronic and may involve various reactions of bone. It can produce radiopaque lesions such as those seen in focal sclerosing osteomyelitis, chronic diffuse sclerosing osteomyelitis, or Garré's osteomyelitis. The brief discussion here will be limited to a reaction that involves lysis of bone.

Osteomyelitis is an inflammatory reaction of the bone marrow that clinically produces pus. The organisms are usually staphylococci and streptococci, but others such as actinomycetes (*Actinomyces israelii*) may be the cause (see Fig. 12–2). The organisms may be introduced as a result of periapical inflammation or fracture or by hematogenous spread from another site. Patients who are immunosuppressed by steroid therapy or other chemotherapy and severely debilitated patients, such as uncontrolled diabetics, are prone to osteomyelitis. When the jaws are involved, patients with Paget's disease and osteopetrosis are more susceptible.

Clinically, pain is sometimes an acute symptom, and expansion of bone is rarely present.

The presence of one or several purulent fistulous tracts and redness of the overlying mucosa are fairly consistent findings. The unresolved acute condition may give rise to chronic osteomyelitis, which is by far the more common occurrence. Treatment consists of long-term antibiotics. Chronic osteomyelitis may be difficult to resolve; thus culture and sensitivity tests are extremely useful. Nuclear scans with ^{69}gallium and ^{99}technetium have been helpful in monitoring progress. Hyperbaric oxygen therapy is a useful adjunct, especially when anaerobic bacilli have been identified. Surgical debridement and removal of sequestrae may be necessary in extensive, tenacious cases.

RADIOGRAPHIC FEATURES (Figs. 12–1 and 12–2)

In acute cases, the radiographic features may not be evident, and minimal bone destruction is seen. In chronic cases, however, the radiographic features are ominous. The classic lesion involves multifocal areas of moth-eaten bone consisting of diffuse zones of bone destruction and an altered trabecular pattern in a generally rarified area with ragged, poorly defined borders. This condition resembles a specific type of chronic osteomyelitis known as osteoradionecrosis (see following section). There may be areas of bony sequestration in chronic osteomyelitis, but these are relatively small compared with those sometimes seen in osteoradionecrosis. Chronic osteomyelitis also resembles many of the primary and metastatic malignancies of the jaws.

OSTEORADIONECROSIS

BRIEF OVERVIEW

Osteoradionecrosis is a peculiar type of osteomyelitis that may only affect bone that has been previously exposed to therapeutic irradiation. It is said to develop as a sequela of the following triad of etiologic factors: previous therapeutic irradiation, trauma, and infection. The basic underlying factor is a compromised blood supply due to radiation-induced fibrosis of the blood vessels; in the jaws, the mandible is much more frequently involved owing to its lack of an adequate collateral blood supply. In the series reported by Dreizen and associates, approximately one in five dentate patients developed osteoradionecrosis, whereas less than 5 per cent of edentulous patients developed the condition. The time of greatest susceptibility was within two years of completion of radiation therapy.

Osteoradionecrosis occurs in two subtypes: superficial and deep. The superficial type may be controlled with a topical paste containing zinc peroxide, carboxymethyl cellulose, and hydrogen peroxide. The deep type is treated in the same manner with the addition of the following adjunctive measures: systemic antibiotic administration, gentle removal of loose bone spicules or sequestrae, and flushing with mild, warm solutions of hydrogen peroxide, salt, or soda. Hydrogen peroxide perfusion of the extremities and hyperbaric oxygen therapy have produced encouraging results for tenacious cases of osteoradionecrosis and chronic osteomyelitis.

Management of osteoradionecrosis is almost always difficult, and prevention is to be greatly encouraged. Daily five-minute applications of a 1% sodium fluoride gel containing plaque-disclosing solution and subsequent brushing and flossing are of paramount importance. Avoidance of extractions and other sources of trauma, such as ill-fitting prostheses, is very important.

RADIOGRAPHIC FEATURES (Fig. 12–3)

Osteoradionecrosis may often begin as a superficial rarefaction of the crestal bone in the mandible in an edentulous area. Other areas of rarefaction may develop in association with periodontal disease or periapical inflammation of pulpal origin or at the site of tooth extraction. If not controlled, which is often the case, the areas of rarefaction spread to eventually involve large portions of the mandible. A typical moth-eaten pattern of bone is seen, with poorly defined, ragged borders, enlarged and irregular trabecular spaces, and, often, evidence of bony sequestration. Management is extremely difficult, and the single most important factor in prevention is educating the patient on what he must do and emphasizing that these instructions must be followed for the rest of his life. Osteoradionecrosis may develop 20 years and more after therapeutic irradiation of the mandible.

Text continued on page 311

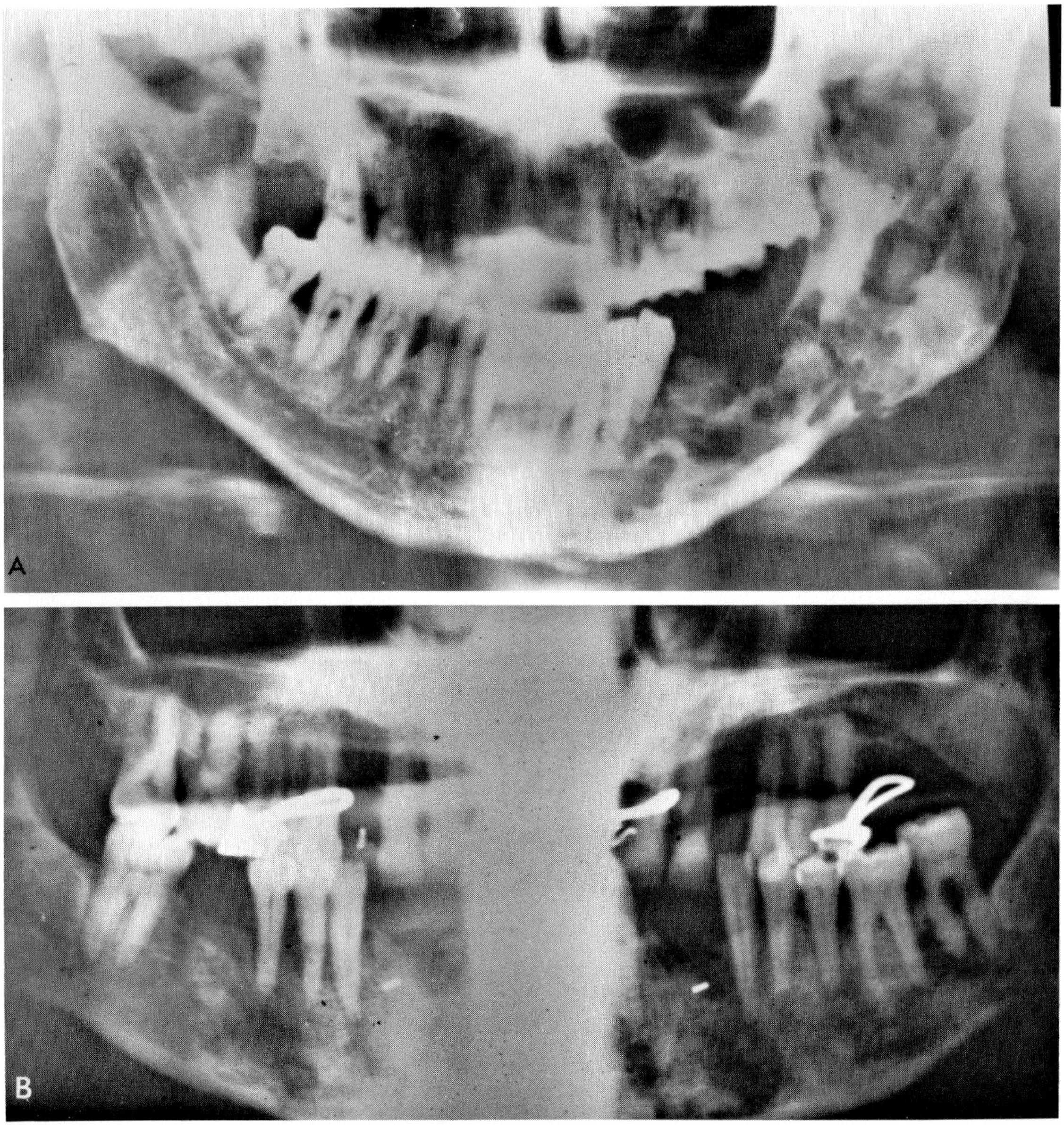

Figure 12–1. Chronic osteomyelitis. **A.** Note the pathologic fracture of the mandible. **B.** Note the moth-eaten pattern bilaterally in the mandible and the ragged, poorly defined borders of the affected areas.

Illustration continued on opposite page

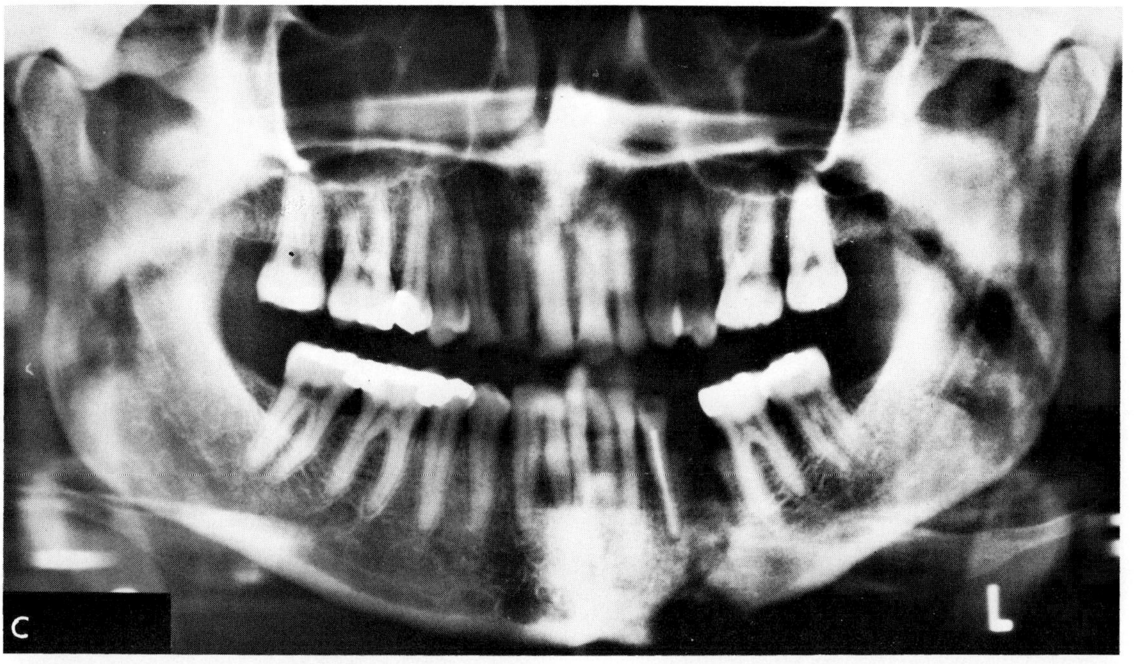

Figure 12–1 *Continued* **C.** This condition developed as a complication of a fracture in the left mandibular bicuspid area. The fracture was undiagnosed, and treatment consisted of endodontic therapy of the cuspid and removal of the loose first bicuspid. (**A** courtesy of Dr. Chris Nortjé, University of Stellenbosch, Tygerberg, South Africa. **C** courtesy of Dr. Birgit Junfin Glass, San Antonio, TX.)

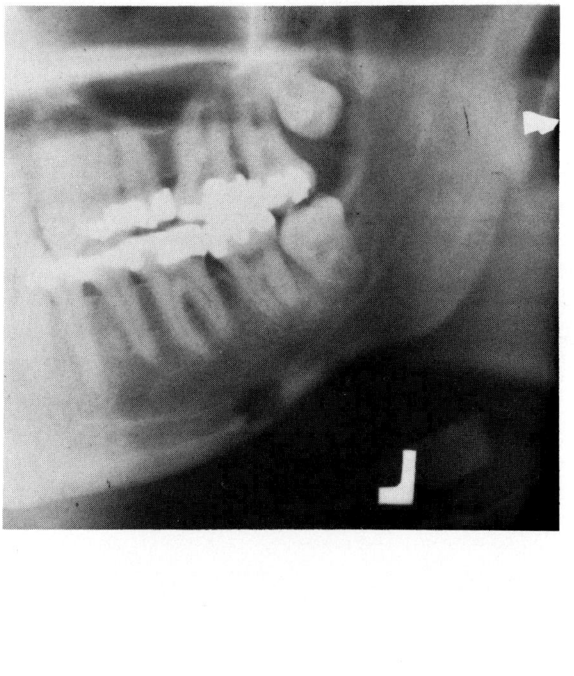

Figure 12–2. Actinomycotic osteomyelitis.

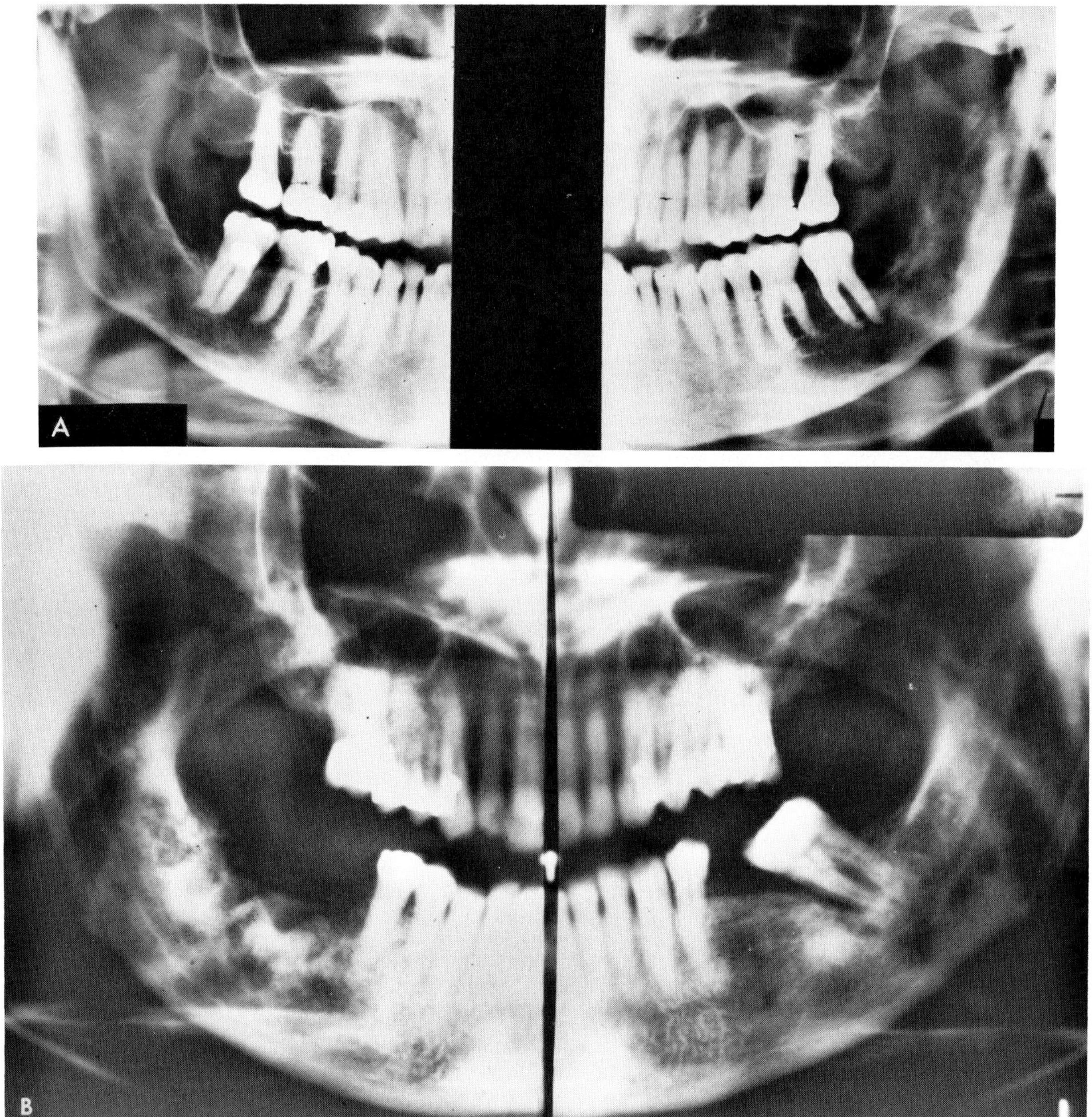

Figure 12–3. Osteoradionecrosis. **A.** Note the pathologic fracture of the coronoid process in this 75-year-old female, whose condition developed following the removal of the erupted lower left third molar. **B.** The condition is bilateral in the mandible of this 51-year-old female. (**A** courtesy of Dr. Philip Boyne, Loma Linda, CA. **B** courtesy of Dr. Doug Stoneman, Toronto, Canada.)

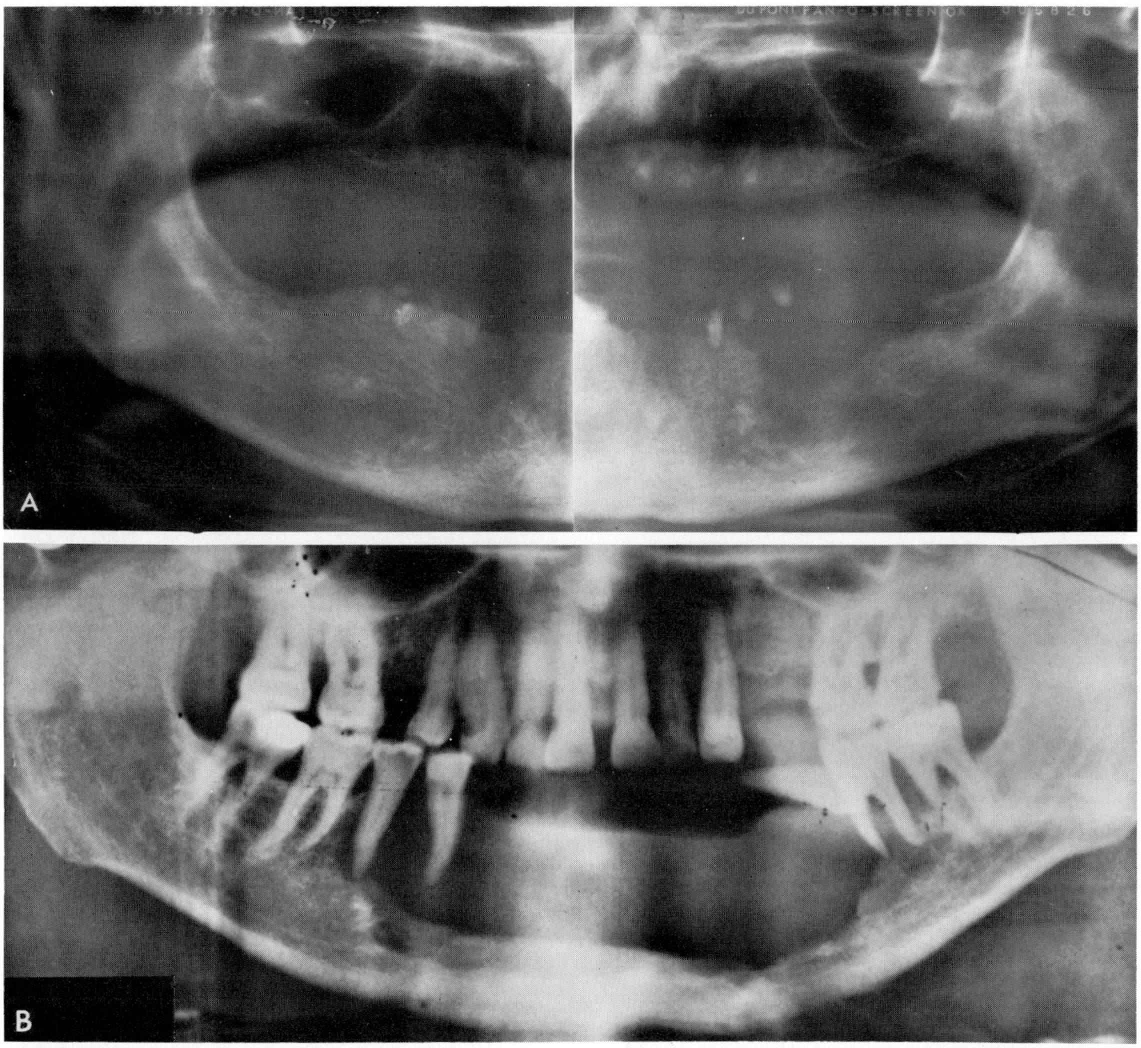

Figure 12–4. Gingival carcinoma. **A.** Note the cupped-out appearance of the crest of the alveolar ridge in the left body of the mandible, with floating root tips within the proliferating soft tissue mass. Courtesy of Drs. Frank Sammis, Jr. and Carlos Portales, San Antonio, TX. **B.** Courtesy of Dr. Gus Pappas, Columbus, OH.

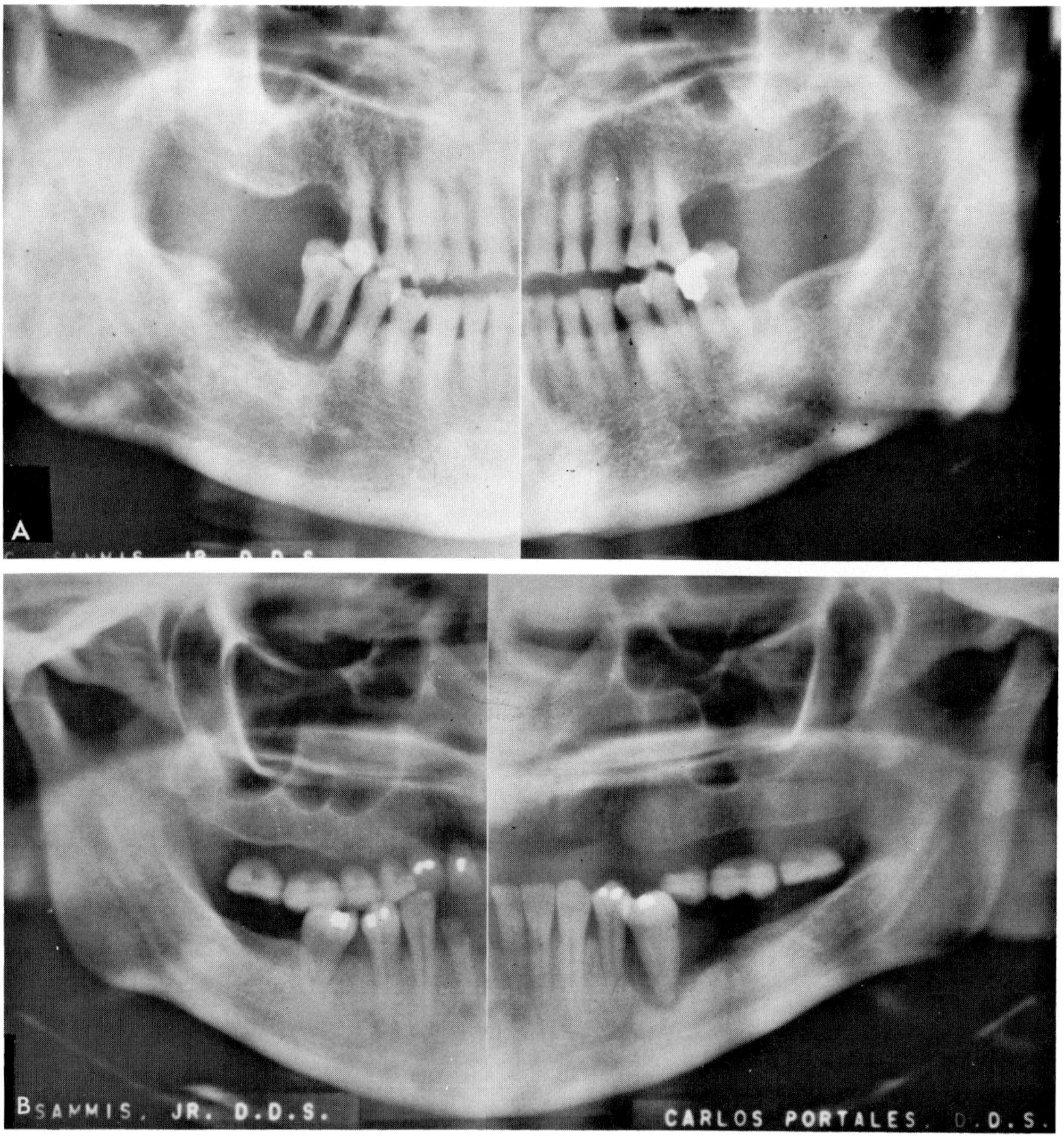

Figure 12–5. Floating tooth. **A.** Owing to gingival carcinoma. **B.** Owing to periodontal disease. (Figure 12–5 courtesy of Drs. Frank Sammis, Jr. and Carlos Portales, San Antonio, TX.)

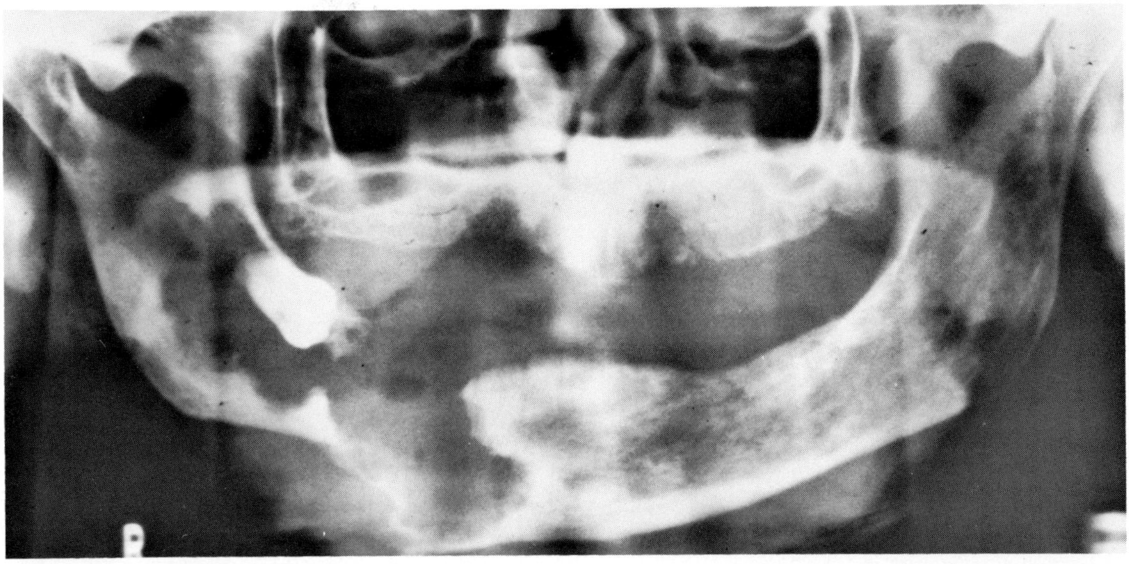

Figure 12–6. Primary intra-alveolar carcinoma arising in a follicular cyst. This 79-year-old male had been edentulous for 55 years, never wore a denture, never smoked, and rarely consumed alcohol. Note the pathologic mandibular fracture.

PRIMARY INTRA-ALVEOLAR EPIDERMOID CARCINOMA (Intra-alveolar Squamous Cell Carcinoma)

BRIEF OVERVIEW

Epidermoid carcinoma is of unknown etiology but has been seen in association with alcoholism, smoking, poor oral hygiene, and other factors. It may arise centrally within the jaws, in which case it is referred to as primary (as opposed to metastatic) intra-alveolar (central) carcinoma. Most frequently, it arises in the mucosa, often that overlying the jaws, and is referred to by the tissue involved, e.g., gingival carcinoma. With carcinoma of surface tissue origin, bony involvement, when present, consists of localized invasion of the underlying alveolar bone. Invasion of the maxillary sinus may also occur. Carcinoma of central bone origin may arise from epithelial remnants in the periodontal ligament or from previously existing central epithelium-containing lesions such as odontogenic cysts. Central epidermoid carcinoma may also arise in existing epithelial lesions, such as a follicular cyst. The condition may be asymptomatic or painful and may mimic localized periodontal disease. Paresthesia is an important clinical symptom. Enlarged, nontender regional nodes may be present. Based on a limited number of cases, surgical resection seems to be the most acceptable mode of treatment, at least with localized lesions.

RADIOGRAPHIC FEATURES (Figs. 12–4 to 12–7)

Intra-alveolar carcinoma may resemble any benign epithelial lesion. With proliferation of more malignant cells, bone destruction becomes more rapid and random. The lesion may become very large, with cortical destruction and pathologic fracture. One of the earliest and most characteristic signs of malignancy is the lack of a well-defined border, be it corticated or not. Generally, resorption or displacement of teeth is not a feature for two reasons: (1) central carcinoma tends to grow too rapidly and to be too destructive to produce these features; (2) it tends to grow around obstructions such as teeth rather than displace them, as invasion probably occurs along the path of least resistance.

The lesion of peripheral origin may present a cupped-out appearance of the alveolar crest in an edentulous area, with varying degrees of distinctiveness of the border from smooth and benign in appearance to moderately rough and ragged at the borders. Larger areas of involvement may show complete destruction of the alveolar bone with only the inferior cortex intact. Within the fungating friable soft tissue

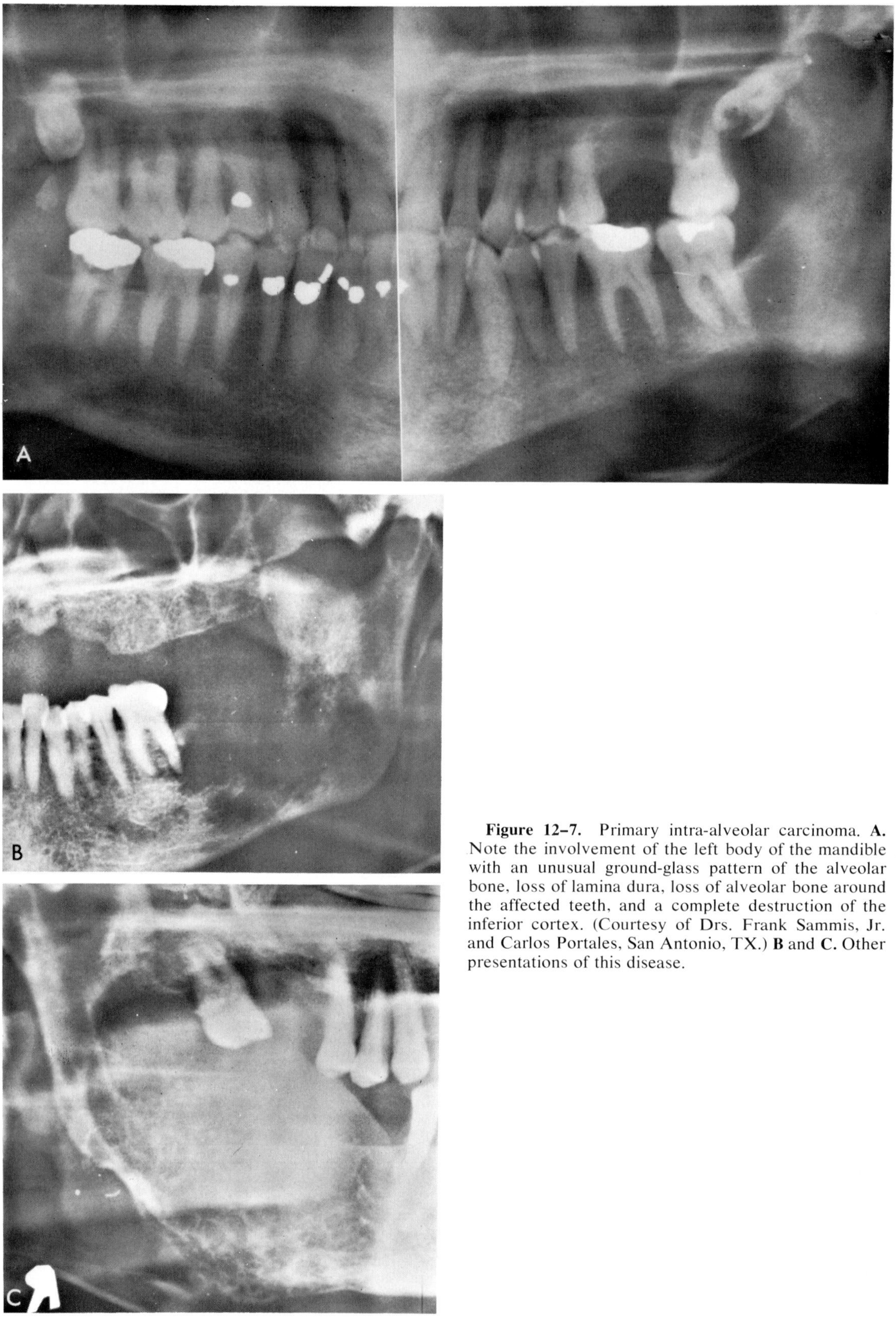

Figure 12–7. Primary intra-alveolar carcinoma. **A.** Note the involvement of the left body of the mandible with an unusual ground-glass pattern of the alveolar bone, loss of lamina dura, loss of alveolar bone around the affected teeth, and a complete destruction of the inferior cortex. (Courtesy of Drs. Frank Sammis, Jr. and Carlos Portales, San Antonio, TX.) **B** and **C.** Other presentations of this disease.

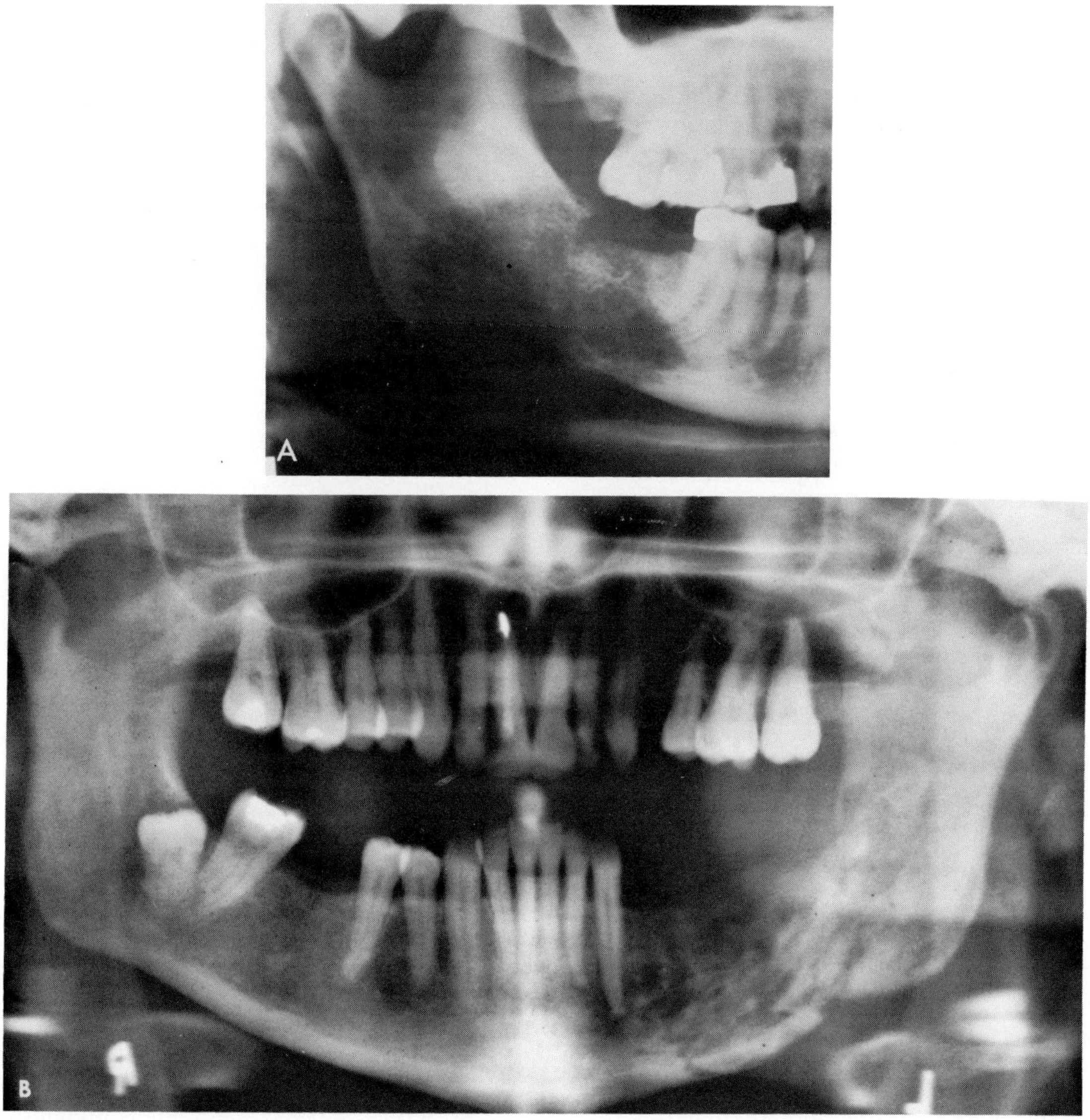

Figure 12–8. Metastatic adenocarcinoma, breast. (**A** Courtesy of Dr. Stanley Lovestedt, Rochester, MN.)

mass, floating teeth may be evident, and some teeth may have fallen out spontaneously (see Fig. 12–4).

METASTATIC CARCINOMA

BRIEF OVERVIEW

Metastatic or secondary carcinoma is second only to primary carcinoma of the jaws in frequency of occurrence of all malignant intraoral lesions. The most common malignancies to metastasize to the jaws are from primary sites in the breast, lung, kidney, thyroid, prostate, colon, and stomach. Since the path of metastasis is usually hematogenous, it is difficult to explain how large malignant cells can bypass both the hepatic and lung microcirculations to eventually end up in the jaws, usually the mandible. One theory postulates that metastasis occurs via Batson's plexus, the major portion of which is located in the paravertebral area. These vessels contain no valves, so that blood may flow to and from the viscera and other primary locations of metastatic lesions to distant sites, bypassing both the hepatic and heart-lung circulations. Along with other anatomic sites, Batson's plexus both supplies and drains the jaws and possibly accounts for many metastases to the jaws from distant primary lesions. Metastatic lesions may be asymptomatic or painful. They may present as localized unexplained periodontal disease, and paresthesia is a common symptom.

One method of detecting bony metastases before they appear on radiographs is through the use of nuclear scans. ^{99}Technetium MDP scans may show bone involvement with as little as 30 per cent bone destruction, whereas standard radiographs may require as much as 60 per cent bone destruction to show bone involvement. Metastatic disease may also be detected with lymphangiography, especially malignancies of the reticuloendothelial system. Metastatic disease, especially if multifocal, is best treated by surgery, radiation therapy and chemotherapy in varying combinations.

RADIOGRAPHIC FEATURES (Figs. 12–8 and 12–9)

There are no specific features of metastatic carcinoma, although generally the lesions tend to be diffusely radiolucent with poorly defined, ragged borders. Some metastatic tumors tend to produce radiopaque or mixed lucent/dense bone lesions, principally those of the prostate and thyroid glands and of the breast.

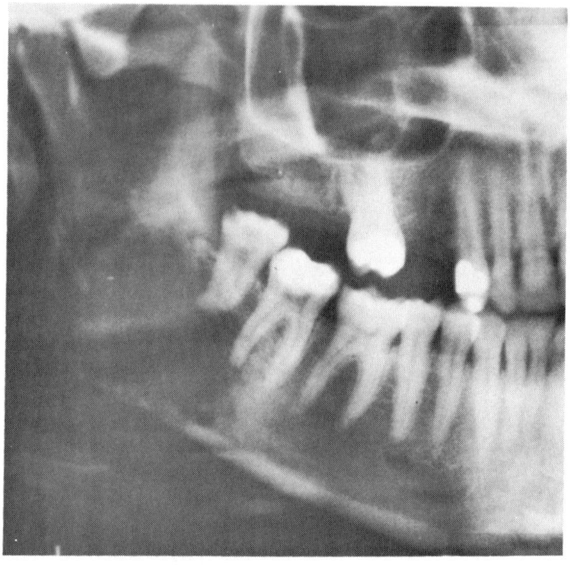

Figure 12–9. Metastatic carcinoma, cervix. The patient was 28 years old.

HISTIOCYTOSIS-X GROUP

BRIEF OVERVIEW

The histiocytosis-X group consists of the following related conditions: Letterer-Siwe disease, Hand-Schüller-Christian disease, and eosinophilic granuloma. These are disorders of the reticuloendothelial system and have been subclassified as the nonlipid reticuloendothelioses.

Letterer-Siwe disease (acute disseminated histiocytosis X) occurs primarily in infants and children up to the age of five years. It is considered to be the acute manifestation of the histiocytosis-X group. The onset of symptoms is usually rapid, and the course is often fatal. Males and females are equally affected. The initial complaint is usually a skin rash resembling diaper rash. The skin lesions are distributed over the trunk, scalp, and extremities. The rash is initially maculopapular and eventually becomes ulcerative and hemorrhagic. Other early signs include otitis externa, purulent discharge from the eyes, a high fever ranging from 101 to 105°F, malaise, and irritability. Other findings include splenomegaly, hepatomegaly, lymphadenopathy, respiratory and gastrointestinal tract involvement, and, eventually, anemia, bleeding disorders, and other hematologic problems owing to destruction of the reticuloendothelial system. Oral findings are usually seen later in the course of the disease and consist primarily of epulislike lesions on the gingiva and localized areas of thick, boggy, edematous gingivae, which respond poorly to

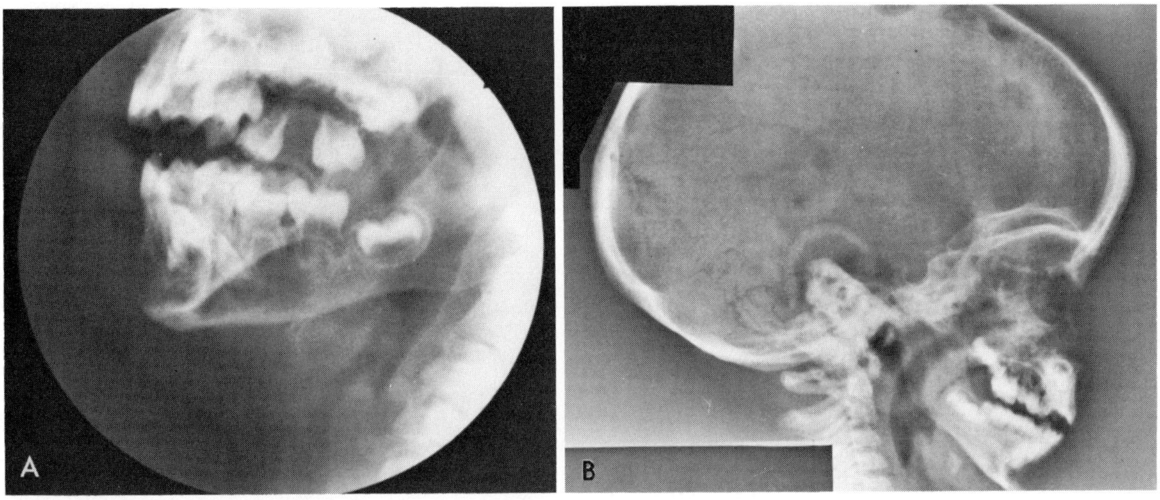

Figure 12–10. Letterer-Siwe disease. **A.** Note the separation of the maxillary primary molars caused by maxillary involvement in this 2½-year-old child with an 18 month history of the disease. **B.** Note the multiple radiolucent areas in the skull of the same patient.

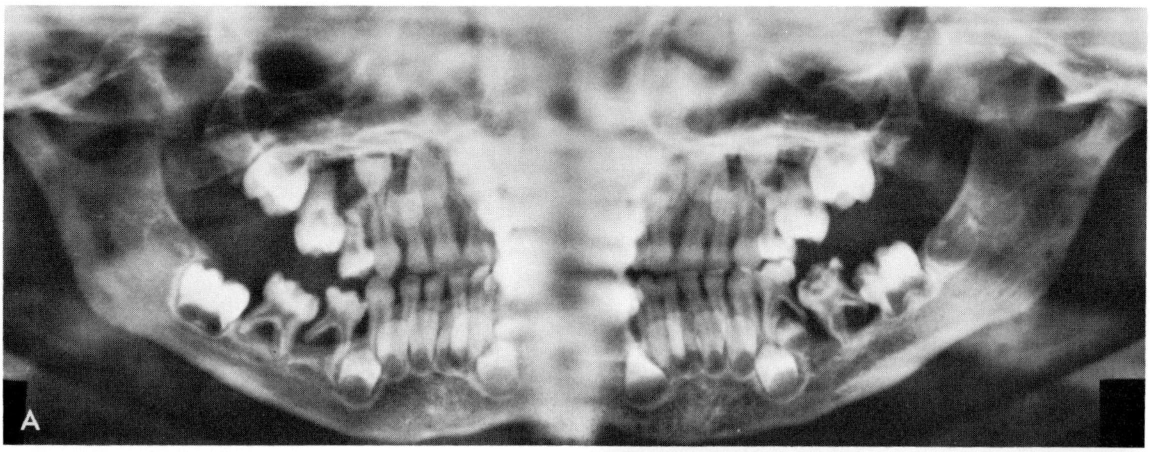

Figure 12–11. Hand-Schüller-Christian disease. **A.** Note the bilateral involvement in this 4½-year-old child with a previous history of Letterer-Siwe disease. **B.** Note the skull lesions in the same patient.

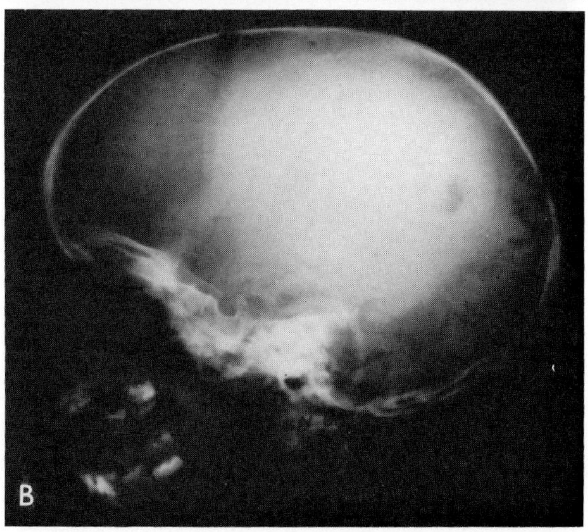

ordinary periodontal therapy. Bony involvement of the skeleton, skull, or jaws is rarely seen in the earlier stages of the disease. Although mortality is high and fatality is rapid, some cases respond to treatment combining radiotherapy, chemotherapy, and surgery. Some responsive cases may evolve into the more chronic sub-type known as Hand-Schüller-Christian disease.

Hand-Schüller-Christian disease (chronic disseminated histiocytosis X) primarily affects children after the age of three years but may affect infants, adolescents, and adults. This is the chronic manifestation of the histiocytosis-X group. The condition is more common in males, with a predilection of three to one over females. Although the main features of this condition resemble those of Letterer-Siwe disease, they tend to be less rapid in onset and less severe in degree, and there is less organ involvement. Skin rash, splenomegaly, hepatomegaly, lymphadenopathy, and hematologic involvement may be present in milder forms. Later complications consist of the classic triad of skull lesions, exophthalmos, and diabetes insipidus. The presenting complaint often involves the oral cavity and consists of generalized thick, edematous, hemorrhagic gingivae and mobile teeth. There may be areas of gingival necrosis, and a fetid breath odor is often present. Bone involvement invariably occurs and includes the skeleton, skull, and jaws. Although the prognosis remains poor, some patients respond to treatment combining radiotherapy, chemotherapy, and surgery. Therapy results in a protracted chronic course; nevertheless, mortality remains relatively high. The prognosis is best when the lesions are localized in bone and decreases with increasing degrees of organ and visceral involvement. Some cases may evolve into the more localized sub-type known as eosinophilic granuloma.

Eosinophilic granuloma (histiocytosis X localized in bone) primarily affects older children and young adults and has a predilection for males. It is most frequently localized to one

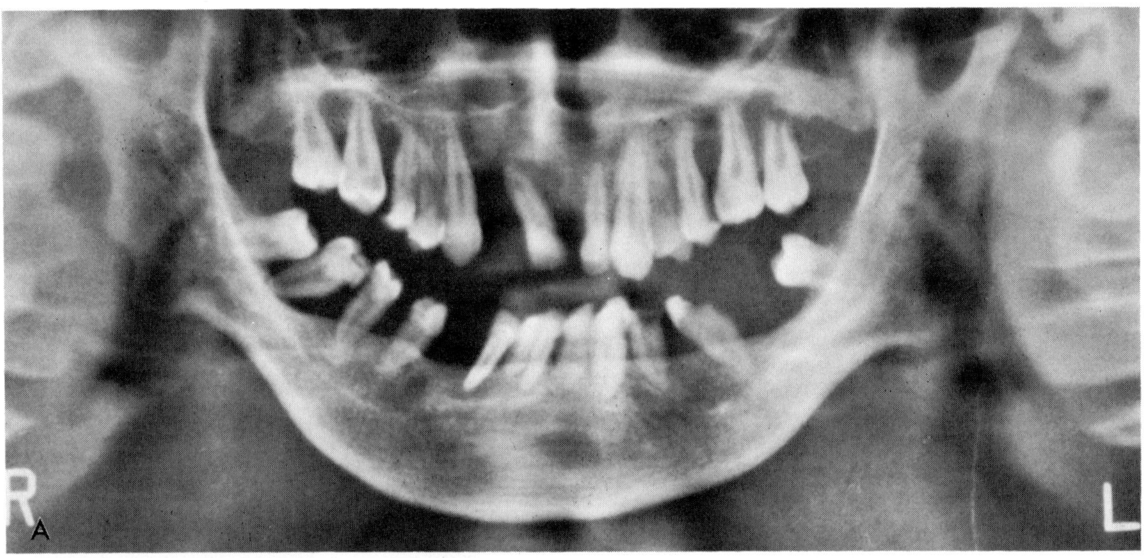

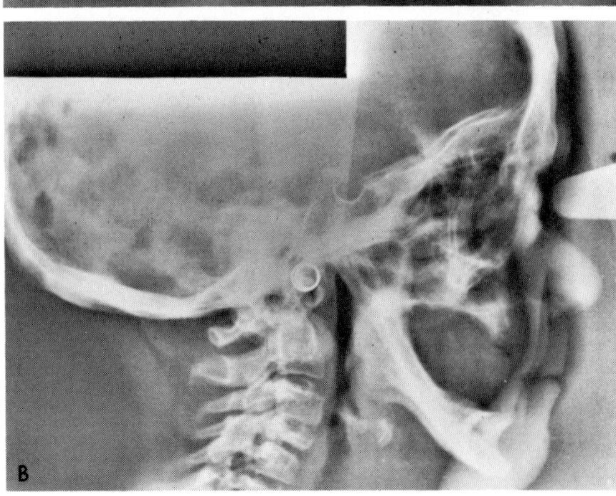

Figure 12–12. Hand-Schüller-Christian disease. **A.** Involvement of the jaws in a 15-year-old patient with an eight-year history of the disease treated by chemotherapy and radiation. **B.** Note the skull involvement and the loss of teeth in the same patient at age 16. (Figure 12–12 courtesy of Dr. Roberto Valencia, Mexico City, Mexico.)

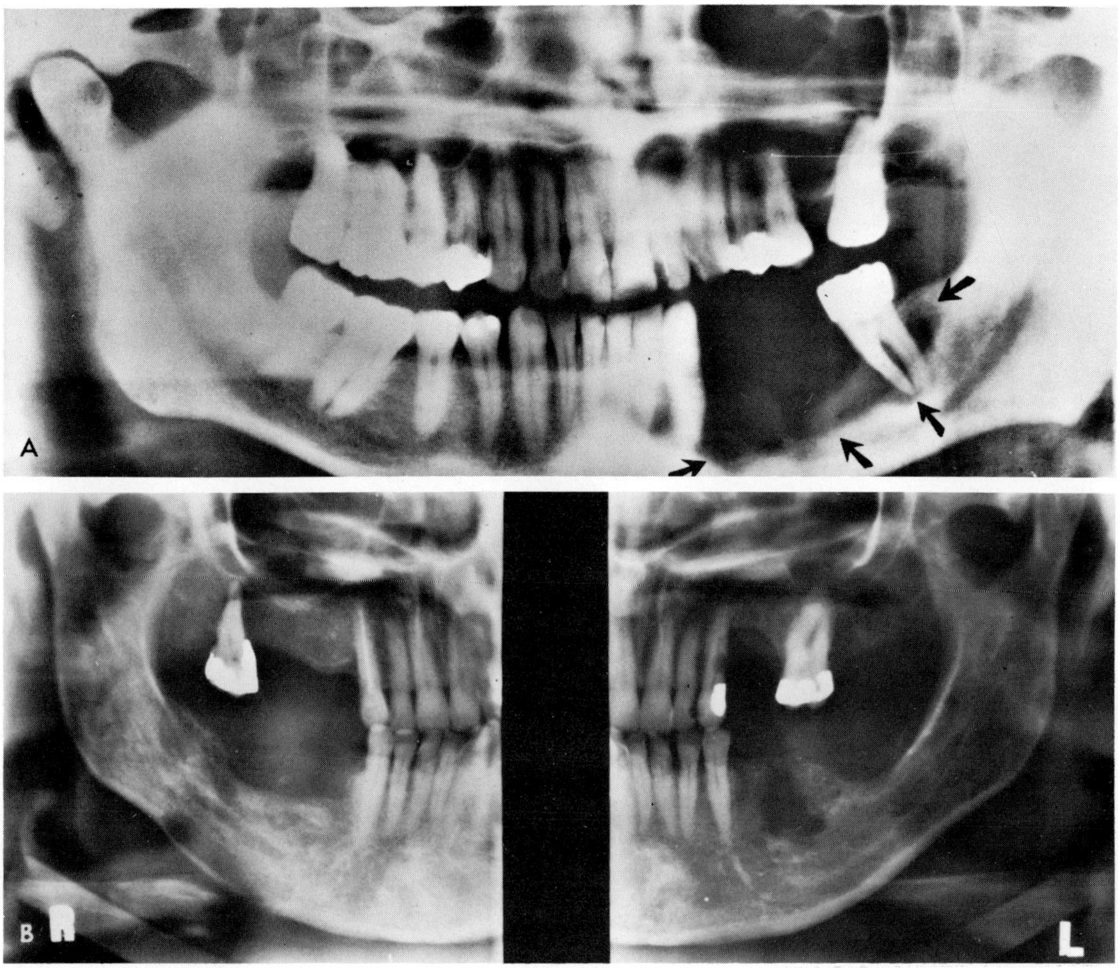

Figure 12–13. Eosinophilic granuloma. **A.** courtesy of Dr. Gus Pappas, Columbus, OH. **B.** courtesy of Dr. Stanley Lovestedt, Rochester, MN.

bone and is referred to as monostotic, although polyostotic forms also occur. This is considered the benign manifestation of the group. Visceral and organ involvement does not occur, however, soft tissue extension of the underlying granulomatous bony lesions is possible. Thus, epulislike lesions and localized areas of thick, boggy, edematous gingivae with separation and mobility of involved teeth are seen. Treatment usually consists of surgical excision or curettage, sometimes supplemented with low doses of radiation therapy in the 300- to 600-rad range. The prognosis is excellent, particularly in the monostotic form.

RADIOGRAPHIC FEATURES

(Figs. 12–10 to 12–13)

Letterer-Siwe disease rarely manifests bony involvement until late in its course. When it does occur, the long bones may be involved. There may be one or several punched-out lesions in the skull, and involvement of the jaws usually consists of a localized loss of alveolar bone around one or several teeth, separation of teeth, and, rarely, one or more central, poorly defined radiolucent areas.

Hand-Schüller-Christian disease invariably includes bony involvement, particularly of the skull and jaws. Other skeletal lesions may be seen in the long bones, pelvis, and ribs. The skull involvement consists of multiple punched-out radiolucencies producing a geographic skull. Involvement of the jaws consists of a generalized loss of alveolar bone resembling advanced periodontal disease, floating teeth, premature loss of primary and permanent teeth, evidence of stunted growth and delayed development of the permanent dentition when the developing teeth are within the portal of the radiation, and central lytic lesions, particularly in the mandible.

Eosinophilic granuloma only involves bone and more typically the flat bones. The long

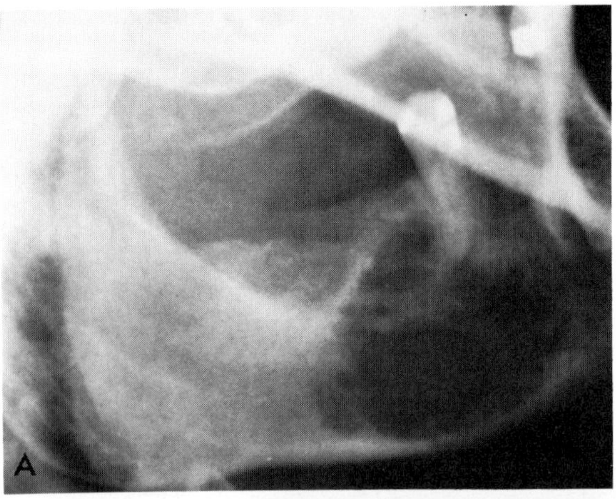

Figure 12–14. Multiple myeloma. **A.** Courtesy of Dr. Stanley Lovestedt, Rochester, MN. **B.** Note the pathologic right mandibular fracture. (**B** courtesy of Dr. Chris Nortjé, University of Stellenbosch, Tygerberg, South Africa.) **C** and **D.** Multiple punched out radiolucencies in the skull.

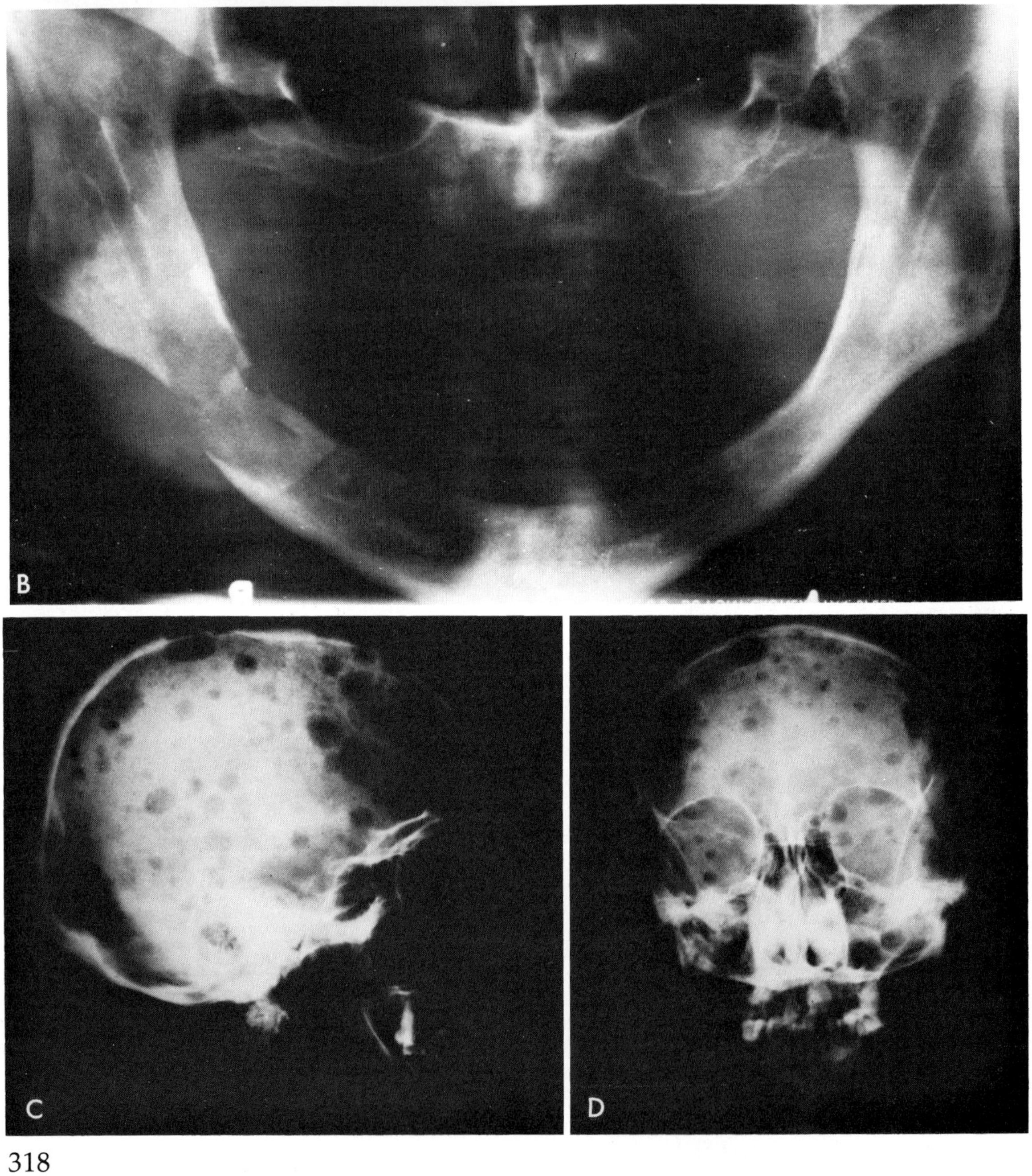

bones are radiographically characterized by destruction of the central medullary region with expansion of the shaft. Lesions localized to the cranial vault, ilium, and other flat bones consist of sharply demarcated punched-out radiolucent areas. When the jaws are involved there may be localized areas of alveolar bone destruction resembling advanced periodontal disease, floating teeth, and cupped-out edentulous areas resembling those seen in peripheral carcinoma of the jaw. Central radiolucent lesions may also be seen in the body of the mandible and in the ramus area.

MULTIPLE MYELOMA (Plasma Cell Myeloma)

BRIEF OVERVIEW

Multiple myeloma is a malignant disorder characterized histologically by the presence of atypical plasma cells. This disease affects many bones, but the skull and jaws are often involved. Adults over the age of 40 years are most frequently affected. Bone pain, paresthesia, and pathologic fracture may be seen. In the jaws, the lesions are more often located in the mandible in the molar-ramus area. Like eosinophilic granuloma, epulistype soft tissue lesions may develop. Clinically, serum hyperglobulinemia produces a reversed albumin-globulin ratio, an increase in total serum protein, and Bence Jones protein in the urine. Radiation therapy and chemotherapy are helpful but usually not curative.

RADIOGRAPHIC FEATURES (Fig. 12–14)

Generally, the skull lesions are described as multiple punched-out radiolucencies; the mandibular lesion in Figure 12–14 is typical of jaw lesions. The lesions of multiple myeloma tend to be well delineated but without any cortical outline. Perforation of the cortex is more common than expansion. In a case reported by Ramon and associates, the primary manifestation of their mandibular lesion was a very distinct sunray radiographic pattern. Multiple punched-out skull lesions are highly characteristic.

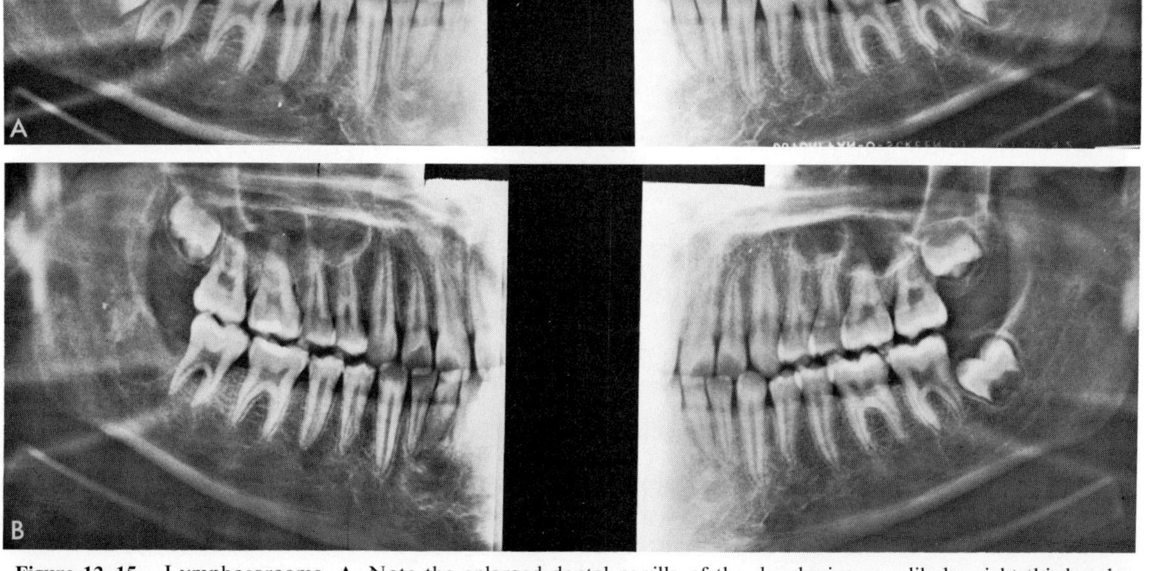

Figure 12–15. Lymphosarcoma. **A.** Note the enlarged dental papilla of the developing mandibular right third molar. Compare the right and left sides. The patient presented with odontalgia. **B.** One month after removal of the third molar. A large, fungating, soft tissue mass was present clinically, apparently growing out of the socket of the extracted third molar.

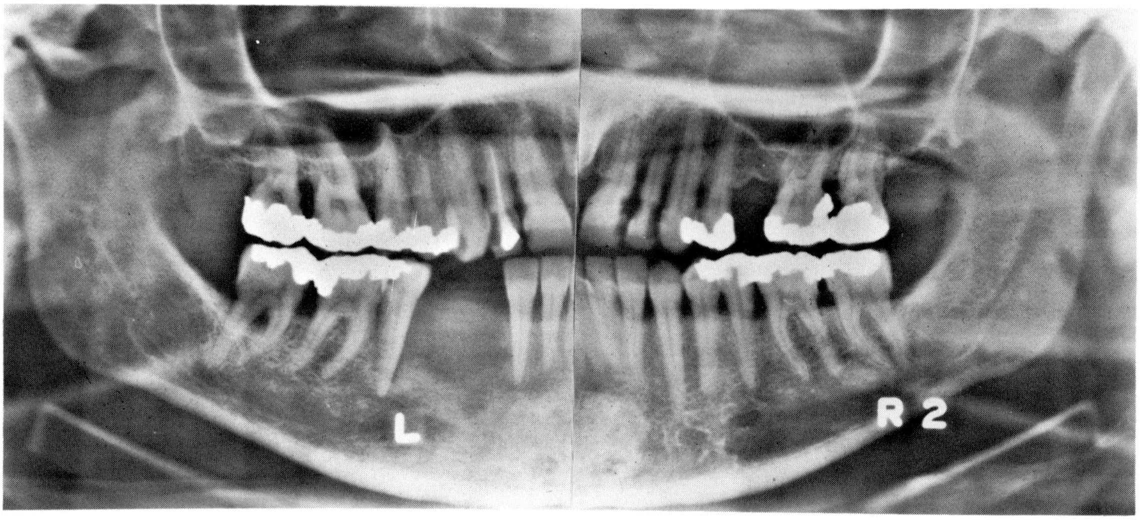

Figure 12–16. Fibrosarcoma. (Courtesy of Dr. E. A. Scott, St. Louis, MO.)

LYMPHOSARCOMA (Diffuse Lymphocytic Non-Hodgkin's Lymphoma)

BRIEF OVERVIEW

The lymphosarcoma is a malignant lymphoma characterized by an abnormal proliferation of lymphocytes or their precursors. These occur more frequently in males over 50 years of age but may occur in children and adolescents. Generally, the disease primarily affects a lymph node, but extranodal jaw involvement is possible. Radiation therapy only delays the inevitable fatality.

RADIOGRAPHIC FEATURES (Fig. 12–15)

Although the number of jaw lesions are relatively few, there may be odontalgia or loosening of the teeth. After extraction, a soft tissue tumor mass may proliferate at a rather rapid and alarming rate at the extraction site.

FIBROSARCOMA

BRIEF OVERVIEW

Fibrosarcoma is a malignant neoplasm of fibrous connective tissue origin and may occur at any location where this tissue is found. Younger to middle-aged adults are most commonly affected. Some fibrosarcomas arise from previously existing fibrous dysplasia and Paget's disease, although these more frequently give rise to osteo- or chondrosarcomas. In the jaws, they may arise in the periosteum or the periodontal ligament, and early lesions may resemble localized periodontal disease. Epulis-like growths may bulge out onto the gingiva from the bone.

RADIOGRAPHIC FEATURES (Fig. 12–16)

There are no pathognomonic findings in fibrosarcoma. This lesion may be a poorly defined radiolucency, central in the jaws. It may begin by resembling localized periodontal disease with an increase in size of the periodontal membrane space along one side of the tooth and may eventually produce one or several floating teeth in the area.

BURKITT'S LYMPHOMA (African Jaw Lymphoma, American Burkitt's Lymphoma)

BRIEF OVERVIEW

Burkitt's lymphoma was once thought to occur only in Africa; it is now known to occur in many places, including the United States, but remains a rare occurrence in this country. It almost exclusively affects children and may etiologically be associated with the Epstein-Barr virus. These children usually develop a rapidly enlarging facial swelling, with loosening of the teeth. Abdominal involvement sometimes occurs, and, in America, Burkitt's lymphoma is primarily an abdominal disease. The disease is usually managed with chemotherapy with varying degrees of success.

RADIOGRAPHIC FEATURES (Fig. 12–17)

Early signs of Burkitt's lymphoma include the separation of the teeth by the tumor mass. A similar separation is sometimes seen in the histiocytosis-X group of diseases. This is followed by rapid loosening and migration of adjacent teeth. Bony involvement usually consists of an expansile lesion, which may perforate the cortex and produce a poorly defined moth-eaten pattern.

HISTIOCYTIC LYMPHOMA (Reticulum Cell Sarcoma)

BRIEF OVERVIEW

This malignant neoplasm has been classified as one of the non-Hodgkin's lymphomas. The disease primarily affects men over the age of 50 and may arise in the pharyngeal and tonsillar areas of the head and neck. When the soft tissues of the oral cavity are involved, the disease usually manifests as a chronic inflammatory process or periodontal disease. There may be fever, malaise, weight loss, hyperhidrosis, and pruritus. There may be cranial nerve palsies involving the ocular, trigeminal, and facial nerves. Firm, enlarged, discrete, nontender, and fixed regional lymph nodes may be present. Treatment consists of radiation therapy with or without chemotherapy. The prognosis is poor.

RADIOGRAPHIC FEATURES

There are no radiographic changes that are specifically limited to this disease. When the mandible is involved, there may be direct extension and erosion of an area secondary to soft tissue involvement. When the lesion arises pri-

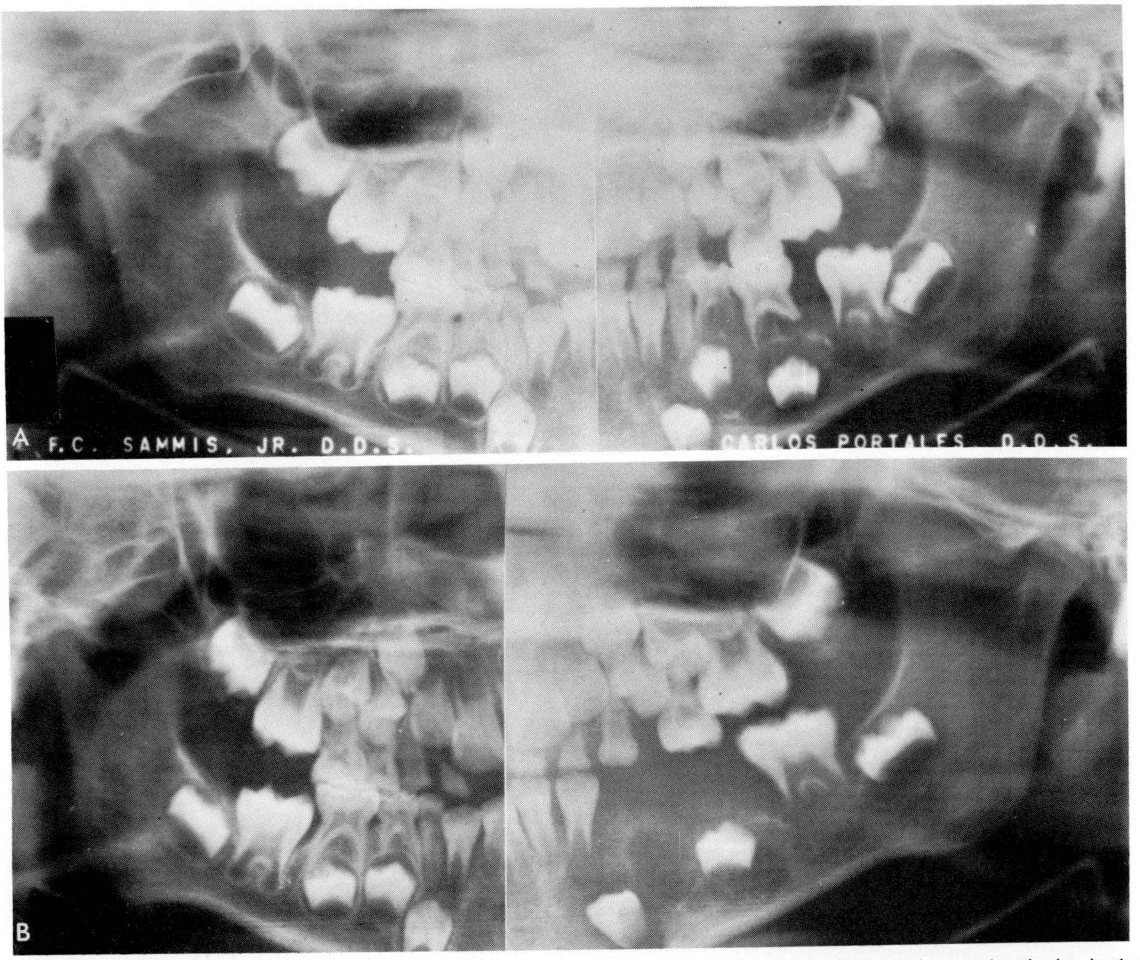

Figure 12–17. Burkitt's lymphoma. **A.** This five-year-old child presented with an epulislike lesion on the gingiva in the mandibular left first bicuspid area. **B.** One month after biopsy. (Figure 12–14 courtesy of Drs. Frank Sammis, Jr. and Carlos Portales, San Antonio, TX.)

marily in bone, it is often a diffuse radiolucency, with poorly defined borders or a moth-eaten appearance. Small radiopaque foci, thin lacy striae, and evidence of cortical expansion with perforation may be present. Subperiosteal new bone formation may occur in mandibular lesions, and complete opacification of the maxillary sinus is sometimes seen in maxillary lesions. Pathologic mandibular fractures may occur.

EWING'S SARCOMA

BRIEF OVERVIEW

Ewing's sarcoma is an extremely rare malignant neoplasm of bone, whose cell of origin remains unknown. The condition is more common in males and mainly affects children and young adults. Onset sometimes resembles an inflammatory condition, with facial swelling, low-grade fever, and an elevated white blood count. Ominous symptoms of paresthesia, anesthesia, and facial neuralgia are often present. Although the long bones are mainly affected, the jaws are involved in about 10 per cent of cases, the mandible being the most frequently affected site. Treatment usually consists of radiation therapy with or without surgery and chemotherapy. The prognosis remains extremely poor.

RADIOGRAPHIC FEATURES

Due to the paucity of cases, the radiographic features of this condition remain variable. The most common presentation probably consists of a prominent central radiolucency with poorly defined borders. Other variants include a predominantly radiopaque response resembling the multiple sclerotic masses seen in chronic diffuse sclerosing osteomyelitis, Paget's disease, or multiple cementomas. A subperiosteal reaction, characterized by the deposition of successive layers of new bone often referred to as onion skinning, is also highly suggestive of Ewing's sarcoma and greatly resembles the subperiosteal reaction seen in Garré's osteomyelitis and in the early subperiosteal proliferation sometimes seen in osteogenic sarcoma and, rarely, reticulum cell sarcoma. The peripheral aspect of the neoplasm sometimes produces a trabecular pattern, which has been discussed as sun ray in appearance, similar to that sometimes seen in osteogenic sarcoma, chondrosarcoma, some hemangiomas, certain complex odontomas, and, in rare instances, multiple myeloma.

REFERENCES

Reference Texts

Eversole, L. R.: **Clinical Outline of Oral Pathology.** Philadelphia: Lea & Febiger, 1978, pp. 213–215, 218–219.

Shafer, W. G., Hine, M. K., and Levy, B. M.: **A Textbook of Oral Pathology**, 3rd Edition. Philadelphia: W. B. Saunders, 1974, pp. 156–158, 174–180, 199–201, 261–263, 453–454, 586–587.

Wood, N. K., and Goaz, P. W.: **Differential Diagnosis of Oral Lesions.** St. Louis: C. V. Mosby, 1975, pp. 376–386.

Selected References

Aresenean, J. C., Canellos, G. P., Banks, P. M., et al.: American Burkitt's lymphoma: A clinicopathologic study of 30 cases. I: Clinical factors relating to prolonged survival. **Am. J. Med. 58**:314, 1975.

Banks, P. M., Arseneau, J. C., Gralnick, H. R., et al.: American Burkitt's lymphoma: A clinicopathologic study of 30 cases. II. Pathologic correlations. **Am. J. Med. 58**:322, 1975.

Baker, R. D., D'Onofrio, E. D., Corio, R. J., et al: Squamous-cell carcinoma arising in a lateral periodontal cyst. **Oral Surg. 47**:495, 1979.

Borghelli, R. F., Barros, R. E., and Zampieri, J.: Ewing sarcoma of the mandible: Report of a case. **J. Oral Surg. 36**:473, 1978.

Cline, R. E., and Stenger, T. G.: Histiocytic lymphoma (reticulum cell sarcoma): Report of five cases. **Oral Surg. 43**:422, 1977.

Domboski, M. L.: Eosinophilic granuloma of bone manifesting mandibular involvement. **Oral Surg. 50**:116, 1980.

Dreizen, S., Daly, T. E., Drane, J. B., and Brown, L. R.: Oral complications of cancer radiotherapy. **Postgrad. Med. 61**:85, 1977.

Eversole, L. R., Sabes, W. R., and Rovin, S.: Aggressive growth and neoplastic potential of odontogenic cysts with special reference to central epidermoid and mucoepidermoid carcinomas. **Cancer 35**:270, 1975.

Hartman, K. S.: Histocytosis X: A review of 114 cases with oral involvement. **Oral Surg. 49**:38, 1980.

Huvos, A. G., Higinbotham, N. L., and Miller, T. R.: Bone sarcomas arising in fibrous dysplasia. **J. Bone Joint Surg.** (Am) **54**:1047, 1972.

Murray, C. G., Daly, T. E., and Zimmerman, S. O.: The relationship between dental disease and radiation necrosis of the mandible. **Oral Surg. 49**:99, 1980.

Onvigbo, W. I. B.: Batson's theory of vertebral venous metastasis: A review. **Oncology 32**:145, 1975.

Ramon, Y., Oberman, M., Horowitz, I., Freeman, A., and Tadmor, R.: A large mandibular tumor with a distinct radiological "sun-ray effect," as the primary manifestation of multiple myeloma. **J. Oral Surg. 36**:52, 1978.

Rapoport, A., Sobrinho, J.deA., de Carvalho, M. B., Magrin, J., de Queiroz Costa, F., and Quadros, J. V.: Ewing's sarcoma of the mandible. **Oral Surg. 44**:89, 1977.

Sanders, B.: Current concepts in the management of osteomyelitis of the mandible. **J. Oral Med. 33**:40, 1978.

Sedano, H. O., Cernea, P., Hosxe, G., and Gorlin, R. J.: Histiocytosis-X, Clinical, radiologic and histologic findings with attention to oral manifestations. **Oral Surg. 27**:760, 1969.

Soskoline, S.: Observations on the pathogenesis of primordial cysts. **Br. Dent. J. 123**:321, 1967.

Terrill, D. G., Lee, A., LeDonne M. A., and Nusbaum, T. O.: American Burkitt's lymphoma in Pittsburgh, Pennsylvania. **Oral Surg. 44**:411, 1977.

Chapter 13
Periapical Radiopacities

IDIOPATHIC OSTEOSCLEROSIS
CONDENSING OSTEITIS
HYPERCEMENTOSIS
PERIAPICAL CEMENTAL DYSPLASIA
BENIGN CEMENTOBLASTOMA
BENIGN OSTEOBLASTOMA
CENTRAL CEMENTO-OSSIFYING FIBROMA

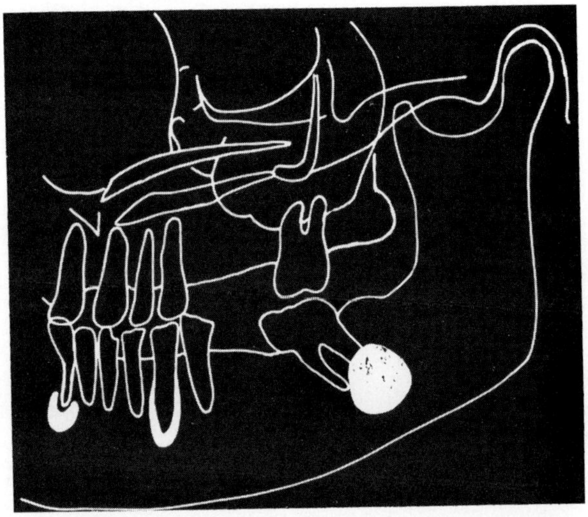

IDIOPATHIC OSTEOSCLEROSIS (Focal Periapical Osteopetrosis)

BRIEF OVERVIEW

Idiopathic osteosclerosis is considered under periapical radiopacities because it is important to distinguish this condition from other lesions in this section, especially condensing osteitis. Idiopathic osteosclerosis is usually located in the mandibular molar and bicuspid areas, and the associated tooth is usually vital. The condition may be associated with endodontically treated teeth and probably represents bone scar or a healed condensing osteitis. The patient is asymptomatic. Idiopathic osteosclerosis may be seen in association with primary teeth and may be located between teeth, in the jaws beyond the periapical area, in edentulous areas, and in the socket areas of previously extracted teeth.

RADIOGRAPHIC FEATURES (Figs. 13–1 and 13–2)

The associated tooth is usually vital, and its radiopacity is of the same density as cortical bone. The radiopaque area, although well defined, is in direct apposition with the surrounding bone with no intervening radiolucent area. There is usually no resorption or obliteration of the associated root. There may be several areas involved in the same patient.

CONDENSING OSTEITIS (Chronic Focal Sclerosing Osteomyelitis)

BRIEF OVERVIEW

Condensing osteitis is most often associated with the apex of a nonvital tooth. It is a periapical reaction to a pulpal inflammation in

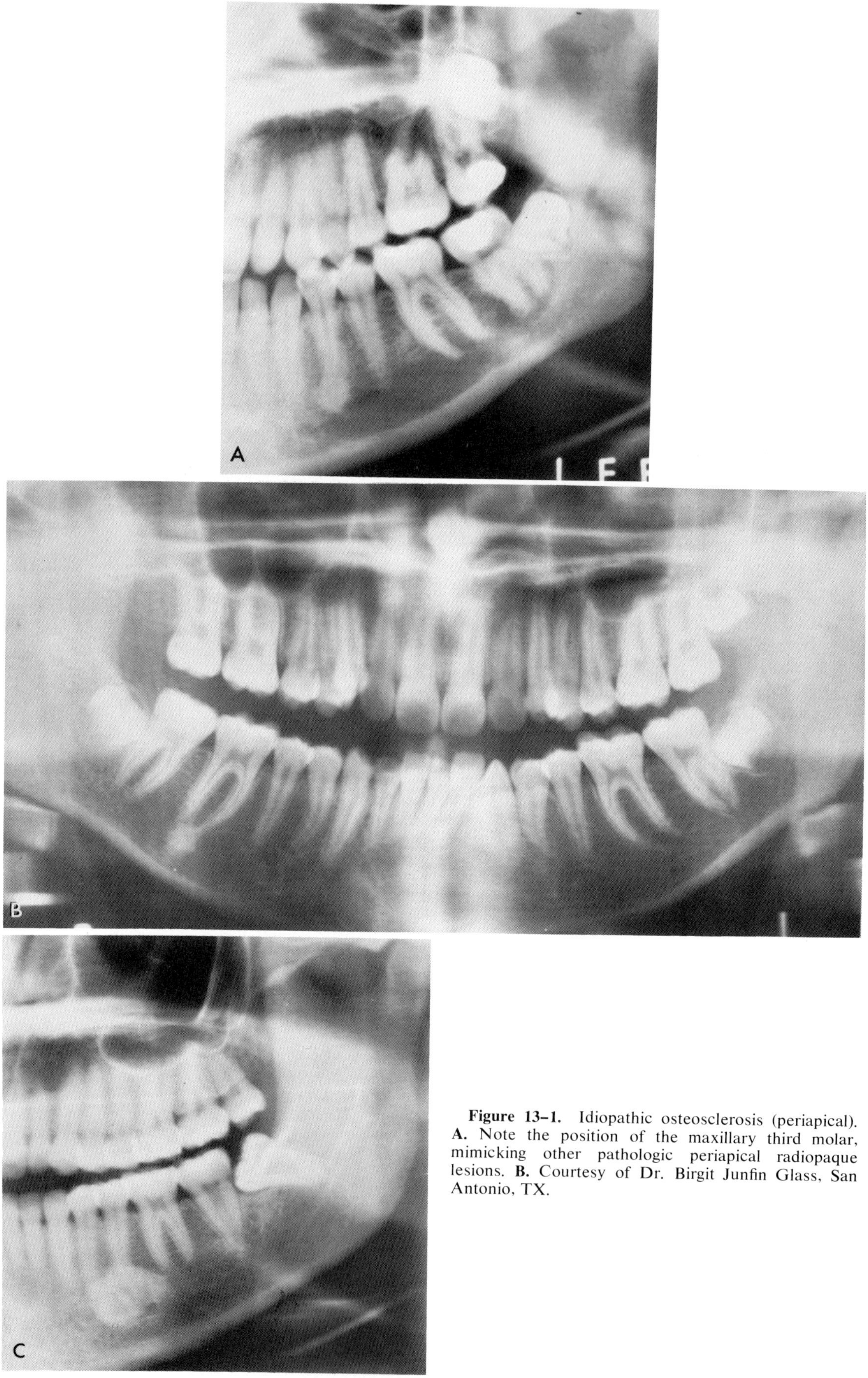

Figure 13–1. Idiopathic osteosclerosis (periapical). **A.** Note the position of the maxillary third molar, mimicking other pathologic periapical radiopaque lesions. **B.** Courtesy of Dr. Birgit Junfin Glass, San Antonio, TX.

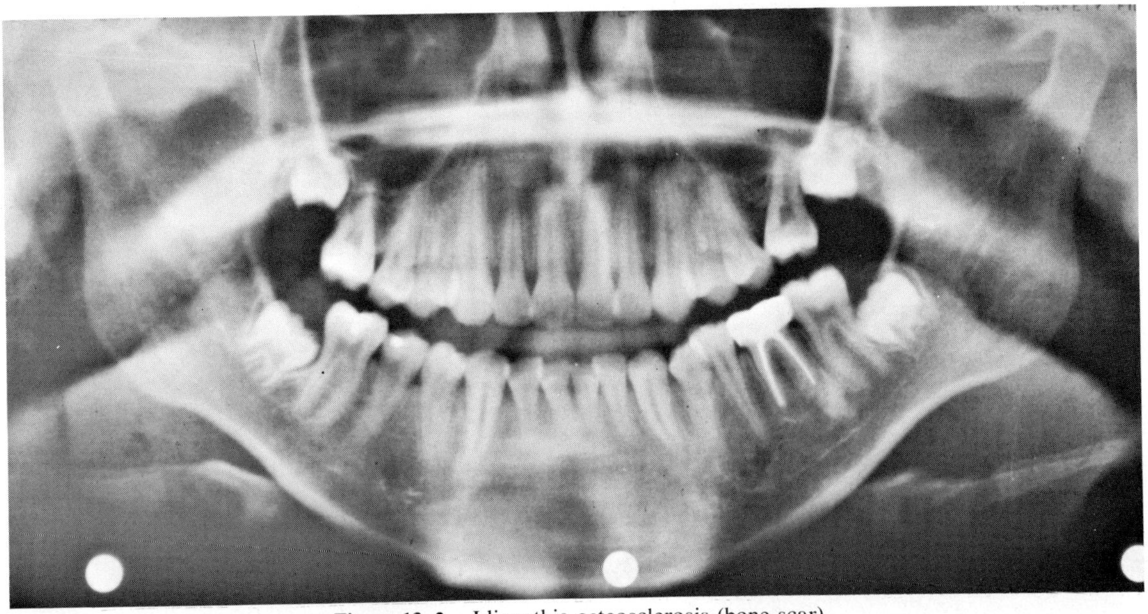

Figure 13–2. Idiopathic osteosclerosis (bone scar).

which reactive bone is produced. Lysis of bone, producing a periapical radiolucency, is the more common reaction. Condensing osteitis probably represents an exuberant attempt at repair, characterized by the deposition of bone in response to inflammation. Since this is usually associated with nonvital pulps of long standing, the condition is most often asymptomatic. Treatment of the involved tooth is required. A sclerotic area may remain at the apex of the endodontically treated tooth or as a central radiopacity in the healed edentulous area previously occupied by the apical region of the affected tooth.

RADIOGRAPHIC FEATURES (Fig. 13–3)

In condensing osteitis, the tooth may be obviously nonvital radiographically. Additionally, the tooth may contain a deep restoration, a large restoration, or a crown, and there may be evidence of caries, redecay, or secondary dentin formation. There may be a radiolucent area at the apex of the involved tooth separating it from the radiopaque area. The radiopaque area may vary in size and density, and it is usually in direct apposition with the surrounding bone. It is most frequently seen in association with mandibular premolars and molars.

HYPERCEMENTOSIS

BRIEF OVERVIEW

Hypercementosis is an excessive deposition of secondary cementum on the roots and is of unknown etiology. Although often idiopathic, it may be associated with periapical inflammation, periodontal disease, lack of opposing occlusion, or transplanted teeth. The condition is generalized in Paget's disease and Gardner's syndrome. Affected teeth may be difficult to extract.

RADIOGRAPHIC FEATURES (Fig. 13–4)

On panoramic radiographs, bulbous, slightly more opaque roots may be noted in the more advanced cases, especially at the apical third. The dentinal outline within the cementum is extremely difficult to see. Subsequent identification (using periapical films) of the dentinal outline of the root within the cemental mass is an important step in ruling out an ordinary bulbous-shaped root that has normal cementum or, less frequently, an early lesion of benign cementoblastoma, in which case the dentinal outline is usually lost within the proliferating cemental mass. The teeth are vital in all cases, unless coincidentally nonvital owing to caries. Apart from the factors previously discussed, hypercementosis is of no clinical significance.

PERIAPICAL CEMENTAL DYSPLASIA (Cementoma)

BRIEF OVERVIEW

This condition is thought to arise from the periodontal ligament and is of unknown and

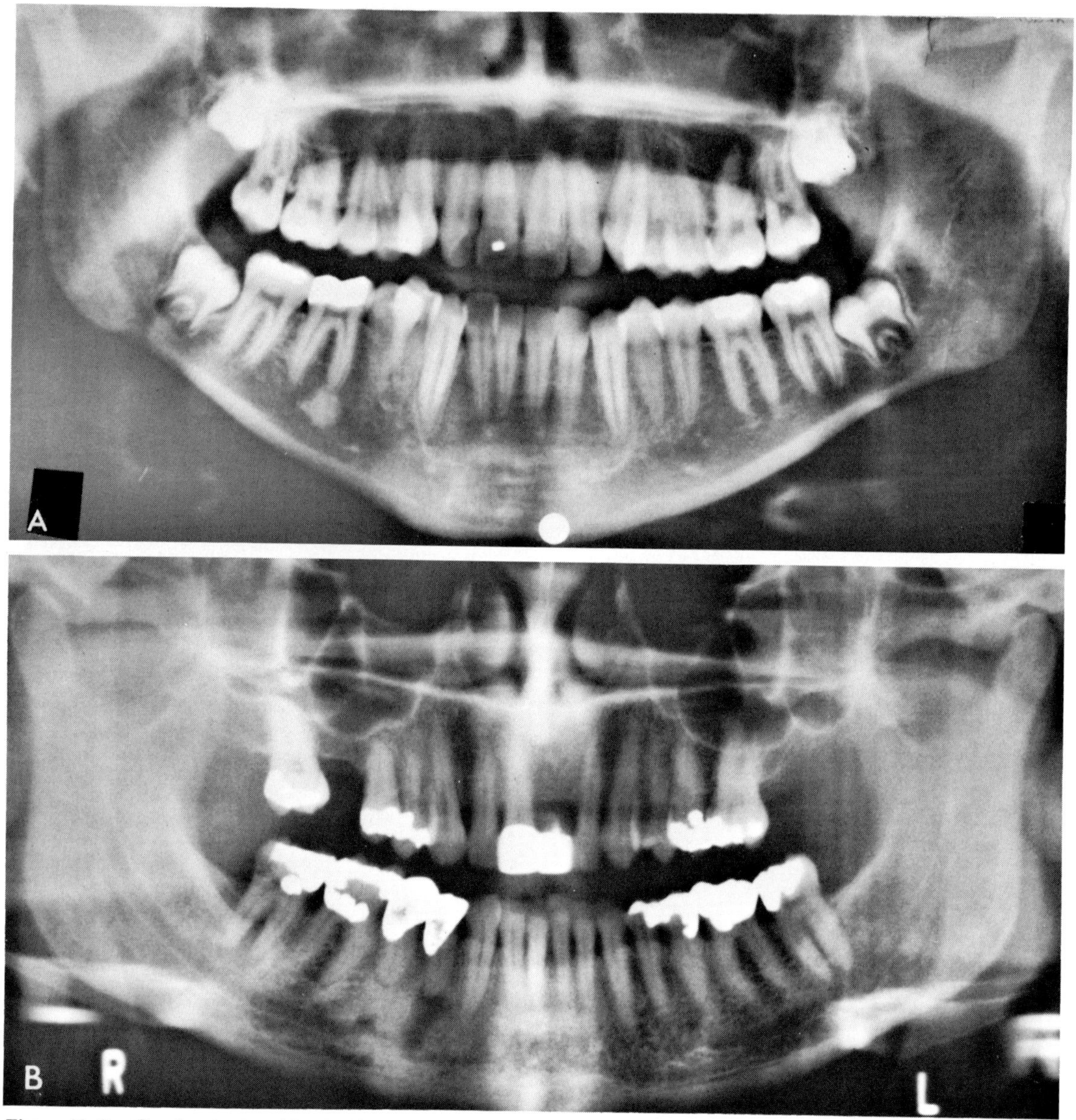

Figure 13–3. Condensing osteitis. **A.** The mandibular right first molar was nonvital. **B.** Both mandibular right bicuspids were nonvital. **B** illustrates both osteoproliferative and osteolytic responses to pulpal inflammation in two adjacent teeth. (Figure 13–3 courtesy of Dr. Steven Bricker, San Antonio, TX.)

much debated etiology. It is most frequently seen in middle-aged black females at the apices of vital lower anterior teeth. Cementomas may be seen in any adult and may involve other vital teeth, particularly molars. They are asymptomatic, and expansion is not a feature. Cementomas are thought by some to be reactive lesions, and the appearance of residual multiple cementomas in edentulous jaws is radiographically identical to the appearance of chronic diffuse sclerosing osteomyelitis, also known as florid cemento-osseous dysplasia. Periapical cemental dysplasia is a self-limiting condition and usually requires no treatment.

RADIOGRAPHIC FEATURES (Figs. 13–5 and 13–6)

The lesions of periapical cemental dysplasia may be single or multiple and may be radiolucent, radiopaque, or mixed. The authors have considered these lesions in the radiopaque section because the mature lesion presents in this manner. However, in the early osteolytic stage, the lesion is radiolucent and resembles a periapical radiolucency of pulpal origin. In the intermediate cementoblastic stage, there are islands of calcified material within the radiolucent area. Usually the periodontal membrane

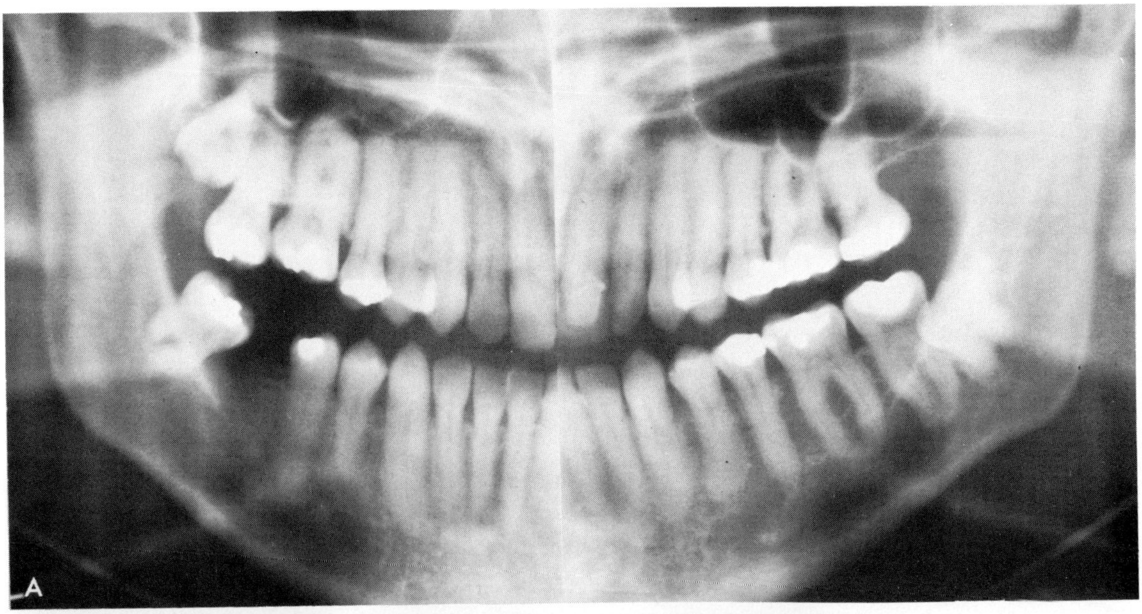

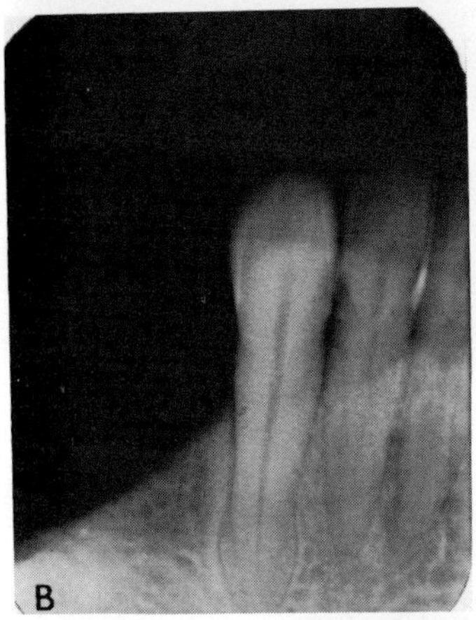

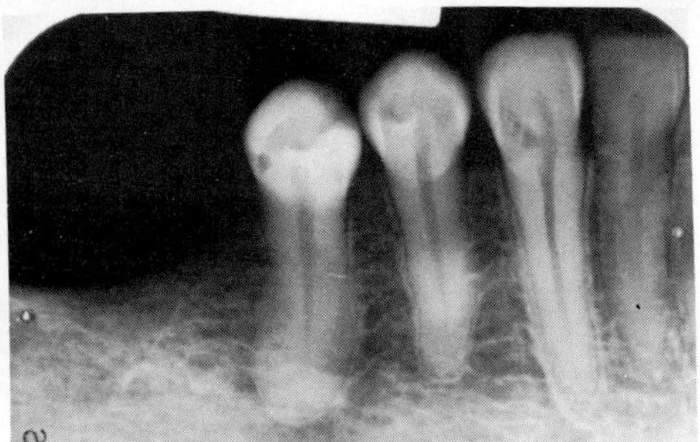

Figure 13–4. Hypercementosis. **A.** Note the difficulty in discerning this condition, which is present bilaterally on the mandibular cuspids and bicuspids. **B** and **C.** Periapical views in two additional patients.

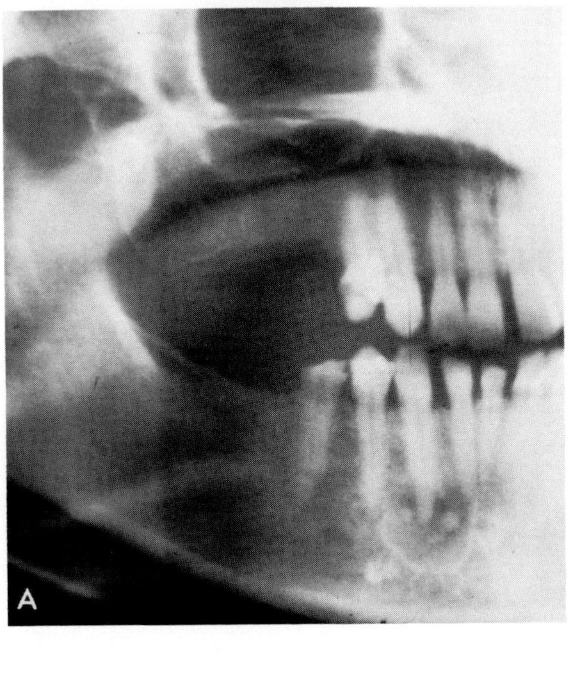

Figure 13–5. Solitary periapical cemental dysplasia. **A.** Mixed radiolucent-radiopaque stage. **B.** Radiopaque stage or Stage III, mature stage.

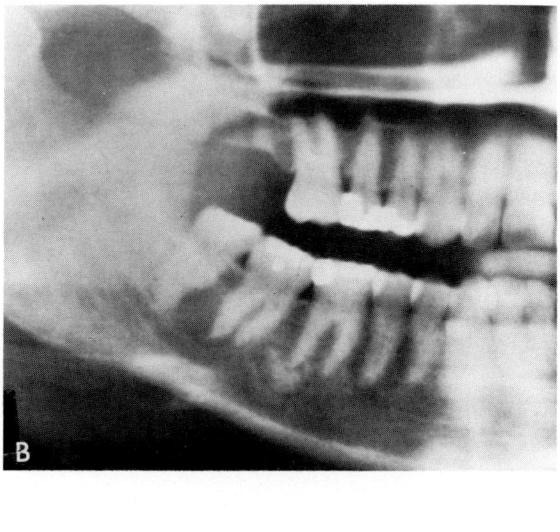

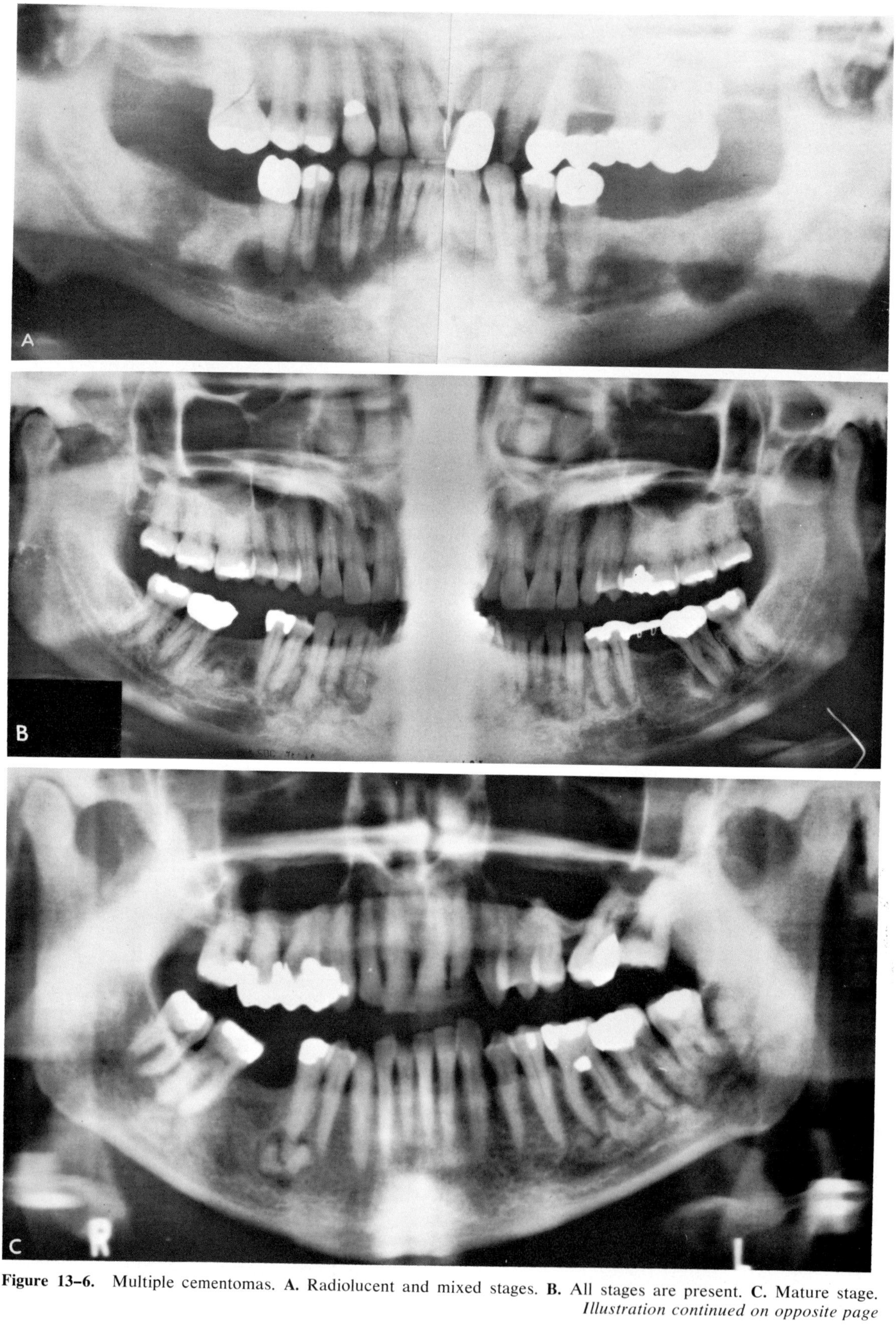

Figure 13–6. Multiple cementomas. **A.** Radiolucent and mixed stages. **B.** All stages are present. **C.** Mature stage.
Illustration continued on opposite page

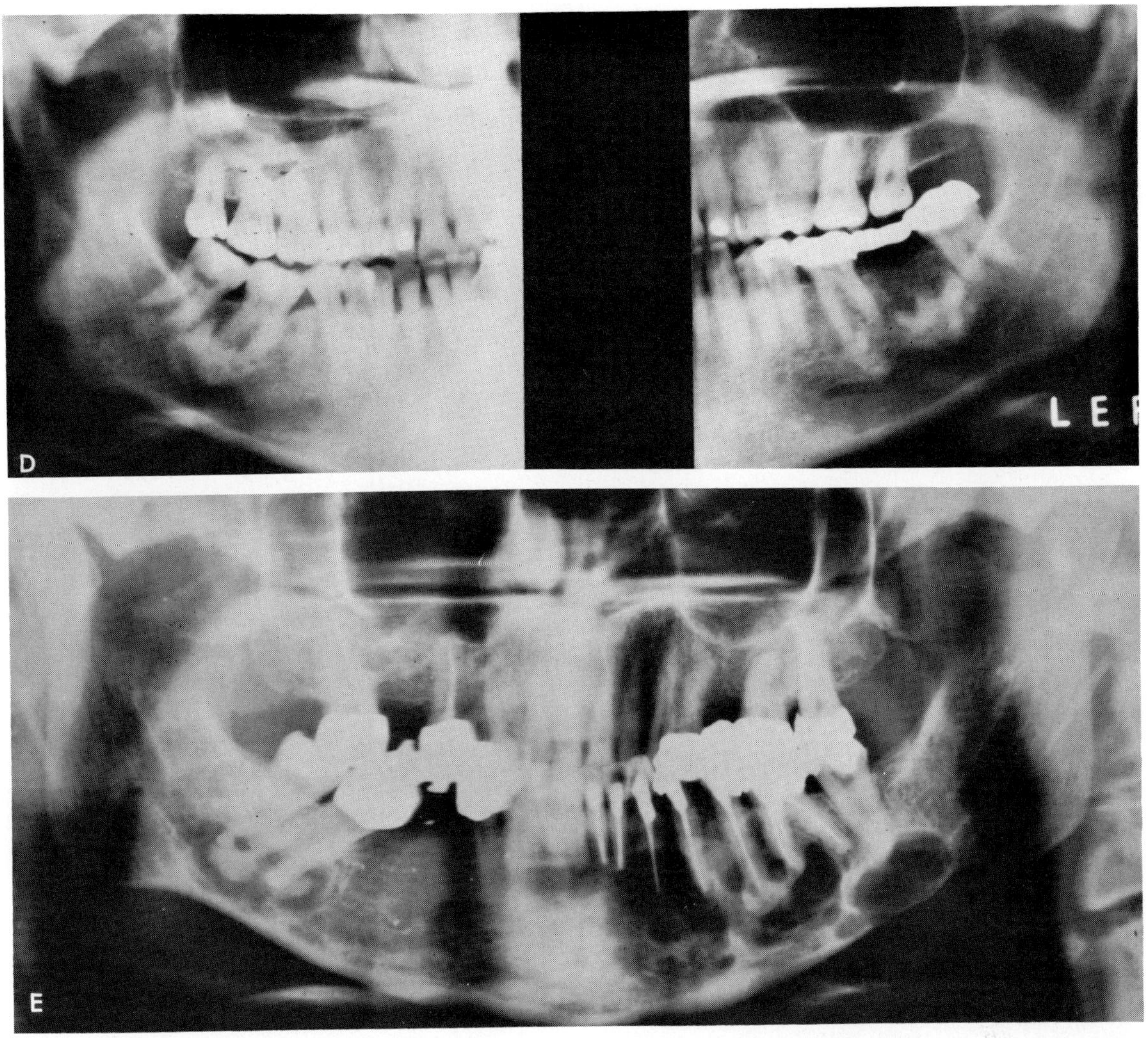

Figure 13–6 *Continued* **D.** Note the residual mature cementoma beneath the bridge pontic. **E.** An unusual presentation. (**B** and **E** courtesy of Dr. Gus Pappas, Columbus, OH. **C** courtesy of Dr. Richard Morse, San Antonio, TX.)

persists between the radiopaque area and the apex of the vital tooth in the mature lesion. The outer rim of the lesion may be radiopaque and probably represents an area of reactive bone. Therefore, the mature lesion may present a targetlike concentric arrangement of radiolucent and radiopaque areas. The outermost rim may be radiopaque, followed by a radiolucent ring, followed by the central opaque cemental mass as seen in Figure 13–5B. It is important to remember that the teeth are vital unless coincidentally nonvital as a result of caries or other causes. The dentinal outline of the root may be easily seen.

In edentulous areas, especially when symptomatic and when sequestration of radiopaque material is apparent, it may be necessary to distinguish this lesion from the condition known as chronic diffuse sclerosing osteomyelitis (also known as florid cemento-osseous dysplasia). This latter condition also affects middle-aged black females, but, unlike cementomas, it may require both surgical and antibiotic treatment. Some consider florid cemento-osseous dysplasia to be an inflamed cementoma.

BENIGN CEMENTOBLASTOMA (True Cementoma)

BRIEF OVERVIEW

The benign cementoblastoma affects teenagers and young adults. The associated teeth are vital, and the most commonly affected tooth is

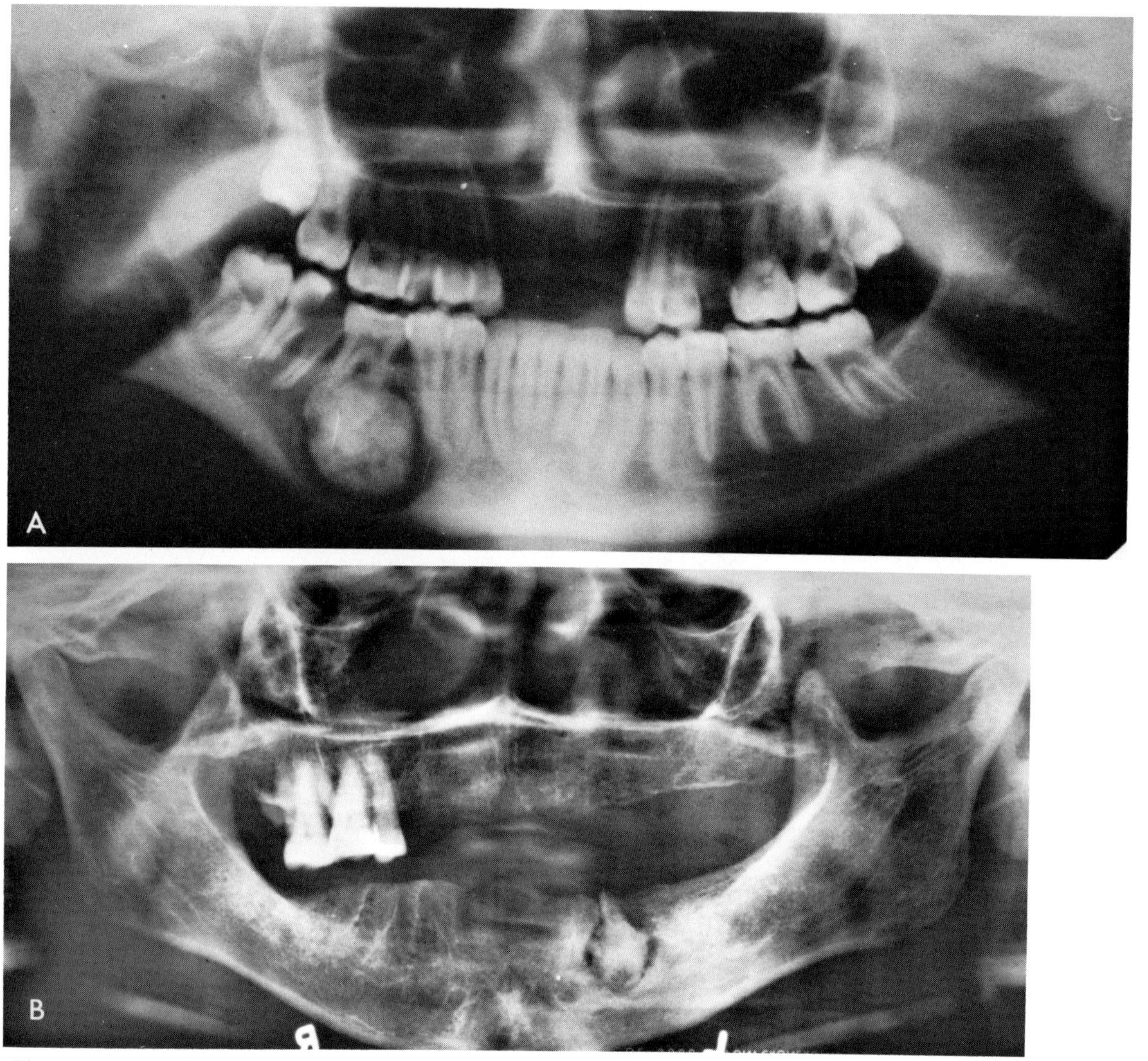

Figure 13–7. Benign cementoblastoma. (Courtesy of Dr. Chris Nortjé, University of Stellenbosch, Tygerberg, South Africa.)

the mandibular first molar. Affected teeth are usually asymptomatic. This lesion may become large and may expand the bone. Considered to be a true neoplasm, although benign, this lesion should be completely excised because of its unlimited growth potential. Usually, the affected tooth must also be removed because of the rigid, inseparable attachment of the neoplasm to the roots.

RADIOGRAPHIC FEATURES (Fig. 13–7)

In the early stages, the benign cementoblastoma is radiolucent. As the lesion matures it becomes mixed with radiopaque foci of cementoblastic material. The mature lesion is characteristic and presents the following features. The radiopaque mass is at the apex of a vital tooth, usually the mandibular first molar. It is of fairly even density and is usually round with buccal and lingual expansion in the larger nickel-sized lesion. Its outer periphery is often well delineated by a thin radiolucent band, but the involved root or roots appear continuous with the mass with no band of separation. In this case, the obliteration of the root is partly due to the opacity of the lesion but mainly due to partial resorption of the involved roots within the mass. Displacement of adjacent teeth is not a usual feature.

BENIGN OSTEOBLASTOMA

BRIEF OVERVIEW

The benign osteoblastoma is included here to contrast it with other similar lesions. This condition is most frequently seen in male children and adolescents at the apices of vital teeth. Although rare in the jaws, there may be a predilection for the maxilla. The presenting features include moderate pain and expansion in the affected area. This lesion should be completely excised.

RADIOGRAPHIC FEATURES (Fig. 13–8)

Although the lesion may be radiolucent in the earlier stages, its expansile nature gives it a tendency to be radiopaque on discovery. The radiopacity is often mottled in appearance, with a density just a little greater than that of bone. The outer margins may not be distinct. Resorption of the involved roots and displacement of adjacent teeth are features. The occlusal aspect of the lesion may extend beyond and above the normal level of alveolar bone. This is a rather alarming and ominous feature when seen radio-

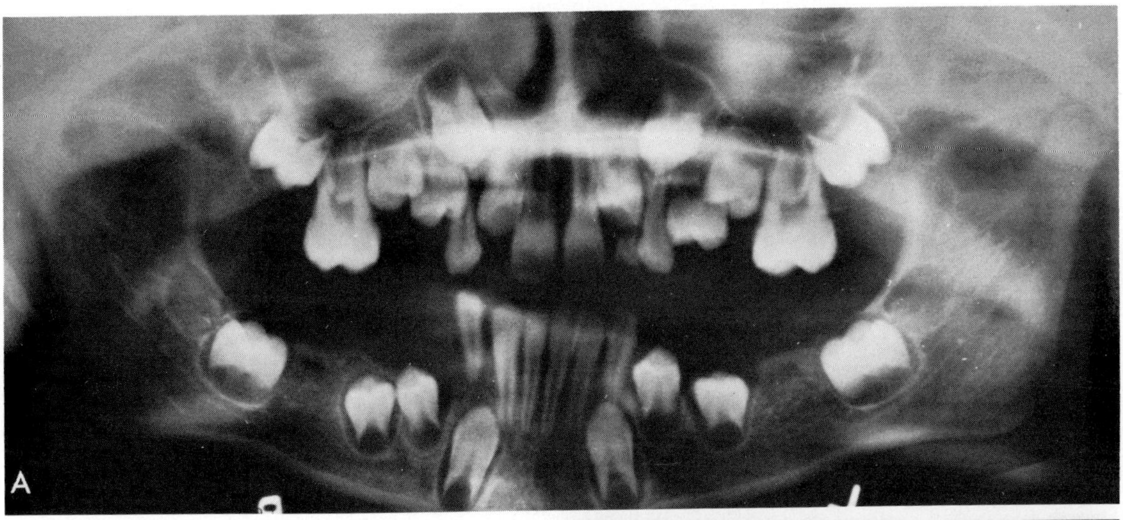

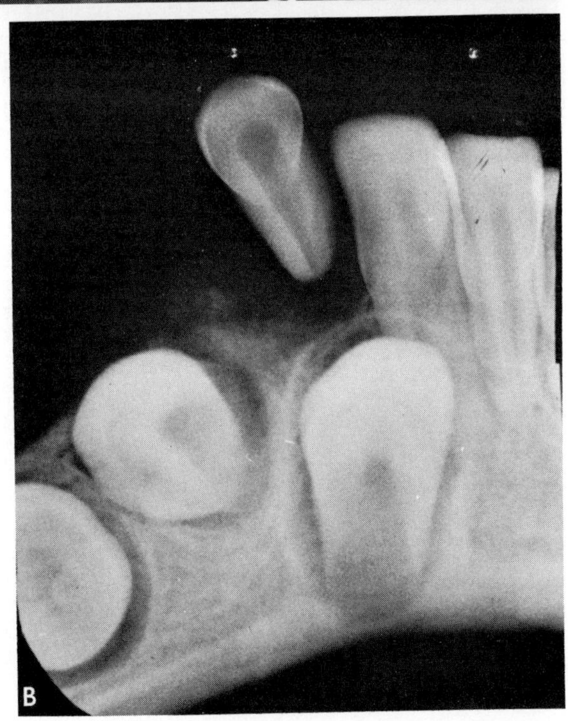

Figure 13–8. Benign osteoblastoma, Note that this early-stage lesion is radiolucent, although displacement of adjacent teeth has already occurred. (Courtesy of Dr. Chris Nortjé, University of Stellenbosch, Tygerberg, South Africa,)

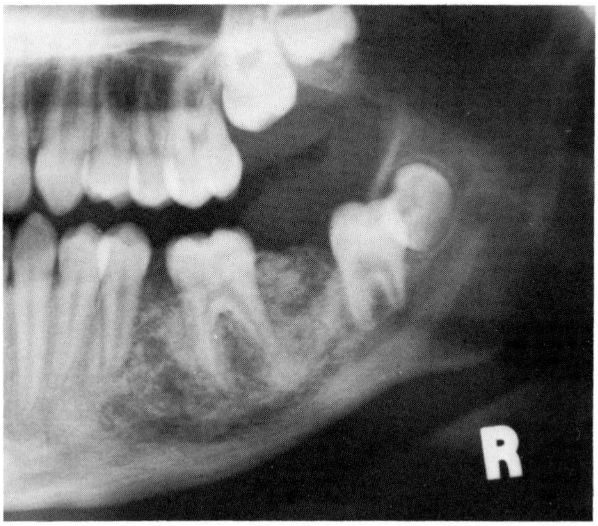

Figure 13–9. Correlation between radiographic and histologic features. Histologically, a definitive diagnosis of many benign fibro-osseous lesions may be difficult to make. However, some of these conditions have very distinct and even pathognomonic radiographic features. This case illustrates the importance of correlating the radiographic and histopathologic findings. This lesion was diagnosed histologically as **benign cementoblastoma,** whereas the radiographic features are more consistent with those of **benign osteoblastoma.** (Courtesy of Dr. Stanley A. Lovestedt, Rochester, MN.)

graphically, as it is sometimes seen with sarcomas such as osteogenic sarcoma.

This lesion should not be confused with the **osteoid osteoma**, which may be very painful. The osteoid osteoma occurs in young people, and the pain is usually reported to be relieved by aspirin. The osteoid osteoma is rare in the jaws and is not a periapical lesion. It is said to occur most frequently in close proximity to the cortex of the inferior border of the mandible in the first and second molar areas. The lesion consists of a radiolucency surrounded by a sclerotic rim of bone. The radiolucency usually undergoes calcification, producing a central ra-

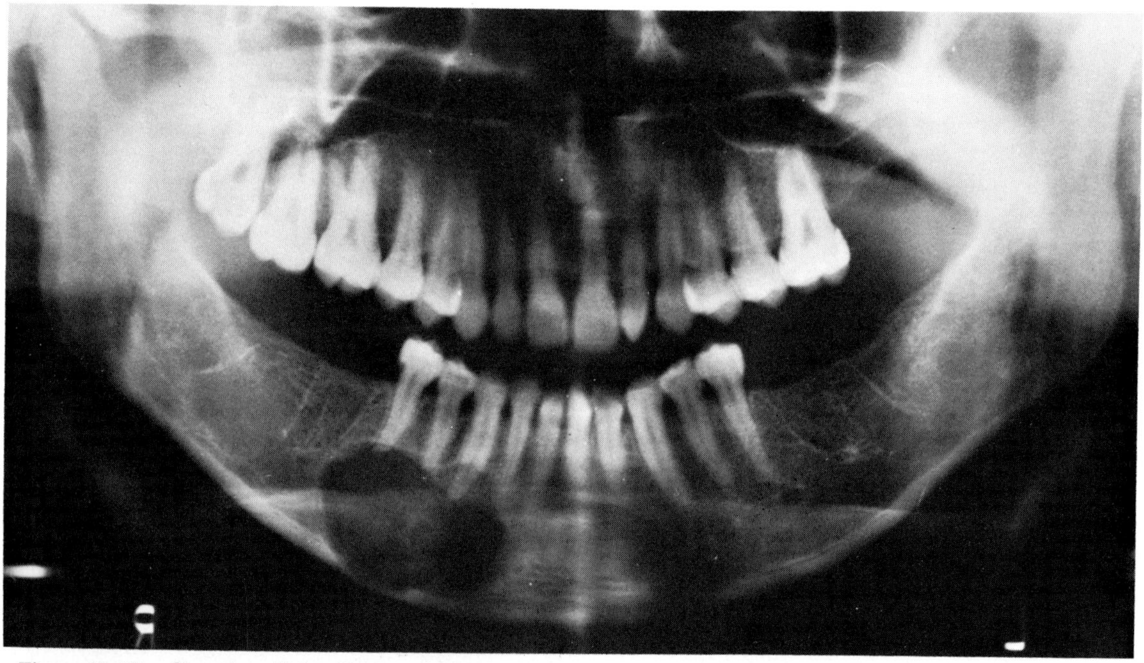

Figure 13–10. Central ossifying fibroma. This early lesion has achieved a rather large size without evidence of calcification. (Courtesy of Dr. Chris Nortjé, University of Stellenbosch, Tygerberg, South Africa.)

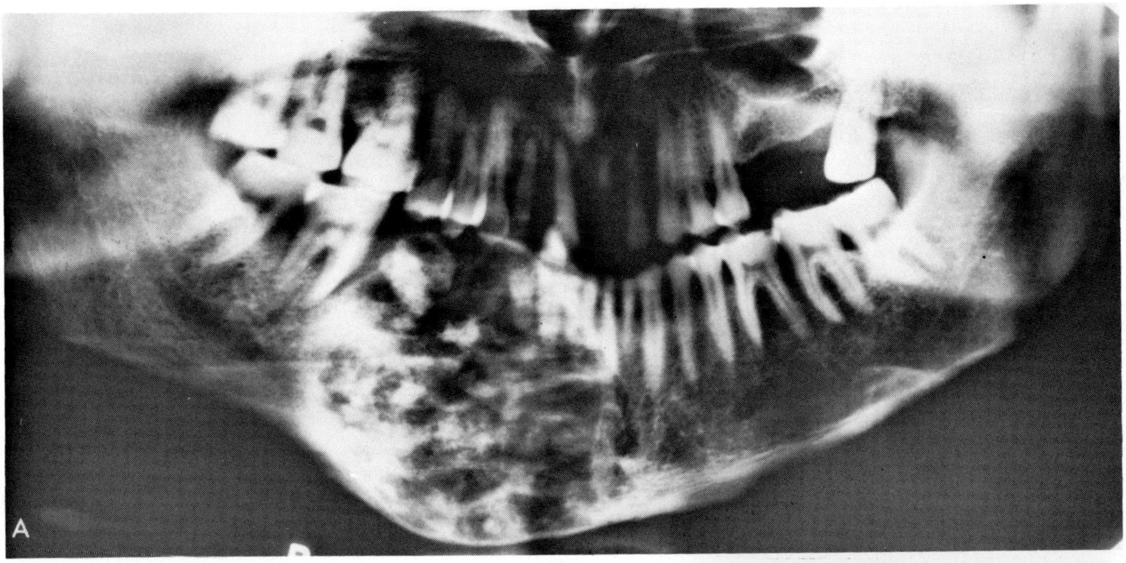

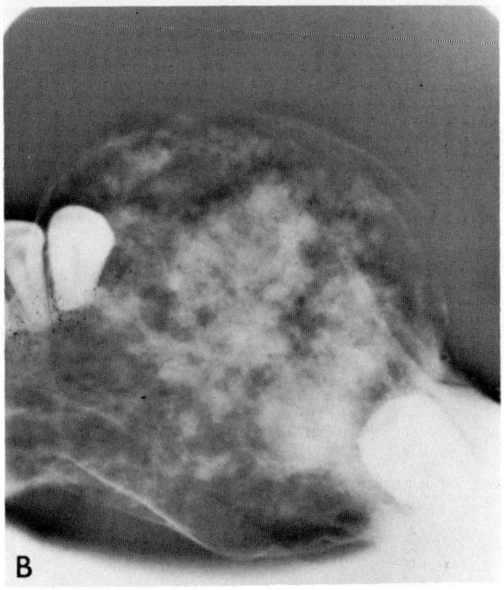

Figure 13–11. Central cemento-ossifying fibroma. (Courtesy of Dr. Chris Nortjé, University of Stellenbosch, Tygerberg, South Africa.)

diopacity surrounded by a radiolucent band. It rarely exceeds 1 cm in diameter. The treatment is surgical excision.

CENTRAL CEMENTO-OSSIFYING FIBROMA (Central Cementifying Fibroma, Central Ossifying Fibroma)

BRIEF OVERVIEW

This condition is separate and distinct from the central odontogenic fibroma previously mentioned under multilocular radiolucencies. This fibro-osseous lesion of periodontal ligament origin occurs more commonly in young adults and often involves the mandible in the area of the molar teeth. The lesion is slow growing and asymptomatic. There may be clinical evidence of bony expansion and abnormal spacing between the teeth in the area. The lesion should be excised, and the recurrence rate is low.

RADIOGRAPHIC FEATURES (Figs. 13–10 to 13–12)

The mature lesion presents as a well-demarcated, ball-like radiopacity, which may cause a bulging out or expansion of the inferior border of the mandible and displacement of

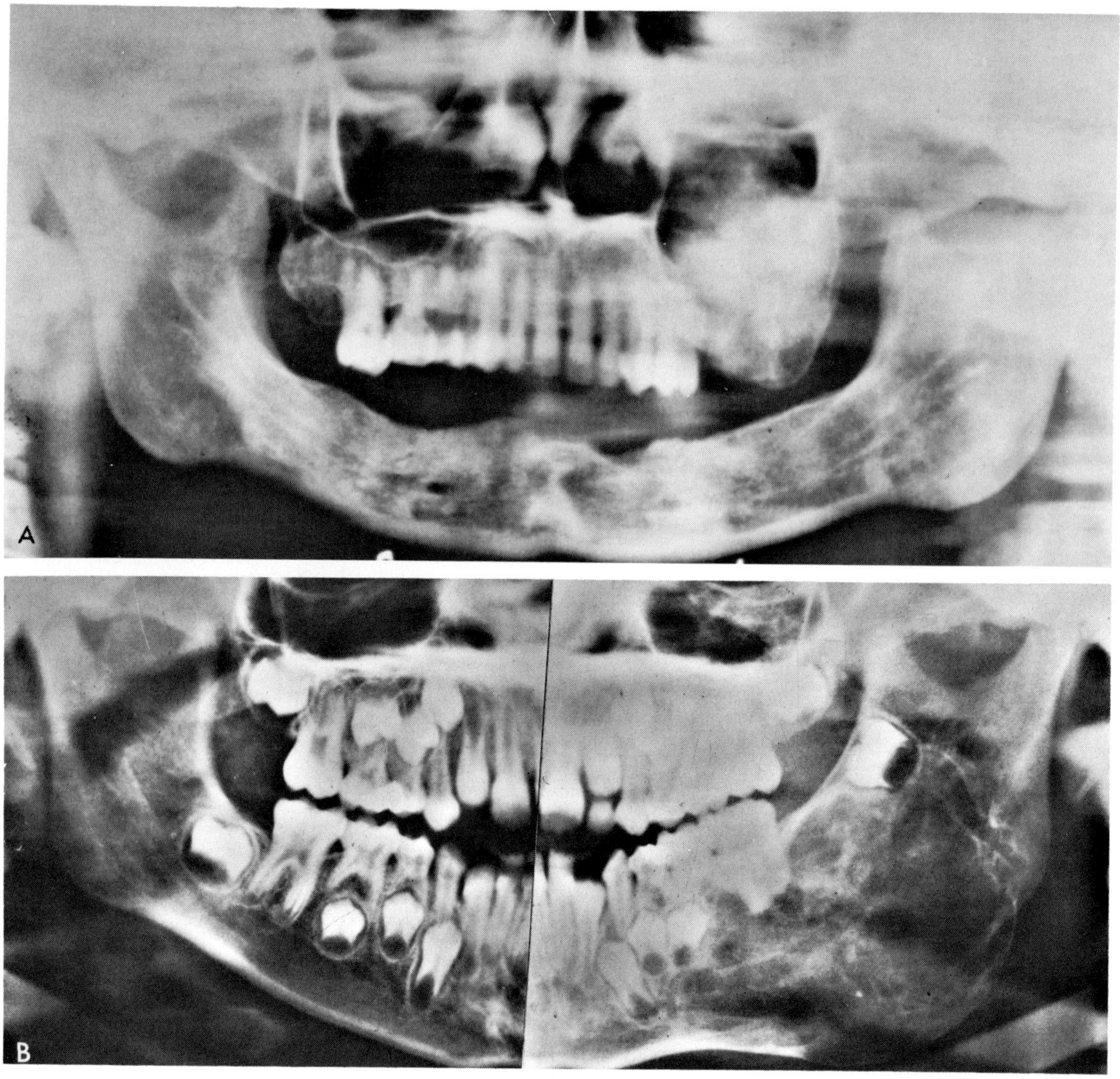

Figure 13–12. Central cementifying fibroma. **A.** Courtesy of Dr. Gus Pappas, Columbus, OH. **B.** Courtesy of Dr. Donald Steed, San Antonio, TX.

adjacent teeth. There are, however, a number of radiographic variants for this lesion. It usually begins as a radiolucency and may achieve a large size during this stage, sometimes producing a multilocular appearance. In the intermediate stage the deposition of cementum, bone, or both in the central area may give rise to radiopaque foci. Displacement of teeth is a fairly consistent feature in any of the stages. Root resorption and obliteration of the root outline are not common.

REFERENCES

Reference Texts

Eversole, L. R.: **Clinical Outline of Oral Pathology.** Philadelphia: Lea & Febiger, 1978, pp. 225–228.

Shafer, W. G., Hine, M. K., and Levy, B. M.: **A Textbook of Oral Pathology,** 3rd Edition. Philadelphia: W. B. Saunders, 1974, pp. 153–154, 267–271, 301–303, 455–456, 637.

Stafne, E. C., and Gibilisco, J. A.: **Oral Radiographic Diagnosis,** 4th Edition. Philadelphia: W. B. Saunders, 1975, pp. 25–27, 128–134.

Wood, N. K., and Goaz, P. W.: **Differential Diagnosis of Oral Lesions.** St. Louis: C. V. Mosby, 1975, pp. 481–492.

Selected References

Cherrick, H. M., King, O. H., Lucatorto, F. M., and Suggs, D. M.: Benign cementoblastoma. **Oral Surg. 37**:54, 1974.

Corio, R. L., Crawford, B. E., and Schaberg, S. J.: Benign cementoblastoma. **Oral Surg. 41**:524, 1976.

Fader, M., Kline, S. N., Spatz, S. S., and Zubrow, H. J.: Gardner's syndrome and a new dental discovery. **Oral Surg. 15**:153, 1962.

Larsson, A., Borsberg, O., and Sjogren, S.: Benign

cementoblastoma — Cementum analogue of benign osteoblastoma? **J. Oral Surg. 36**:299, 1978.

Melrose, R. J., Abrams, A. M., and Mills, B. G.: Florid osseous dysplasia. A clinical pathologic study of 34 cases. **Oral Surg. 41**:62, 1976.

Regezi, J. A., Kerr, D. A., and Courtney, R. M.: Odontogenic tumors: Analysis of 706 cases. **J. Oral Surg. 36**:775, 1978.

Reinagen, W., and Prein, J.: Benign osteoblastoma. **Oral Surg. 39**:279, 1975.

Waldron, C. A., and Giansanti, J. S.: Benign fibro-osseous lesions of the jaws: A clinical radiologic-histologic review of 65 cases. Part II: Benign fibro-osseous lesions of periodontal ligament origin. **Oral Surg. 35**:340, 1973.

Waldron, C. A., Giansanti, J. S., and Browand, B. C.: Sclerotic cemental masses of the jaws (so-called chronic sclerosing osteomyelitis, sclerosing osteitis, multiple enostosis and gigantiform cementoma). **Oral Surg. 39**: 590, 1975.

Chapter 14

Separate, Single, or Multiple Radiopacities

RADIOPACITIES ASSOCIATED WITH THE JAWS
- Exostosis
- Enostosis
- Osteosclerosis
- Osteoma
- Chondrosarcoma
- Osteosarcoma
- Foreign Bodies
- Root Fragments
- Odontoma
- Ameloblastic Odontoma
- Garré's Osteomyelitis

RADIOPACITIES OUTSIDE THE JAWS
- Rhinoliths, Antroliths, Sialoliths
- Soft Tissue Calcifications
- Eagle's Syndrome

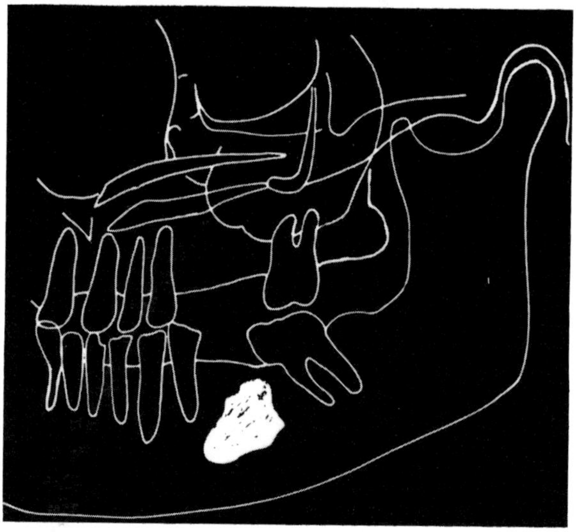

RADIOPACITIES ASSOCIATED WITH THE JAWS

EXOSTOSIS

BRIEF OVERVIEW

Exostoses are bony outgrowths from the outer cortex of the maxilla and mandible. The **torus palatinus** is an exostosis that occurs in the midline of the palate, whereas the **torus mandibularis** appears on the lingual aspect of the mandible in the cuspid-bicuspid area. Except for the torus palatinus, which is a midline structure, exostoses tend to be bilateral and may be lobulated. Clinically, the mucosa is usually intact unless coincidentally traumatized. Exostoses may be composed entirely of cortex like compact bone or there may be a central nidus of spongy bone surrounded by an outer layer of compact bone. The distinction between exostosis, enostosis, osteosclerosis, and osteoma is one of location and description, since the histologic features of these entities are identical.

RADIOGRAPHIC FEATURES (Figs. 14–1 to 14–3)

The torus palatinus is a single midline structure; however, on panoramic films it usually appears as a bilateral radiopacity, often superimposed on both maxillary sinuses, sometimes appearing to fill the entire sinus. One important distinguishing feature is that the anterior aspect of the torus may extend beyond the anterior boundaries of the maxillary sinus.

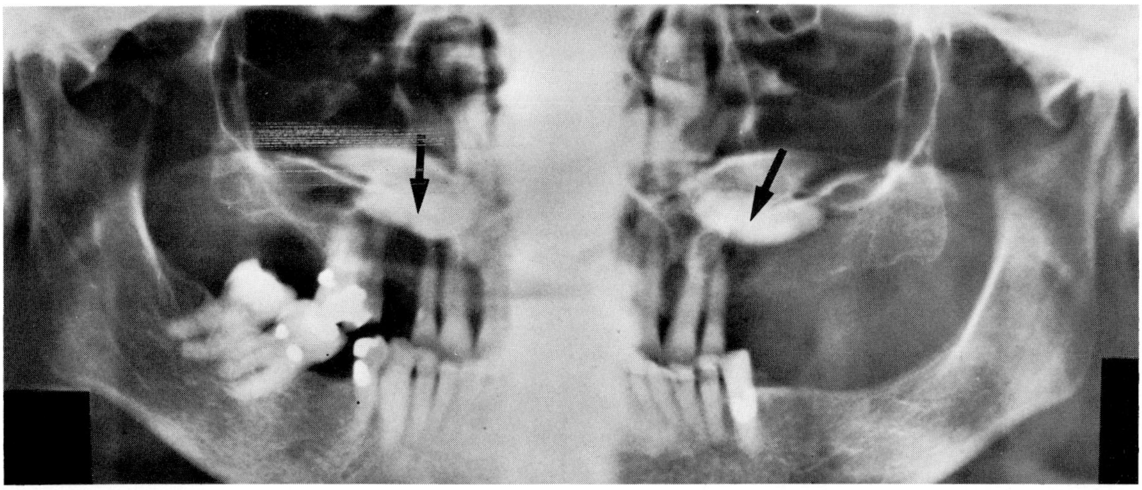

Figure 14–1. Exostosis. Torus palatinus. Note that the use of the SLOB (Same on Lingual (palatal). Opposite on Buccal) rule and movement of the observer's eye confirms the location of this structure on the palatal side. (Courtesy of Dr. Gus Pappas, Columbus, OH.)

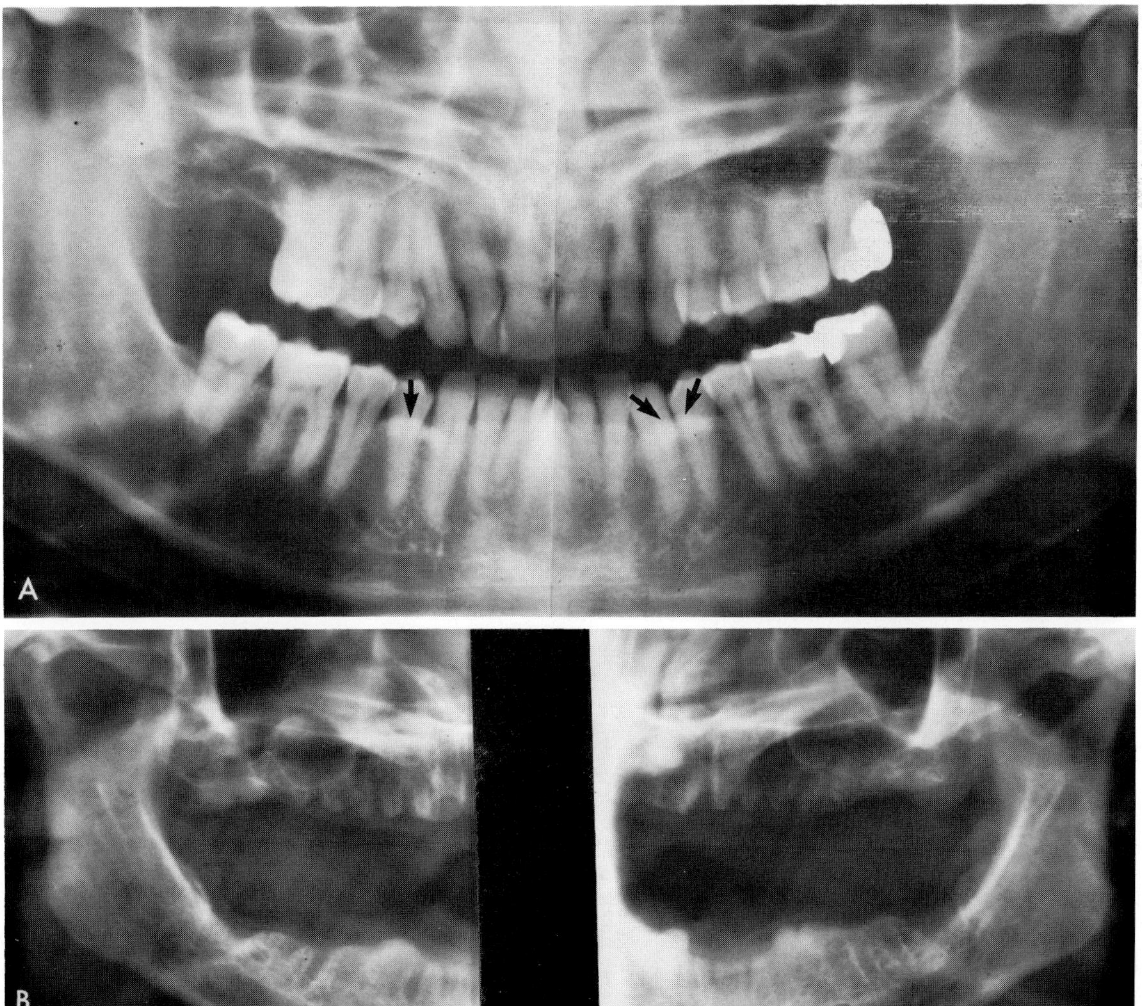

Figure 14–2. Exostoses. Mandibular tori.

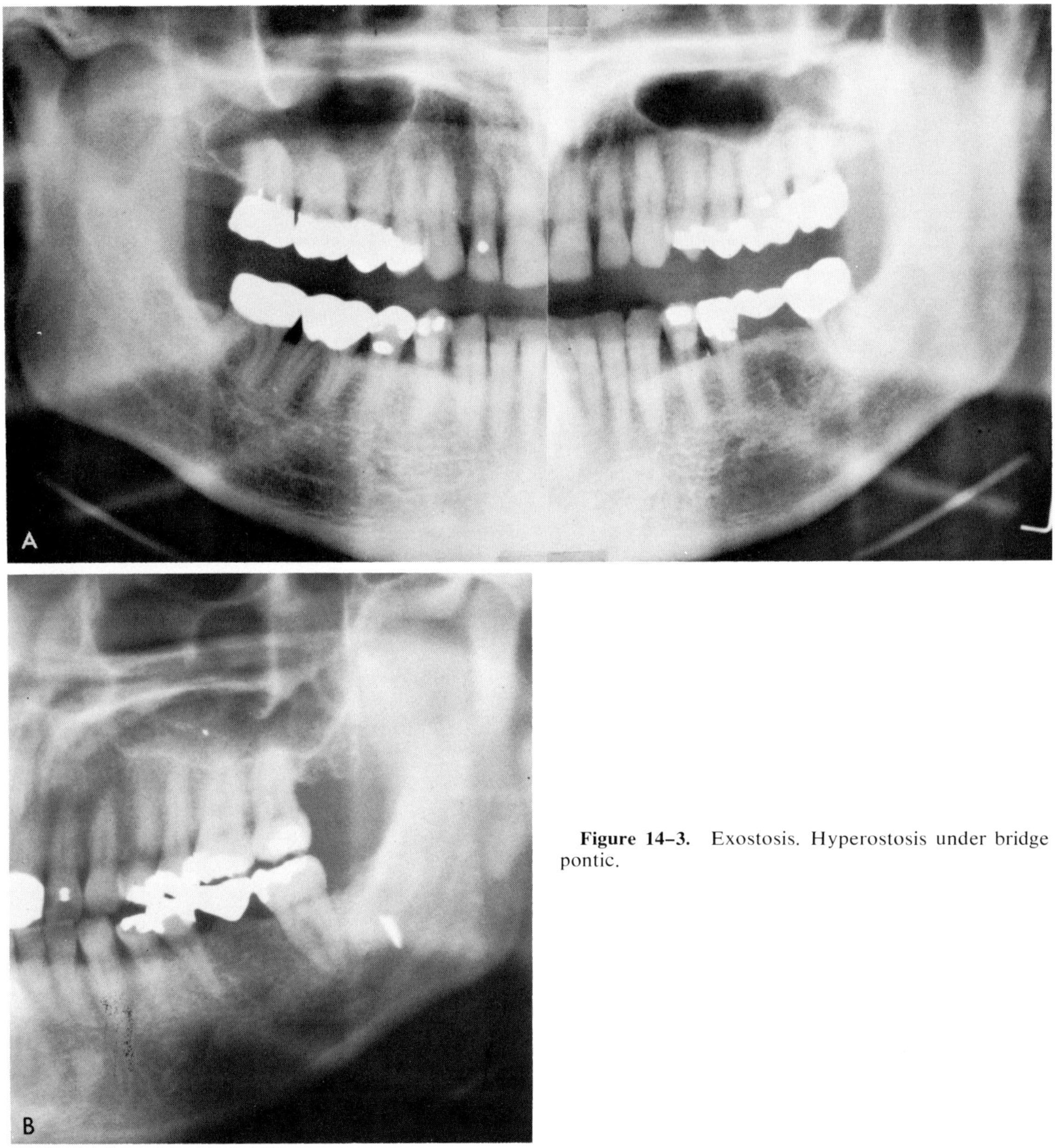

Figure 14–3. Exostosis. Hyperostosis under bridge pontic.

The dense, opaque, midline soft tissue outline of the nose should not be mistaken for a torus palatinus.

The torus mandibularis is often indistinct in panoramic films; its extreme lingual location is often outside the focal trough, and it is, therefore, not visualized. When present on panoramic films, mandibular tori are usually high up on the alveolar process and appear as round, ovoid, or crescent-shaped radiopacities superimposed on the roots of the mandibular cuspid and/or bicuspids. They may be single, lobulated, or multiple and are usually bilateral. Their position high up on the ridge is partly due to their anatomic location and partly due to the angulation (–7 to –15°) of the cone of most panoramic machines. This negative vertical angulation tends to project all structures slightly higher up than they actually are.

One type of exostosis is the so-called **hyperostosis under a bridge pontic**. This is not present when the bridge is placed but develops subsequently. Its etiology is unknown. It may require removal if it enlarges sufficiently to impinge on the pontic and interfere with home care. In this situation, the overlying mucosa may become inflamed, and the patient may complain of pain.

ENOSTOSIS

BRIEF OVERVIEW

Although the existence of enostosis as a separate entity is questioned by some individuals, it is mentioned here simply for completeness. Enostosis refers to an inward growth of compact bone or a mixture of compact and cancellous bone from the inner aspect of the buccal or lingual cortical plate. According to Worth, it occurs more frequently in the mandibular cuspid-bicuspid area, below the apices of these teeth.

RADIOGRAPHIC FEATURES (Fig. 14–4)

The radiographic features of enostosis are indistinguishable from those of osteosclerosis. The distinction is academic, since neither condition requires treatment nor is there any histologic difference between them.

OSTEOSCLEROSIS (Focal Osteopetrosis, Bone Scar, Sclerotic Bone, Socket Sclerosis, Osteopetrotic Scar)

BRIEF OVERVIEW

Osteosclerosis is an area of denser than normal bone. The etiology of this condition remains obscure; some cases represent the bone scar of a healed focal sclerosing osteomyelitis (condensing osteitis), some cases develop in the socket area as an exuberant attempt at repair and are known as socket scleroses, and some cases develop below the tooth-bearing areas and are not associated with any previous known inflammatory or traumatic episode. These areas are all referred to as osteosclerosis by most clinicians, although others, such as Worth, refer to them as enostosis. Suffice it to say that when the sclerotic bone is intimately associated with the apex of a tooth, the condition must be distinguished from focal sclerosing osteomyelitis. This distinction and others have been previously discussed with periapical radiopacities. The mandible is more frequently involved than the maxilla. Osteosclerosis is painless and nonexpansile and does not require treatment.

One important distinction not previously discussed is the significance of **socket sclerosis**. According to Burrell and Goepp, socket sclerosis is probably not found in children, and its presence may be an early sign of gastrointestinal disorders, particularly malabsorption disturbances, or renal disease, especially nephritis and nephrosis.

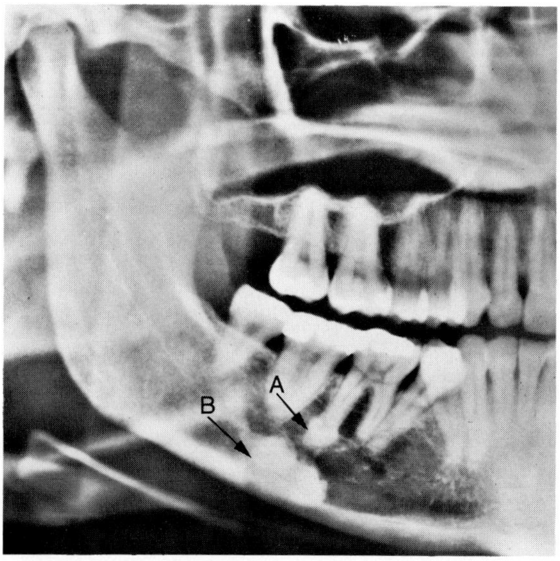

Figure 14–4. Enostosis. A. Periapical idiopathic osteosclerosis. B. Radiopacity compatible with enostosis.

RADIOGRAPHIC FEATURES (Figs. 14–5 to 14–7)

Osteosclerosis consists of round or irregularly shaped radiopaque areas. These appear to be contiguous with the surrounding bone with no radiolucent rim intervening. The areas do not tend to enlarge over the years. Osteosclerosis may be located between teeth, at the apices of teeth, beyond the apices of teeth, and in edentulous areas. When several lesions are present in the same quadrant, especially in edentulous cases, the condition may be difficult to distinguish from chronic diffuse sclerosing osteomyelitis, multiple periapical cemental dysplasias, and Paget's disease on the basis of the panoramic radiograph alone.

Socket sclerosis occurs uniquely in the socket area of previously extracted permanent teeth. A lack of resorption of the lamina dura is the earliest sign. Socket sclerosis begins at the base of the socket and works its way up along the walls, until the entire area previously occupied by the tooth is uniformly opaque and sharply demarcated from the remaining bone by the persistent cortical outline of the socket.

OSTEOMA

BRIEF OVERVIEW

There is some debate as to whether the osteoma is a true neoplasm of bone or if it is simply a developmental anomaly or a variant of

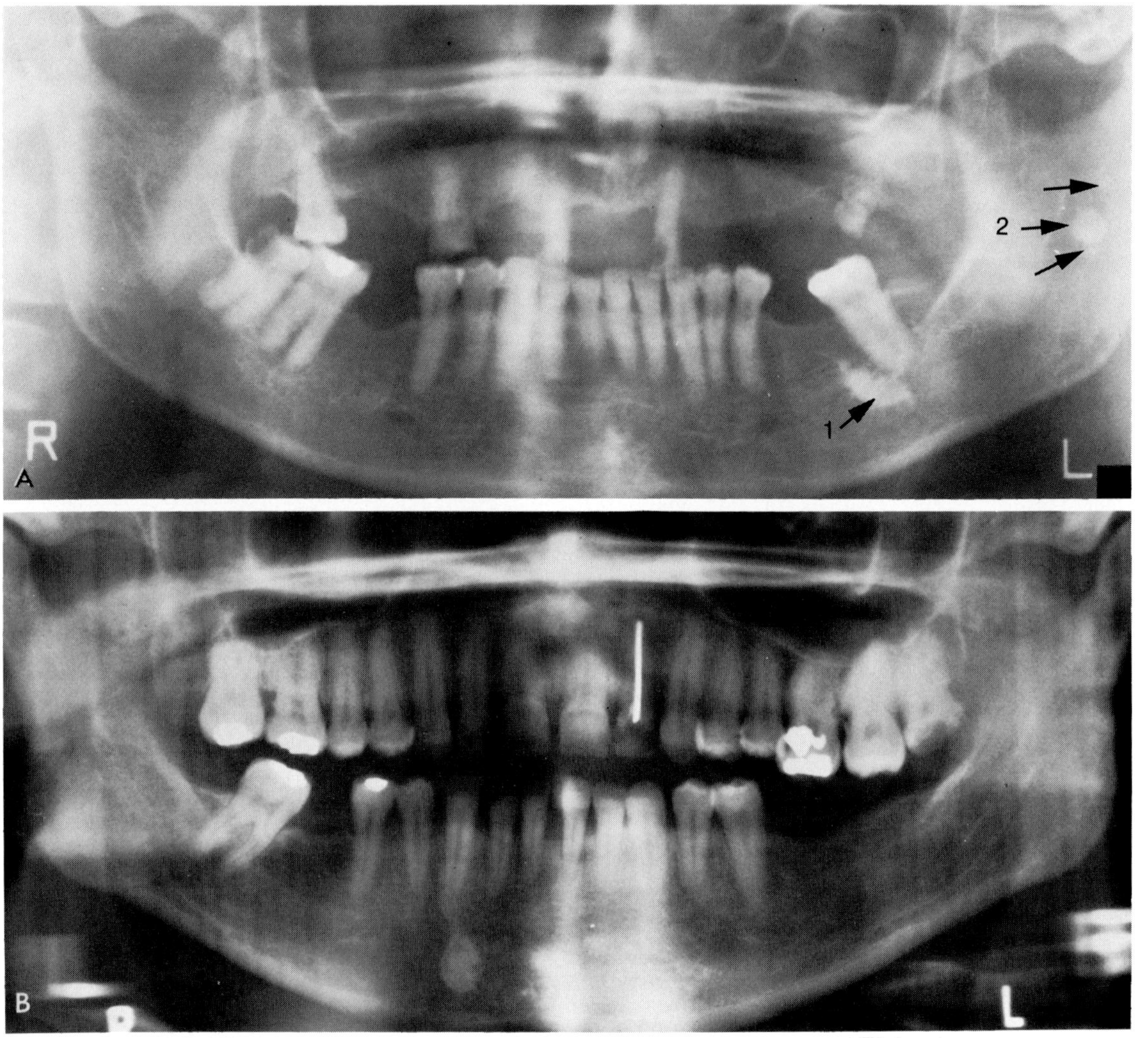

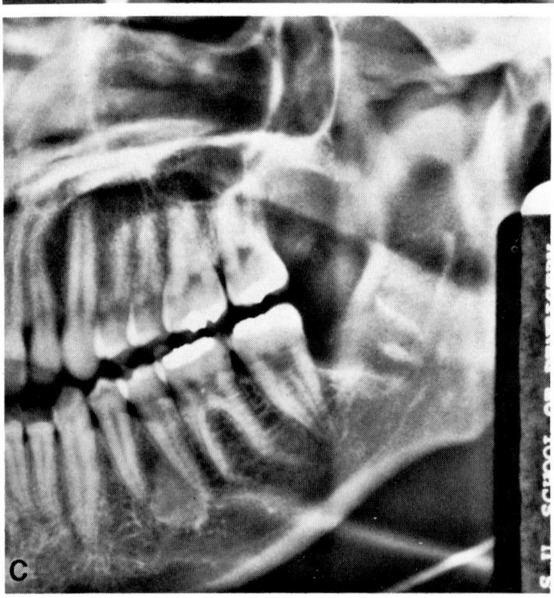

Figure 14–5. Osteosclerosis. **A.** 1. Osteosclerosis. 2. Single or possible multiple radiopacities, which in this area are more likely to consist of parotid salivary calculi or other soft tissue calcifications such as tonsilliths. **B** and **C.** Additional presentations of this condition,

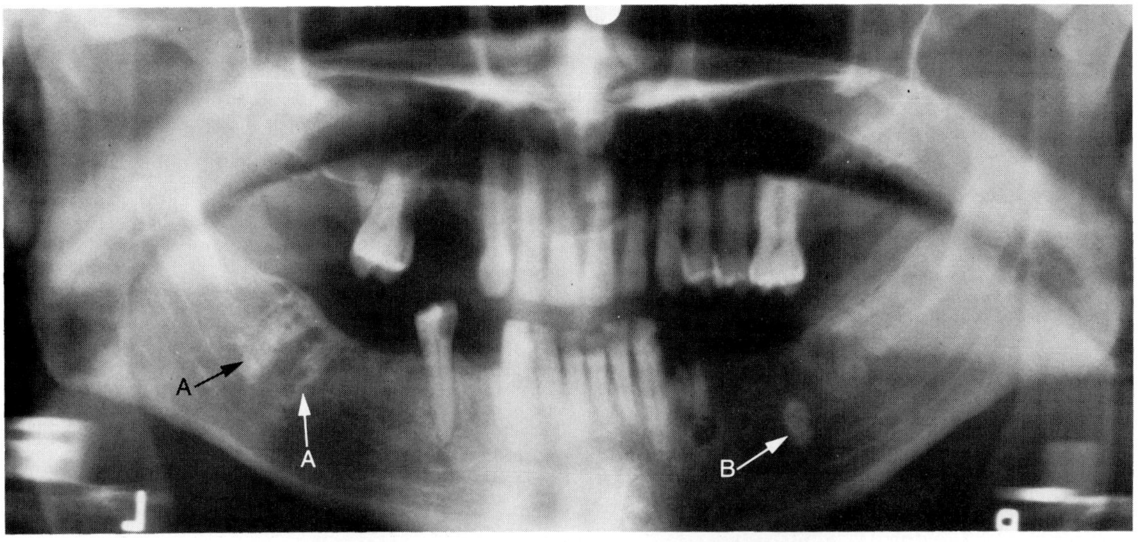

Figure 14–6. A. Socket sclerosis. B. Osteosclerosis.

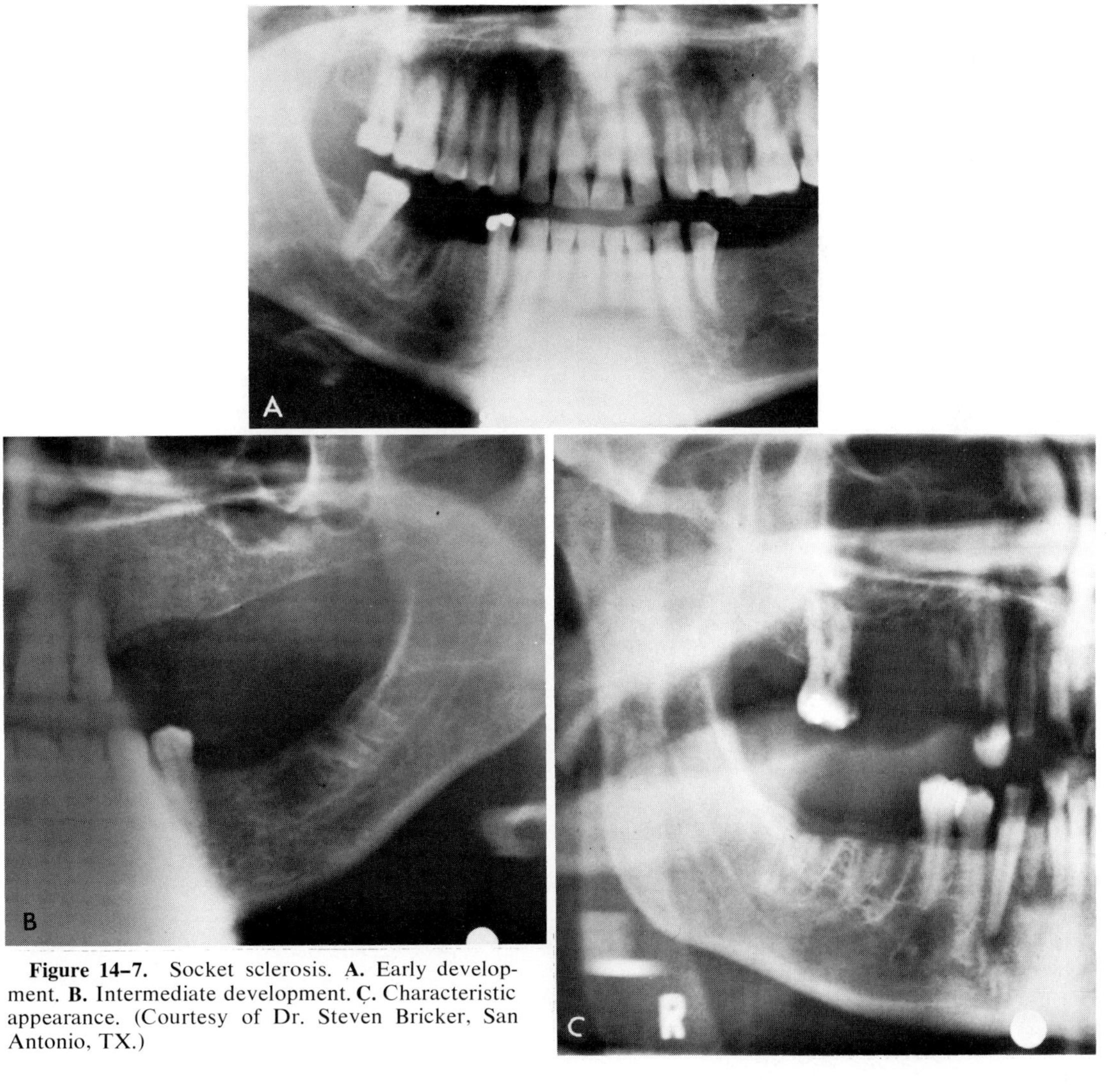

Figure 14–7. Socket sclerosis. **A.** Early development. **B.** Intermediate development. **Ç.** Characteristic appearance. (Courtesy of Dr. Steven Bricker, San Antonio, TX.)

exostosis, enostosis, or osteosclerosis. All of these conditions are identical histologically, and the distinction between them is one of location and description. The osteoma may be located on the outer periosteal surface of the jaws or it may be located endosteally. Osteomas may also be seen in the frontal or maxillary sinuses and in the region of the condyle and may also be located entirely in soft tissue. In a recent review of the literature, Schneider, Dolinsky, and Grodjesk could find only 12 previously reported solitary peripheral osteomas of the jaws. Eleven of the twelve cases occurred in the mandible; three were located in the condylar area. One maxillary osteoma was in the antrum. The presence of osteomas and unerupted supernumerary teeth should alert the clinician to the possible coexistence of **Gardner's syndrome.** Osteomas may be removed when they interfere with normal function or for esthetics when they are sufficiently large to cause a deformity.

RADIOGRAPHIC FEATURES (Fig. 14–8)

Osteomas are usually well-defined, extremely dense radiopacities. They are often round or oval in shape, may be lobulated, tend to have smooth peripheral outlines, and may achieve large proportions. Some may also have a central radiolucent core with a trabecular pattern. When in the periosteal location, they may extend beyond or outside the peripheral outline of the involved bone, whereas in the endosteal location they usually remain within the peripheral outline of the involved bone but may show expansion. In the endosteal location, osteomas may be radiographically indistinguishable from enostoses, osteosclerosis, and chronic diffuse sclerosing osteomyelitis.

A second endosteal manifestation may show diffuse radiopaque mottling of the involved bone over an entire quadrant or even involving the whole bone. In this case, the condition must be distinguished from osteopetrosis, chronic diffuse sclerosing osteomyelitis, and some forms of fibrous dysplasia. A description of the osteomas of Gardner's syndrome may be found in Chapter 7 under Hyperdontia.

CHONDROSARCOMA (Chondrogenic Sarcoma)

BRIEF OVERVIEW

The distinction between chondrosarcoma and chondroblastic osteosarcoma is often histologically difficult yet important as the chondrosarcoma in the jaws is invariably fatal, whereas the chondroblastic osteosarcoma in the jaws may have a 25 to 40 per cent five-year survival rate. Chondrosarcoma occurs mainly in adults over 30 years of age, and, although it is a slow-growing lesion, surgical intervention may stimulate hematogenous metastasis.

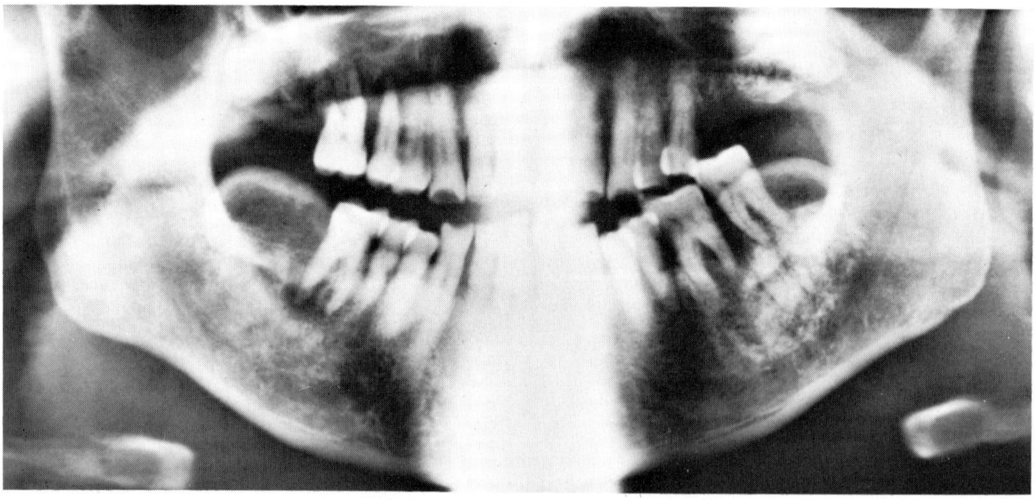

Figure 14–8. Peripheral and central osteomas. Right side: Note the central trabecular pattern and the outer rim of cortical bone. Left side: Note the peripheral portion and underlying central portion, which is producing a diffuse, mottled radiopacity. Proliferation of the osteoma may be the cause of the extrusion of the two molars. Both peripheral osteomas were located on the lingual surface. (Courtesy of Dr. Richard Morse, San Antonio, TX.)

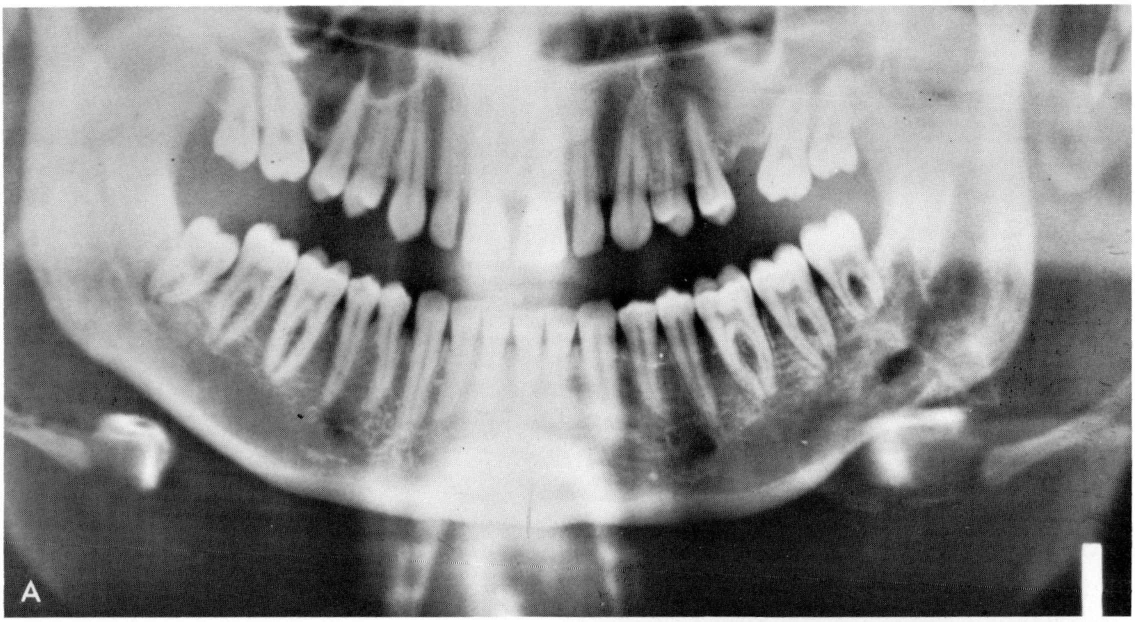

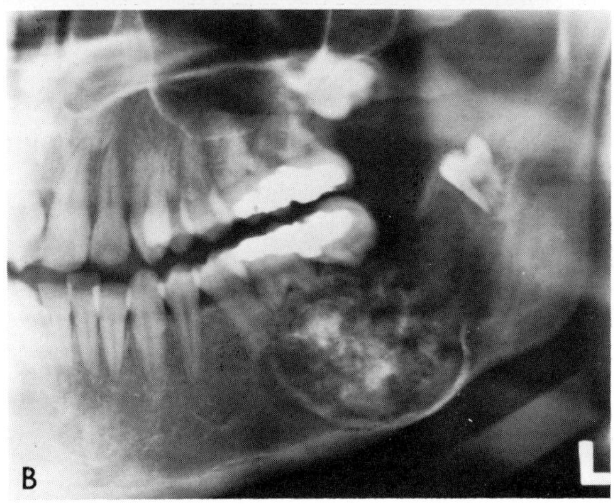

Figure 14–9. Chondrosarcoma. **A.** Courtesy of Dr. Gus Pappas, Columbus, OH. **B.** Courtesy of Dr. Stanley Lovestedt, Rochester, MN.

RADIOGRAPHIC FEATURES (Fig. 14–9)

The chondrosarcoma is a slow-growing tumor, and its radiographic features may resemble those of the chondroma. The lesion generally begins as a radiolucency and soon develops foci of calcification. The calcification may take on a mottled or a linear appearance suggestive of the sunray pattern of some osteosarcomas. The lesion, although often asymtomatic, is usually locally expansile and destructive. Root resorption is often a feature when teeth are present, and displacement of unerupted teeth may occur in younger individuals. The radiographic borders of the chondrosarcoma are usually poorly defined, and early wide excision is recommended. Like osteosarcoma, many early lesions show a smooth but asymmetrical widening of the entire periodontal membrane space about one or several teeth.

OSTEOSARCOMA (Osteogenic Sarcoma)

BRIEF OVERVIEW

Since the osteosarcoma has three histologic sub-types (fibroblastic, chondroblastic, and osteoblastic), this presents some diagnostic problems for the oral pathologist. Of more significance to oral radiologists is the fact that the osteosarcoma may be predominantly sclerosing

1
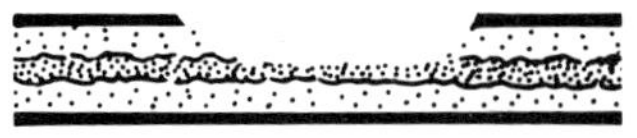

Bone destruction with no periosteal new bone formation.

2
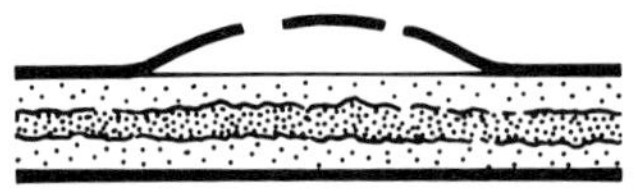

Thin layer of new bone deep to periosteum, but with discontinuities. This is usual, but not invariable; no bone destruction here, but usually present.

3
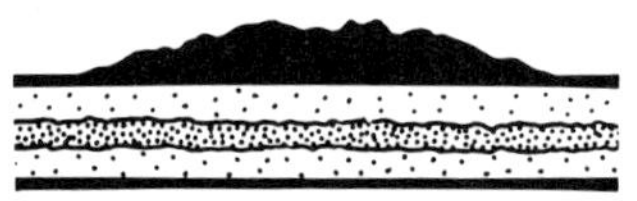

Irregular mass of subperiosteal new bone, usually associated with some bone loss.

4
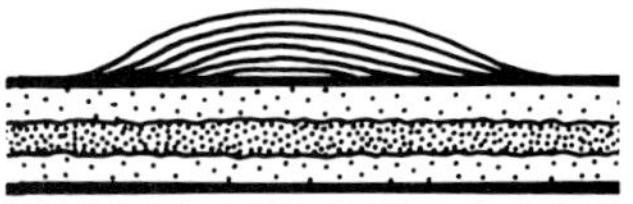

Laminated subperiosteal new bone formation, as is found often in inflammatory conditions.

5
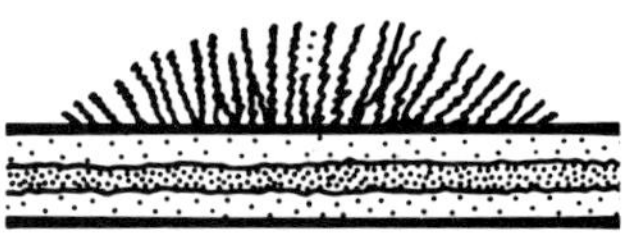

Radiating bony spicules, often regarded as periosteal reaction, but actually a change within tumor itself.

6
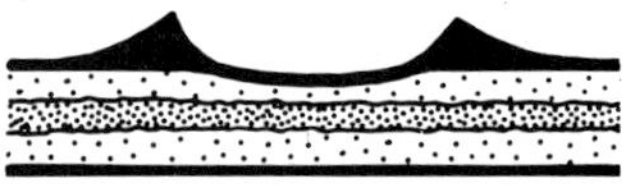

Codman's triangle, an appearance highly suggestive of osteogenic sarcoma. Tumor strips periosteum from bone and new bone is laid down between tumor and attachment of periosteum to bone.

Figure 14–10. Various periosteal reactions in osteogenic sarcoma. (Courtesy of Dr. H. M. Worth, Vancouver, Canada.)

or predominantly lytic in appearance. This lesion occurs most frequently in the long bones, especially the tibia and femur. When the jaws are affected, the most common site is the mandible, with a slight predilection for males in the fourth decade. A previous history of trauma is often present, and symptoms include swelling, pain, paresthesia, and loosening of teeth. There may be a coexistence of Paget's disease or a previous history of radiation therapy for a benign lesion such as fibrous dysplasia. Treatment consists of wide surgical excision.

RADIOGRAPHIC FEATURES (Figs. 14–10 to 14–12)

The lesion is classically described as a radiopacity in the mandibular molar-ramus area in which there is a characteristic sunray arrangement of the neoplastic trabeculae at the periphery. This arrangement is said to occur in about 25 per cent of cases. Early lesions may present an asymptomatic localized symmetric widening of the periodontal ligament space involving one or several teeth. This widening is due to sarcomatous involvement of the periodontal ligament and is similar in appearance to several isolated teeth as seen in scleroderma or acrosclerosis. The sclerosing lesion may be diffusely radiopaque, resembling chronic diffuse sclerosing osteomyelitis or Paget's disease of bone, or there may be radiolucent areas interspersed with radiopaque areas. The lytic variant may produce a poorly defined or moth-eaten radiolucent area resembling chronic osteomyelitis or metastatic disease. In most instances there is expansion, and the border may be poorly defined in one or more areas.

According to Worth, a number of periosteal reactions may be seen in association with osteosarcoma including a cupping out of subperiosteal cortical bone; a thin, bulging, opaque, noncontinuous line of new bone beneath the periosteum; an irregular sclerotic mass of subperiosteal new bone; and multiple laminations of subperiosteal new bone formation at the peripheral margin of the tumor mass. Multiple views supplementing the panoramic radiograph are important, as the identification of any one of these periosteal reactions in association with the central radiographic changes is a critical step in establishing a differential diagnosis, since the central bone changes are in themselves highly nonspecific and may resemble a variety of other lesions.

FOREIGN BODIES

BRIEF OVERVIEW

Foreign metallic objects within the hard and soft tissues in the region of the jaws are easily identified when seen on panoramic films. Because of the focal trough, however, a lack of foreign bodies on panoramic film does not necessarily rule out their presence. Foreign bodies include various dental materials and instruments, the most common of these being

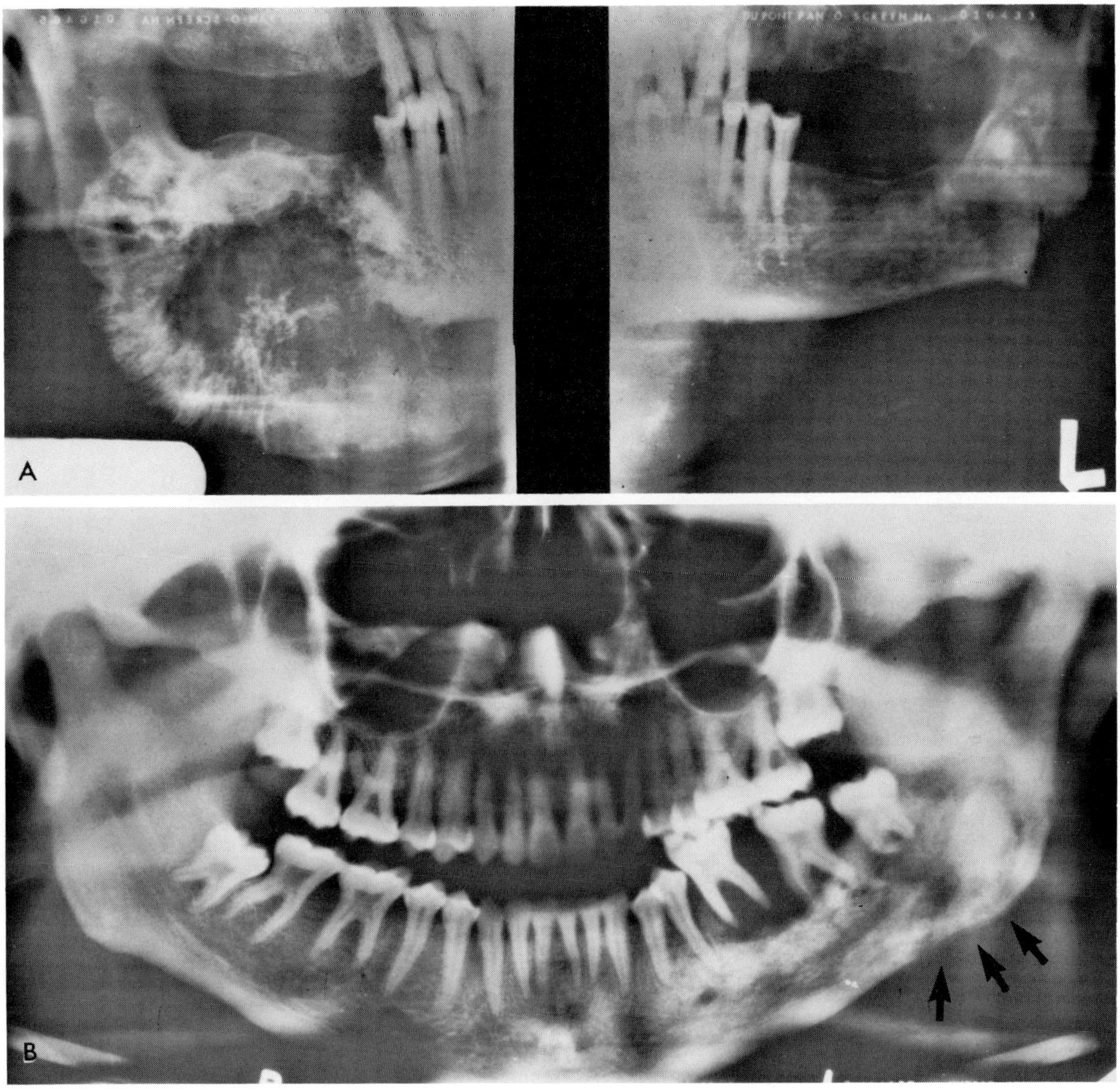

Figure 14–11. Osteogenic sarcoma. **A.** Courtesy of Dr. Doug Stoneman, Toronto, Canada. **B.** Lytic variant. Note the faint periosteal reaction at the inferior border of the mandible (arrows). (Courtesy of Dr. Chris Nortjé, University of Stellenbosch, Tygerberg, South Africa.)

amalgam, which often drops into the socket during the extraction of a tooth. Others include gutta percha, silver points, broken dental instruments, and needles. Additionally, shotgun pellets, bullets, and other metallic fragments are seen. Leaded glass from automobiles can also be identified. Any number of other foreign objects may be visualized such as radon seeds, nose jewelry, and hearing aids. Questioning the patient often helps identify the nature of the object. Objects located in soft tissue, when superimposed on bony structures, will appear to be embedded in bone. Use of the buccal-object rule and other localization techniques is helpful. Characteristic linear ghost images of metallic objects may be seen on the contralateral side. Evidence of reactivity of bone in association with a foreign object warrants further investigation and possible removal of the object.

RADIOGRAPHIC FEATURES (Figs. 14–13 to 14–19)

The radiographic features vary with the nature of the object. Ghost images are not always present. The authors have included a representative sampling of commonly encountered foreign bodies.

Text continued on page 350

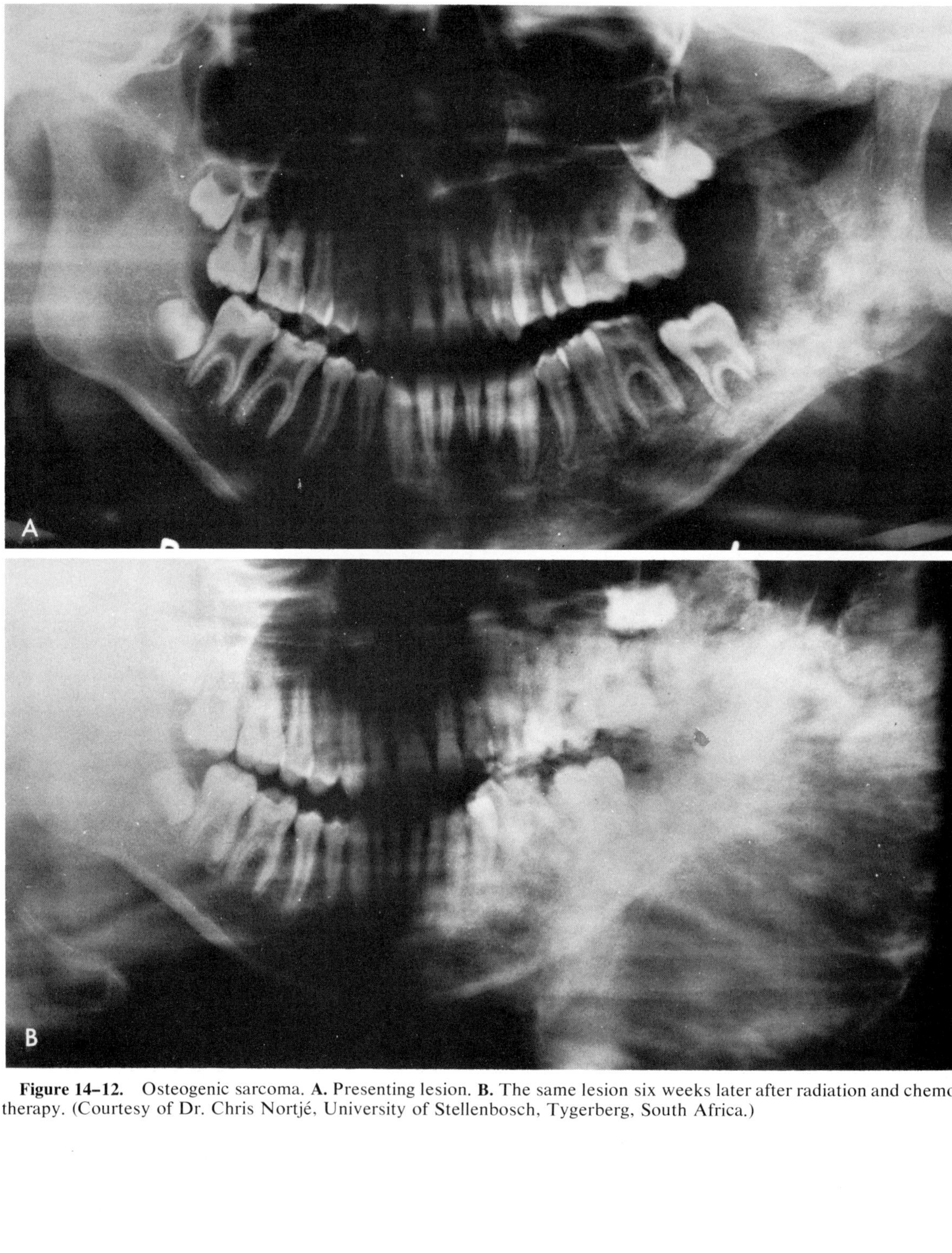

Figure 14–12. Osteogenic sarcoma. **A.** Presenting lesion. **B.** The same lesion six weeks later after radiation and chemotherapy. (Courtesy of Dr. Chris Nortjé, University of Stellenbosch, Tygerberg, South Africa.)

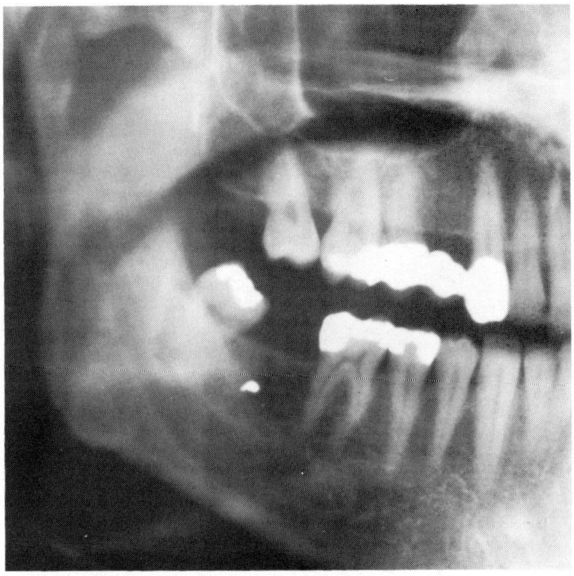

Figure 14–13. Amalgam fragment.

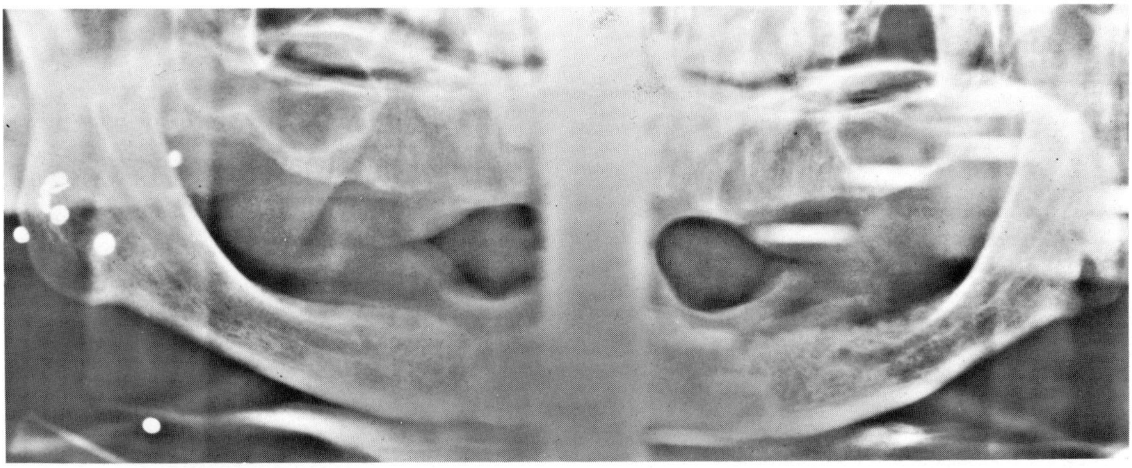

Figure 14–14. Buckshot. Note the linear horizontal ghost images on the left side.

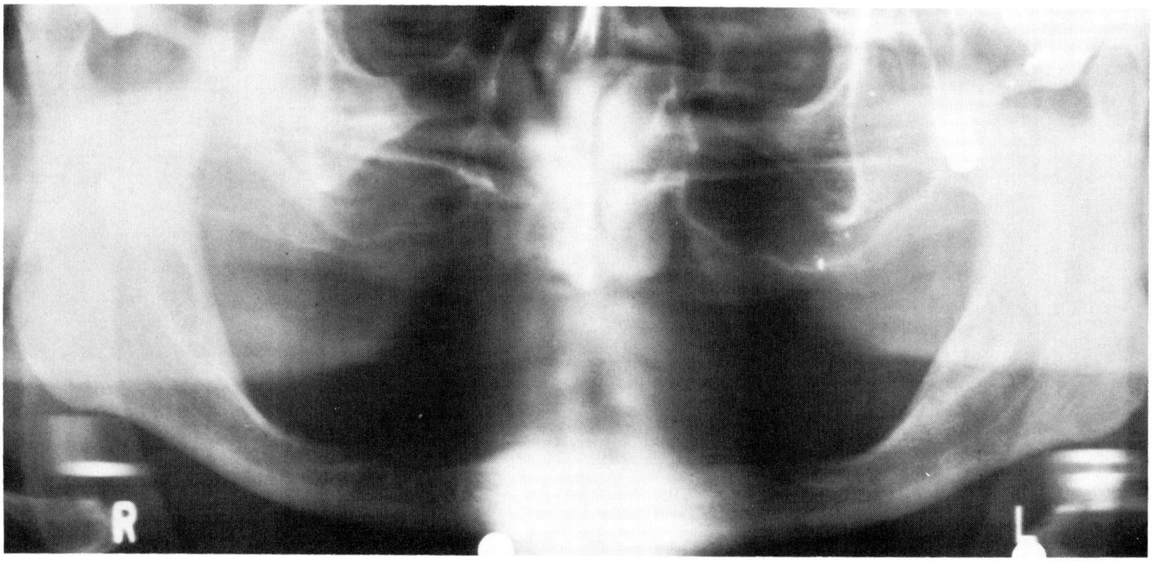

Figure 14–15. Bullet. Note that the bullet struck the left zygomatic arch and subsequently lodged between the posterior wall of the maxillary sinus and the lateral pterygoid plate, just beneath the pterygomaxillary fissure.

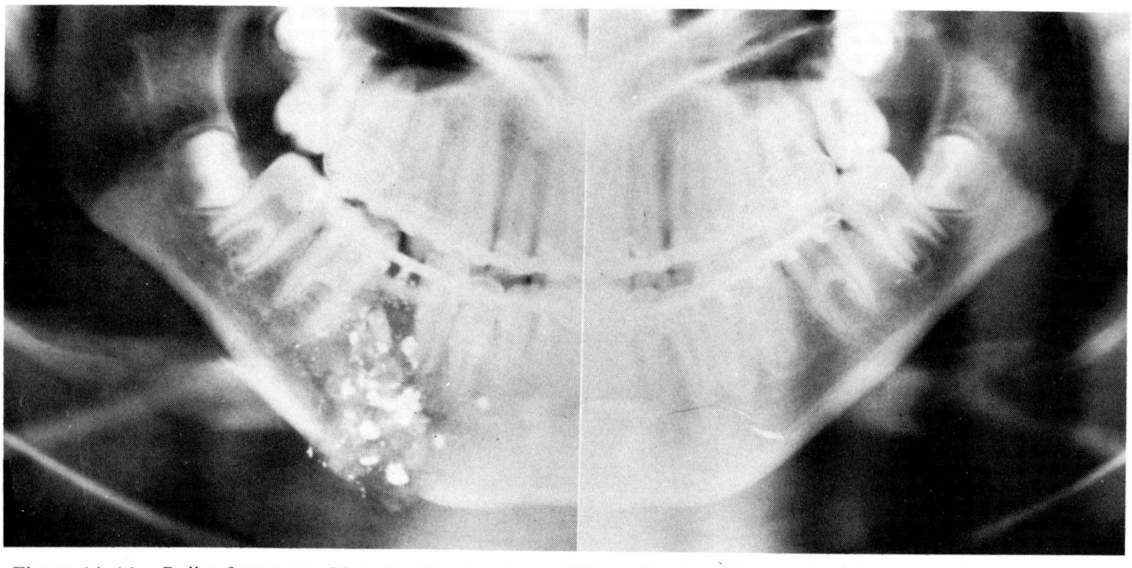

Figure 14–16. Bullet fragments. Note the fractured mandible at the site of impact in this 12-year-old boy. (Courtesy of Drs. Frank Sammis, Jr. and Carlos Portales, San Antonio, TX.)

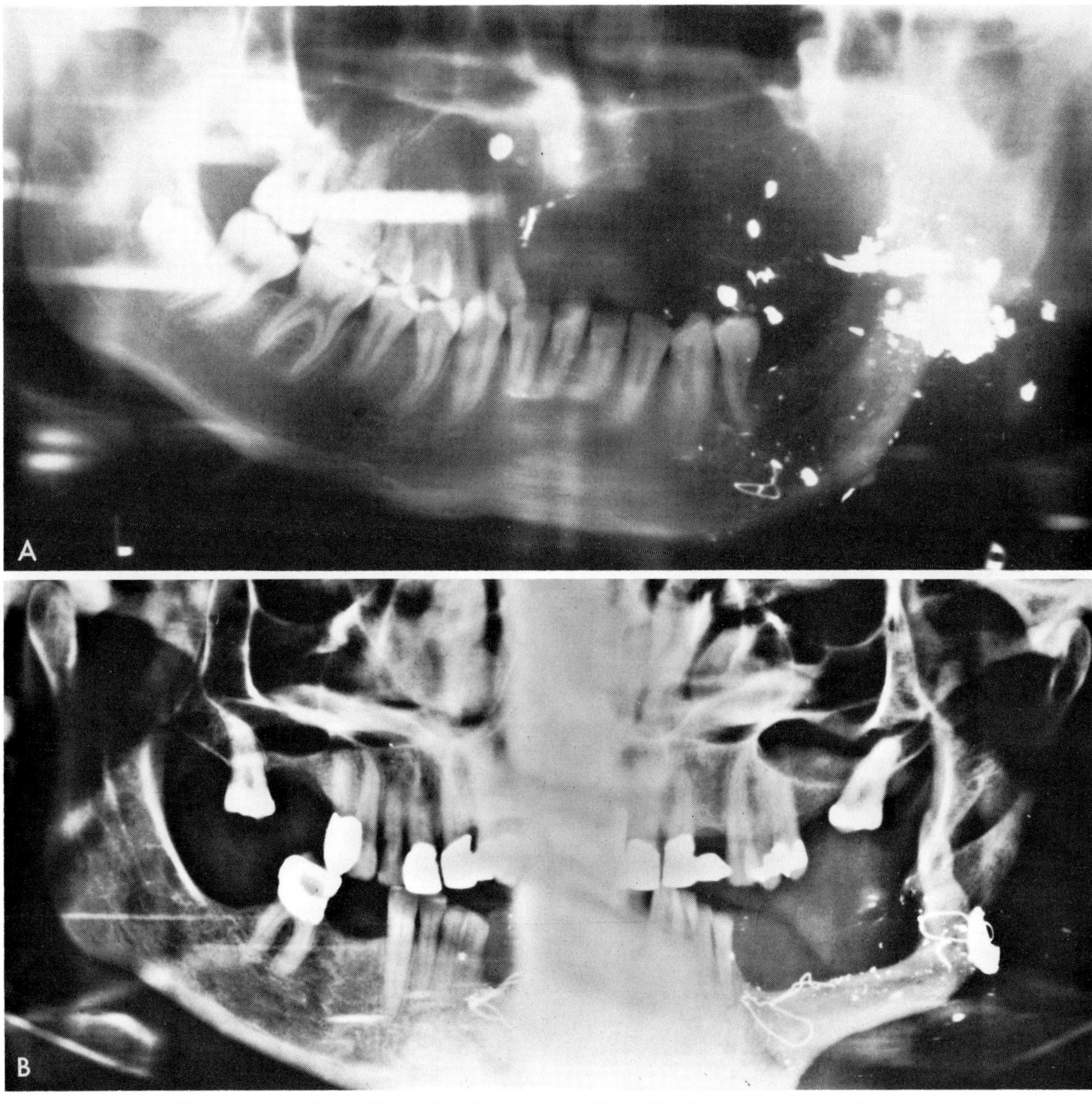

Figure 14–17. Shotgun wound. **A.** The patient is 14 years old. **B.** Healed gunshot wound.

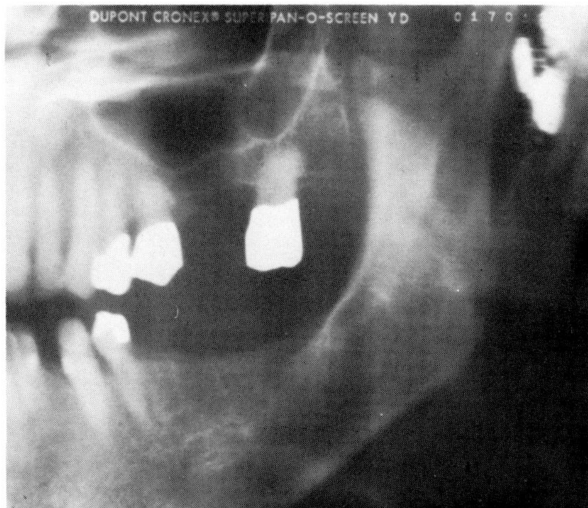

Figure 14–18. Hearing aid.

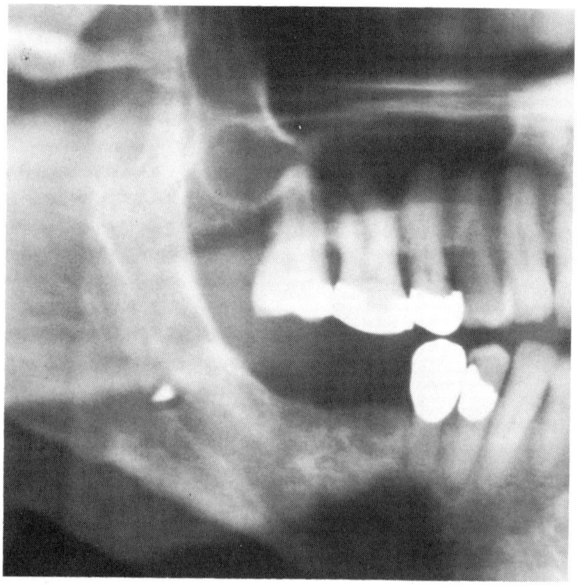

Figure 14–19. Foreign body. The associated radiolucency is an indication for possible removal. The location of the object in close proximity to the mandibular canal warrants further localization procedures preoperatively.

ROOT FRAGMENTS

BRIEF OVERVIEW

Root fragments are seen in areas previously occupied by teeth. They may occasionally be seen in the maxillary sinus. Root fragments of primary teeth may be present, especially mesial and distal to the second bicuspid roots. These may occur idiopathically in one, several, or all quadrants in the same individual, and their presence is not necessarily an indication of iatrogenic dentistry or a previous difficult extraction. Retained root tips that extend to or beyond the crest of the ridge should probably be removed surgically, especially if a prosthesis is planned. If the root tip is buried in bone and if there is no radiographic or clinical evidence of associated pathology, it may be left alone and observed periodically.

RADIOGRAPHIC FEATURES (Figs. 14–20 to 14–22)

Classically, root tips are distinguished from the radiographic appearance of socket sclerosis and osteosclerosis by the presence of a periodontal membrane space and a root canal space. When the root tip is completely ankylosed and if the root canal space has been obliterated, it may be difficult to distinguish a root tip from socket sclerosis or osteosclerosis. It is important to make this distinction with additional intraoral periapical films, since root tips contiguous with the crest of the ridge should be extracted, whereas socket sclerosis need not be treated. It is important to recognize socket sclerosis, as it may be associated with intestinal malabsorption and renal problems.

Root tips in the maxillary sinus can sometimes be identified by their shape and by the presence of a root canal space. Over the years, root fragments in the sinus may serve as a nidus

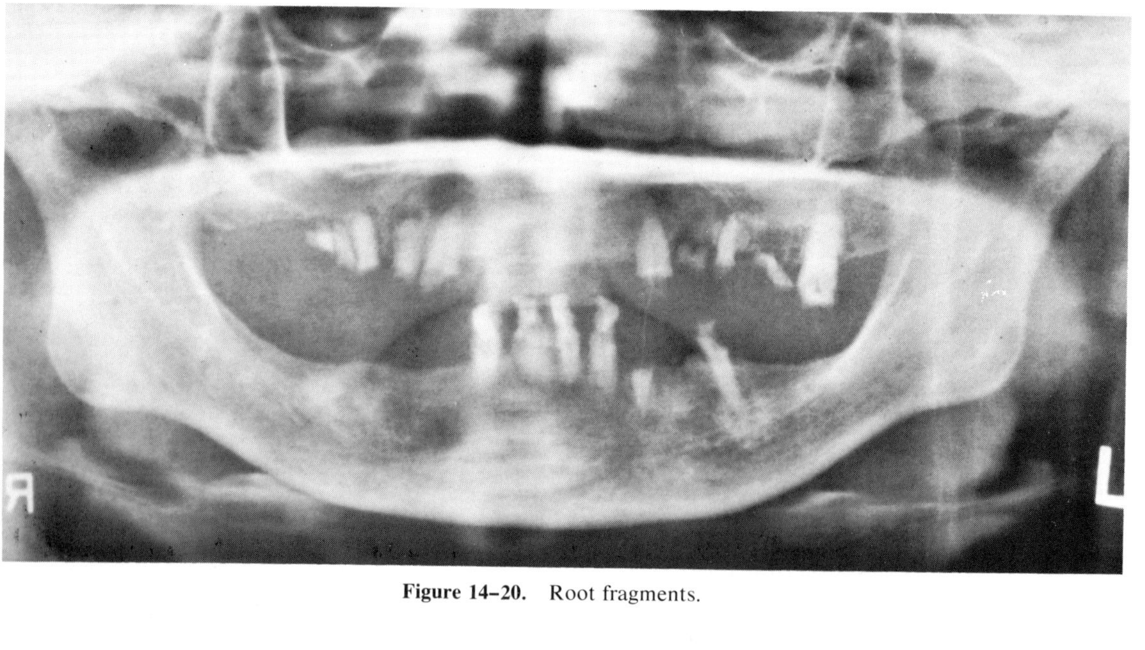

Figure 14–20. Root fragments.

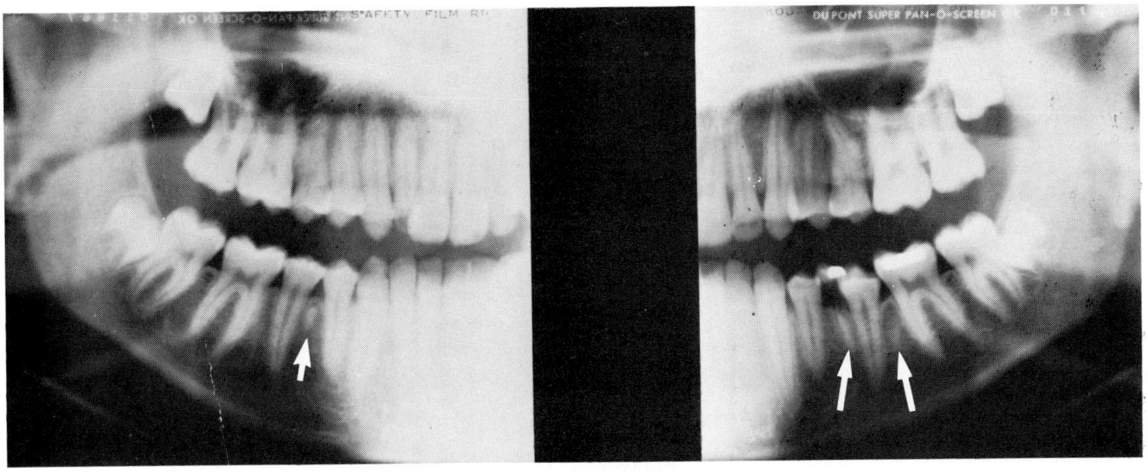

Figure 14–21. Retained primary root tips.

for antrolith formation. Root fragments in the maxillary antrum may resemble antroliths, small osteomas, or superimposed soft tissue calcifications such as phleboliths, miliary osteomas, and calcified scars.

ODONTOMA

BRIEF OVERVIEW

The odontoma occurs mainly during the ages of tooth development, including third molars. According to an analysis of 706 odontogenic tumors by Regezi, Kerr, and Courtney, 67 per cent were odontomas, making this the most common odontogenic neoplasm in their series. This neoplasm is capable of elaborating dental tissues such as dentin, pulp, and cementum. Additionally, the presence of enamel or enamel matrix is required to differentiate this condition from a dentinoma, which is a much less common occurrence.

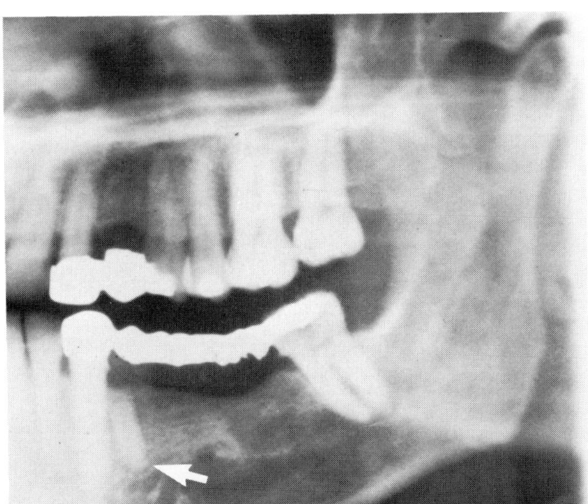

Figure 14–22. Retained root tip.

Odontomas have been separated into two types: **compound odontoma,** which may produce toothlike structures, and **complex odontoma**, which produces a jumbled mass of dental tissues that do not resemble teeth.

RADIOGRAPHIC FEATURES (Figs. 14–23 to 14–26)

The compound odontoma usually consists of a central area containing several to dozens of toothlike shapes. These are usually surrounded by a 2- to 3-mm radiolucent area, which corresponds to the follicular sac. The complex odontoma consists of a hodge-podge of radiopaque material that is usually a single homogenous mass. At times this homogenous mass may have a sunray or sunburst pattern of radiating radiopaque lines. Odontomas are often associated with impacted teeth, particularly third molars. Odontomas have erupted in rare instances. In a recent review of 149 cases, Budnick reported that 67 per cent of odontomas occurred in the maxilla. He also reported a marked predilection for compound odontomas in the anterior maxilla, whereas complex odontomas tend to occur in the posterior jaws.

Like a developing tooth, odontomas may be radiolucent in the early stages; they then develop small foci of radiopaque material as enamel and dentin are elaborated, and the foci become predominantly radiopaque in the mature lesion.

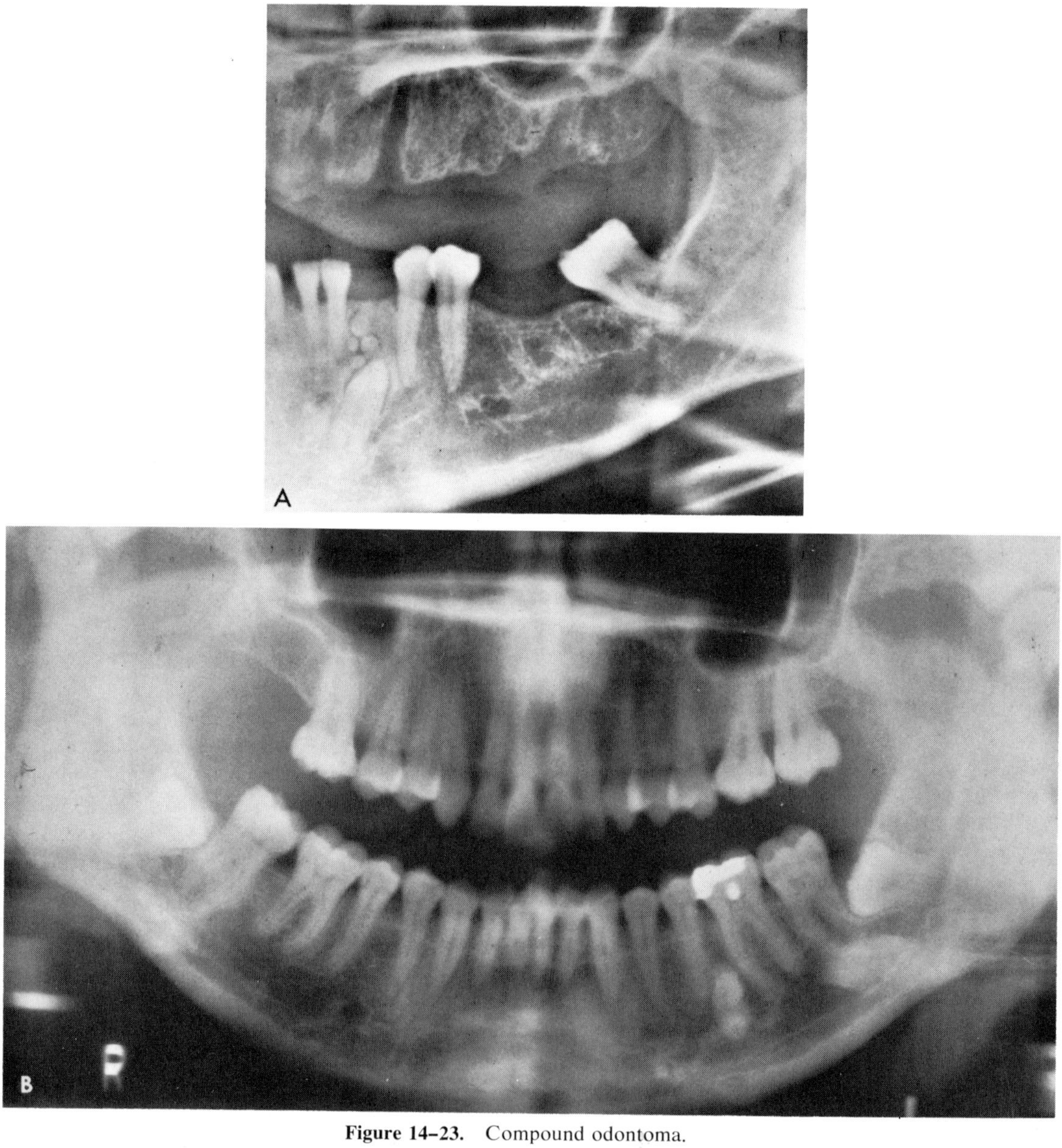

Figure 14–23. Compound odontoma.

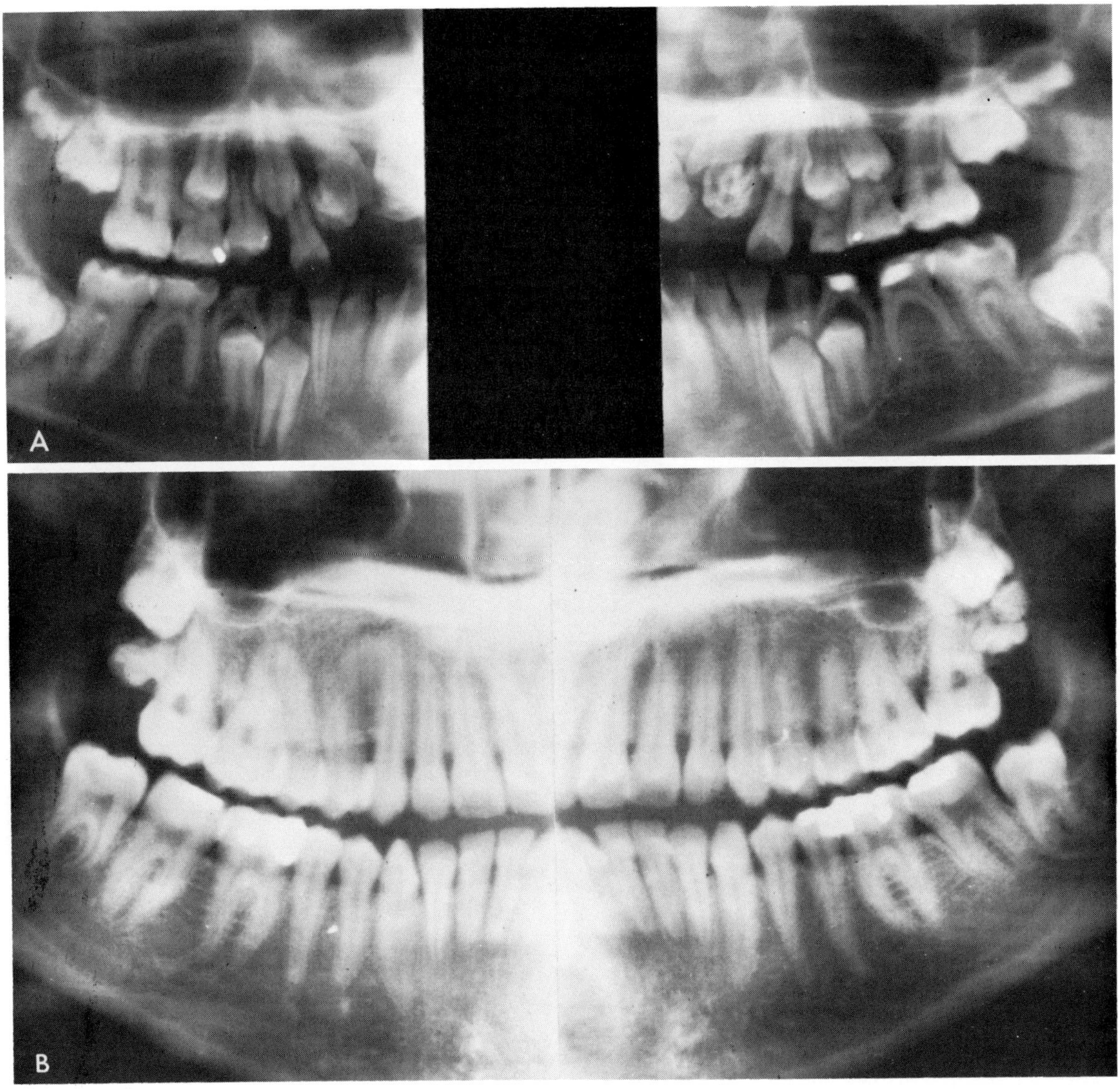

Figure 14–24. Bilateral compound odontomas.

Figure 14–25. Developing complex odontoma. (Courtesy of Dr. Gus Pappas, Columbus, OH.)

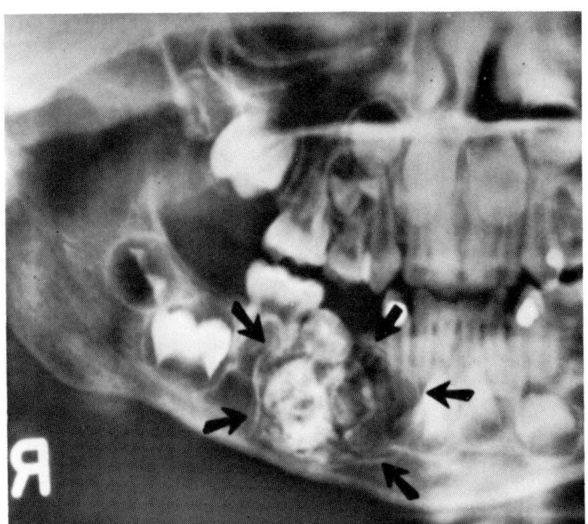

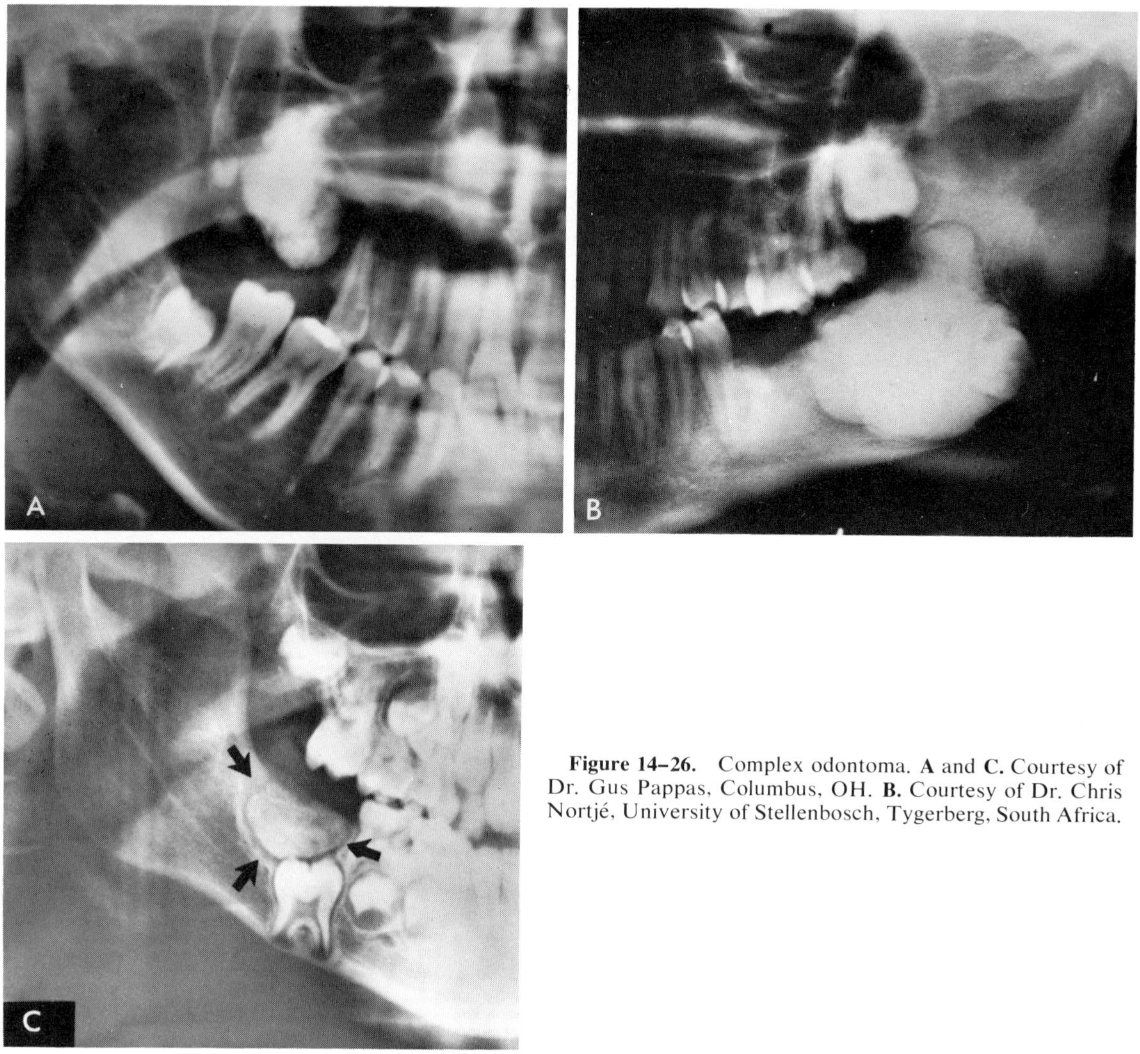

Figure 14–26. Complex odontoma. **A** and **C.** Courtesy of Dr. Gus Pappas, Columbus, OH. **B.** Courtesy of Dr. Chris Nortjé, University of Stellenbosch, Tygerberg, South Africa.

Small, squashed radiolucent lines seen within the complex homogenous mass probably represent pulp tissue spaces and may resemble the parallel striae seen in some hemangiomas. Some odontomas may be radiographically indistinguishable from other odontogenic neoplasms such as ameloblastic odontoma, ameloblastic fibro-odontoma, ameloblastic fibrodentinoma, Pindborg tumor (when calcified), and adenomatoid odontogenic tumor (when calcified). The latter two conditions also may be associated with impacted teeth.

AMELOBLASTIC ODONTOMA (Odontoameloblastoma)

BRIEF OVERVIEW

Although the occurrence of this lesion is infrequent, it is mentioned here to emphasize the fact that this neoplasm should always be considered in the differential diagnosis of an odontoma. The ameloblastic odontoma probably occurs more frequently in the mandible in children. When left untreated, the lesion may be expansile, and some pain may develop. Since this lesion behaves like an ameloblastoma, the philosophy of treatment and subsequent radiographic follow-up should be the same as that for an ameloblastoma.

RADIOGRAPHIC FEATURES (Fig. 14–27)

This lesion may resemble a compound odontoma, a complex odontoma, a pericoronal radiolucency with flecks of calcification, a multilocular radiolucency, or a central radiolucency with varying degrees of calcification. Larger lesions tend to be expansile and more destructive looking with scalloped or infiltrating bor-

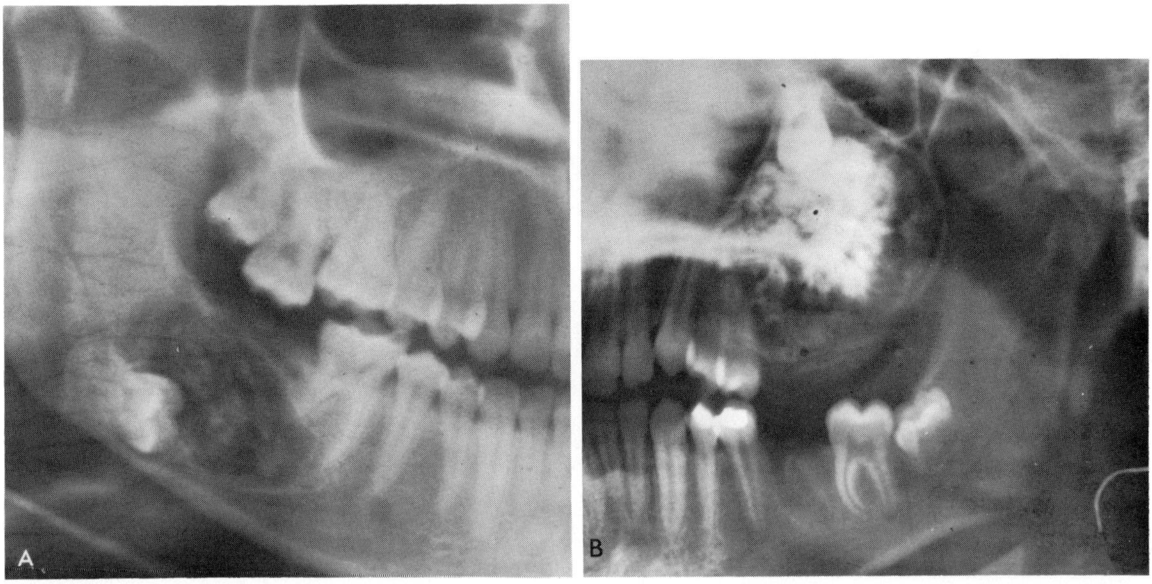

Figure 14–27. Ameloblastic odontoma. **A.** Note that the criss-cross radiolucent lines on the right ramus are artifacts. **B.** Courtesy of Dr. Doug Stoneman, Toronto, Canada.

ders. The radiolucent component may become much more prominent than the radiopaque component in larger lesions. Certainly, a clinical impression of cystic odontoma, especially in the mandible of a young patient, should lead one to include this lesion in the differential diagnosis.

GARRÉ'S OSTEOMYELITIS (Proliferative Periostitis, Garré's Periostitis)

BRIEF OVERVIEW

The most common type of periostitis is Garré's osteomyelitis, and the eponym is probably a misnomer. Perhaps a more appropriate term might be **juvenile periostitis of the mandible**. The condition occurs mainly in children up to adolescence and almost exclusively affects the mandible. There is usually a pulpally involved mandibular first molar or an infected operculum associated with an erupting first or second permanent molar. There is often a bone-hard facial swelling on the affected side, and there is characteristically no depth to the mucobuccal fold adjacent to the affected area. There may be a low-grade fever, but pain is not usually a feature. The pathogenesis consists of subperiosteal new bone deposition stimulated by the inflammatory process. Treatment consists of extraction of the offending tooth or management of the operculitis. In either case, supplementation with antibiotic therapy may be helpful. In no instance has endodontic therapy ever been reported to have been attempted as a treatment for this condition. Resolution usually occurs within one year.

Periostitis may also occur in adults secondary to osteomyelitis or tuberculous or syphilitic involvement of the jaws or as a result of the use of nonsterile surgical instruments. A periosteal reaction may also occur in association with certain neoplasms such as Ewing's sarcoma or osteogenic sarcoma.

RADIOGRAPHIC FEATURES (Fig. 14–28)

Juvenile periostitis produces a characteristic laminated pattern of radiopaque layers of varying density and thickness at the inferior border of the mandible, often described as an onion-skin pattern. The peripheral outline is usually evenly convex in shape. Characteristically, there is an absence of expansion or destruction of the underlying cortical bone of the inferior border of the mandible. An abscessed mandibular first molar or primary molar is most often present. A similar onion-skin pattern may be seen in Ewing's sarcoma, a rapidly fatal disease, which tends to occur in the same age group and may present clinically as a rapidly enlarging unilateral facial swelling. Similar findings may also be present in association with osteosarcoma. Other central bony findings, suggesting the presence of a neoplasm, are usually present in Ewing's sarcoma and osteosarcoma.

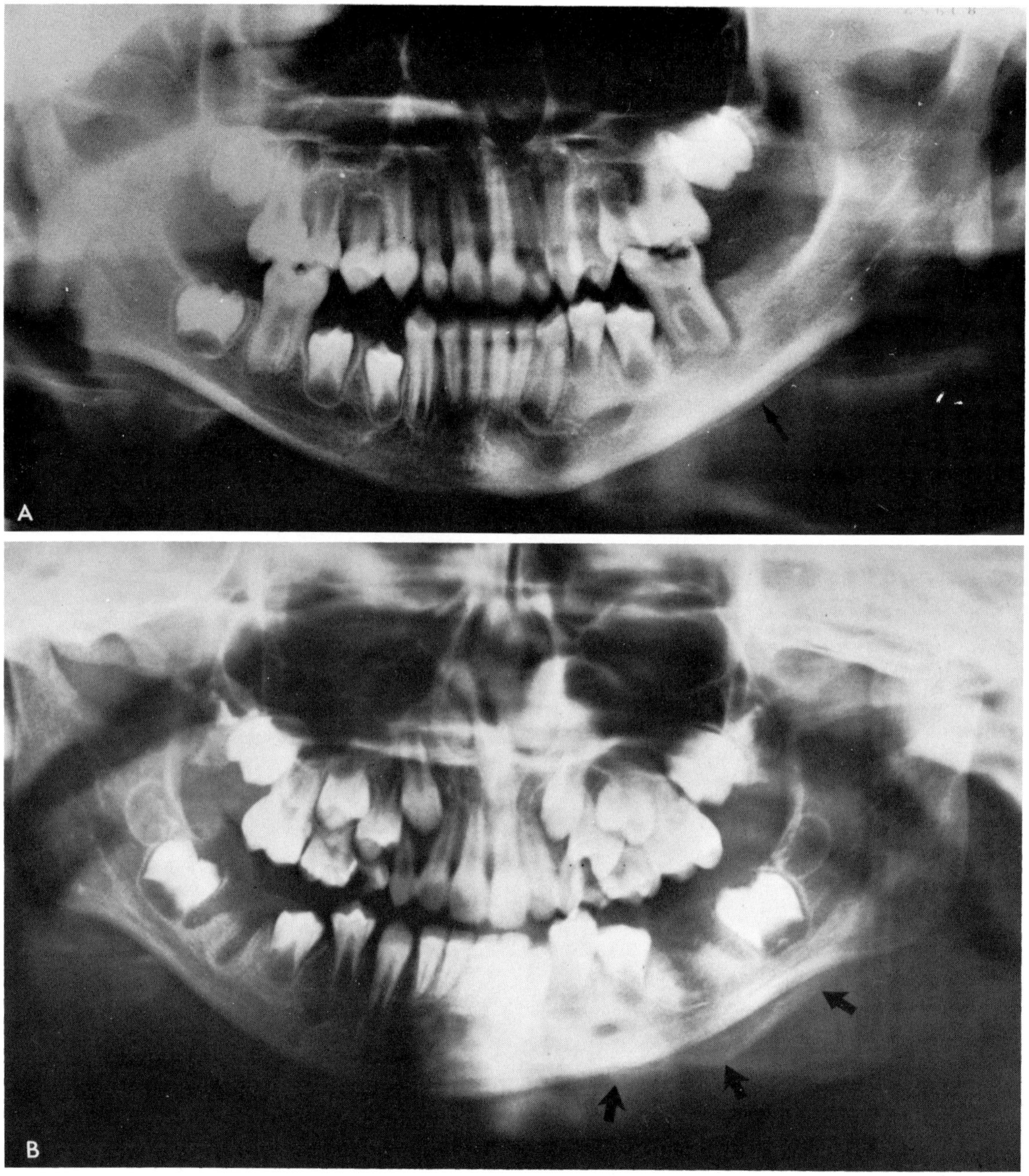

Figure 14–28. Garré's osteomyelitis. **A.** Courtesy of Dr. Chris Nortjé, University of Stellenbosch, Tygerberg, South Africa. **B.** The source of inflammation was an abscessed lower left first permanent molar, which has been extracted. No further treatment was necessary. (Courtesy of Dr. Gus Pappas, Columbus, OH.)

RADIOPACITIES OUTSIDE THE JAWS

RHINOLITHS, ANTROLITHS, SIALOLITHS

BRIEF OVERVIEW

Rhinoliths, antroliths, and sialoliths are calcified masses in the nasal cavity, maxillary antrum, and major or minor salivary glands, respectively. Antroliths may, upon occasion, block the osteum of the maxillary sinus, preventing normal sinus drainage. Sialoliths may, on occasion, block salivary gland secretions. When these calcified masses are associated with symptoms, they should be removed. When salivary calculi are located in the hilum of the involved gland, their removal will usually necessitate removal of the gland. Salivary calculi located in the duct of the gland may sometimes be removed without sacrificing the gland. When counseling patients concerning the removal of a major salivary gland it is important to note that the three pairs of major salivary glands together produce approximately 50 per cent of the total volume of saliva, and the minor salivary glands produce the remaining 50 per cent.

RADIOGRAPHIC FEATURES (Figs. 14–29 to 14–32)

A rhinolith is a round or ovoid opaque mass in the nasal cavity. When seen on panoramic films, it may resemble an osteoma or a migrated tooth. The supernumerary mesiodens, when inverted, may sometimes erupt into the floor of the nose and resemble a rhinolith.

Antroliths are often small, ovoid, opaque masses and may resemble retained roots, osteomas, migrated third molars, or superimposed soft tissue calcifications. These are further discussed in Chapter 16.

Submaxillary sialoliths may be superimposed upon the mandible and may resemble osteomas, osteosclerosis, or soft tissue calcifications buccal or lingual to the mandible such as a calcified lymph node or phlebolith. When located in the hilum of the gland, they are usually seen at the inferior border of the mandible in the third molar-ramus area. They may or may not appear to contact the mandible. Parotid calculi are usually seen about halfway up on the ramus and may be multiple. Suspected salivary calculi should be further studied with sialography, a procedure in which panoramic radiography may be used. Radiolucent, poorly calcified calculi and mucous plugs are best visualized by sialography. The presence of calcified salivary calculi cannot be ruled out by panoramic films alone, since the stone may not fall within the focal trough of the machine used.

SOFT TISSUE CALCIFICATIONS

BRIEF OVERVIEW

It is the authors' contention that soft tissue calcifications are seen much less frequently in panoramic radiography, once again due to the fact that it is the deeper bony structures that tend to be visualized within the sharply depicted layer. However, they can and do occur, and the authors will present a brief summary.

Phleboliths are calcified thrombi and are most likely to be seen in association with a hemangioma. Other dystrophic calcifications include calcified lymph nodes and may be a sign of previous disease such as tuberculous lymphad-

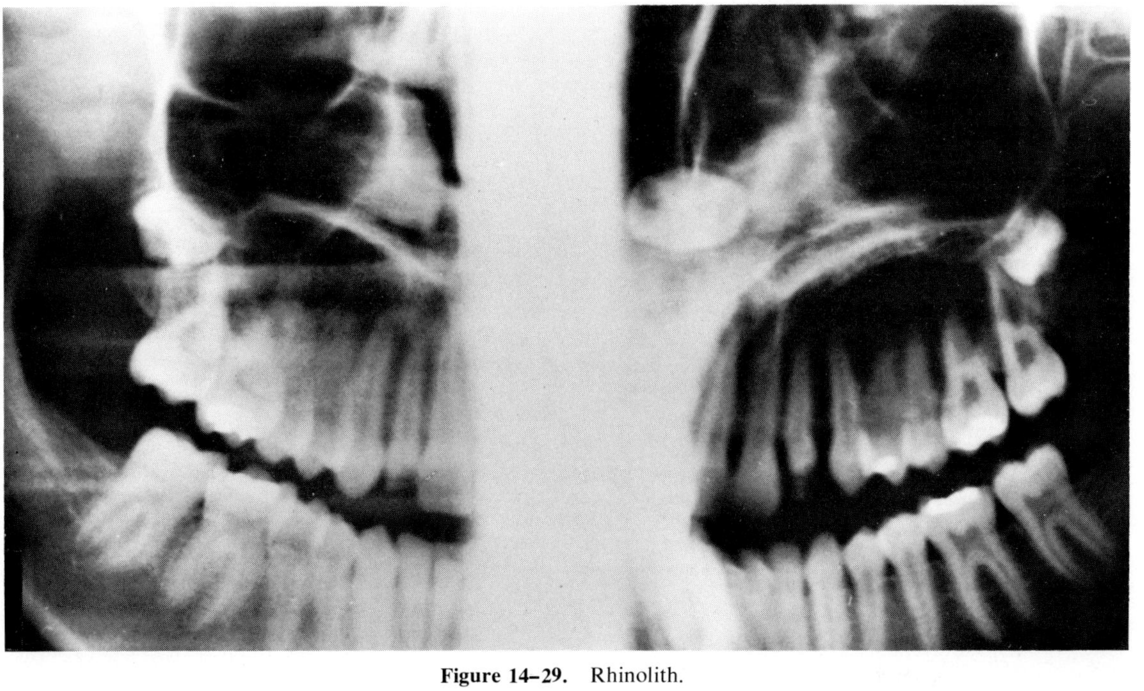

Figure 14–29. Rhinolith.

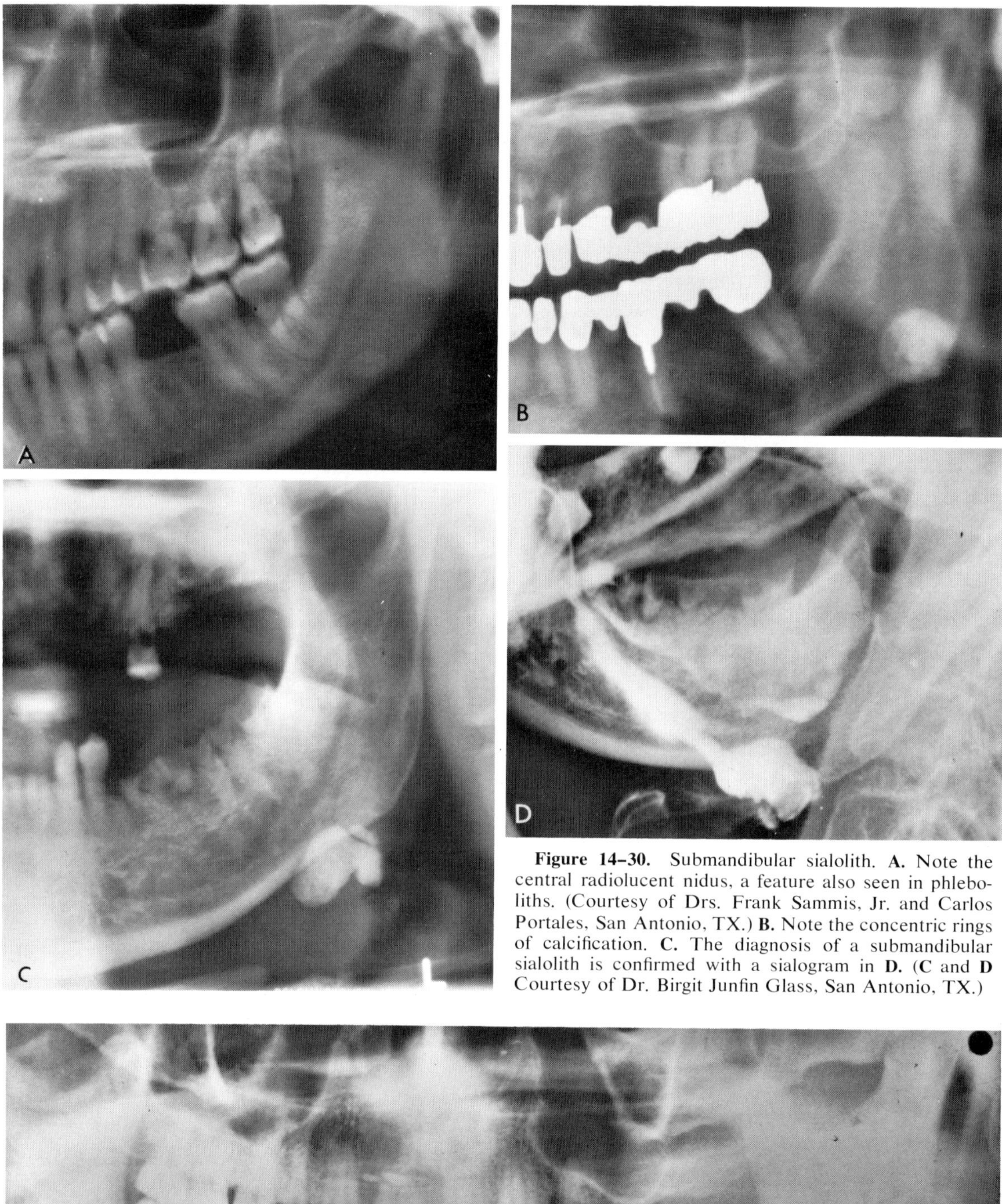

Figure 14–30. Submandibular sialolith. **A.** Note the central radiolucent nidus, a feature also seen in phleboliths. (Courtesy of Drs. Frank Sammis, Jr. and Carlos Portales, San Antonio, TX.) **B.** Note the concentric rings of calcification. **C.** The diagnosis of a submandibular sialolith is confirmed with a sialogram in **D.** (**C** and **D** Courtesy of Dr. Birgit Junfin Glass, San Antonio, TX.)

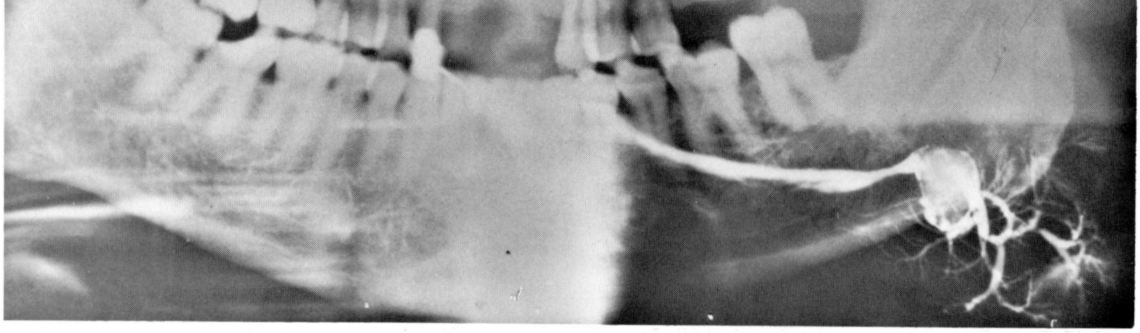

Figure 14–31. Panoramic sialogram diagnostic of a submandibular sialolith. Note the linear ghosting of the sialographic image on the contralateral side. (Courtesy of Dr. Gus Pappas, Columbus, OH.)

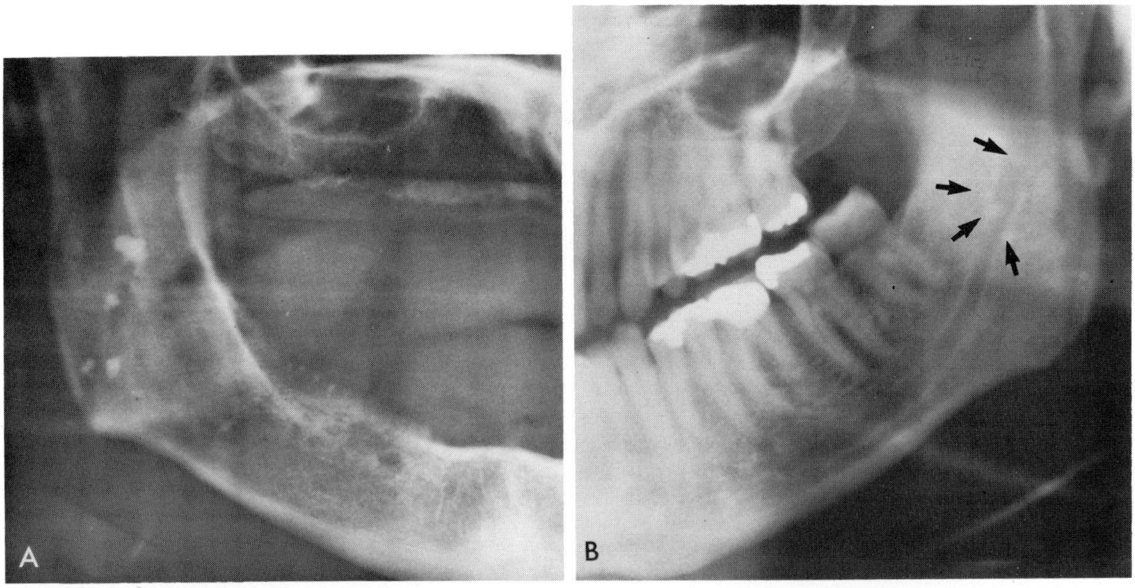

Figure 14–32. Parotid calculi. **A.** Courtesy of Dr. Gus Pappas, Columbus, OH.

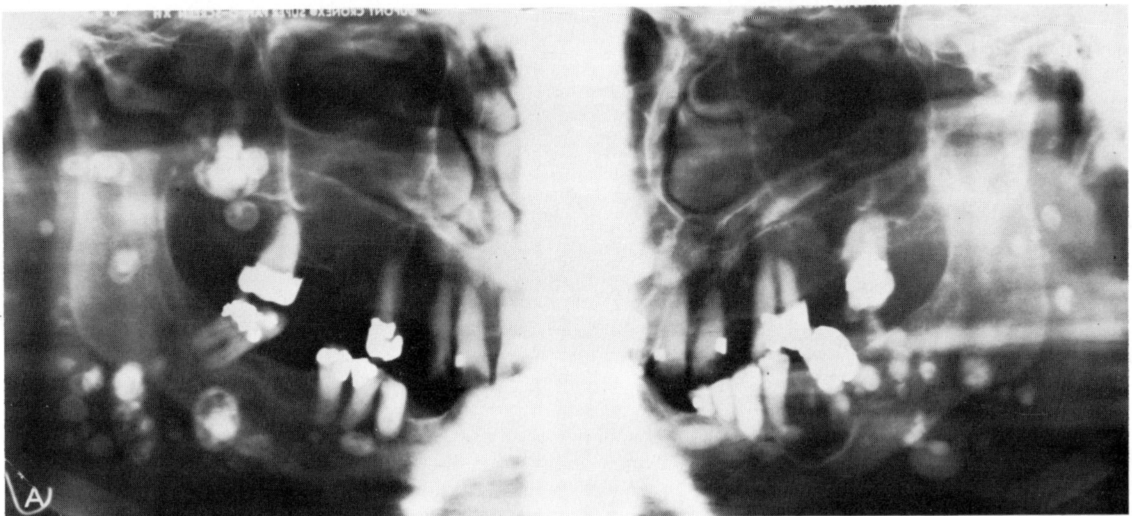

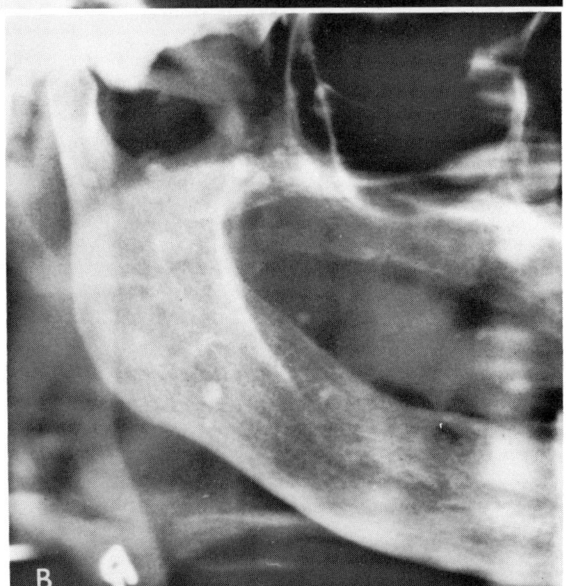

Figure 14–33. Phleboliths. **A.** Courtesy of Dr. Charles Calder, Dansville, NY; Eastman Kodak Co., Rochester, NY. **B.** Associated with a hemangioma. (Courtesy of Dr. Doug Stoneman, Toronto, Canada.)

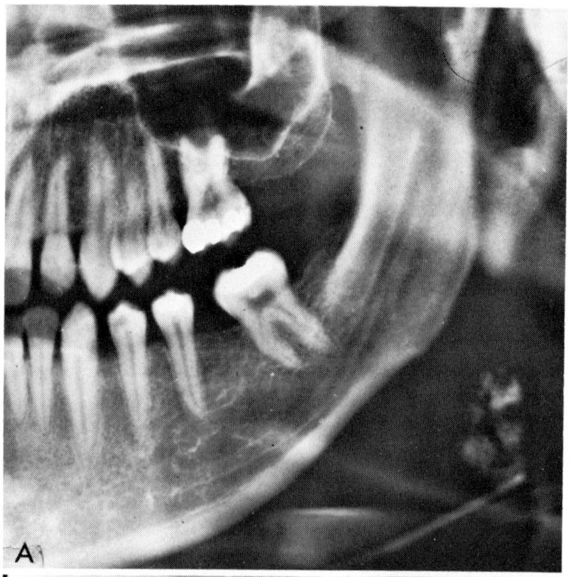

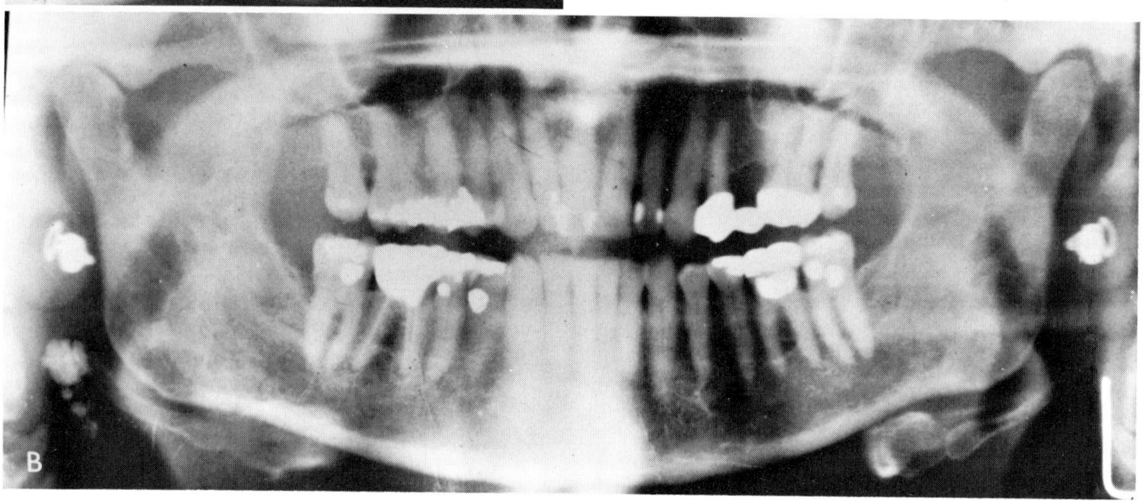

Figure 14–34. Calcified lymph nodes. **A.** Note the cauliflowerlike appearance. **B.** Note the chainlike arrangement. (**B** courtesy of Dr. Doug Stoneman, Toronto, Canada.)

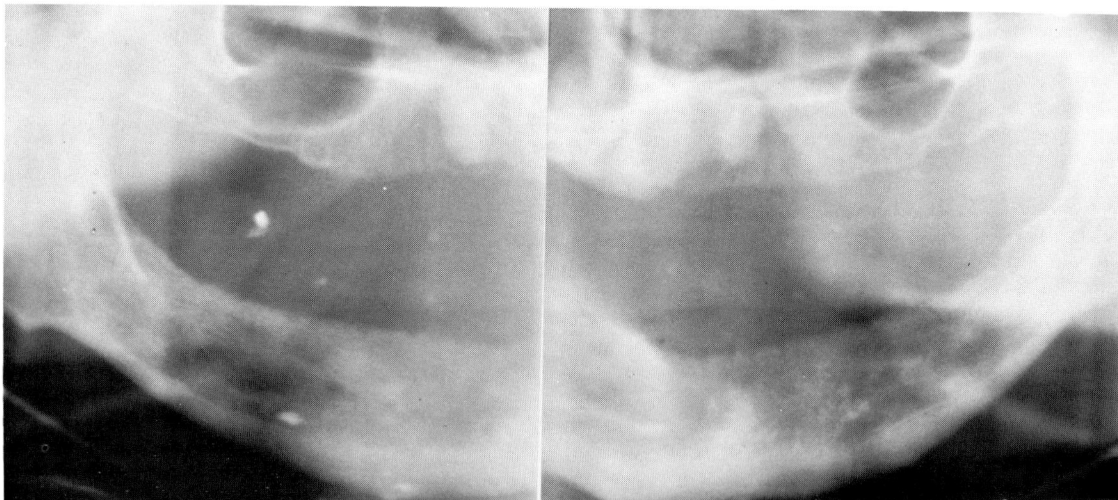

Figure 14–35. Soft tissue calcifications. Origin undetermined.

enitis (scrofula). Others include calcified epidermoid and sebaceous cysts and scars and may be associated with Gardner's syndrome.

Calcified blood vessels may also be seen and occur in association with arteriosclerosis obliterans and renal osteodystrophy (secondary hyperparathyroidism) and also occur idiopathically.

Other conditions that produce small nodular calcifications include cysticercosis, multiple miliary osteomas of the skin, and calcified acne scars. Traumatic myositis ossificans is a calcification of poorly understood etiology that may occur in muscle following trauma and may resemble a large osteoma or even osteogenic sarcoma in some cases.

RADIOGRAPHIC FEATURES (Figs. 14–33 to 14–36)

Some calcifications, such as phleboliths and salivary calculi, may present a targetlike appearance of concentric rings of calcification.

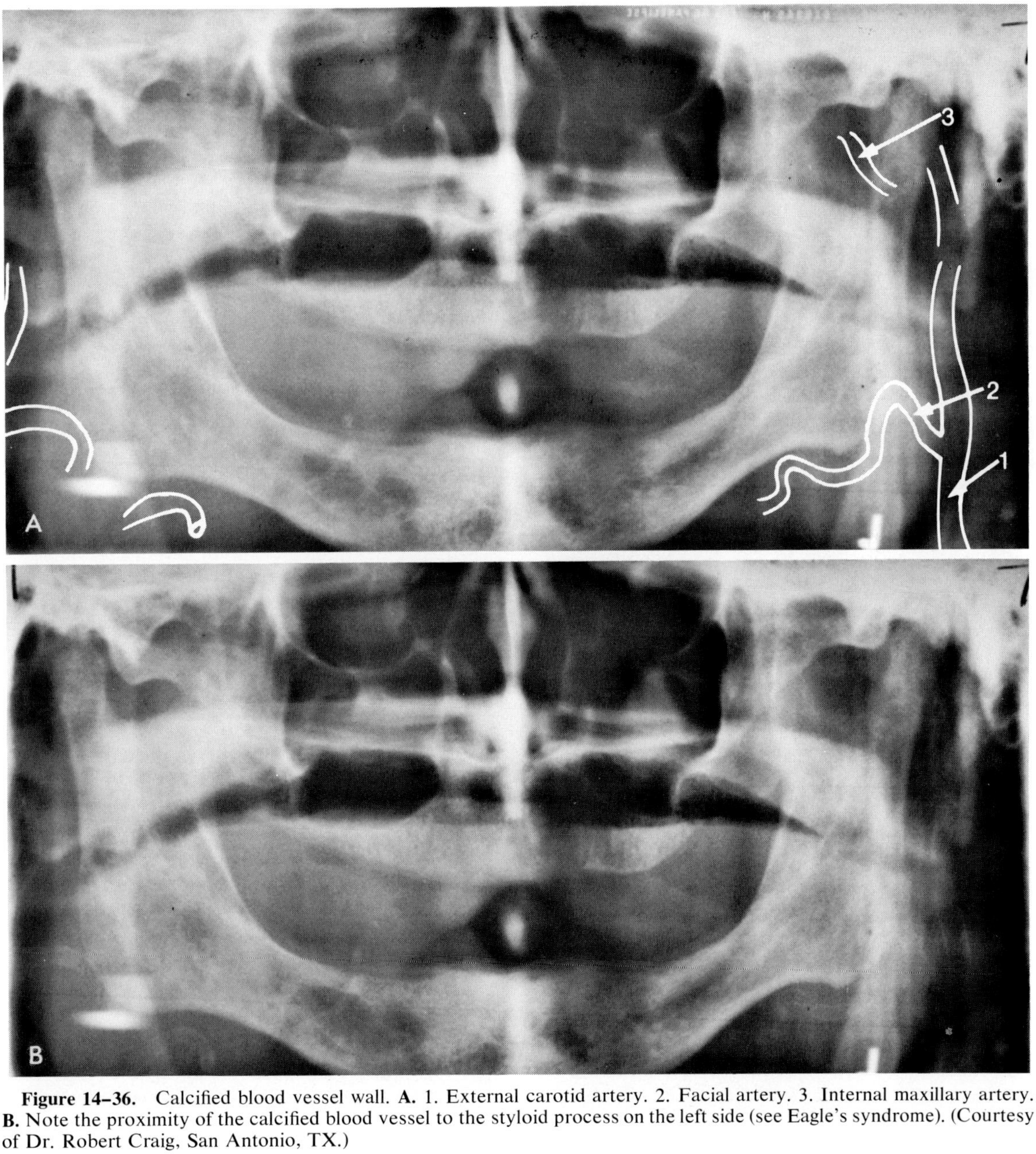

Figure 14–36. Calcified blood vessel wall. **A.** 1. External carotid artery. 2. Facial artery. 3. Internal maxillary artery. **B.** Note the proximity of the calcified blood vessel to the styloid process on the left side (see Eagle's syndrome). (Courtesy of Dr. Robert Craig, San Antonio, TX.)

Calcified lymph nodes may be cauliflowerlike in shape and multiple in a chainlike arrangement. Multiple small calcifications resembling grains of rice might lead one to suspect cysticercosis, calcified acne lesions, or multiple miliary osteomas of the skin. Calcified blood vessels are striking when they are well visualized. Most soft tissue calcifications are nonspecific and may mimic frank pathology. They should be identified more specifically by further clinical and radiographic procedures. The most important of these to recognize is the phlebolith, which usually has a radiolucent center, may have concentric rings, and may be multiple. The presence of a phlebolith should alert the clinician to the possible coexistence of a hemangioma or other central or peripheral vascular lesions.

EAGLE'S SYNDROME (Elongated Styloid Process Syndrome, Styloid Process–Carotid Artery Syndrome, Stylohyoid Syndrome, Styloid Process Neuralgia)

BRIEF OVERVIEW

The eponym Eagle's syndrome describes a symptom complex that may be referable to an elongated styloid process or a mineralized stylohyoid or stylomandibular ligament. The condition will be discussed in detail here because it

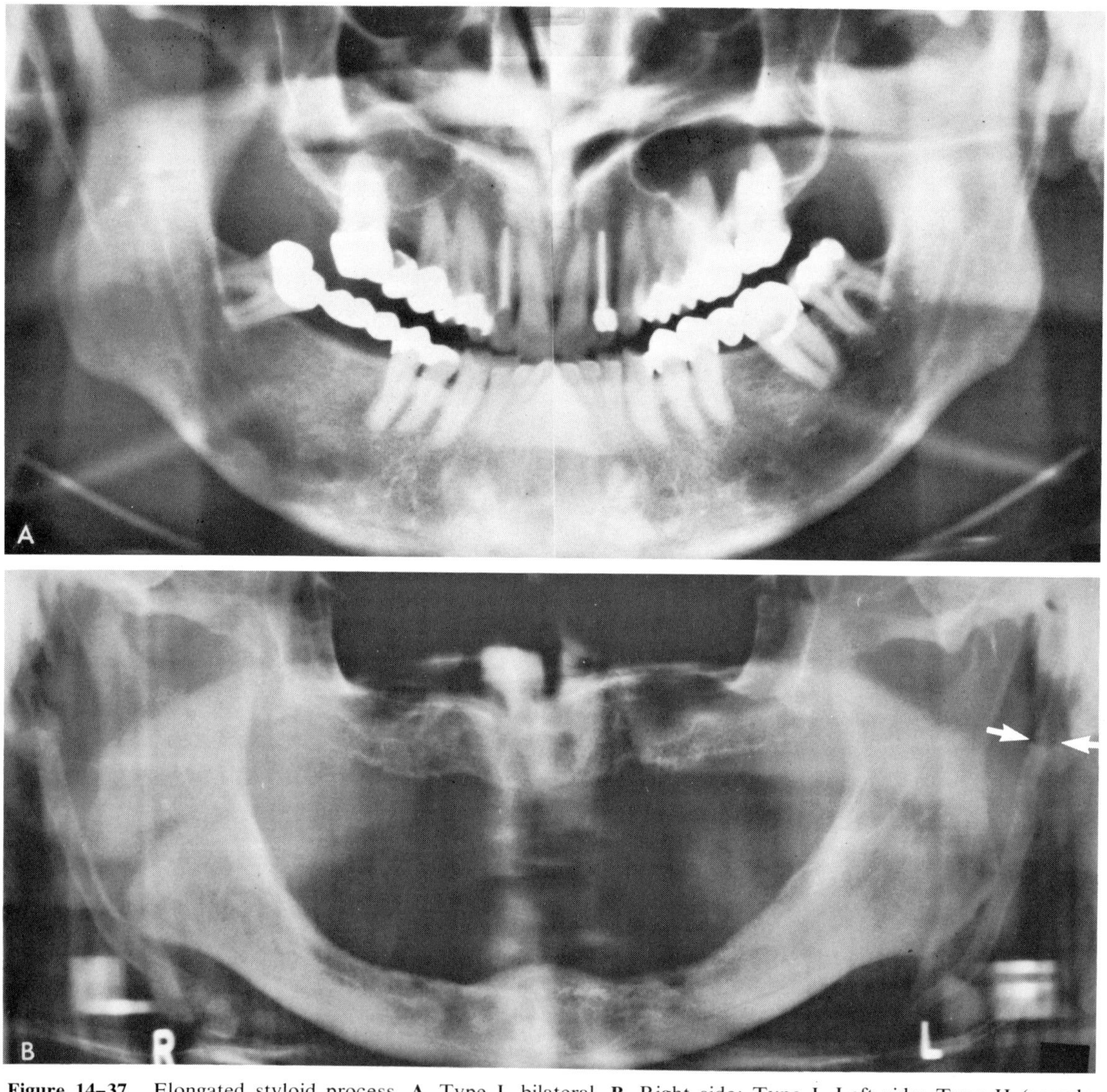

Figure 14–37. Elongated styloid process. **A.** Type I, bilateral. **B.** Right side: Type I. Left side: Type II (pseudoarticulated).

Illustration continued on opposite page

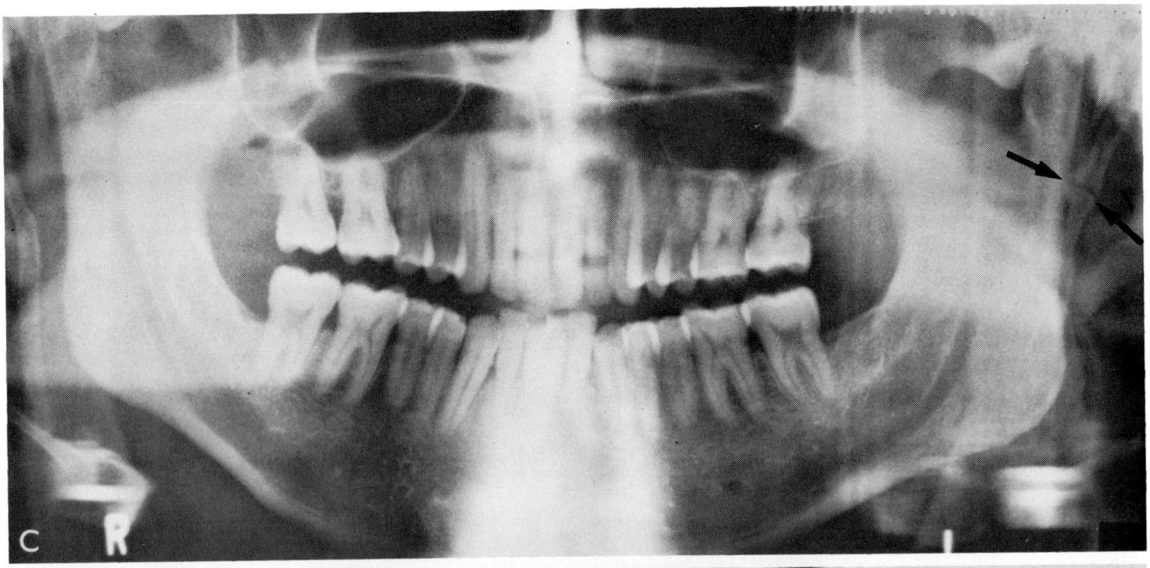

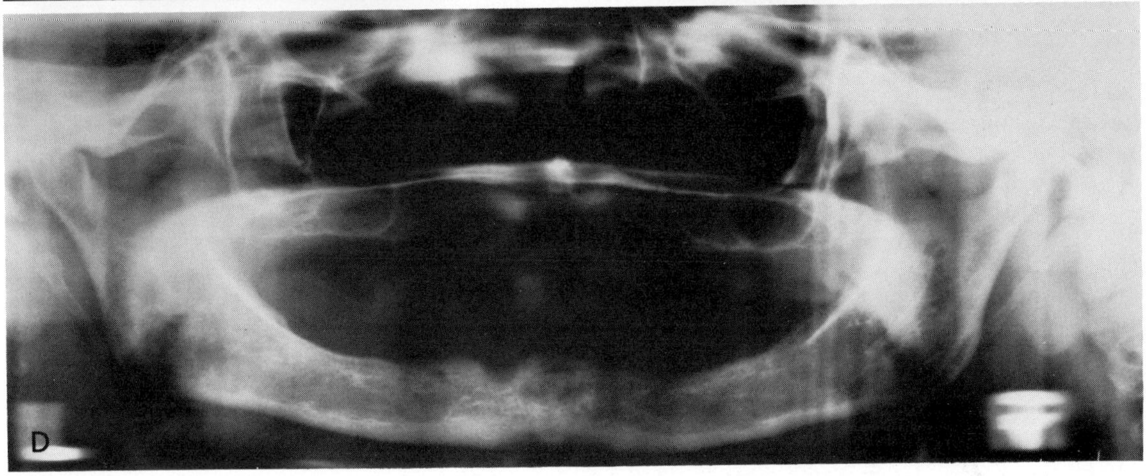

Figure 14–37 *Continued* **C.** Right side: Type I. Left side: Type II (pseudoarticulated). **D.** Type III, bilateral (segmented).

is not usually described in the standard dental and otolaryngologic reference texts and also because the mineralized portions of the stylohyoid complex, when present, are well visualized on most panoramic films.

The styloid process is connected to the temporal bone by cartilaginous tissue. The styloid process gives rise to the stylomandibular ligament, which inserts on the medial aspect of the angle of the mandible, and the stylohyoid ligament, which inserts on the lesser horn of the hyoid bone. It is postulated that the styloid process may become elongated by continued growth at its cartilaginous base or may appear to become elongated by mineralization of the stylomandibular or stylohyoid ligaments. An elongated styloid process is said to exist when either the styloid process (in the absence of a mineralized ligament) or the combined lengths of the styloid process (elongated or not) and the mineralized stylomandibular or stylohyoid ligament exceed 30 mm on the panoramic radiograph. The reported incidence of this abnormality has varied between 4 and 28 per cent and has probably been most accurately compiled by Correll and associates at 18 per cent, with over 93 per cent of the cases being bilateral. The percentage of patients who are symptomatic has never been accurately compiled, but it is generally believed to be less than 5 per cent.

The syndrome can probably be broken down into two sub-types, both originally described by Eagle in 1937. In the first instance, symptoms begin immediately post tonsillectomy and are believed to be caused by a fibrous scar, which, when associated with the subjacent elongated styloid process, produces stimulation of the sensory nerve endings of any or all of cranial nerves V, VII, IX, or X. The symptoms include subjective complaints of throat pain, which the patient attributes to improper postsurgical healing, a sensation of a foreign body such as a fish bone stuck in the throat, pain on swallowing, and, frequently, referred pain to the ear on the affected side. A clinical finding of tenting or a firm bulge in the tonsillar fossa is sometimes present. Firm resistance is met when the tonsillar fossa is palpated, and palpation usually elicits the patient's symptoms.

In the second case as originally cited by Eagle, the elongated styloid process produces impingement on or compression of the internal or external carotid artery. The symptoms are thought to be produced mainly by irritation of the rich sympathetic nerve supply to the walls of the carotid arteries, producing referred pain in the areas supplied by these vessels. Additionally, when the external carotid artery is involved, regional carotidynia, tinnitus, pain in the anterior cervical triangle, or pain on turning the head may be noted. When the internal carotid artery is affected, headaches in the orbital area and other sites supplied by this vessel may be present. Other symptoms include transitory dizziness or lightheadedness, cervical pain, a sensation of a frequent need to swallow, and other painful symptoms. The differential diagnosis, depending on the symptoms, includes glossopharyngeal neuralgia, sphenopalatine neuralgia or Sluder's syndrome, histamine cephalgia or cluster headaches, migraine headaches, carotidynia, myofascial pain–dysfunction (MPD) or the temporomandibular joint (TMJ) syndrome, impacted third molars, and other conditions associated with dysphagia, otalgia, and/or tinnitus. Treatment usually consists of surgical excision of the excessive mineralized portion of the stylohyoid complex, usually via an intraoral approach at the tonsillar fossa. It is interesting to note that although the condition is usually bilateral, paradoxically, the symptoms are almost invariably unilateral.

RADIOGRAPHIC FEATURES (Fig. 14–37)

An elongated styloid process, as previously mentioned, measures in excess of 30 mm on the panoramic radiograph. The elongated styloid process may present in any one of three basic subtypes. **Type I** consists of an apparently elongated styloid process whose radiographic integrity is uninterrupted throughout its length. **Type II** occurs when the styloid process is apparently joined to the mineralized stylomandibular or stylohyoid ligament by a single pseudoarticulation, which is usually located superior to a level tangential to the inferior border of the mandible, the overall picture being one of an apparently articulated elongated styloid process. **Type III** consists of either short or long noncontinuous portions of the styloid process or interrupted segments of mineralized ligament. In either case, two or more segments are seen, with the interruptions either above or below the level of the inferior border of the mandible or both. The overall appearance is one of a segmented mineralized stylohyoid complex. Owing to the position of the patient's head when the film is exposed, the calcified stylomandibular ligament cannot be definitively distinguished from an incompletely mineralized stylohyoid ligament. The mineralized stylohyoid ligament may be distinguished more definitively when it is seen to extend below the inferior border of the mandible or when its attachment to the inferior cornu of the hyoid bone is seen. All three types are believed by the authors to be capable of producing the symptoms of Eagle's syndrome. Additionally, there are no radiographic features that can be used to identify or distinguish symptomatic from nonsymptomatic elongated styloid processes.

REFERENCES

Reference Texts

Eversole, L. R.: **Clinical Outline of Oral Pathology**. Philadelphia: Lea & Febiger, 1978, pp. 231–232, 243–245, 247–248, 249–250.

Shafer, W. G., Hine, M. K., and Levy, B. M.: **A Textbook of Oral Pathology**, 3rd Edition. Philadelphia: W. B. Saunders, 1974, pp. 44, 151–152, 156, 165–170, 276–278, 458–461.

Stafne, E. C., and Gibilisco, J. A.: **Oral Radiographic Diagnosis**. Philadelphia: W. B. Saunders, 1975, pp. 135–146, 189–196, 358–364.

Wood, N. K., and Goaz, P. W.: **Differential Diagnosis of Oral Lesions.** St. Louis: C. V. Mosby, 1975, pp. 506, 509–511, 516, 518–519, 521–525, 528–530.

Worth, H. M.: **Principles and Practice of Oral Radiologic Interpretation.** Chicago: Year Book Medical Publishers, 1963, pp. 176, 233–237, 271, 563–578.

Selected References

Arlen, M., Tollefsen, H. R., Huvos, A. G., et al.: Chondrosarcoma of the head and neck. **Am. J. Surg. 120**:456, 1971.

Budnick, S. D.: Compound and complex odontomas. **Oral Surg. 42**:501, 1976.

Burrell, K. H., and Goepp, R. A.: Abnormal bone repair in jaws, socket sclerosis: A sign of systemic disease. **J.A.D.A. 87**:1206, 1973.

Correll, R. W., Jensen, S. L., Taylor, J. B., and Rhyne, R. R.: Mineralization of the stylohoid-stylomandibular ligament complex. A radiographic incidence study. **Oral Surg. 48:**286, 1979.

Farman, A. G., Kohler, W. W., Nortjé, C. J., and Van Wyk, C. W., Cementoblastoma: Report of a case. **J. Oral Surg. 37**:198, 1979.

Franklin, C. D., and Pindborg, J. J.: The Pindborg tumor: A review and analysis of 113 cases. **Oral Surg. 42**:753, 1976.

Gardner, D. G., and Mills, D. M.: The widened periodontal ligament of osteosarcoma of the jaws. **Oral Surg. 41**:652, 1976.

Grossman, J. R., and Tarsitano, J. J.: The styloid-stylohyoid syndrome. **J. Oral Surg. 35**:555, 1977.

Lichty, G., Langlais, R. P., and Aufdemorte, T.: Garré's osteomyelitis: Literature review and case report. **Oral Surg. 50**:309, 1980.

Miller, A. S., Lopez, C. F., Pullon, P. A., and Elzay, R. P.: Ameloblastic fibro-odontoma: Report of seven cases. **Oral Surg. 41**:354, 1976.

Plezia, R. A., Mintz, S. M., and Colligaro, P.: Myositis ossificans traumatica of the masseter muscle: Report of a case. **Oral Surg. 44**:351, 1977.

Ramon, Y., Oberman, M., Horowitz, I., Freedman, A., and Todmor, R.: A large mandibular tumor with a distinct radiological "sun-ray effect" as the primary manifestation of multiple myeloma. **J. Oral Surg. 36**:52, 1978.

Regezi, J. A., Kerr, D. A., and Courtney, R. M.: Odontogenic tumors: Analysis of 706 cases. **Oral Surg. 36**:771, 1978.

Schneider, L. C., Dolinsky, H. B., and Grodjesk, S. E.: Solitary peripheral osteoma of the jaws: Report of case and review of literature. **J. Oral Surg. 38**:452, 1980.

Seeliger, J. E., and Reynecke, J. P.: The calcifying odontogenic cyst: Report of a case. **J. Oral Surg. 36**:469, 1978.

Small, I. A., Shandler, H., Husain, M., and Haskell, D.: Gardner's syndrome with an unusual fibro-osseous lesion of the mandible. **Oral Surg. 49**:477, 1980.

Smith, S. N., and Farman, A. G.: Osteomyelitis with proliferative periostitis (Garré's osteomyelitis). **Oral Surg. 43**:315, 1977.

Turney, J. A., and Fonseca, R. J.: The anatomy of the internal maxillary artery in the pterygopalatine fossa: Its relationship to maxillary surgery. **J. Oral Surg. 38**:92, 1980.

Chapter 15

Generalized or Diffuse Radiopacities Involving One or More Quadrants

CHRONIC DIFFUSE SCLEROSING OSTEOMYELITIS
FIBROUS DYSPLASIA
OSTEOPETROSIS
PAGET'S DISEASE OF BONE
HYPERPARATHYROIDISM
DOMINANT CRANIOMETAPHYSEAL DYSPLASIA
van BUCHEM'S DISEASE

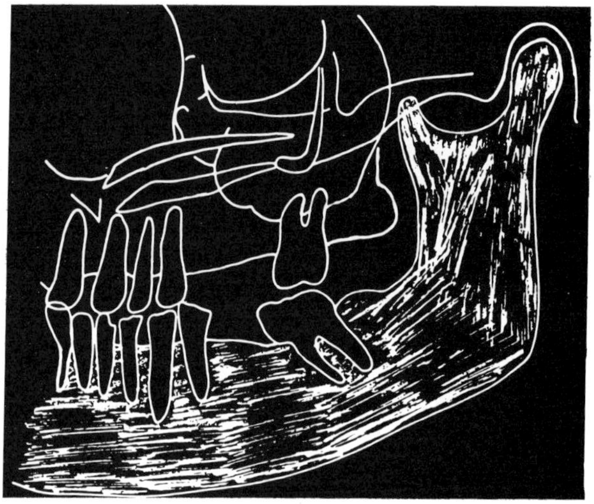

CHRONIC DIFFUSE SCLEROSING OSTEOMYELITIS (Florid Cemento-osseous Dysplasia, Sclerosing Cemental Masses of the Jaws, Diffuse Cementosis, Gigantiform Cementomas)

BRIEF OVERVIEW

Chronic diffuse sclerosing osteomyelitis is probably inherited as an autosomal dominant trait and is usually seen in middle-aged black females, most frequently in the mandible in edentulous areas. It is seen only in the jaws.

The condition probably represents a proliferation of cementum or bone in response to a low-grade infection of long standing, most often of previous pulpal or periodontal origin. Although this condition is often asymptomatic, it sometimes becomes acute, with mild pain and inflammation of the overlying mucosa. Fistulous tracts may be seen, and there may be evidence of bony sequestration. Expansion is not a usual feature but may occur. A frequent presenting complaint is pain or discomfort beneath a complete or partial denture base. Long-term antibiotic treatment, preferably based on culture and sensitivity tests, followed by conservative sequestrectomy may be required to control the condition. Future acute episodes are possible.

RADIOGRAPHIC FEATURES (Fig. 15–1)

In the dormant stage, the radiographic findings may be identical to those of multiple mature cementomas and very similar to those of

Figure 15–1. Chronic diffuse sclerosing osteomyelitis. **A.** Multiple areas occurred in all four quadrants. (Courtesy of Dr. Gus Pappas, Columbus, OH. **B.** After sequestrectomy in the maxillary anterior area. (Courtesy of Drs. Frank Sammis, Jr. and Carlos Portales, San Antonio, TX.) **C.** Note the evidence of sequestration in the maxillary left cuspid–bicuspid area. Compare the more minimal areas of periapical involvement with the more diffuse radiopacity in the mandibular right edentulous area. (Courtesy of Dr. Gus Pappas, Columbus, OH. **D.** Courtesy of Dr. Chris Nortjé, University of Stellenbosch, Tygerberg, South Africa.)

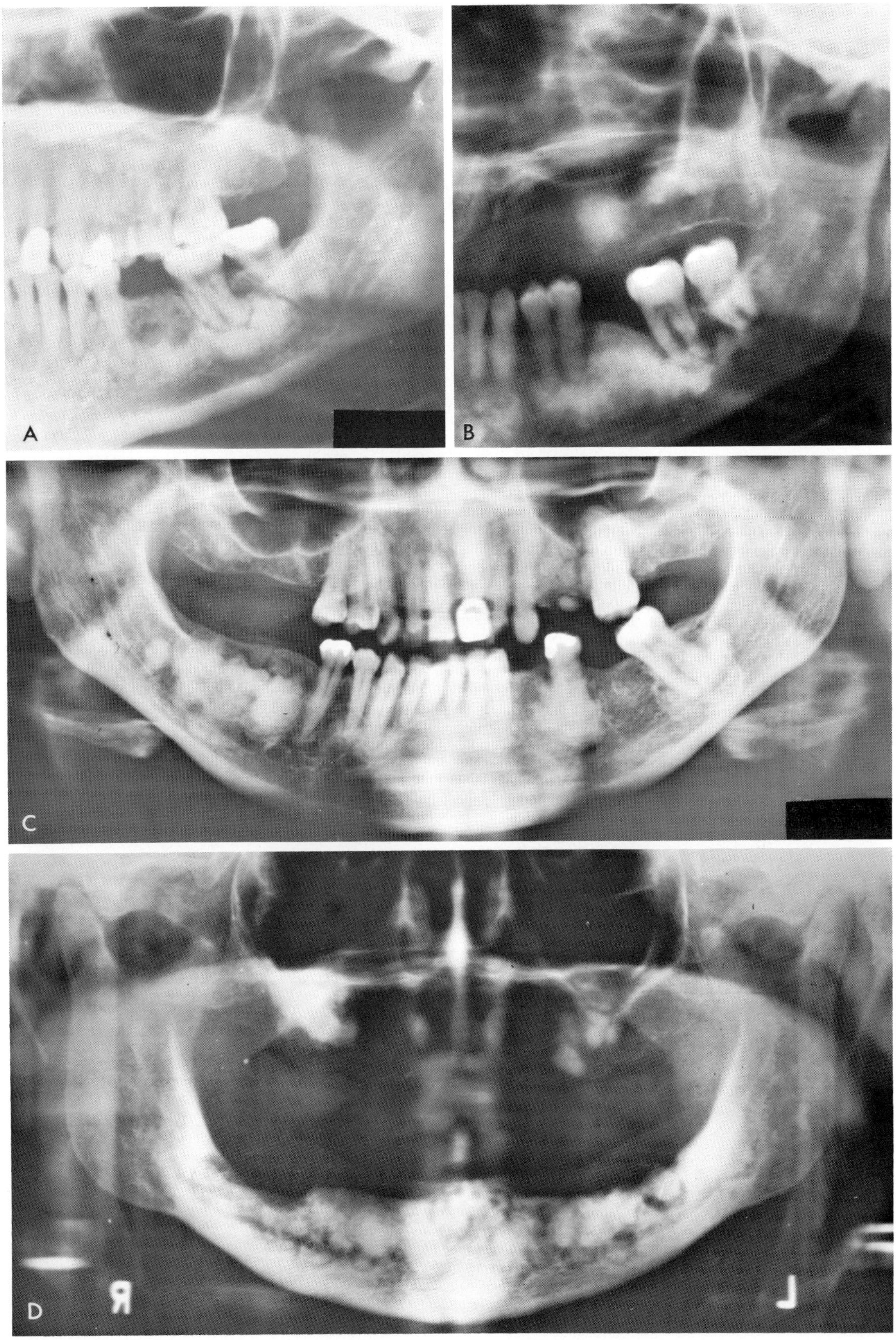

Figure 15–1. *See legend on opposite page*

Paget's disease. These features include uniformly radiodense masses resembling cotton wool, which may be multiple and separate or contiguous. One, several, or all quadrants may be involved, with edentulous mandibular areas being the most frequently involved. There is usually no radiolucent line separating affected and unaffected areas (an important distinguishing feature), in contrast to the targetlike radiolucent and radiopaque appearance of multiple cementomas. Definitive diagnosis can sometimes only be made by biopsy upon the identification of chronic inflammatory elements as well as other findings.

The condition is more easily identified in an acute episode. Radiographically, there may be evidence of sequestration of some of the sclerotic, dense, bonelike material, and there may be a diffuse radiolucent area in this region between the radiopaque mass and the normal bone.

FIBROUS DYSPLASIA

BRIEF OVERVIEW

Fibrous dysplasia is a condition of unknown etiology. It has been subdivided into polyostotic and monostotic types. Both types may affect the jawbones. The polyostotic type has been further subdivided into Jaffe-Lichtenstein syndrome, which includes café au lait spots on the skin and involvement of several bones, and Albright's syndrome. The latter sub-type is

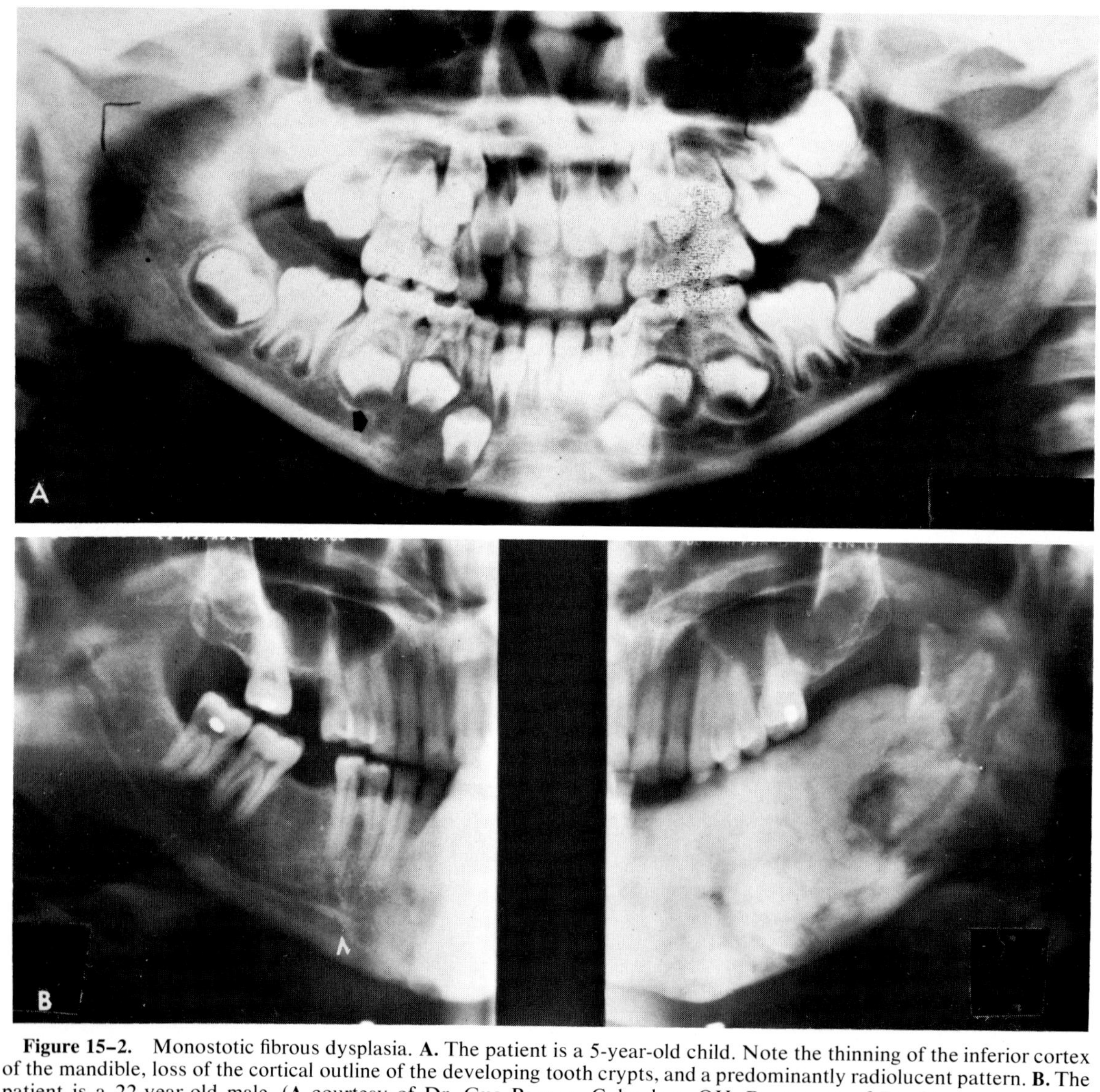

Figure 15–2. Monostotic fibrous dysplasia. **A.** The patient is a 5-year-old child. Note the thinning of the inferior cortex of the mandible, loss of the cortical outline of the developing tooth crypts, and a predominantly radiolucent pattern. **B.** The patient is a 22-year-old male. (**A** courtesy of Dr. Gus Pappas, Columbus, OH. **B** courtesy of Dr, Stanley Lovestedt, Rochester, MN.)

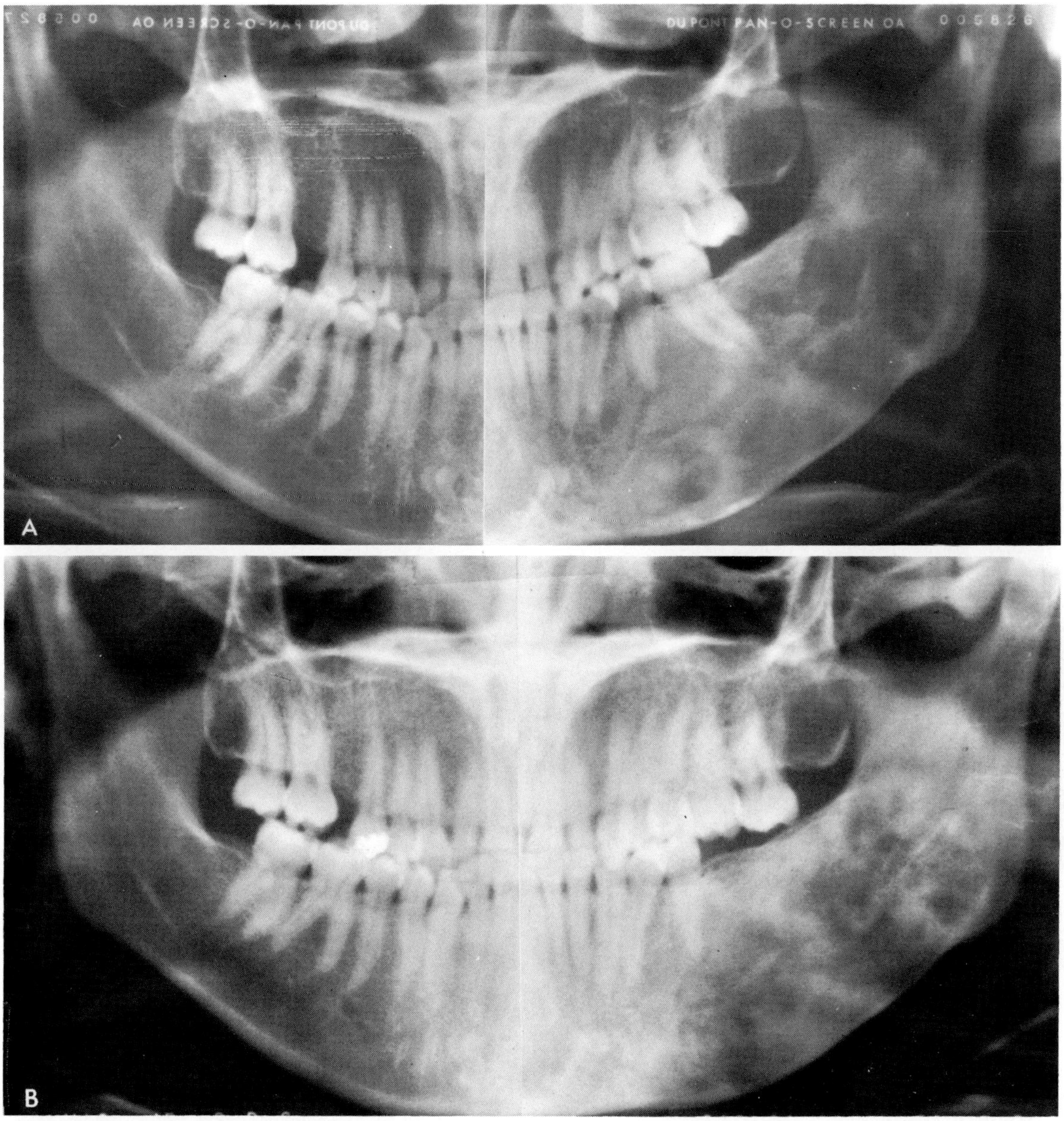

Figure 15–3. Monostotic fibrous dysplasia. **A.** Present since age 11, the patient is now 44. **B.** The patient at age 49. (Figure 15–3 courtesy of Drs. Frank Sammis, Jr, and Carlos Portales, San Antonio, TX.)

similar to Jaffe-Lichtenstein syndrome (café au lait spots are present), but bony involvement is more generalized, and various endocrine disturbances occur. The least severe type of fibrous dysplasia is the monostotic type, in which only one bone is affected.

In all types of fibrous dysplasia, onset is often during childhood. Surgical intervention should be avoided in the earlier stages. All forms of the disease may undergo malignant transformation into a sarcoma, usually osteosarcoma. Radiotherapy of fibrous dysplasia increases the probability of malignant transformation.

The presence of café au lait spots clinically should alert the clinician to the possibility of an existing polyostotic fibrous dysplasia, Jaffe-Lichtenstein or Albright's syndrome, cherubism, von Recklinghausen's disease (neurofibromatosis), neuropolyendocrine syndrome (Sipple's syndrome), or an idiopathic finding.

RADIOGRAPHIC FEATURES (Figs. 15–2 and 15–3)

Fibrous dysplasia may present in a variety of radiographic manifestations. The mature lesion is a diffuse radiopacity involving one or more quadrants of the jaws. This fibro-osseous condition of idiopathic but apparently nonperiodontal origin may present as a radiolucency, often in the mandible, but with poorly defined borders. It may also be radiolucent with islands of calcification or a homogenous dense radiopacity involving a whole quadrant or more. Expansion may be evident, especially in the more mature lesion, thus producing facial deformity. During one phase of the disease, fibrous dysplasia may present as a ground-glass, orange-peel, or salt-and-pepper trabecular pattern with a loss of the associated lamina dura and must be distinguished from primary and secondary hyperparathyroidism, Paget's disease, and craniometaphyseal dysplasia, all of which may manifest this same radiographic picture. Thinning of the cortex is an early feature in all types of fibrous dysplasia. Perforation of the cortex and periosteal proliferation are not usually seen.

OSTEOPETROSIS (Marble Bone Disease, Albers-Schönberg Disease)

BRIEF OVERVIEW

This condition is said to exist in two forms: a malignant recessive type, which manifests very early in life and is incompatible with long-term survival beyond early adulthood; and a benign dominant type, which is often not recognized until adulthood and is compatible with a normal

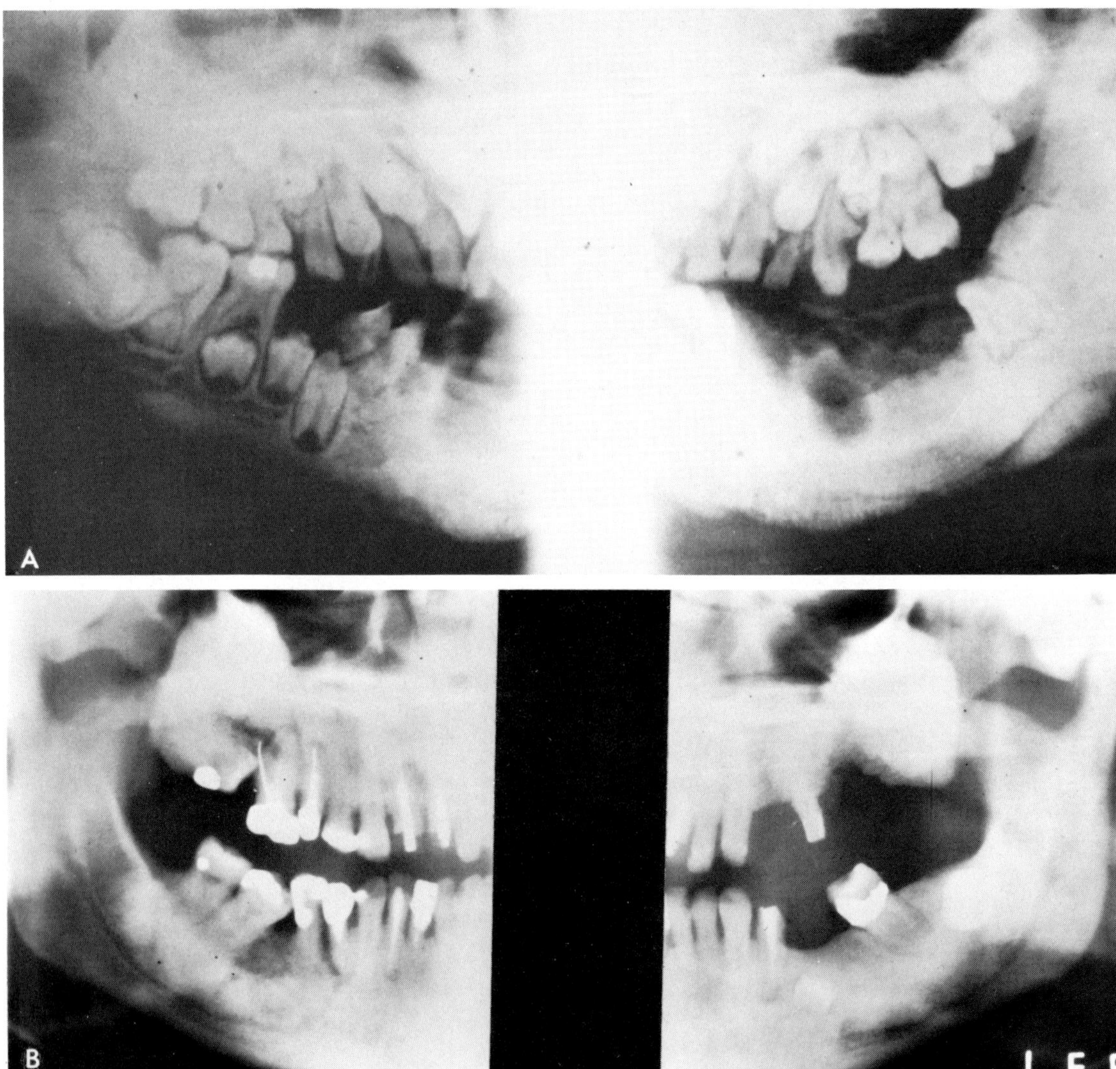

Figure 15–4. Osteopetrosis. **A.** The patient is a 10-year-old child. **B.** Note the bilateral involvement of both jaws and several impacted or unerupted teeth.

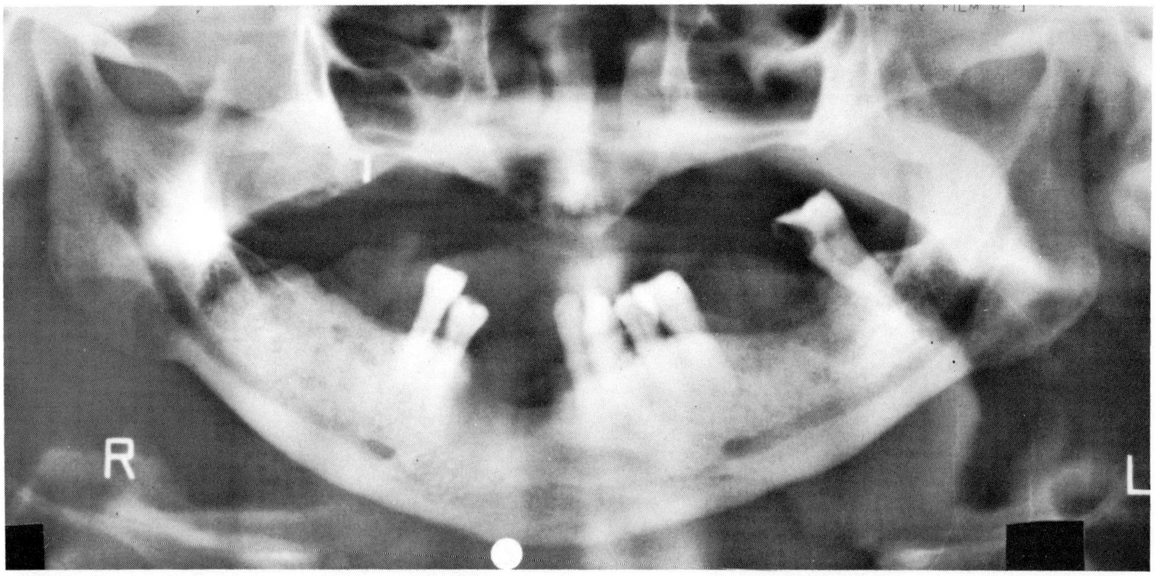

Figure 15–5. Possible osteopetrotic involvement of the mandible. The patient is an asymptomatic 70-year-old male. (Courtesy of Dr. Steven Bricker, San Antonio, TX.)

life span. Features common to both types include varying degrees of anemia, susceptibility to infection, cranial nerve involvement owing to narrowing of the foraminae, bone pain, and pathologic fractures.

Although the etiology is unknown, one theory postulates a partial failure of osteoclastic resorption of the primary spongiosum, leading to excess deposition of spongy and cortical bone and a narrowing of the marrow spaces. The manifestations of the malignant form are much more severe, whereas the benign form may be completely asymptomatic. Treatment involves management of the side effects of the disease when present. When the jaws are involved, prevention of dental and periodontal infections is important, as osteomyelitis may develop and may be difficult to manage.

RADIOGRAPHIC FEATURES (Figs. 15–4 and 15–5)

The definitive diagnosis of osteopetrosis is based on the overall radiographic picture. When the jaws are involved, there is a fairly uniform increase in density of the affected areas. Involvement is usually diffuse throughout both jaws. Delayed eruption, especially of the permanent teeth, is a fairly consistent feature, and a number of teeth may remain embedded. The clinician should check for any superimposed moth-eaten or radiolucent areas, which represent osteomyelitis or evidence of pathologic fracture. The teeth are said to be more susceptible to enamel hypoplasia and caries. According to Worth, an increased thickness of the lamina dura is a notable finding.

PAGET'S DISEASE OF BONE (Osteitis Deformans, Paget's Disease)

BRIEF OVERVIEW

Paget's disease of bone usually affects adults over the age of 40. The etiology is unknown. Symptoms may include bone pain, headache, and signs of other cranial nerve involvement including visual and hearing disturbances. Pathologic fracture and the development of osteomyelitis are common sequelae. Malignant sarcomatous transformation has been reported in rare instances. The skull, long bones, and vertebral column are often involved, and deformity usually results. When the jaws are affected the maxilla is the more frequent site. Progressive tightening of the dentures or separation of the teeth may be presenting complaints. The disease produces extremely high levels of serum alkaline phosphatase. Thryocalcitonin may be a promising pharmacologic agent in arresting the progress of this disease.

RADIOGRAPHIC FEATURES (Fig. 15–6)

Paget's disease is classified as a generalized radiopacity because this is the appearance of

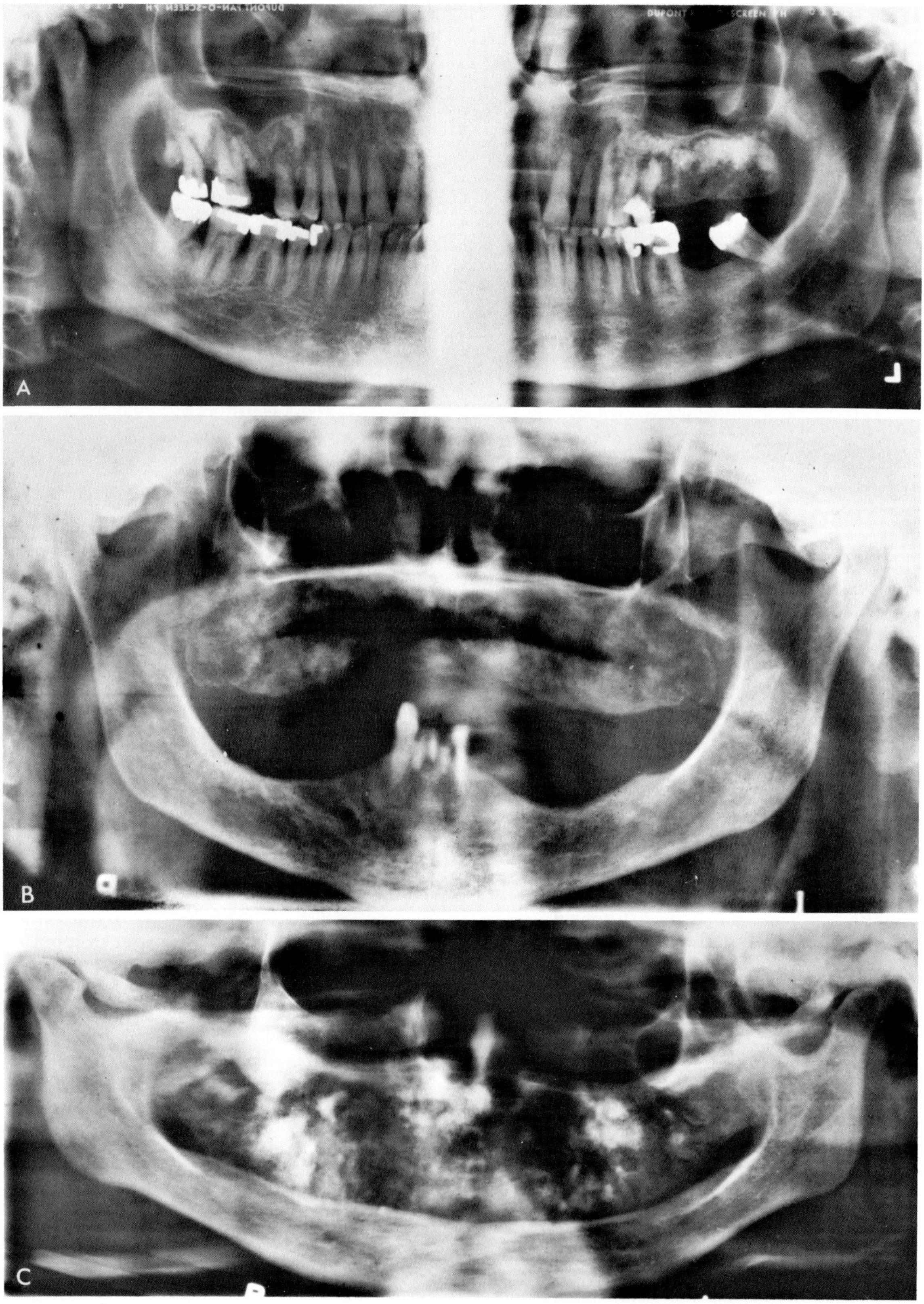

Figure 15-6. Paget's disease. **A.** Note the involvement of the maxilla bilaterally. **B.** Note the diffuse enlargement of the maxilla bilaterally. The radiolucent area represents an air space between the dorsum of the tongue and the palate. **C.** Diffuse involvement of the maxilla.

Illustration continued on opposite page

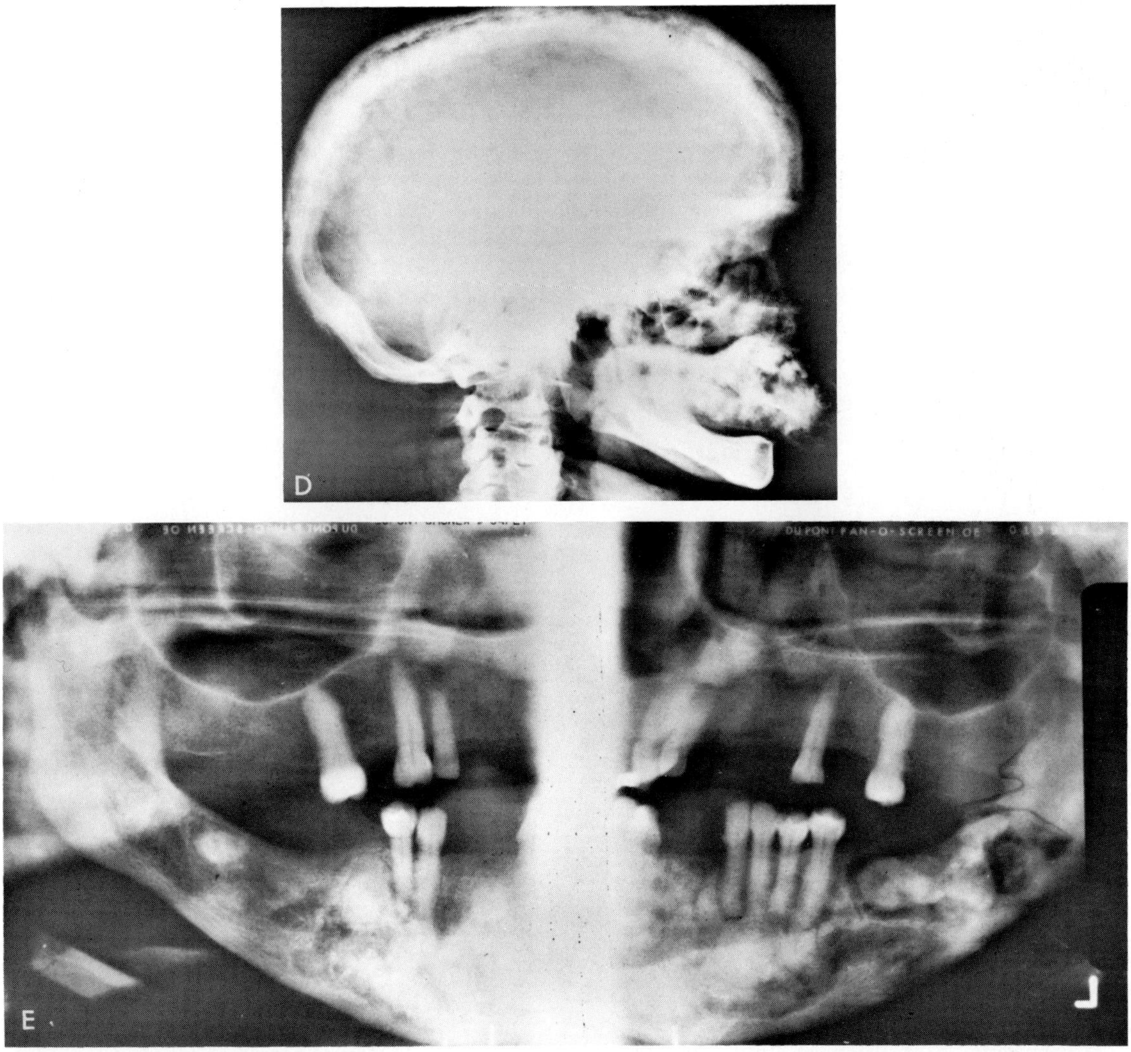

Figure 15–6 *Continued* **D.** Skull and maxillary involvement in the patient in **C. E.** Note the mandibular involvement. (**A** and **B** courtesy of Dr. Doug Stoneman, Toronto, Canada. **C** and **D** courtesy of Dr. Chris Nortjé, University of Stellenbosch, Tygerberg, South Africa. **E** courtesy of Dr. Albert M. Abrams, Los Angeles, CA.)

the mature lesion. There are, however, a number of variants. First, Paget's disease is one of four conditions that may demonstrate a loss of lamina dura and a ground-glass trabecular pattern of the alveolar bone, especially on intraoral periapical films. The other conditions are primary, secondary, and tertiary hyperparathyroidism, fibrous dysplasia, and craniometaphyseal dysplasia. Second, Paget's disease and primary and secondary hyperparathyroidism may also show lesions in the jaws that are radiolucent, mixed radiolucent/radiopaque, or radiopaque.

In Paget's disease, the mature lesion has been described as having a cotton-wool appearance when it involves alveolar bone or skull. These radiopaque masses are not unlike those of the dormant form of chronic diffuse sclerosing osteomyelitis or multiple cementomas. Helpful in distinguishing Paget's disease radiographically is the presence of a generalized hypercementosis and cotton-wool involvement of the skull. Osteogenic sarcoma may arise in areas of bone affected by Paget's disease, usually as a poorly defined radiolucency.

HYPERPARATHYROIDISM (Primary Hyperparathyroidism, Secondary Hyperparathyroidism, Renal Osteodystrophy, Tertiary Hyperparathyroidism)

BRIEF OVERVIEW

Primary hyperparathyroidism is caused by excessive production of parathyroid hormone by the parathyroid glands. This is sometimes caused by hyperplasia of one or more of the four parathyroid glands, most often by a functional adenoma, and rarely by carcinoma. There is usually an elevated serum calcium concentration, but several repeated blood tests may be necessary to demonstrate this. Serum phosphate levels as well as serum alkaline phosphatase and urinary calcium are increased. This disease occurs most frequently in middle-aged females. The brown tumors seen in affected bone are histologically identical to those of central giant cell granulomas. Primary hyperparathyroidism is very suspect in patients over the age of 20 with recurrent central giant cell granulomas, especially multiple lesions. A return of normal bone morphology on radiographic follow-up is used to monitor successful surgical removal of the affected glands.

Secondary hyperparathyroidism or renal osteodystrophy is more common than the primary type and is associated with renal disease. There is spilling of calcium into the urine, producing a hypocalcemia. This results in the stimulation of production and release of parathyroid hormone, which in turn raises the serum calcium to normal or high-normal levels. Hypercalcemia is rarely seen in secondary hyperparathyroidism, and urinary excretion of calcium on a low-calcium diet is elevated. Renal osteodystrophy is seen most frequently in children with severe renal disease but occurs in adults as well.

Tertiary hyperparathyroidism results primarily from renal disease that leads to hyperplasia of the parathyroid glands. This may give rise to a functional adenoma, whence calcium metabolism is affected by the combined effects of renal disease and increased secretion of parathyroid hormone. Similar radiographic changes are seen in all three types of hyperparathyroidism.

RADIOGRAPHIC FEATURES (Figs. 15–7 and 15–8)

One of the earliest radiographic signs of hyperparathyroidism is subperiosteal erosion of cortical bone in the middle phalanges of the hands. This is usually followed by a ground-glass pattern of the alveolar bone, a loss of the lamina dura in affected areas, and a relative increase in the thickness of the periodontal membrane space due to the loss of the lamina dura. Eventually, brown tumors develop, which produce radiolucent lesions in the jaws and the long bones. These areas appear extremely destructive, may have ragged borders, may cause root resorption, and may even extrude adjacent teeth from their sockets. The resorbed portions of the root may protrude into the radiolucent area, a radiographic finding consistent with the presence of a neoplasm. In contrast, when cysts are associated with root resorption, the roots rarely protrude beyond the radiographic boundaries of the lesion. Other radiographic changes may include a loss of the cortical outline of the nasal fossae and around the crypts of developing teeth in children.

The skull changes include an overall grayness with a lack of contrast or sharpness of the vault. There may be some moth-eaten radiolucent areas resembling those changes seen in osteomyelitis, multiple myeloma, and carcinoma. Many of these same changes are seen in renal

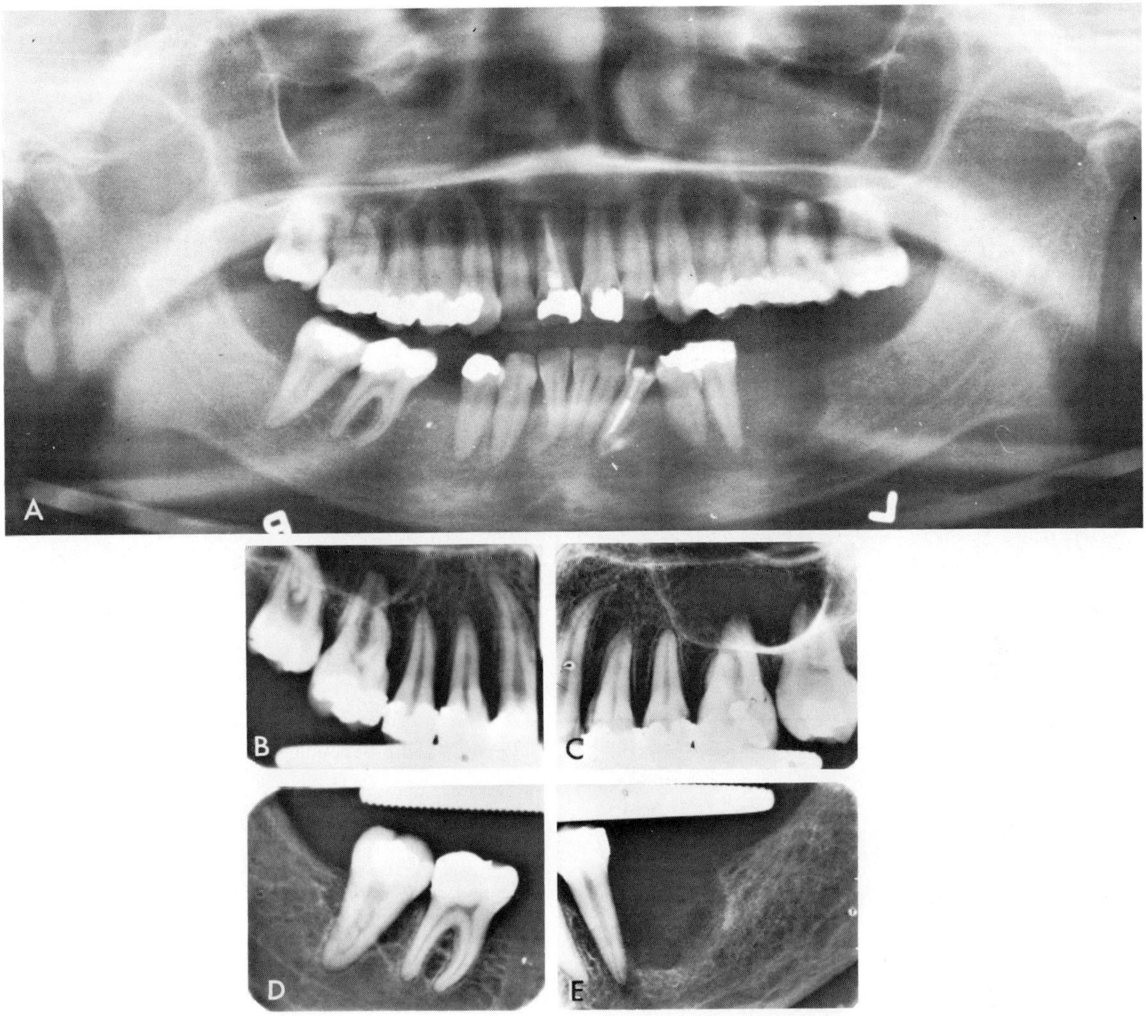

Figure 15–7. Primary hyperparathyroidism. **A.** Note the presence of a brown tumor in the mandibular left bicuspid area. **B, C, D,** and **E.** Bone changes are minimal except in the area of the mandibular left bicuspid, where there is a loss of the lamina dura and a moth-eaten appearance of the alveolar bone. (Figure 15–7 courtesy of Dr. Chris Nortjé, University of Stellenbosch, Tygerberg, South Africa.)

osteodystrophy. According to Worth, the most typical pattern, especially in children, is an overall lack of sharpness and a uniform density of the alveolar bone, a finding that the authors and others describe as ground glass. In children, this pattern may be so dense and uniform as to resemble osteopetrosis. However, there is thickening of the lamina dura in osteopetrosis, whereas in renal osteodystrophy the lamina dura is lost.

At times there are areas of increased bone density, representing a dense ground-glass pattern, adjacent to areas of decreased bone density, representing brown tumors. According to Worth, in cases where there are erupting teeth, eruption appears to be too far advanced for the degree of root development, there may be abnormally large pulps, and very pointed, tapered roots are also apparent. The authors have found that if disease persists, the abnormally large pulps eventually become abnormally small for the patient's age. Some of the skull changes in renal osteodystrophy include calcification of the falx cerebri and the petroclinoid ligament. Changes reminiscent of the cotton-wool pattern seen in Paget's disease are sometimes seen in these children. The hand films may show destruction of the terminal tufts and shortening of the terminal phalanges, much like the changes seen in scleroderma.

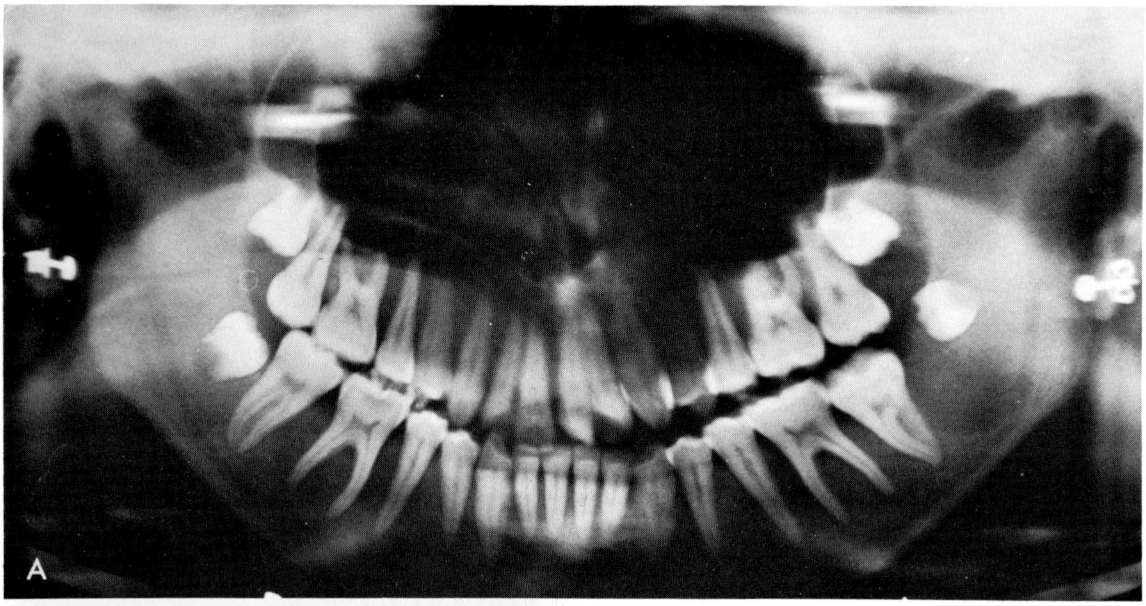

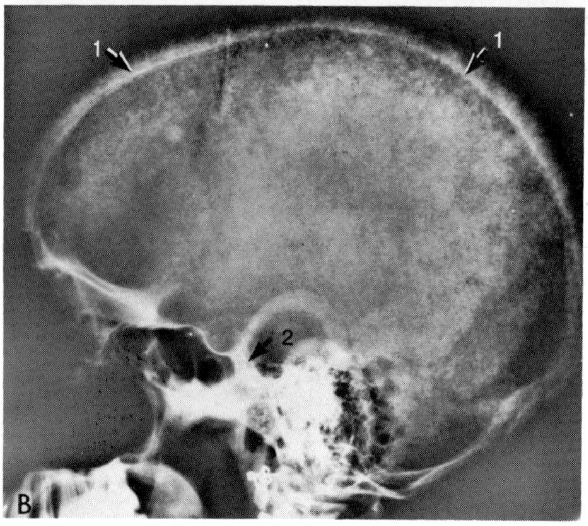

Figure 15–8. Secondary hyperparathyroidism (renal osteodystrophy). **A.** Note the loss of cortical outline about the developing tooth crypt, the displacement of the lower left third molar by a brown tumor, the slightly enlarged root canal spaces and a generalized ground-glass pattern of the alveolar bone in this 18-year-old female. **B.** Note the generalized thinning of the calvarium (1), the generalized salt-and-pepper to cotton-wool appearance of the skull, and calcification of the petroclinoid ligament (2).

Illustration continued on opposite page

DOMINANT CRANIOMETAPHYSEAL DYSPLASIA

BRIEF OVERVIEW

Craniometaphyseal dysplasia has been classified by Gorlin and associates as one of the craniotubular bone dysplasias. They have further subdivided craniometaphyseal dysplasia into dominant and recessive forms. Although the etiology is unknown, craniometaphyseal dysplasia is believed to be caused by a partial failure of osteoclastic resorption of the secondary spongiosum. This is unlike osteopetrosis, in which there is failure of osteoclastic resorption of the primary spongiosum. This causes a tubular defect in the long bones characterized by splayed metaphyses and hyperostosis in the skull and facial bones. The dominant form is characterized by ocular hypertelorism; broadening of the base of the nose; an open mouth resulting from narrowing of the nasal lumen; deafness, usually before puberty; and in rare instances, facial paralysis or defective vision. The clinical characteristics of the recessive form are more severe including facial deformity, blindness, and deafness. In the dominant form there is only mild facial deformity. The dominant and recessive forms of craniometaphyseal dysplasia should be distinguished from other, more severe craniotubular dysplasias including Pyle's disease (metaphyseal dysplasia) and craniodiaphyseal dysplasia.

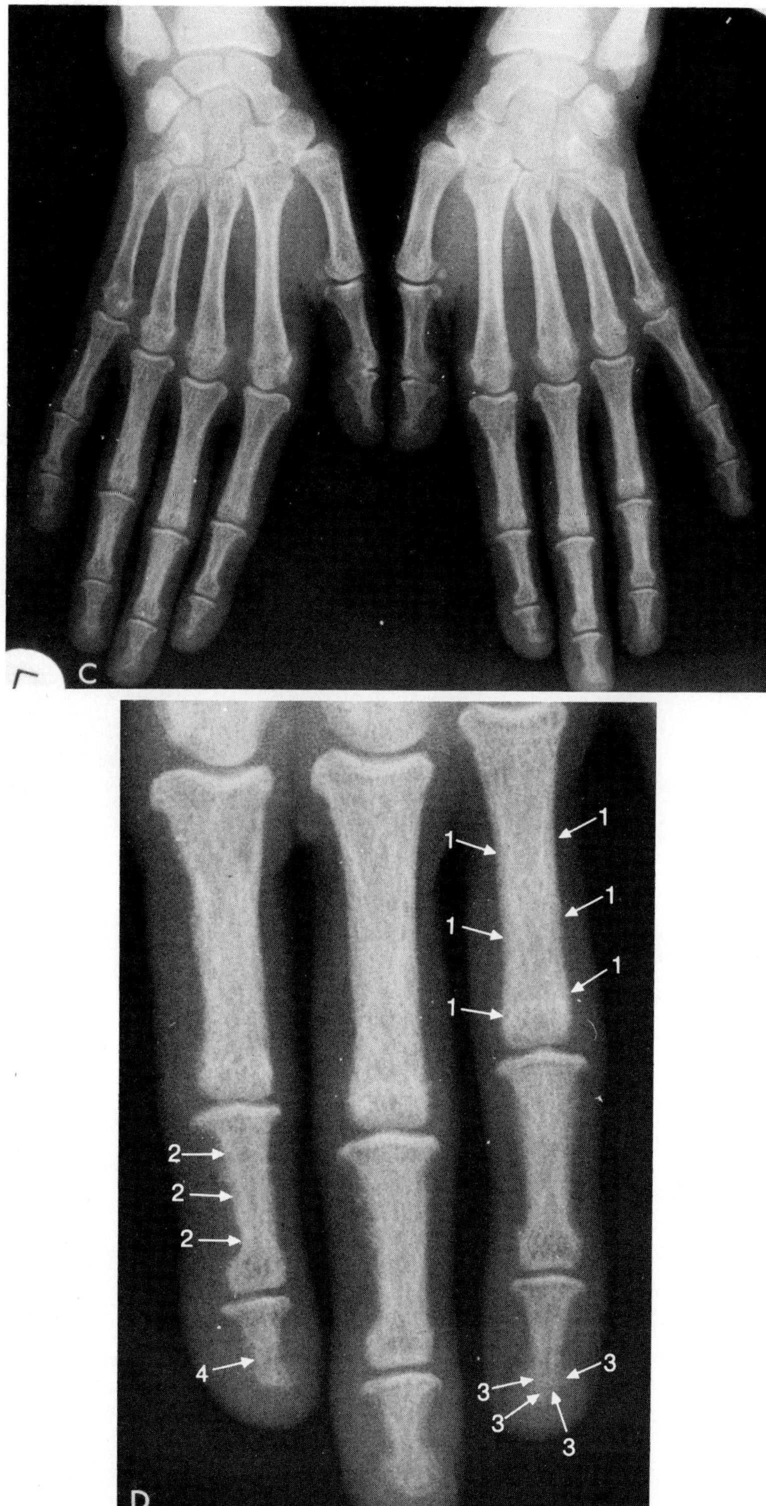

Figure 15–8 *Continued.* **C.** Note the generalized loss of the cortical outline of all of the phalanges, the subperiosteal erosion of the second (middle) phalanges, destruction of the terminal tufts of the distal phalanges, and shortening of the distal phalanges. **D.** Closer view of the phalangeal changes in **C.** 1. Loss of cortical outline of a proximal phalanx. 2. Subperiosteal erosion of the middle phalanx. 3. Destruction of the terminal tuft. 4. Shortening of the distal phalanx. Note the overall indistinctness of the trabecular pattern in the phalanges similar to the changes seen in the skull and jaws. (Figure 15–8 courtesy of Dr. Chris Nortjé, University of Stellenbosch, Tygerberg, South Africa.)

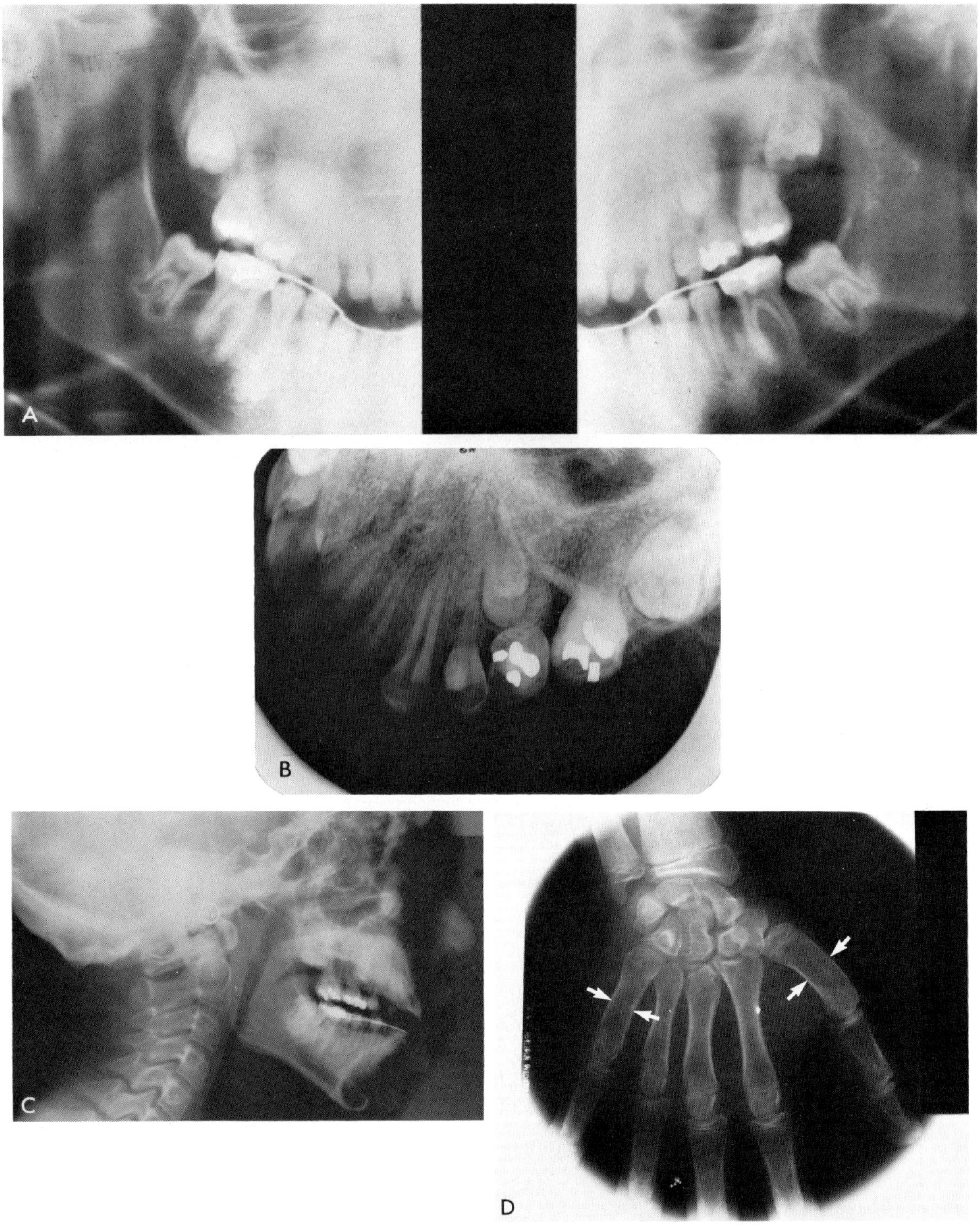

Figure 15–9. Dominant craniometaphyseal dysplasia. The patient is a 15-year-old male. **A.** Several retakes were necessary for most views and, even with maximum KV settings, a good image could not be obtained. **B.** Note that the crowns of the teeth are burnt out owing to the excessive exposure factors required to obtain this image. Note the classic ground-glass pattern and the generalized loss of the lamina dura. **C.** Note the lack of pneumatization of the paranasal sinuses and the absence of mastoid air spaces. The soft tissue outline shows the typical open mouth physiognomy. **D.** The arrows point to the typical tubular defect in the metacarpals, in which a failure of remodeling has resulted in a lack of constriction in the midshaft area.

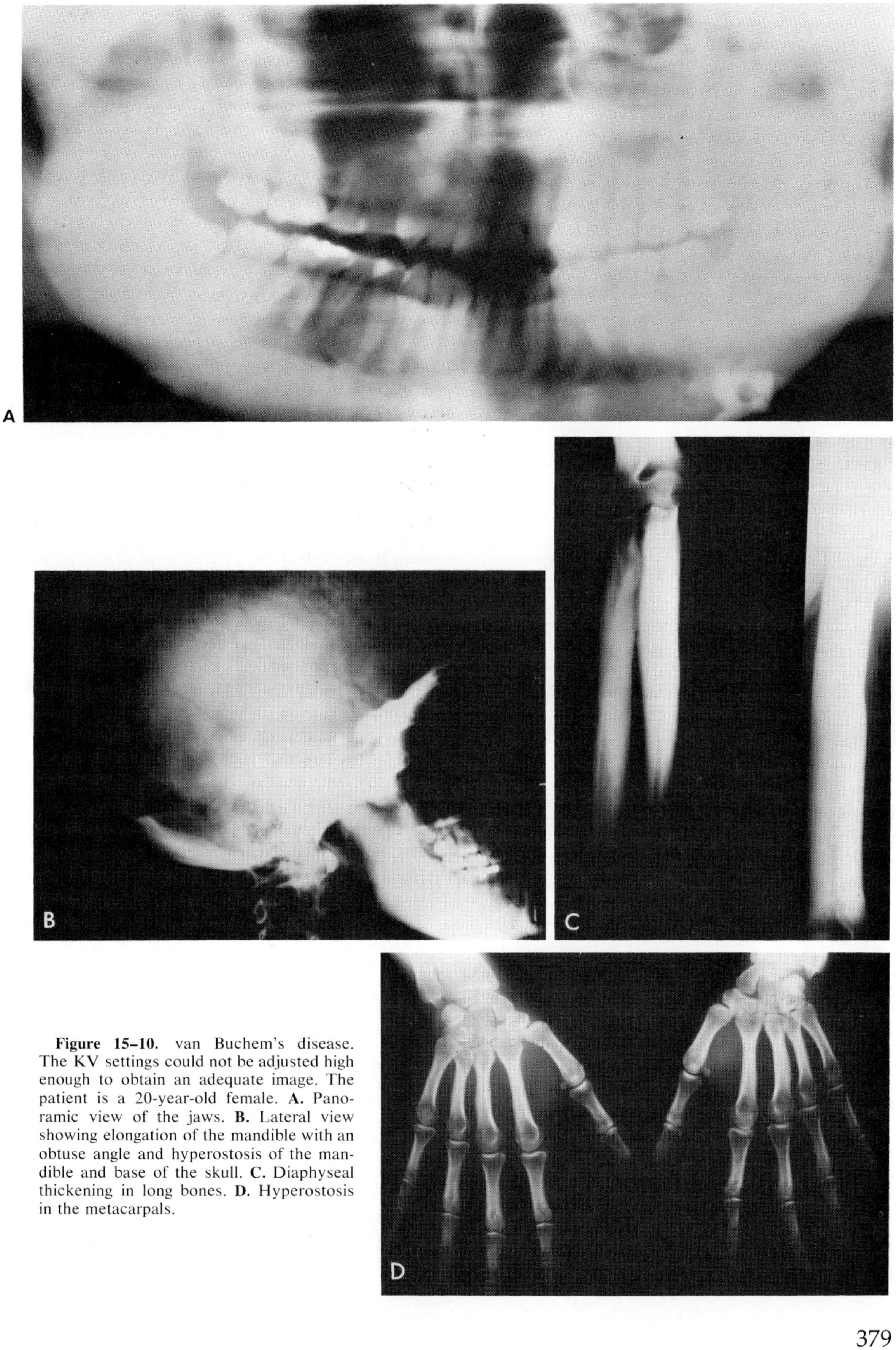

Figure 15–10. van Buchem's disease. The KV settings could not be adjusted high enough to obtain an adequate image. The patient is a 20-year-old female. **A.** Panoramic view of the jaws. **B.** Lateral view showing elongation of the mandible with an obtuse angle and hyperostosis of the mandible and base of the skull. **C.** Diaphyseal thickening in long bones. **D.** Hyperostosis in the metacarpals.

RADIOGRAPHIC FEATURES (Fig. 12–9)

According to Gorlin, Spranger, and Kozalka, the radiographic features include frontal and occipital hyperostosis of the calvarium. The base of the skull is usually sclerotic, with obliteration of the paranasal sinuses and lack of pneumatization of the mastoid air spaces. The long bones have a club-shaped metaphyseal flare and the short tubular bones show a similar lack of remodeling.

van BUCHEM'S DISEASE (Generalized Cortical Hyperostosis)

BRIEF OVERVIEW

Gorlin, Spranger, and Kozalka have classified this disorder as one of the genetic craniotubular hyperostoses, which differ from the craniotubular bone dysplasias of which dominant craniometaphyseal dysplasia is an example. The hyperostoses involve an active overgrowth of bone, whereas the dysplasias involve a defect in bone modeling.

van Buchem's disease is transmitted as an autosomal recessive trait with a variable expressivity. The cortical hyperostosis has been postulated to result mainly from endosteal bone deposition and, when severe, it may occlude the medullary spaces. The clinical features of van Buchem's disease include a characteristic broadening and prominence of the mandible with a normal occlusion, occasional mild exophthalmos, occasional facial paralysis, and visual and hearing difficulties. There are occasional headaches. Growth, development, and intelligence are normal. Alkaline phosphatase levels may be increased from 50 to 250 per cent above normal. There is no increased tendency for fractures. Treatment may be directed at management of the clinical features including orthognathic surgical reconstruction of the mandible.

RADIOGRAPHIC FEATURES (Fig. 15–10)

In the panoramic film, the mandible appears to be generally enlarged to the point of having difficulty in maintaining all areas within the sharply depicted layer. The jaws are uniformly more radiodense, and there may be difficulty in obtaining a good image even with the highest kVp and mAs factors available. In the lateral cephalometric view, the mandible will appear elongated with an obtuse angle and is extremely radiodense, as is the base of the skull. The long bones show diaphyseal thickening, and these bony changes are similar to those found in pachydermoperiostosis and hyperostosis generalisata with striation.

REFERENCES

Reference Texts

Shafer, W. G., Hine, M. K., and Levy, B. M.: **A Textbook of Oral Pathology**, 3rd Edition. Philadelphia: W. B. Saunders, 1974, pp. 456–458, 631–633, 635–640, 640–646.

Wood, N. K., and Goaz, P. W.: **Differential Diagnosis of Oral Lesions**. St. Louis: C. V. Mosby, 1975, pp. 539–546.

Worth, H. M.: **Principles and Practice of Oral Radiologic Interpretation.** Chicago: Year Book Medical Publishers 1963.

Selected References

El Deeb, M., Waite, D. E., and Jaspers, M. T.: Fibrous dysplasia of the jaws: Report of five cases. **Oral Surg. 47**:312, 1979.

Fletcher, P. D., Scopp, I. W., and Hersh, R. A.: Oral manifestations of secondary hyperparathyroidism related to long-term hemodialysis therapy. **Oral Surg. 43**:218, 1977.

Gorlin, R. J., Spranger, J., and Kozalka, M. F.: Genetic craniotubular bone dysplasias and hyperostoses, a critical analysis. **Birth Defects 4**:79, 1969.

Jacobsson, S., and Hollender, L.: Treatment and prognosis of diffuse sclerosing osteomyelitis (DSO) of the mandible. **Oral Surg. 49**:7, 1980.

Melrose, R. J., Abrams, A. M., and Mills, B. G.: Florid osseous dysplasia: A clinical-pathologic study of thirty-four cases. **Oral Surg. 41**:62, 1976.

Mincer, H. H., McGinnis, J. P., and Wyatt, J. R.: Ultrastructure of sclerotic cemental masses. **Oral Surg. 43**:70, 1977.

Obisesan, A. A., Lagundoye, S. B., Daramola, J. O., Ajagbe, H. A., and Oluwasanmi, J. O.: The radiologic features of fibrous dysplasia of the craniofacial bones. **Oral Surg. 44**:949, 1977.

Rubin, P.: **Dynamic Classification of Bone Dysplasias**. Chicago: Year Book Medical Publishers, 1964, pp. 280–296.

Waldron, C. A., Giansanti, J. S., and Browand, B. C.: Sclerotic cemental masses of the jaws (so-called chronic sclerosing osteomyelitis, sclerosing osteitis, multiple enostosis and gigantiform cementoma). **Oral Surg. 39**:590, 1975.

Chapter 16
The Maxillary Sinus

VISUALIZATION OF STRUCTURES

The maxillary sinus begins to develop in utero at about three months, at which time there is an invagination of the epithelium of the lateral wall of the nasal fossa. The maxillary sinus is about the size of a pea at birth and increases in size to adulthood. It is larger than usual when pneumatized by local factors such as allergy, trauma, and frequent colds. It is the largest of the paranasal sinuses, which also include the ethmoid, frontal, and sphenoid sinuses (Fig. 16–1). It is centrally located in the maxilla and consists of an air-filled cavity lined with ciliated pseudostratified columnar epithelium. Its medial wall is the lateral wall of the nasal cavity, its roof is the floor of the orbit, and its floor is the alveolar process of the maxilla. The mucosal lining contains a large number of seromucinous glands on the nasal wall but few on the lateral wall. The floor of the sinus is usually about 1 cm below the level of the floor of the nasal cavity. The floor may also be above the apices of the associated premolars and molars or it may dip down in between their roots, with only a thin layer of cortical bone separating the two.

All of the paranasal sinuses communicate with the nasal cavities and, indirectly, with each other. Their main function is to warm and humidify the inspired air. They also reduce the weight of the facial bones, influence vocalization, and, in prehistoric days, may have been involved in olefaction. The maxillary ostium is located near the top of the maxillary sinus, on the medial wall, about level with the second molar. This is the main opening through which the maxillary sinus drains its secretions into the nasal cavity, at the level of the middle meatus. There is sometimes an accessory opening,

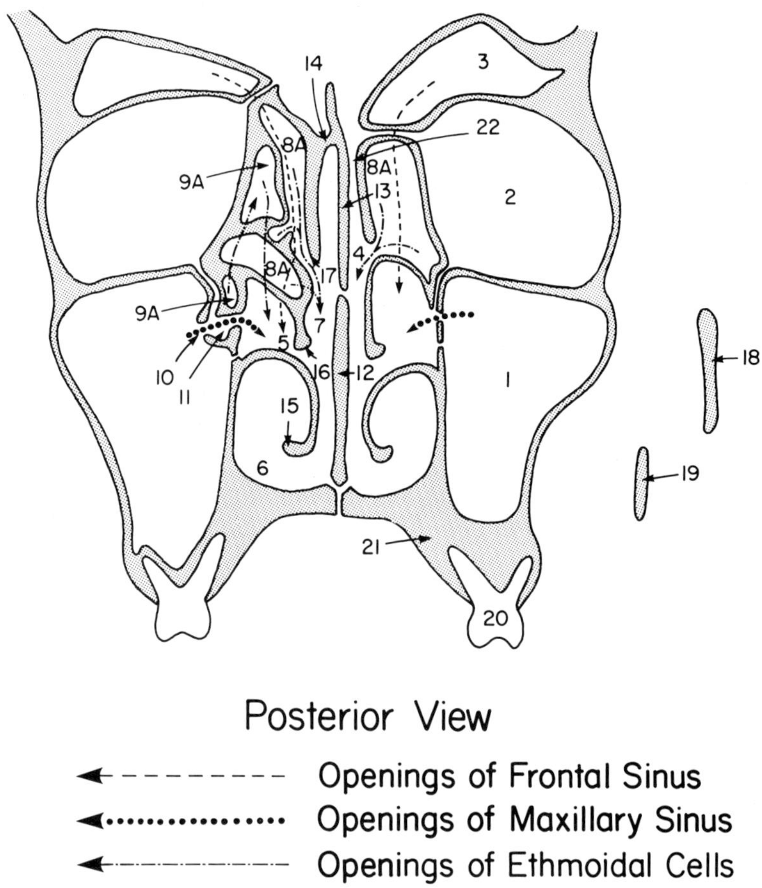

Figure 16–1. Schematic representation of a frontal section of the nasal cavities and surrounding structures. 1. Maxillary sinus. 2. Orbit. 3. Frontal sinus. 4. Superior nasal meatus. 5. Middle nasal meatus. 6. Inferior nasal meatus. 7. Common nasal meatus. 8A. Posterior ethmoid cells. 9A. Anterior ethmoid cells. 10. Maxillary ostium. 11. Ethmoid infundibulum. 12. Vomer. 13. Perpendicular plate of ethmoid bone. 14. Cribriform plate of ethmoid bone. 15. Inferior nasal concha. 16. Middle nasal concha. 17. Superior nasal concha. 18. Zygomatic arch. 19. Coronoid process of mandible. 20. Maxillary second molar. 21, Alveolar process of maxilla. 22. Olfactory fissure. (Adapted from Pernkopf, E.: Atlas of Topographical and Applied Human Anatomy, Vol. 1, Head and Neck. Philadelphia: W. B. Saunders, 1963, p. 126.)

usually posterior and inferior to the main opening.

The authors have included this basic information concerning the paranasal sinuses, particularly the maxillary sinus, because this knowledge is helpful in understanding the conditions they are about to describe. Additionally, and more importantly, the manner in which panoramic radiographs project anatomic structures is unique. Prior knowledge of the correct anatomic interrelationships of the structures is essential to their interpretation on the panoramic view. Knowledge of the projection factors as described in Chapter 2 is also necessary.

Although the maxillary sinus may be studied with panoramic radiographs, the projection method of choice is the Waters' view. Ohba and Katayama found that panoramic views were superior to the Waters' projection in detecting cyst-like densities, whereas the Waters' view was better for demonstrating cloudiness and sclerotic changes in the bony walls. They concluded that both techniques should be included in the standard sinus examination. Also helpful are periapical, occlusal, lateral head, and Caldwell views. The Caldwell view is a nose-to-forehead posteroanterior projection.

NORMAL ANATOMIC STRUCTURES AND VARIATIONS OF NORMAL

In panoramic radiography, the maxillary sinuses are visualized with the standard technique. Additionally, most machines can be adjusted so that the more superior aspects of the antrum can be seen. Also, some manufacturers offer a cassette that is 6 in. wide rather than the standard 5 in. The wider film shows more of the

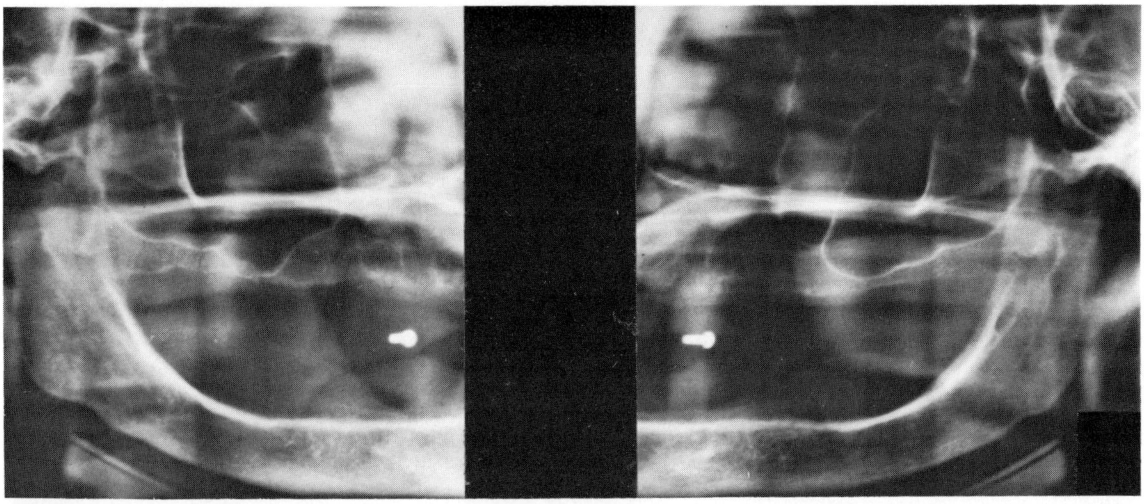

Figure 16–2. Modified standard view. With the chin raised to the horizontal position, much of the sinus may be viewed.

superior aspects of the maxillary sinus than the standard view (Figs. 16–2 and 16–3).

In the panoramic projection of the maxillary sinus, the **body of the zygomatic bone** and the **temporal process of the zygomatic bone**, which is the anterior half of the zygomatic arch, will almost invariably be superimposed on the sinus (Fig. 16–4). The **panoramic innominate line** is a thin, vertical, radiopaque line in the posterior third of the sinus and is so named because it is composed of the panoramic juxtapositioning of two separate bones, the lower half consisting of the thin cortical outline of the posterior surface of the zygomatic process of the maxilla, and the upper half consisting of the thin cortical outline of the posterior surface of the frontal process of the zygoma. The panoramic innominate line is similar to, but different from, the innominate line seen in the Caldwell view, in which the innominate line crosses the outer third of the orbit in an oblique vertical direction and corresponds to a cross section of the squamozygomatic surface of the sphenoid bone. The panoramic innominate line should not be misinterpreted as the posteromedial wall of the maxillary sinus (see Fig. 16–4).

The **pterygomaxillary fossa** is a well-corticated, teardrop-shaped radiolucency, which is outside but immediately adjacent to the posteromedial wall of the maxillary sinus. The posterior portion consists of the anterior cortical outline of the lateral pterygoid plate of the sphenoid bone up to the point where it fuses with the posterior wall of the maxillary sinus, forming the pterygomaxillary fissure. The rounded superior portion consists of the most inferior aspect of the greater wing of the sphenoid bone, which is superimposed on the posteromedial wall of the maxillary sinus. The anterior portion of the fossa is the posterior wall

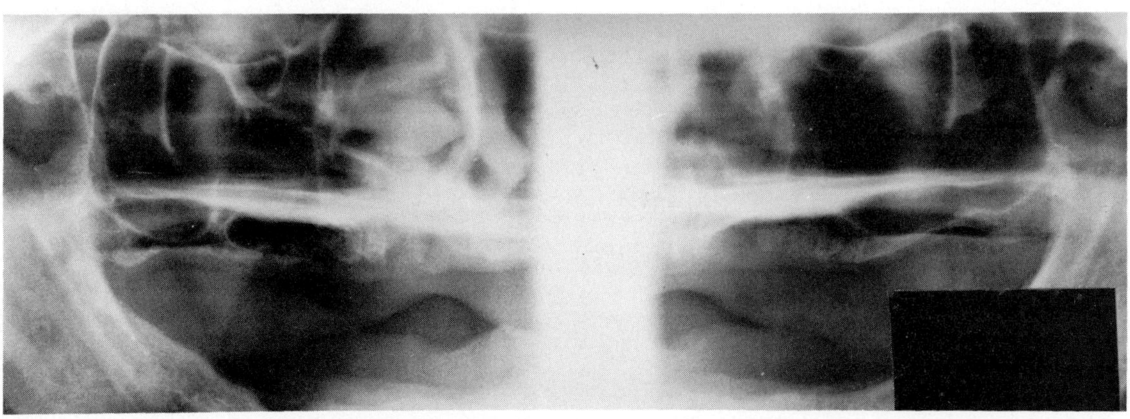

Figure 16–3. Sinus projection.

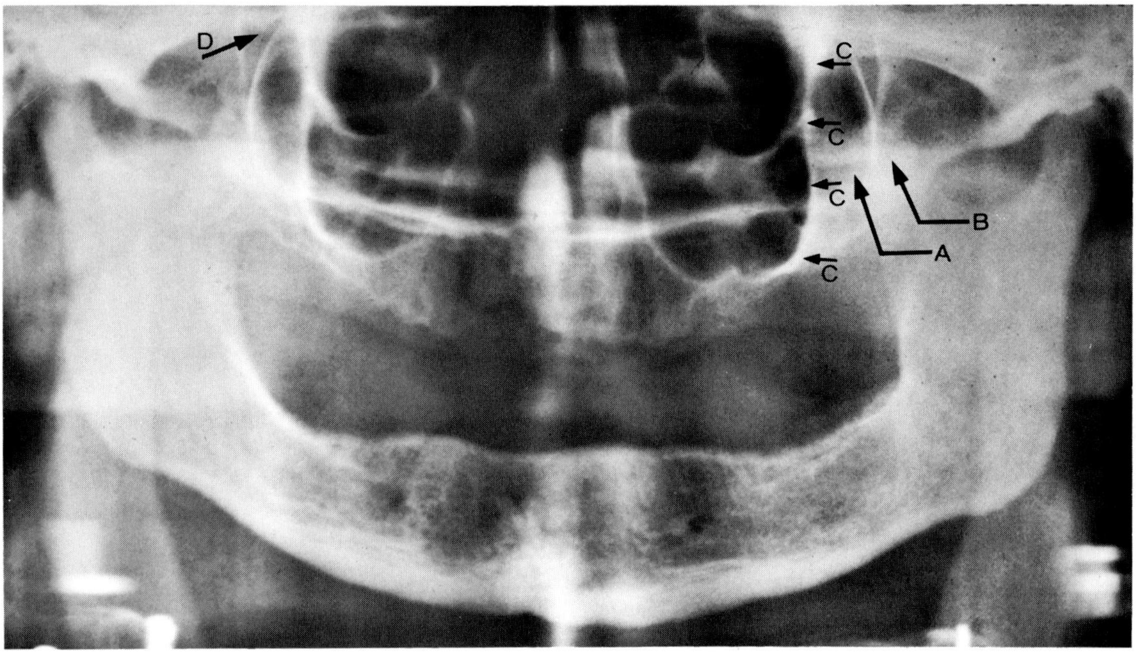

Figure 16–4. Visualization of structures. A. Body of the zygomatic bone. B. Temporal process of the zygomatic bone. C. Panoramic innominate line. D. Pterygomaxillary fossa.

of the maxillary sinus. The pterygomaxillary fossa should not be mistaken for an extra compartment or lobe of the maxillary sinus (see Fig. 16–4).

Spreading horizontally across the entire breadth of the lower third of the maxillary sinus is the double image of the **hard palate (floor of the nose)**. The lower radiopaque line is the actual image, whereas the upper line is the ghost image of the contralateral hard palate. The degree of separation of the two lines depends on the position of the chin. The ghost image moves away from the actual image when the chin is tilted downwards (Figs. 16–5 and 16–6).

The **infraorbital canal** and **infraorbital foramen** may be superimposed in the superior mid-portion of the maxillary sinus (see Fig. 16–5).

When the **dorsum of the tongue** is not placed in intimate contact with the hard palate during

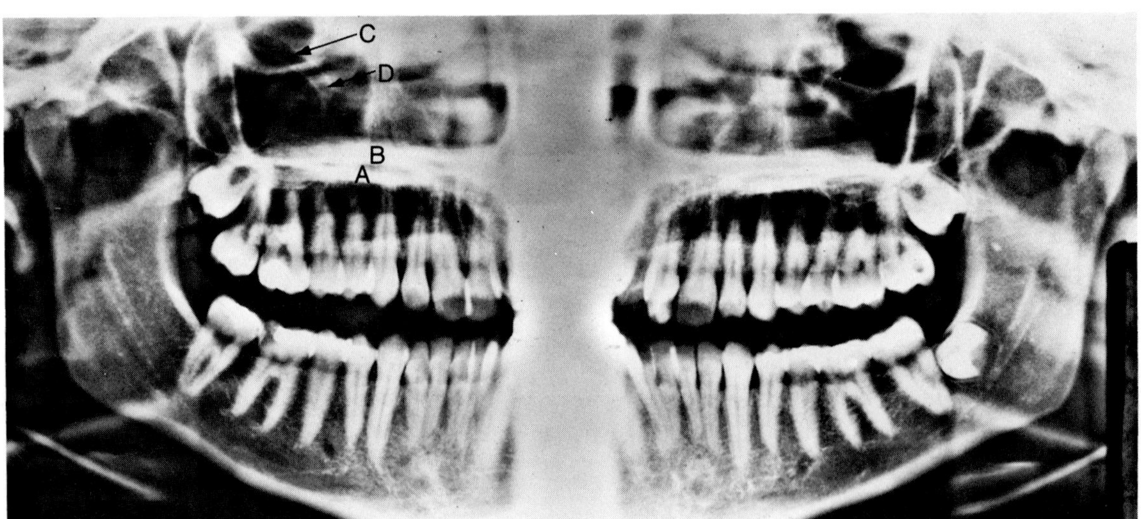

Figure 16–5. Visualization of structures. A. Actual hard palate. B. Ghost of contralateral palate. C. Infraorbital canal. D. Infraorbital foramen.

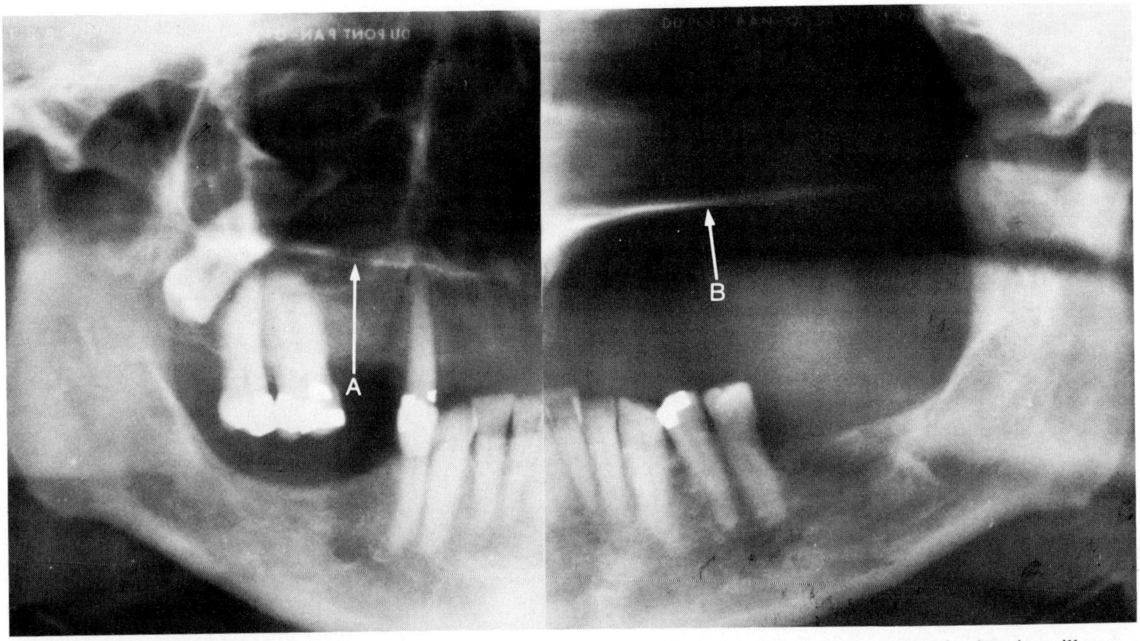

Figure 16-6. Visualization of structures. This is a postoperative film of a patient who received a hemimaxillectomy with removal of the orbit for an antral carcinoma. This film illustrates the actual hard palate on the right side (A) and the ghost image on the left side (B). (Courtesy of Drs. Frank Sammis, Jr. and Carlos Portales, San Antonio, TX.)

exposure, the intervening air will allow the dorsum of the tongue to be visualized as a bilateral, smooth, convex radiopacity in the lower sinus that extends beyond the sinus. The dorsum of the tongue should not be mistaken for a fluid level or a thickening of the mucosal lining (Fig. 16-7).

In certain projections, the soft tissue of the **inferior and middle turbinates** may be projected as a radiopacity that traverses horizontally across the midportion of the maxillary sinus. The radiopaque areas are usually more opaque towards the anterior portion and may extend beyond the anterior boundary of the sinus (see Fig. 16-8).

The **inferior, middle**, and, sometimes, **superior meati** may be projected horizontally across the maxillary sinus as radiolucent lines. These radiolucent lines are not corticated and should not be mistaken for nutrient canals or fracture lines. The inferior meatus is usually just above the hard palate shadow. The meati may outline the turbinate shadow (Figs. 16-8 and 16-9). Additionally, there may be ghosting of the contralateral turbinates and meati. Aside from the radiopaque lines already discussed, the maxillary sinus may be **multicompartmentalized** and may contain a number of thin, radiopaque **bony septae** (see Fig. 16-8).

When **maxillary tori** are present, they are seen as bilateral, dense, radiopaque masses of varying size on the panoramic films. They may extend beyond the inferior or anterior boundaries of the maxillary sinus but do not usually extend above the hard palate. They should not be mistaken for pathologic sinus conditions such as osteomas, fibrous dysplasia, or inflammatory changes (Figs. 16-10 and 16-11).

Pneumatization of the maxillary sinus is said to exist when it is the examiner's impression that the sinus is enlarged by air. This may occur in the presence of all the teeth, in which case the floor of the sinus may dip down in between the roots of the subjacent teeth. More frequently, when teeth have been lost the floor of the sinus may be very close to the crest of the alveolar ridge. Pneumatization, especially when the teeth are present, may be an indication of previous allergic and inflammatory involvement. When pneumatization is present, care should be taken when removing retained or broken root tips and during other surgical procedures, as the root tips may be accidentally displaced into the sinus or an oroantral fistula may be created (Fig. 16-12).

From time to time, a **sinus recess** is encountered. This is a small outpocketing of the wall of the sinus and appears as a radiolucency. When superimposed on the apices of teeth, it should not be misinterpreted as periapical pathology (Fig. 16-13).

Knowledge of these normal structures and

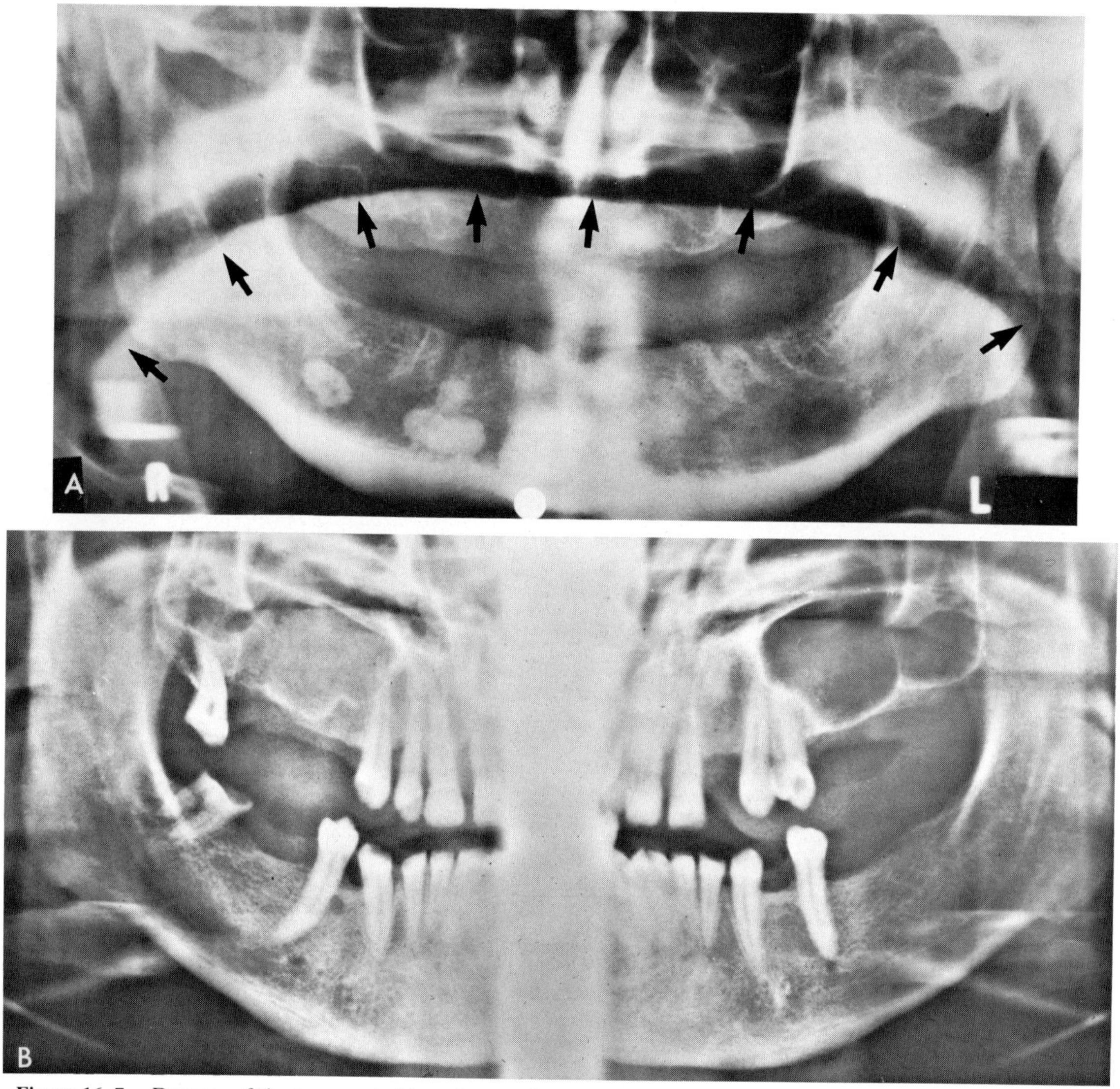

Figure 16–7. Dorsum of the tongue. **A.** Note the excellent visualization of the nasal area and the lateral spreading of the turbinate shadow across the sinus. **B.** Note that the tongue extends beyond the sinuses and causes varying degrees of opacity within the antrum.

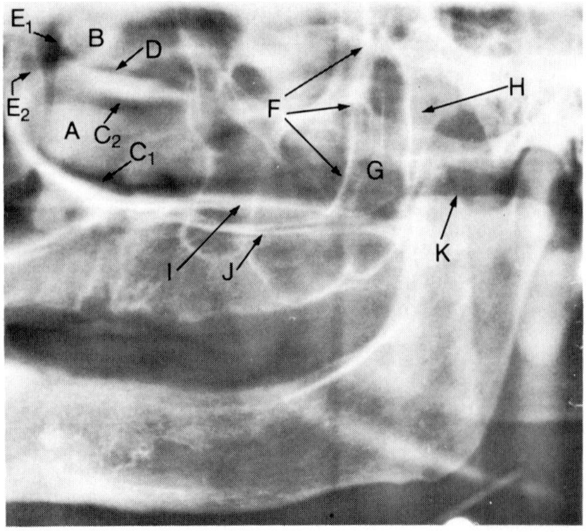

Figure 16–8. Multicompartmentalized sinus. A. Inferior turbinate. B. Middle turbinate. C_1. Inferior meatus. C_2. Ghost image of the contralateral meatus. D. Middle meatus. E_1. Common meatus. E_2. Ghost image of contralateral meatus, F. Panoramic innominate line. G. Body of the zygomatic bone. H. Pterygomaxillary fossa. I. Ghost contralateral hard palate. J. Actual hard palate. K. Dorsum of the tongue.

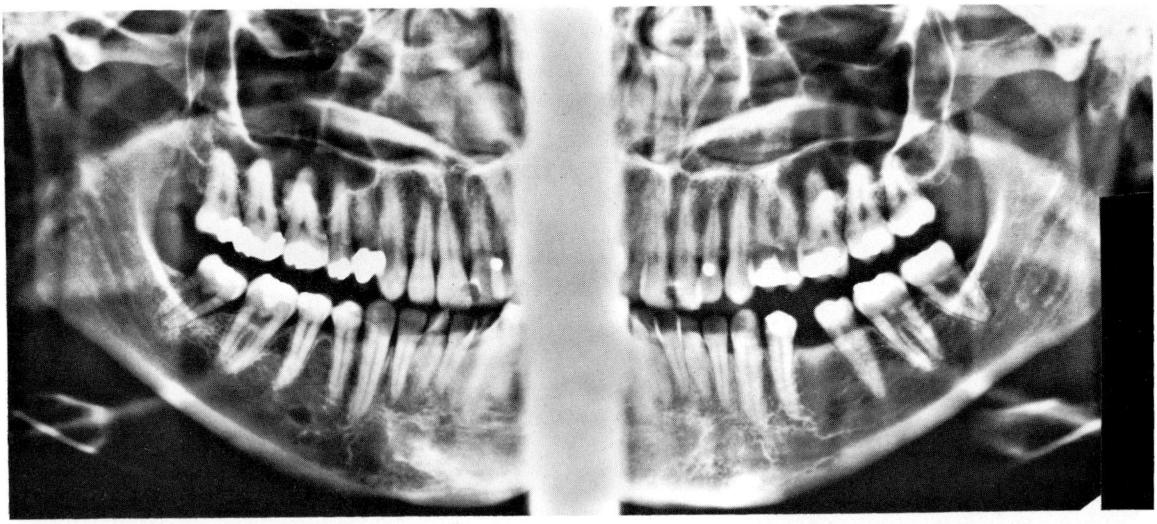

Figure 16–9. Pneumatization. Note that the floor dips down below the level of the apices of the adjacent roots. Note the actual and contralateral images and the ghost images of the turbinates and meati.

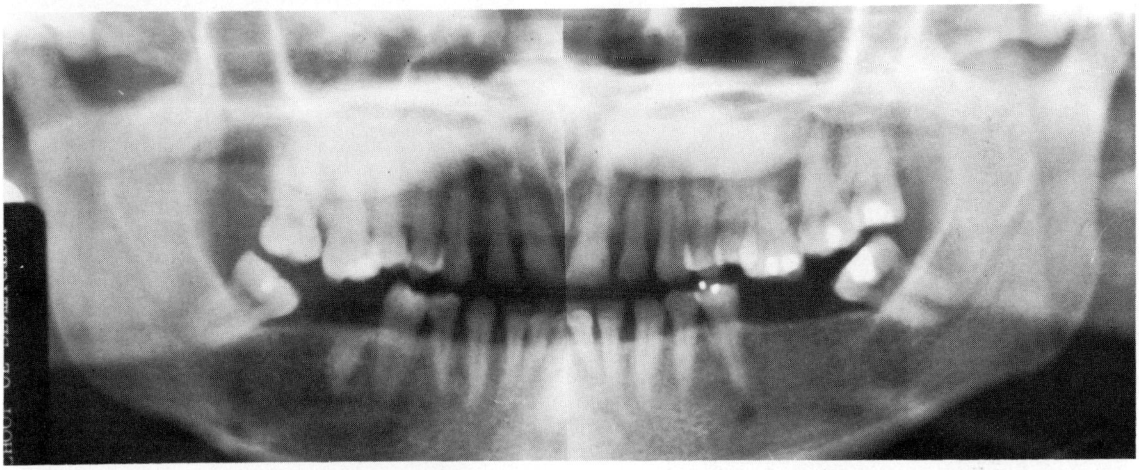

Figure 16–10. Torus palatinus.

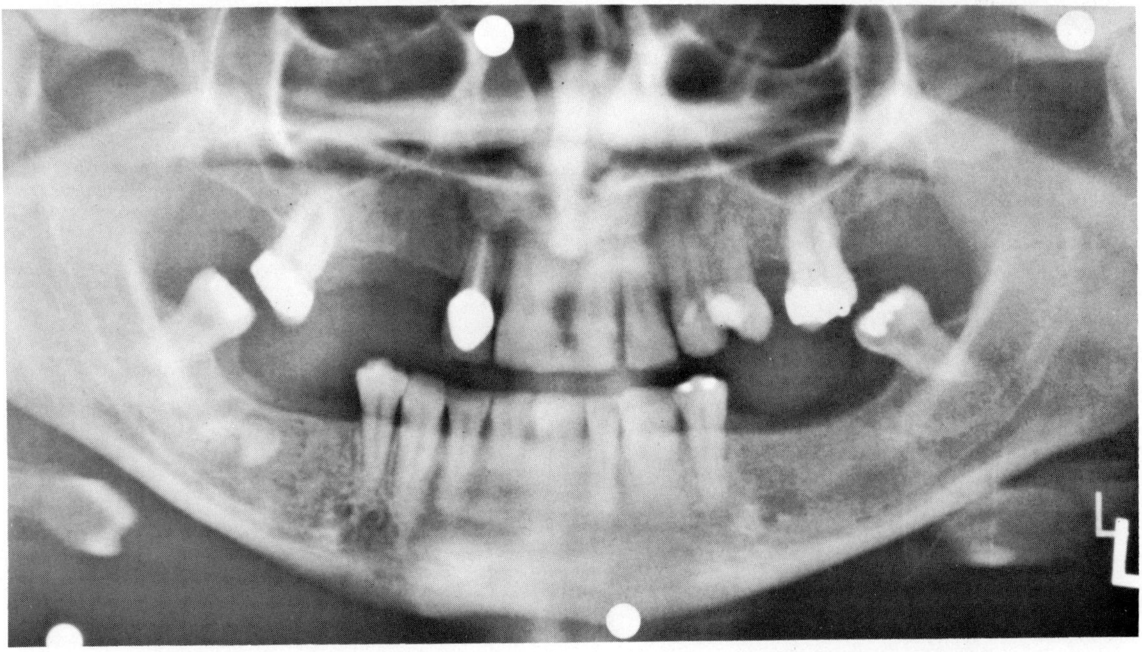

Figure 16–11. Soft tissue of the nose. This should not be mistaken for a torus palatinus.

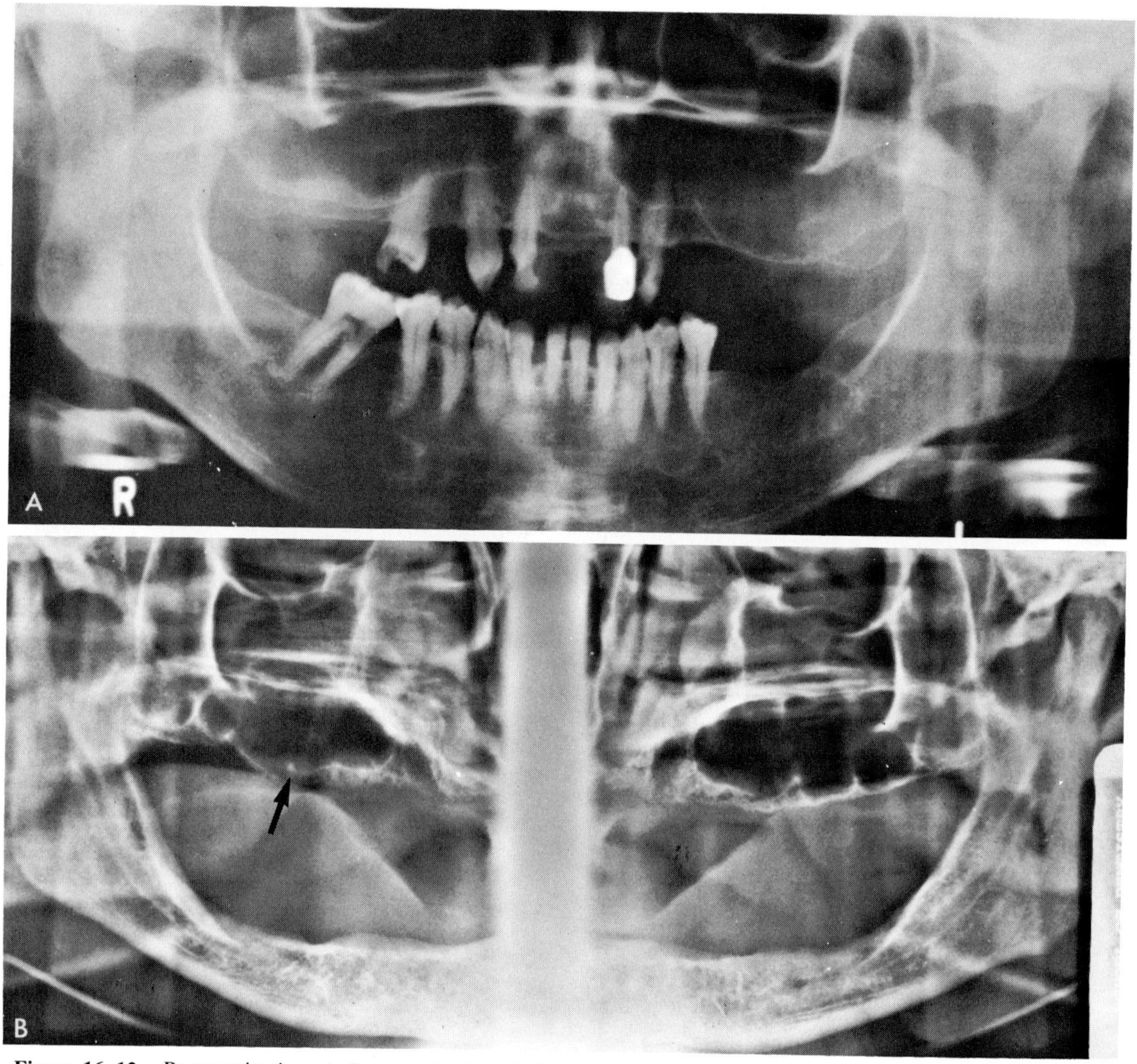

Figure 16–12. Pneumatization. **A.** Pneumatization of the maxillary sinus. **B.** Pneumatization with an oroantral fistula present. Note the loss of continuity of the bony wall of the sinus floor and the thickening of the antral mucosa in the area (arrow).

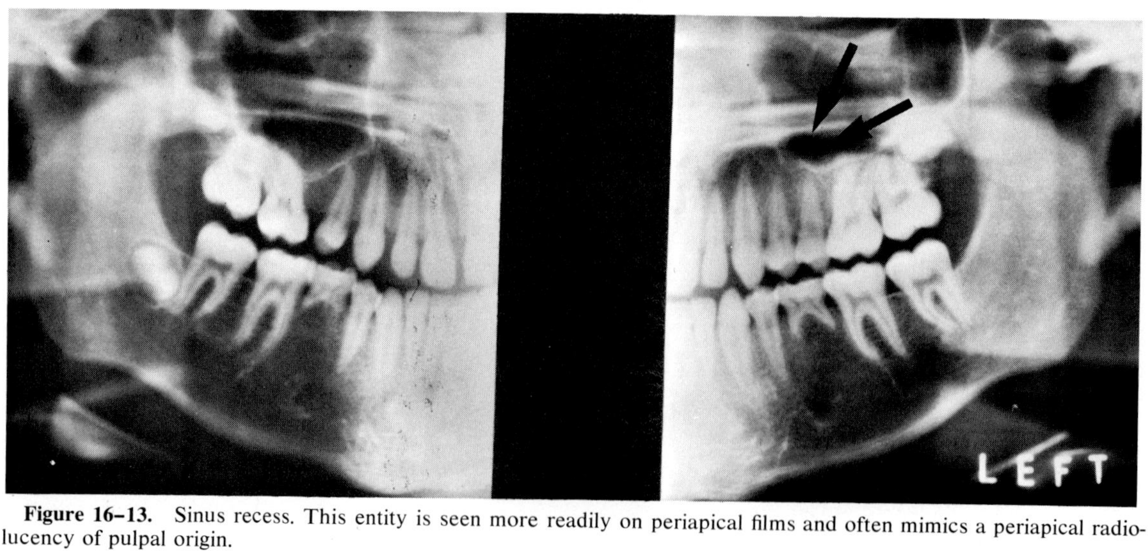

Figure 16–13. Sinus recess. This entity is seen more readily on periapical films and often mimics a periapical radiolucency of pulpal origin.

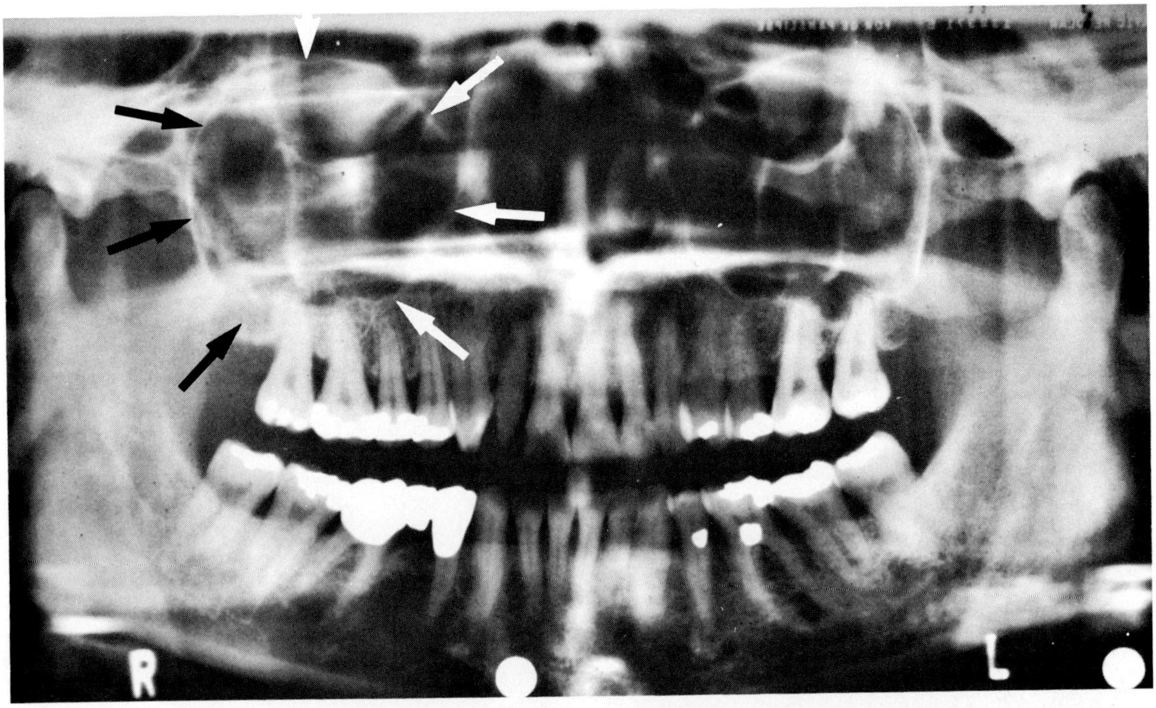

Figure 16–14. Panoramic innominate circle. What bones make up this circle?

their variations is the first and most important step in recognizing an abnormality of the maxillary sinus (Fig. 16–14).

INFLAMMATORY PROBLEMS OF NONDENTAL OR NONPERIODONTAL ORIGIN

The most important sequela of a sinus infection is excessive production of fluids by the mucosal lining. These secretions, as well as other inflammatory products such as pus, accumulate and will not drain until they reach the level of the maxillary ostium. Drainage may be prevented if the swollen sinus mucosa blocks the ostium. In this event, the patient may complain of a unilateral headache and a throbbing, constant pain in the area of the maxillary sinus, which may radiate to the teeth or ears. Toothache is a common presenting symptom. Many of the teeth in the quadrant may be sore and painful to percussion but are found vital on pulp testing. The teeth may be stomp positive, i.e., they are more painful when running, jumping, or descending stairs. The area of the canine fossa is tender to palpation, and the overlying skin may be slightly swollen and red. These symptoms are mainly referable to **acute sinusitis** or **allergic sinusitis.** In the latter case there may also be sneezing, watering of the eyes, or pruritus in the eyelids. Radiographically, when the mucosal lining becomes thickened or hyperplastic, it encroaches upon the airspace and changes from radiolucent to radiopaque. The degree of mucosal thickening may be localized to a single area; more frequently it may involve multiple areas, or it may produce a complete opacification of the sinus (Figs. 16–15 and 16–16).

Additionally, a **fluid level** may be seen. It is always located in the lowest portion of the sinus when the patient is erect. Its upper margin remains parallel to the horizontal plane when a second film is taken with the head tilted. The upper margin of the fluid level is always a straight line and does not follow anatomic contours as does mucosal thickening. A fluid level may be associated with or may be superimposed on other areas of mucosal thickening, which are the source of the abnormal accumulation of fluid (Fig. 16–17).

If the ostium remains blocked, pus may accumulate (**empyema**), and **mucocele, osteomyelitis,** or **antro-oral fistula** may result. The condition may become chronic, and **antral** or **nasal polyps** may develop and cause mechanical blockage of the ostium or of the air flow. Management usually includes decongestants, antibiotics, and antihistamines, depending on the nature and cause of the sinusitis. Surgical intervention, such as nasal antrostomy, may eventually become necessary.

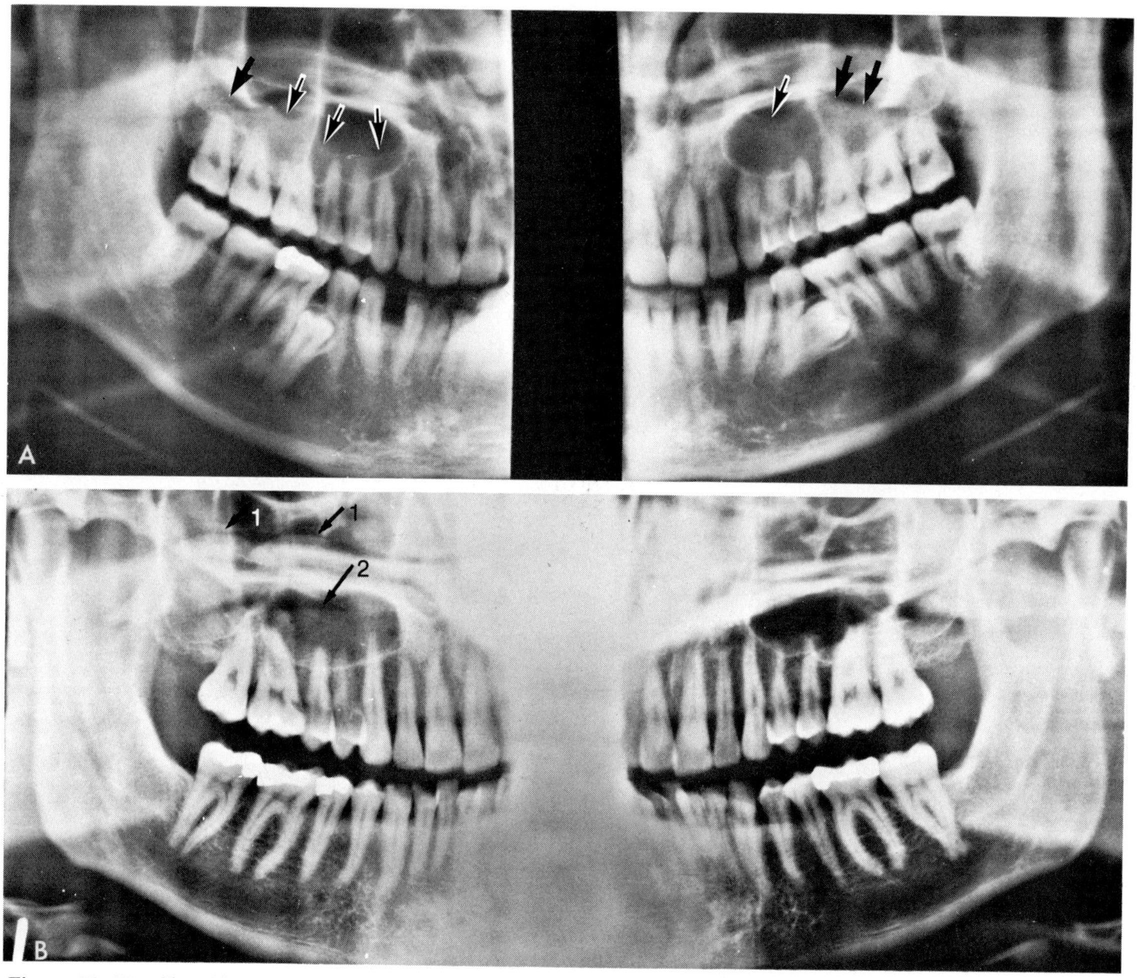

Figure 16–15. Sinusitis. **A.** Note the varying degrees of mucositis of nondental or periodontal origin. **B.** 1. Multiple areas of localized mucosal thickening. 2. Dorsum of the tongue.

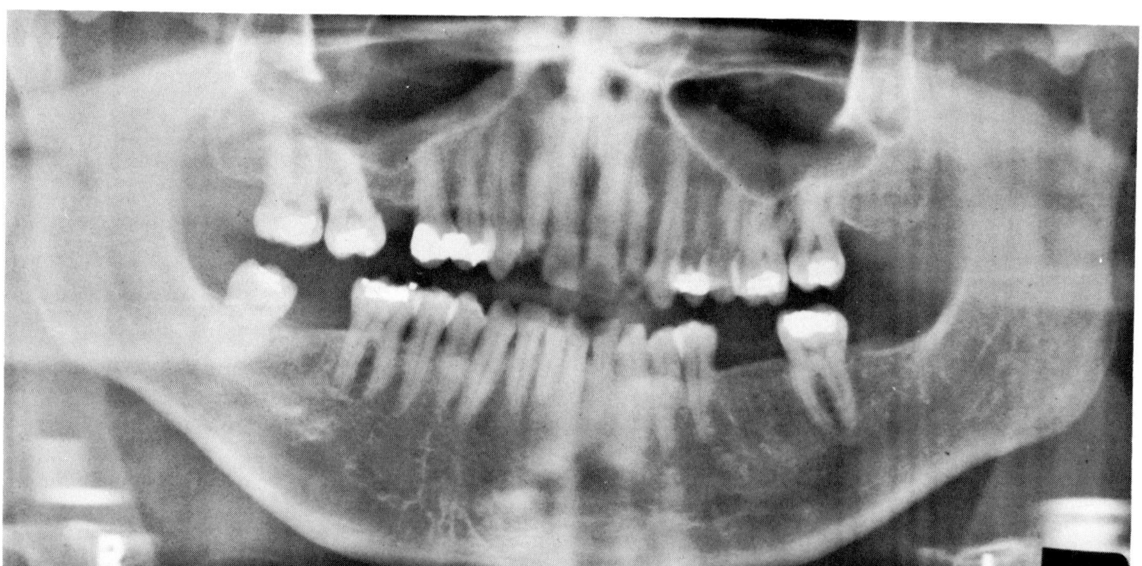

Figure 16–16. Mucositis.

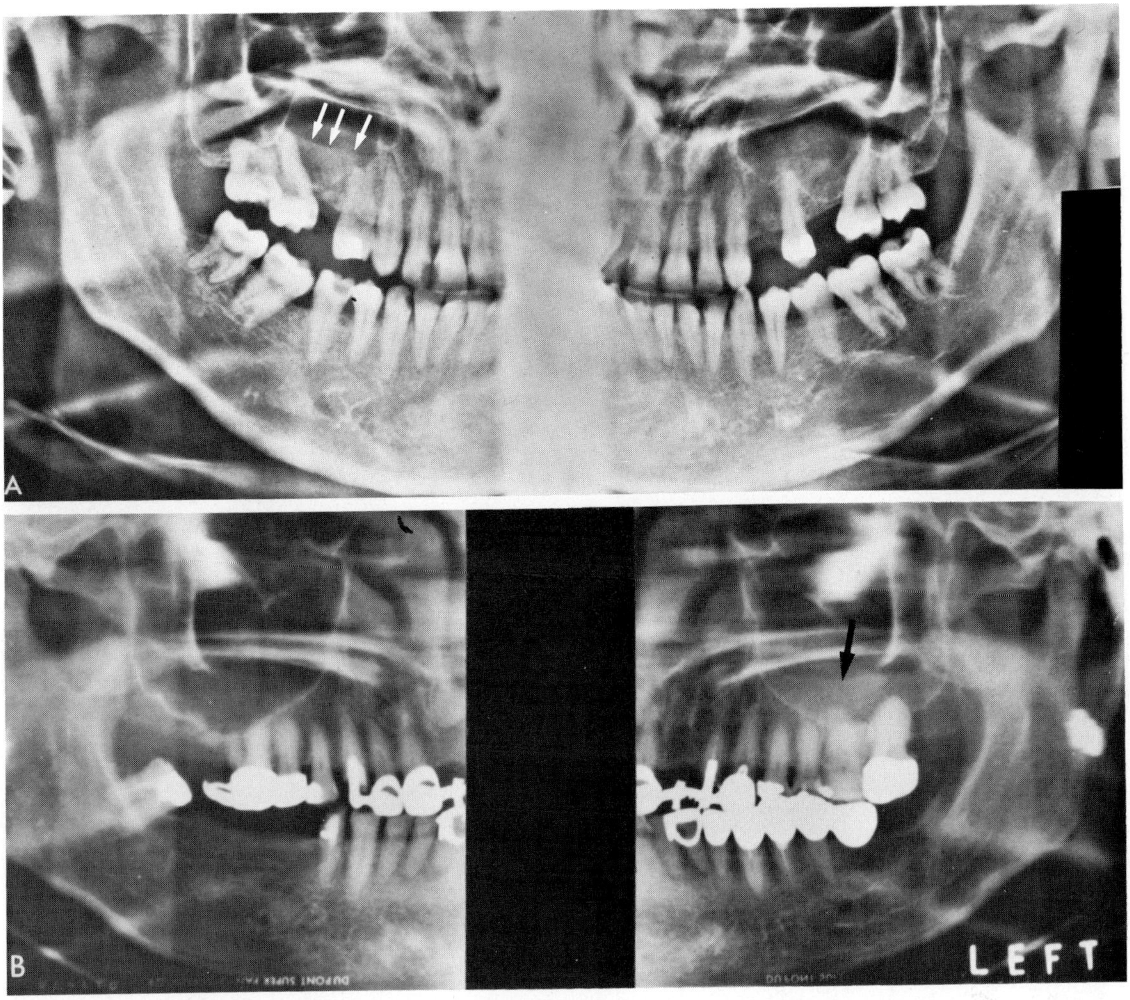

Figure 16–17. Fluid level. **A.** Note the great degree of pneumatization. **B.** The opacity on the right side is the dorsum of the tongue. Note the typical convex outline.

A fungal disease that may affect the paranasal sinuses is **phycomycosis (mucormycosis)**. The organisms enter via the nasal passages into the paranasal sinuses, pharynx, palate, orbit, and brain. This condition is usually a sign of a coexisting debilitating condition, often diabetes. It is also seen in cancer patients, especially those with lymphomas. In phycomycosis there is complete opacification of the sinus, along with involvement of the adjacent tissues. The condition may mimic a primary malignancy of the sinus.

INFLAMMATORY PROBLEMS OF DENTAL OR PERIODONTAL ORIGIN

The usual cause of sinus infection is an organism, commonly bacterial, that is inhaled. In the case of allergic sinusitis, which may accompany an allergic rhinitis, it is the inhaled allergens that cause the problem. In some instances, however, the cause of the sinusitis may be bacterial organisms of pulpal or periodontal origin. In these instances, according to Worth and Stoneman, there are two possible periapical reactions. First, there may be destruction of the periapical lamina dura, periapical alveolar bone, and the cortex of the adjacent sinus floor. There is usually a well-defined periapical radiolucency resulting from the bone destruction. The periosteum may be displaced superiorly by the accumulation of inflammatory elements and may then deposit a layer of new bone, which appears as a thin radiopaque **halo** bulging into the sinus beyond the sinus floor. Others have referred to this as expansion or bowing of the sinus floor (Figs. 16–18 and 16–19). A second

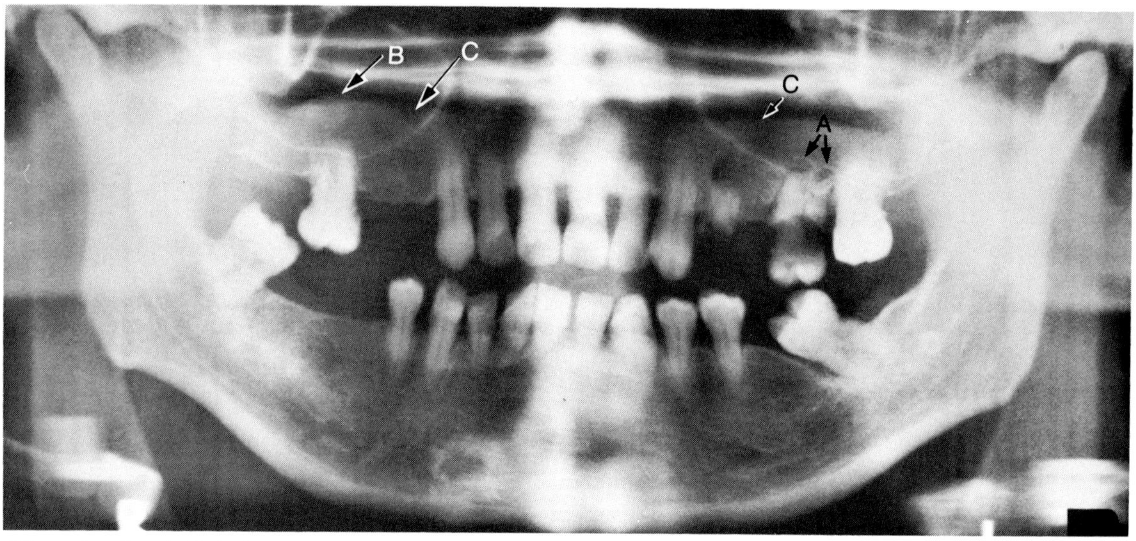

Figure 16–18. A. Halo formation. Any associated mucositis is not seen owing to superimposition of the tongue shadow (C). B. Mucositis. This may be of periodontal origin. C. Dorsum of the tongue.

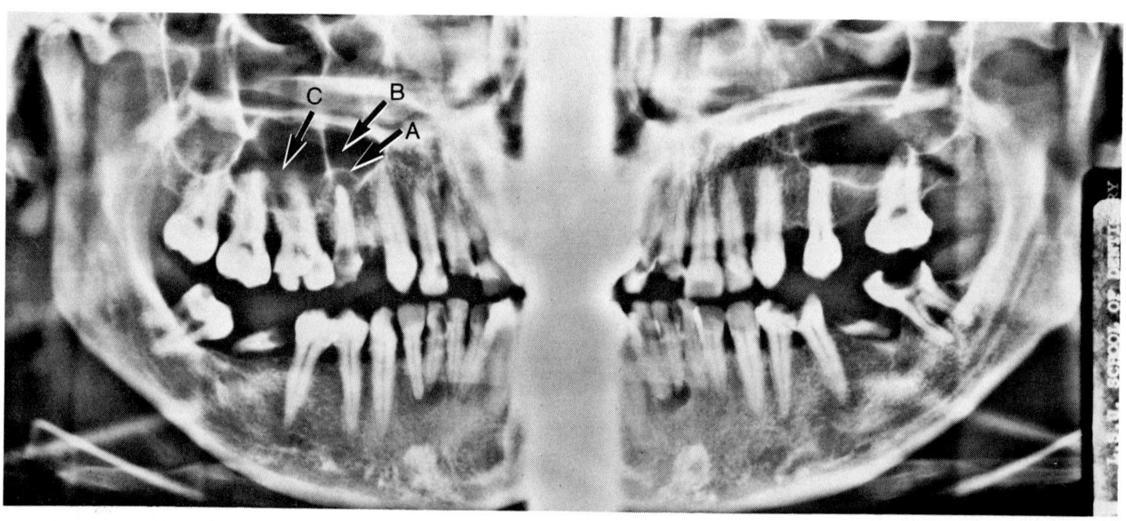

Figure 16–19. Halo formation with mucositis. A. Halo formation. B. Mucositis. C. Dorsum of the tongue.

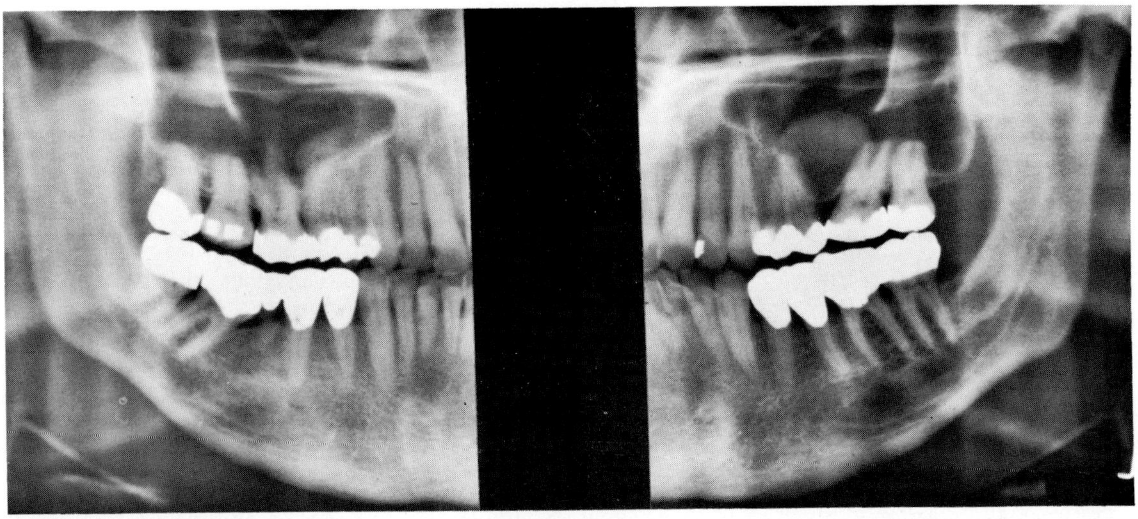

Figure 16–20. Right maxillary sinus. Periapical mucositis. Left maxillary sinus. Mucous retention cyst. The maxillary right second bicuspid was nonvital.

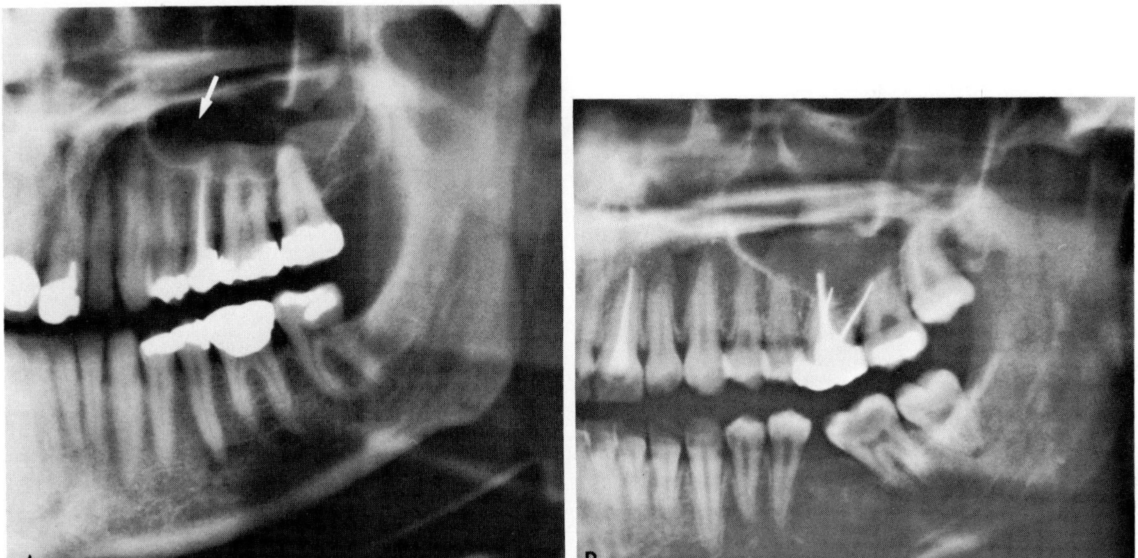

Figure 16–21. Periapical mucositis. **A.** Note the incompletely filled root canal space, the periapical radiolucency, and the faint radiopaque mucositis at the apex. These findings may be indicative of an endodontic failure. **B.** The area is so large that it resembles a mucous retention cyst and is suggestive of an endodontic failure.

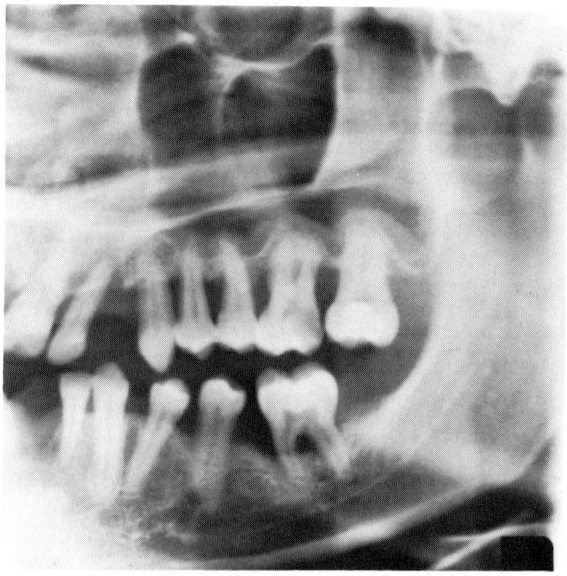

Figure 16–22. Mucositis. Associated with periodontal disease.

type of reaction to periapical inflammation, according to Worth and Stoneman, is one in which there is minimal or no periapical bone destruction. Both the alveolar bone and the antral floor appear relatively normal, but some organisms penetrate the sinus and cause a localized thickening, known as **periapical mucositis** or **inflammatory hyperplasia** of the antral mucosa. This thickening may be markedly pronounced and may resemble a mucous retention cyst. The periapical mucositis may be the only indication of a problematic tooth or an endodontic failure. Pulp tests may be difficult with multiple crowns and large restorations (Figs. 16–20 and 16–21). According to Worth and Stoneman, when the cause of antral mucositis is a tooth, the mucositis is usually localized; when mucositis is seen in association with advanced periodontal disease, the entire antral mucosa of the floor thickens, and halo formation rarely occurs (Fig. 16–22).

Mucositis of dental and periodontal origin is often asymptomatic, and usually the antral lining will return to normal and disappear radiographically with proper endodontic or periodontal treatment.

CYSTIC CONDITIONS

Cystic problems peculiar to the maxillary sinus are subdivided into intrinsic and extrinsic types. **Extrinsic cysts** occur outside the maxillary sinus and encroach upon it as they enlarge. A thin sclerotic border may sometimes delineate the cyst from the remainder of the sinus cavity upon which it has encroached. Any number of cysts previously discussed, such as **periapical cysts, follicular cysts, primordial cysts, odontogenic keratocysts,** and the like, may be involved (Figs. 16–23 and 16–24). Additionally, other neurogenic cystic conditions, such as **encephalocele** and **meningocele**, may involve the sinus. Follicular cysts may occupy the entire maxillary sinus and, in this instance, are difficult to distinguish from the normal sinus space. Evidence of a tooth either close to or within the sinus may be the only sign of a coexisting cyst (Figs. 16–25 and 16–26). The borders of a cystic antrum usually have a smooth, straight outline, whereas the normal sinus floor has a more irregular, undulating outline, with slight discontinuities apparent at the wall. This is an important distinction when the cyst occupies the entire sinus, showing little evidence of its presence. Aspiration will usually yield straw-colored fluid, and subsequent injection of radiopaque contrast medium will remain within the cyst rather than drain out through the ostium.

Another extrinsic cyst is the **surgical ciliated cyst of the maxilla.** This cyst invariably follows a surgical procedure in the maxilla or maxillary sinus, sometimes many years previously. It is considered an implantation cyst along the surgical margin. It is usually a well-defined radiolucency, which may appear to be inside the maxillary sinus but with a corticated peripheral outline. The condition may be vaguely painful, and the pain is difficult to localize. Injection of the sinus with radiopaque material will clearly outline the cyst as being separate from and outside the sinus. Treatment consists of enucleation.

According to Hames and Rakoff, intrinsic cysts are of three basic types. The first type is the **mucous retention cyst** or **cyst of McGregor**, which is thought to be caused by the obstruction and dilatation of the duct of a minor seromucinous gland. This cyst is asymptomatic and appears as a clear, well-defined ball-like or dome-shaped radiopacity in the antrum with no peripheral cortical outline. The sinus is usually clear of all other pathology including expansion and perforation. The mucous retention cyst is self-limiting and regresses spontaneously (Fig. 16–27).

The second type of intrinsic cyst is the **serous retention cyst.** According to Hames and Rakoff,

Text continued on page 400

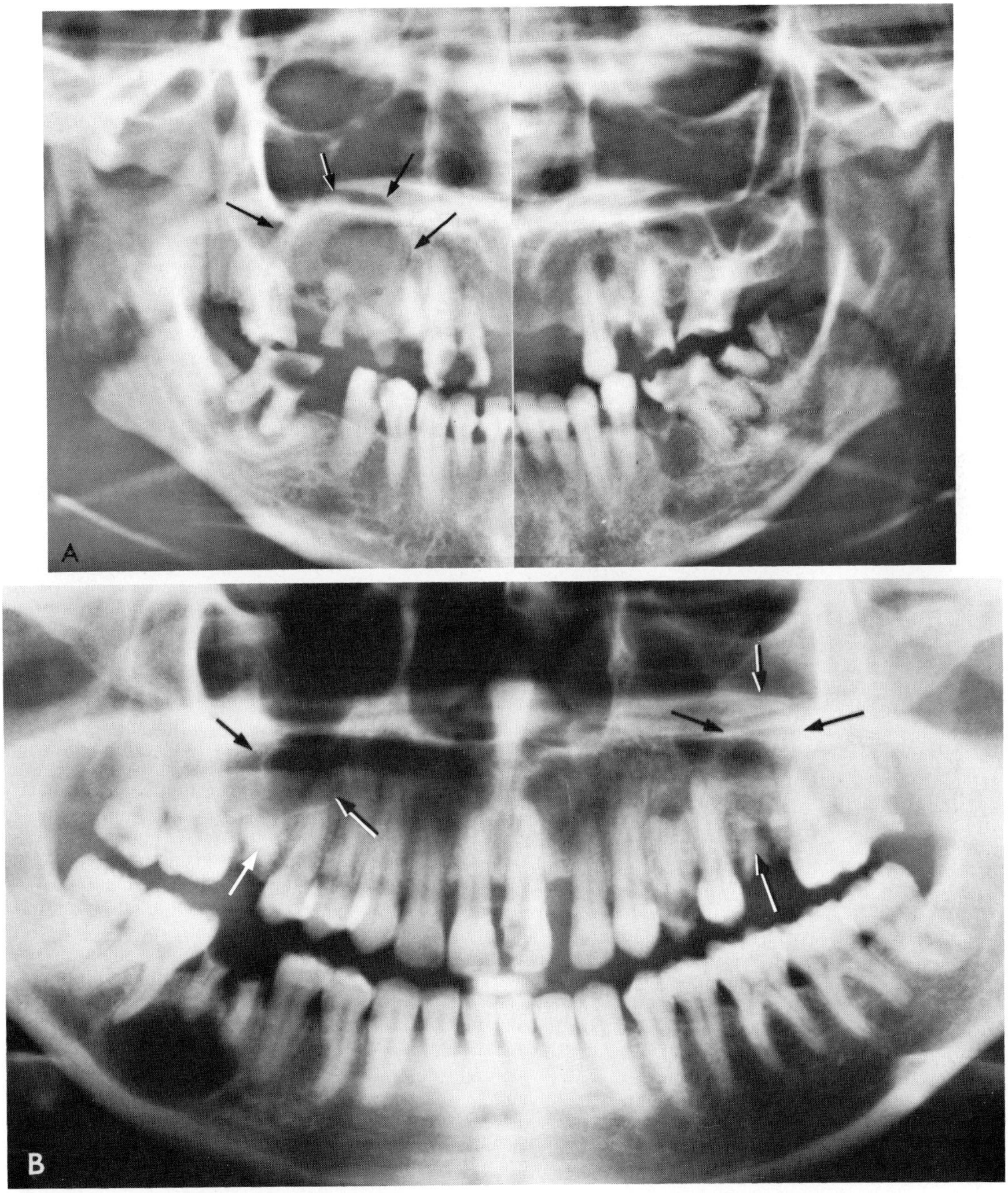

Figure 16–23. Extrinsic cyst: periapical cyst. **A.** Note the impingement upon the right maxillary sinus. **B.** Note the periapical cyst in the maxillary **right** first molar area, which is confined mainly to the maxillary alveolar bone. Compare this with the periapical mucositis of the **left** maxillary first molar.

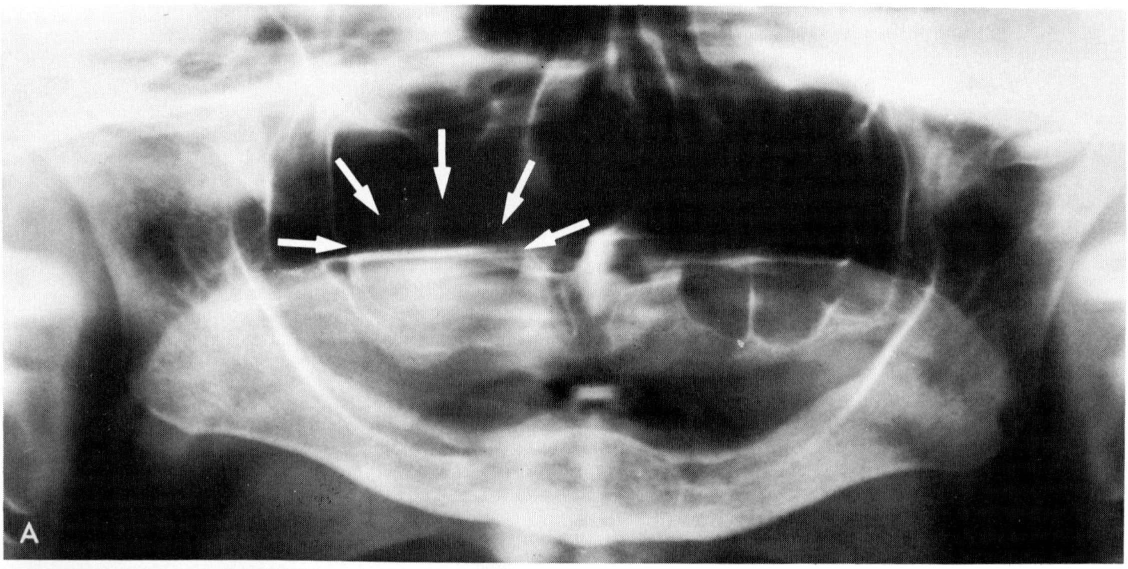

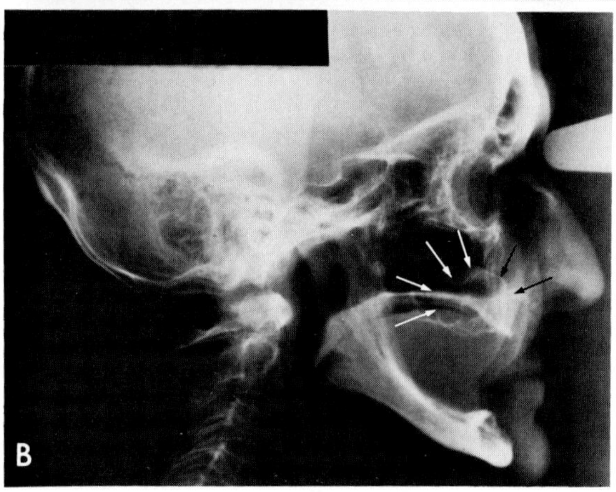

Figure 16–24. Extrinsic odontogenic cyst. **A.** Panoramic view. **B.** Lateral cephalometric view.

Illustration continued on opposite page

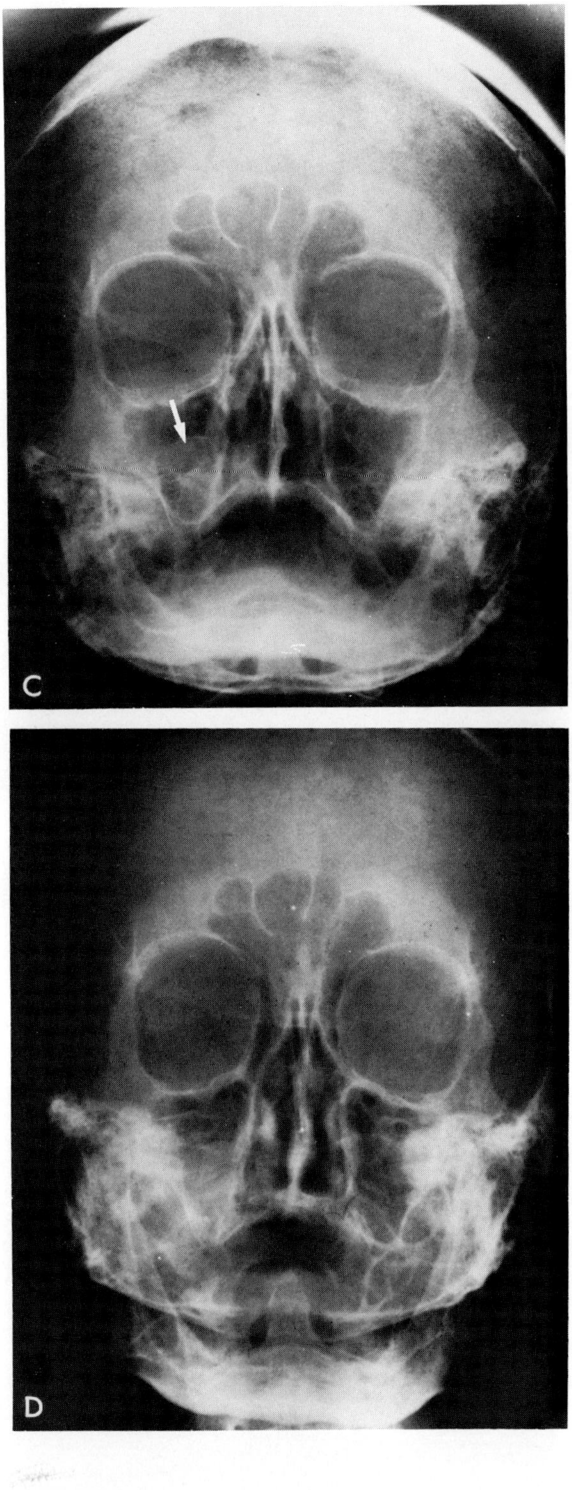

Figure 16–24 *Continued* **C.** Waters' view. **D.** Caldwell view. This 69-year-old female was asymptomatic. A radiopaque dome-shaped radiopacity was noted in the right maxillary sinus on the panoramic film. A notable finding was the well-corticated superior outline, distinguishing this condition from the mucous retention cyst. The lesion proved to be outside the maxillary sinus, with a thin bony wall separating it from the antrum. Histologically, the cyst was lined with odontogenic epithelium, which was nonkeratinizing. (Figure 16–24 courtesy of Dr. Dale Miles, San Antonio, TX.)

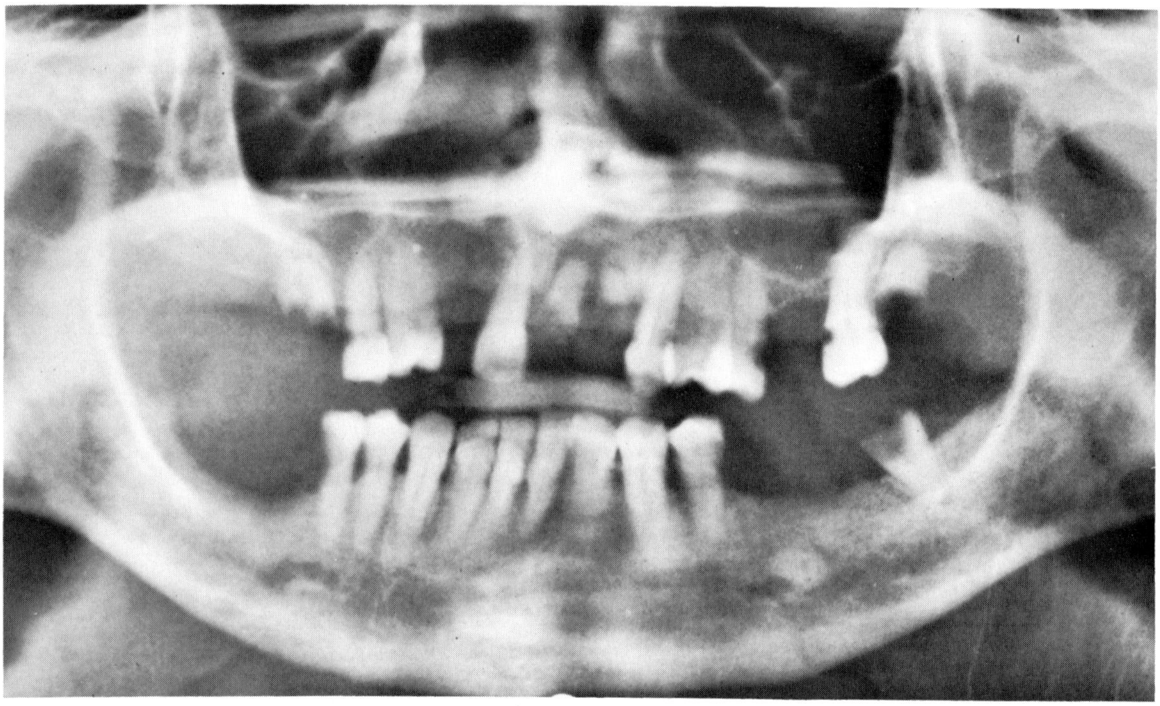

Figure 16–25. Tooth in the right maxillary sinus. No apparent cystic involvement.

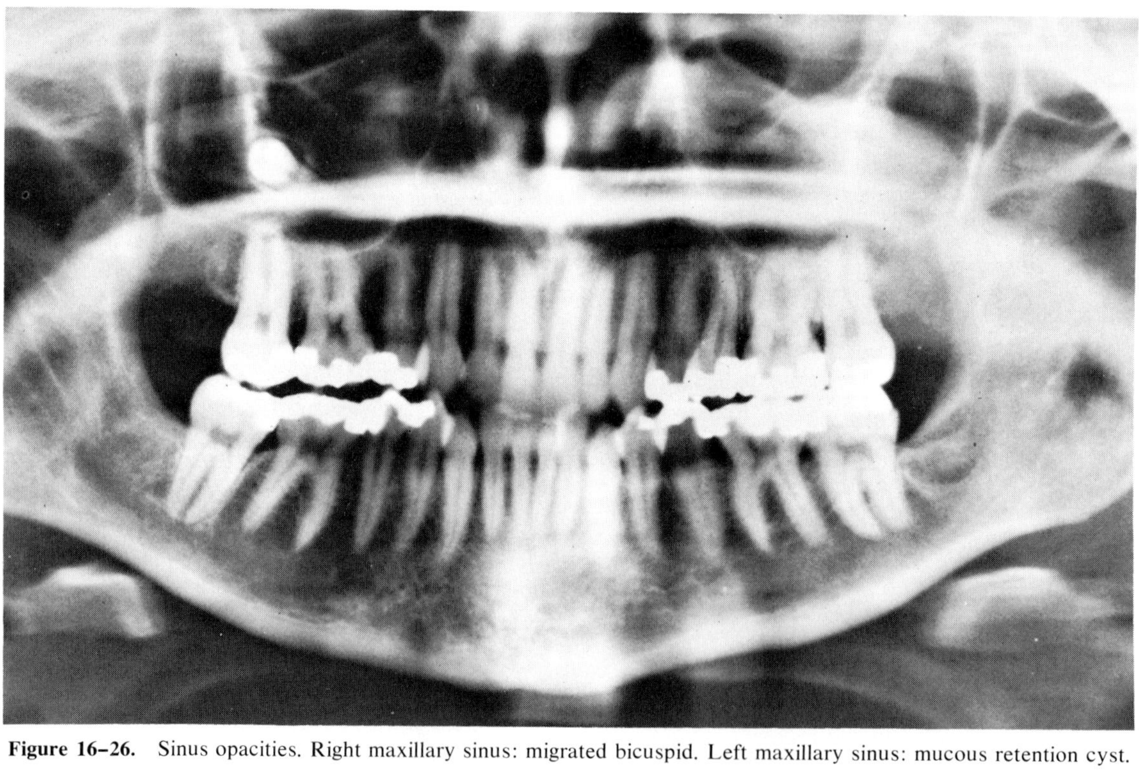

Figure 16–26. Sinus opacities. Right maxillary sinus: migrated bicuspid. Left maxillary sinus: mucous retention cyst.

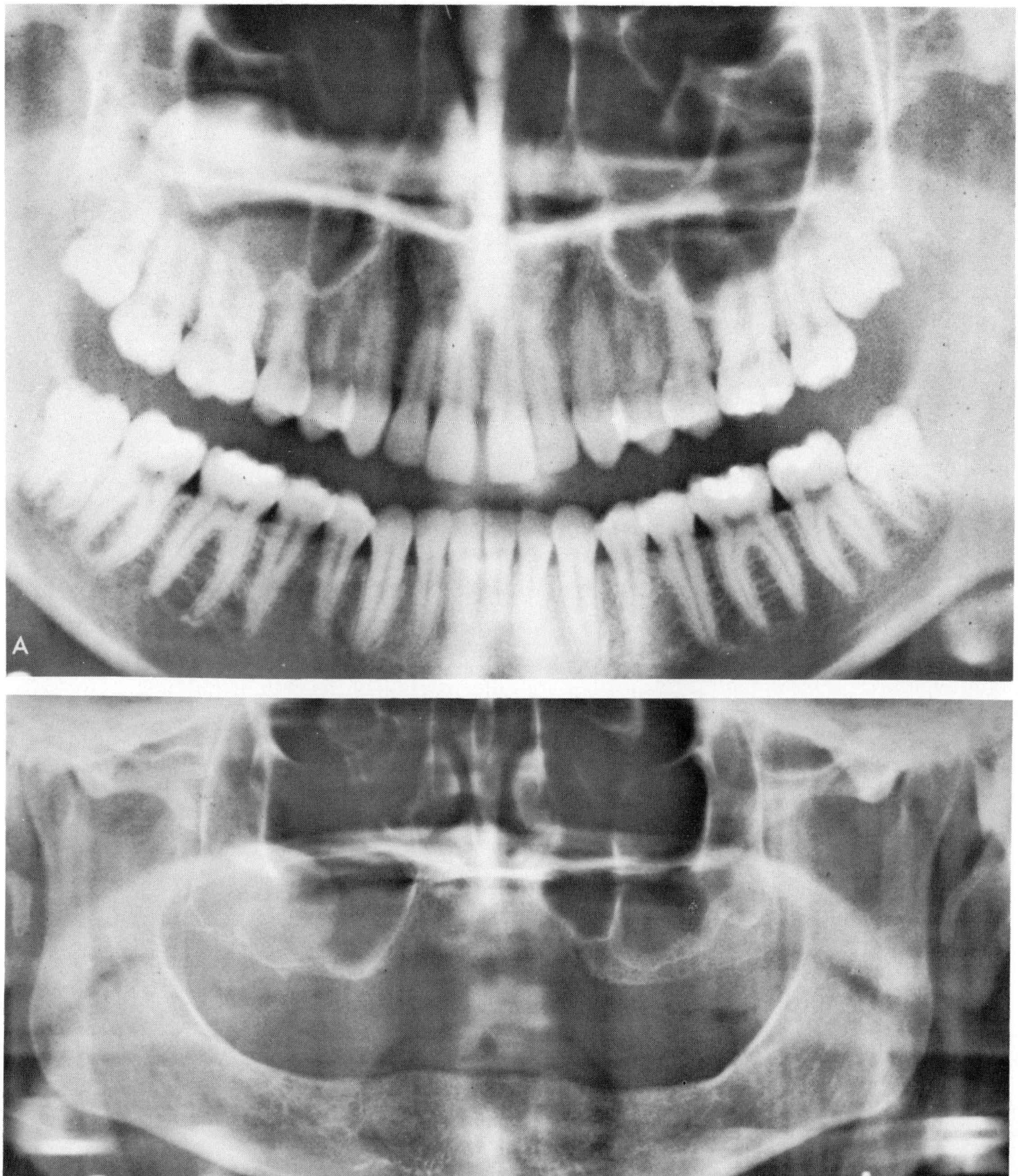

Figure 16–27. Intrinsic cyst: mucous retention cyst. **A.** Note the dome-shaped radiopacity in the right maxillary sinus. Also note the characteristic lack of a cortical outline. **B.** Contrast the mucositis of nondental or periodontal origin in the left antrum with the dome-shaped mucous retention cyst in the right sinus. Note the bilateral pneumatization.

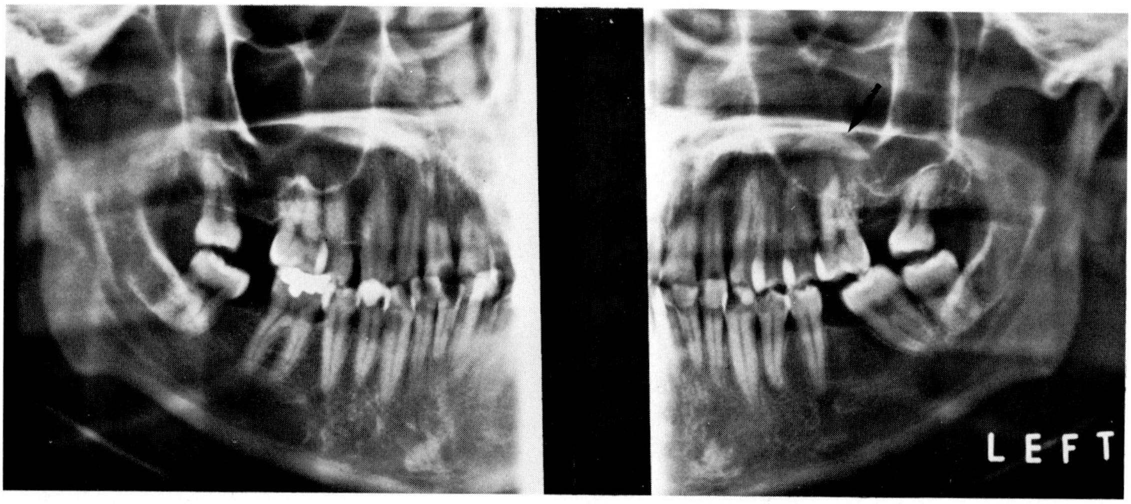

Figure 16–28. Intrinsic cyst: Serous retention cyst (periapical mucositis of periodontal origin). Compare the radiodensity of this area to the mucous retention cyst in Figure 16–27**A.** The authors believe the term periapical mucositis is preferable.

this cyst has no epithelial lining and consists of loculated fluid in the mucoperiosteum, which anchors the overlying sinus mucosa to the bony wall. They further state that these cysts are usually found in the sinus floor, and, unlike the mucous retention cyst, they are thought to be inflammatory in origin. These cysts are often asymptomatic and, according to Hames and Rakoff, require no treatment. The authors are of the opinion that these serous retention cysts are identical to the equally asymptomatic condition referred to by Worth and Stoneman as periapical mucositis, which does require pulpal or periodontal treatment, which brings about resolution. The so-called serous retention cyst is said to be less radiopaque than the mucous retention cyst (Fig. 16–28).

The third type of intrinsic cyst, as outlined by Hames and Rakoff, is the **mucocele**, which, in the paranasal sinuses, is separate and distinct from the mucous retention cyst. The mucocele is described as a gradually expanding collection of fluid within a paranasal sinus initiated by the obstruction of the ostium and typified by expansion and thinning of the sinus walls, with destruction and compression of adjacent structures. The most common sites for mucoceles are the frontal and ethmoid sinuses. Proptosis may occur if the pressure is exerted on the floor of the orbit, or there may be loosening of the

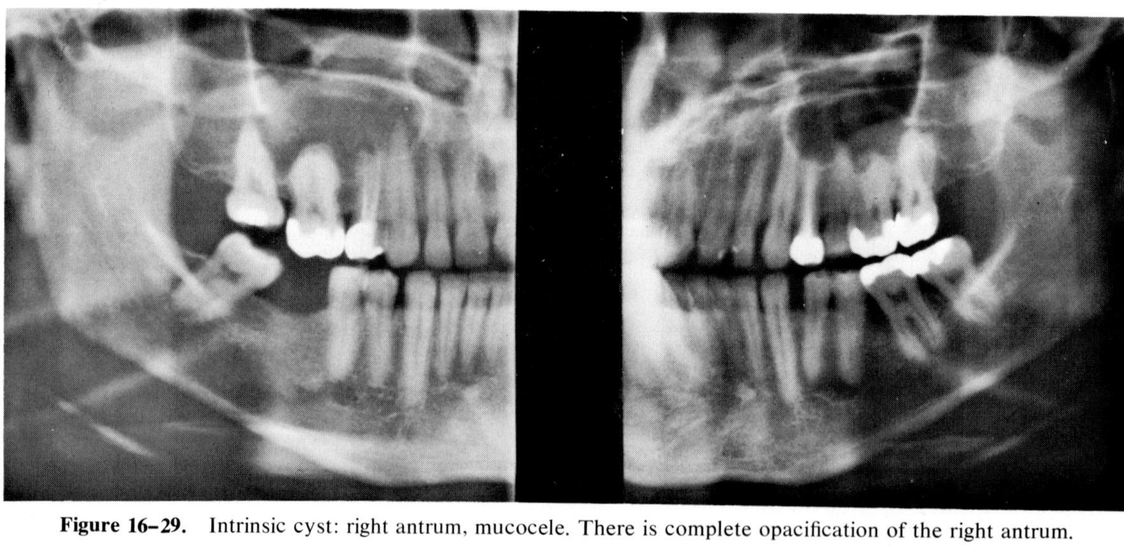

Figure 16–29. Intrinsic cyst: right antrum, mucocele. There is complete opacification of the right antrum.

teeth if the vector of force is directed downward. Radiographically, the sinus is usually totally opaque. The mucocele may be associated with thinning of intact walls, whereas a destructive malignant process usually destroys and eventually perforates the bony walls of the sinus (Fig. 16–29).

TRAUMA AND THE MAXILLARY SINUS

Various **maxillary fractures** involve the nose and paranasal sinuses. Additionally, **fracture of the floor of the sinus** during exodontia may occur. The most common sequela of fracture is acute sinusitis. An **oroantral fistula** may be a further complication. When visible radiographically, the oroantral fistula appears as a discontinuity of the alveolar bone and sinus floor, delineating a communication between the maxillary sinus and the oral cavity (Fig. 16–30). There may be a prolapse of the sinus lining into the oral cavity, which may be seen radiographically as a soft tissue shadow. Chronic sinusitis may be associated with the oroantral fistula, and varying degrees of mucositis may be visible. The oroantral fistula may resemble a breakthrough or a perforation by malignant neoplastic tissue. Treatment usually involves careful surgical closure of the communication. Implantation of foreign bodies, such as teeth and root tips, may act as a nidus for the deposition of calcific salts and results in the formation of **antroliths** or **rhinoliths.** These may or may not be associated with varying degrees of sinus opacification (Figs. 16–31 and 16–32).

A blow to the orbit sometimes produces a **blow-out fracture.** The floor of the orbit, which is the roof of the maxillary antrum, is sometimes very thin. Medially, the bone that separates the orbit from the ethmoid sinus is also thin. The blow creates a momentary increase in intraorbital pressure and causes a fracture or blowout of thin portions of the bony lining of the orbit. According to Hames and Rakoff there are three radiographic findings (best seen in the Waters' view): orbital emphysema, especially with involvement of the ethmoid sinus; partial to complete opacification of the maxillary sinus caused by hemorrhage; and the hanging-drop opacity into the superior portion of the maxillary sinus due to herniation of orbital structures through the fractured orbital floor. Tomographs are sometimes required to verify the clinical impression of a blow-out fracture.

Perhaps the most consistent panoramic finding in association with trauma is the complete opacification of the sinus owing to hemorrhage. This should be considered in the differential diagnosis of sinus opacification, along with mucocele, complete tumorification of the antrum, and opacification due to the superimposition of anatomic structures.

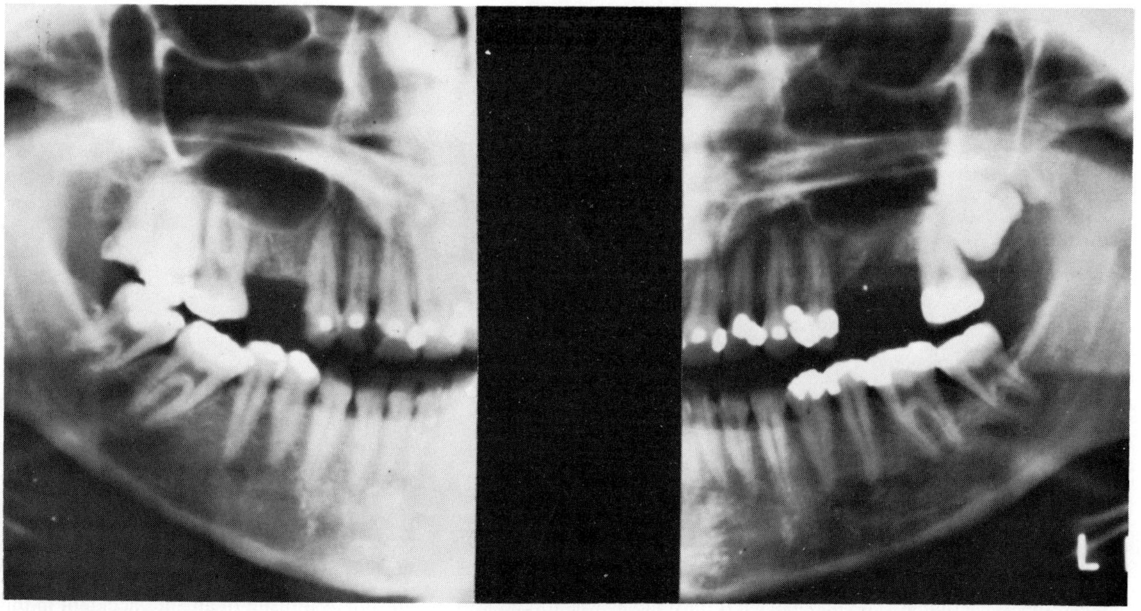

Figure 16–30. Left antrum: oroantral fistula.

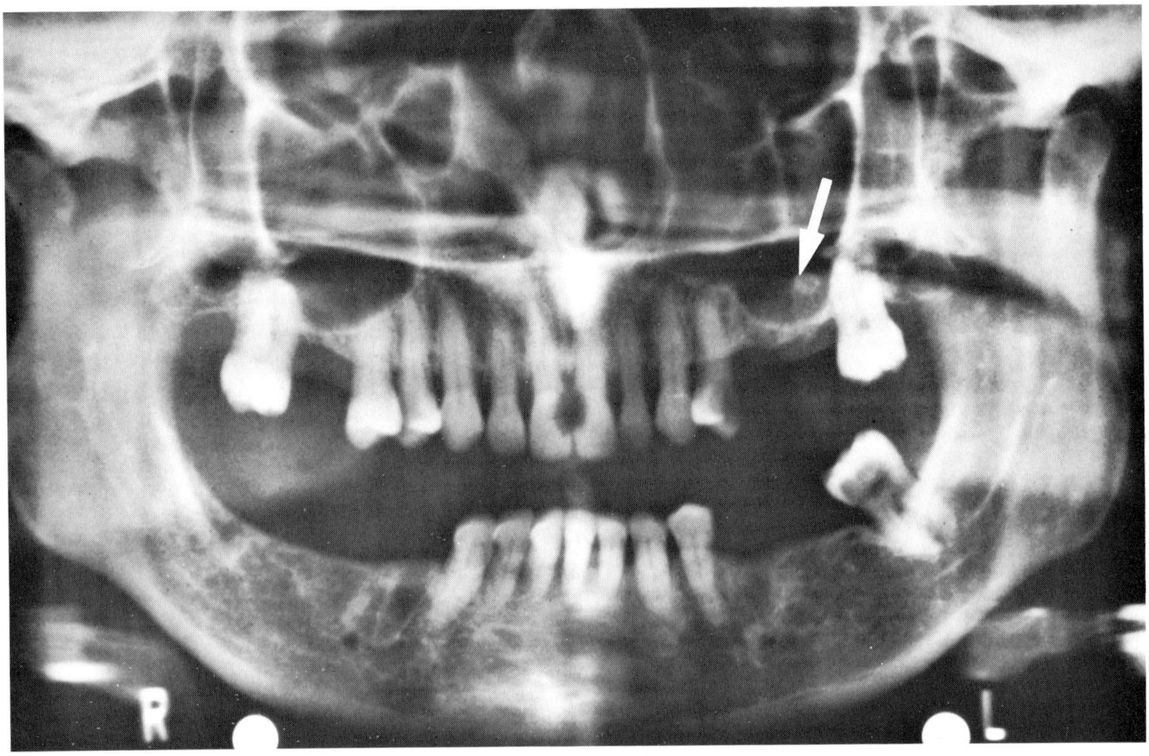

Figure 16–31. Antrolith. The central radiolucency suggests a possible root tip in cross section as the central core. (Courtesy of Dr. Steven Bricker, San Antonio, TX.)

OTHER PATHOLOGIC CONDITIONS AFFECTING THE MAXILLARY SINUS

The object of this section is to illustrate some cases located in or near the maxillary sinus. For a more complete discussion of these disorders please refer to the pertinent sections of the book as they relate to the jaws (Fig. 16–33 to 16–41). These conditions include **antral polyposis, fibrous dysplasia, central giant cell**

Text continued on page 408

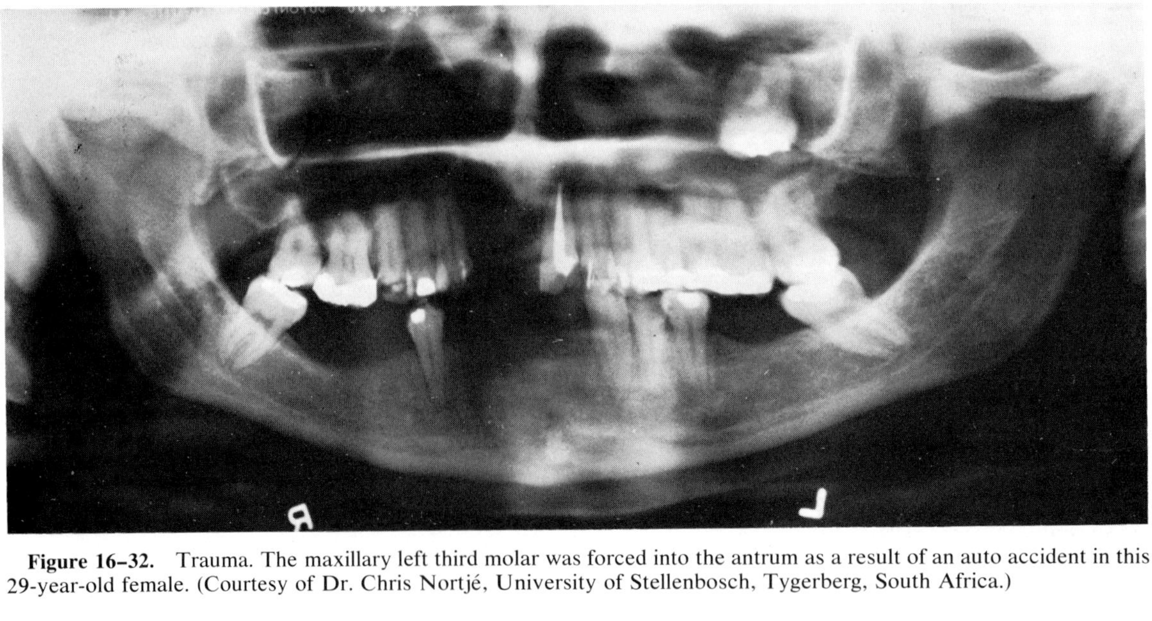

Figure 16–32. Trauma. The maxillary left third molar was forced into the antrum as a result of an auto accident in this 29-year-old female. (Courtesy of Dr. Chris Nortjé, University of Stellenbosch, Tygerberg, South Africa.)

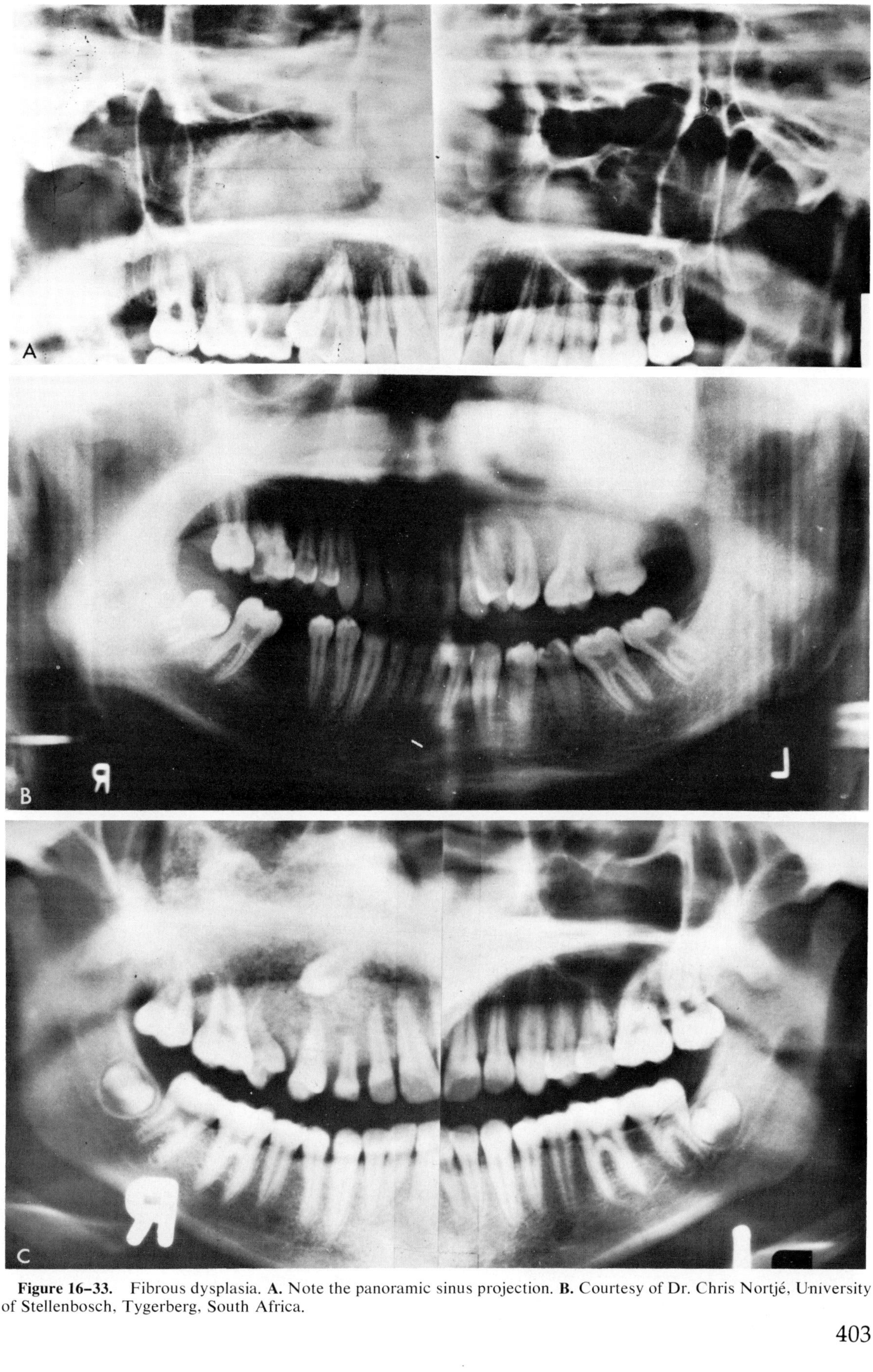

Figure 16–33. Fibrous dysplasia. **A.** Note the panoramic sinus projection. **B.** Courtesy of Dr. Chris Nortjé, University of Stellenbosch, Tygerberg, South Africa.

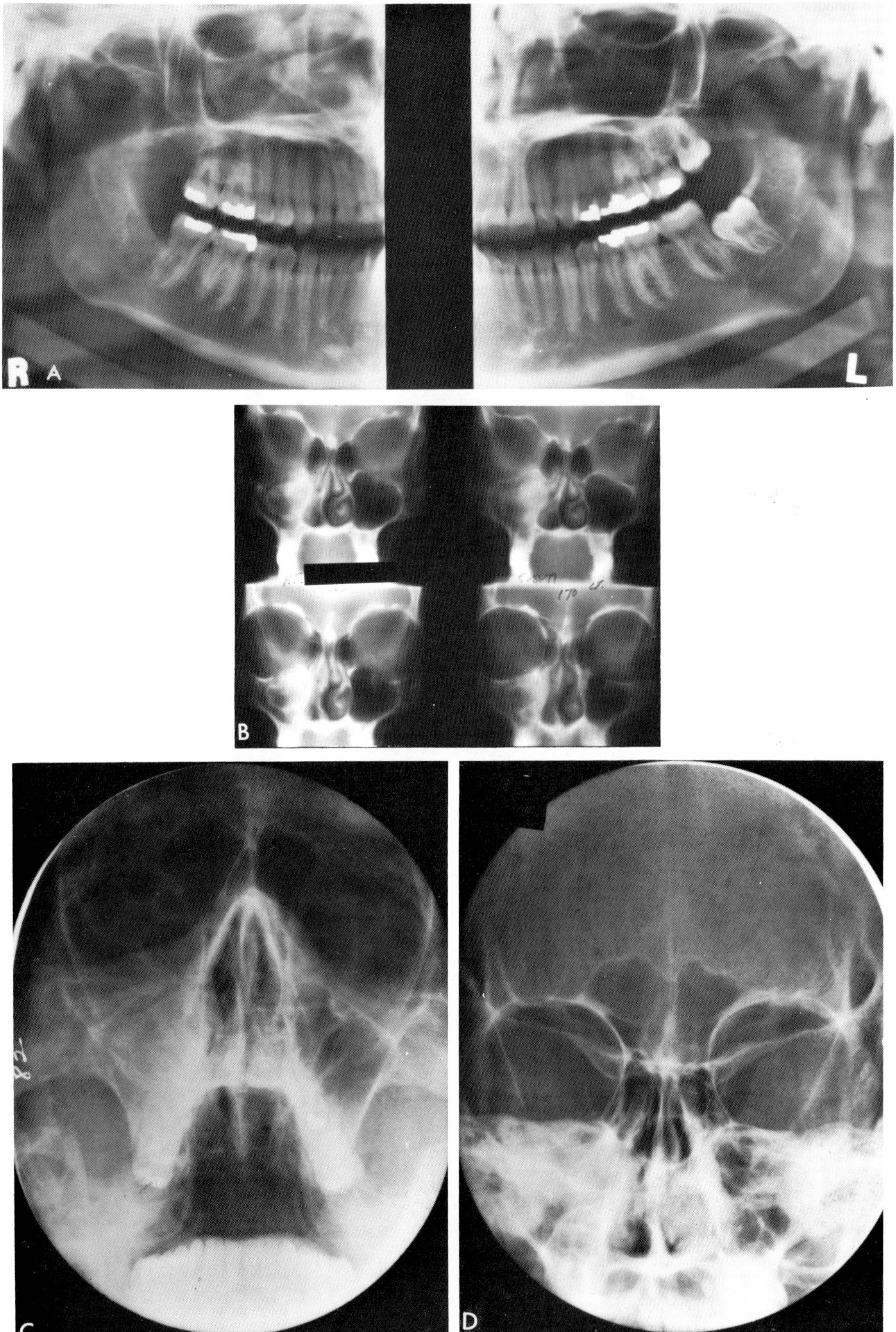

Figure 16–34. Central giant cell granuloma. **A.** Panoramic view showing complete opacification of the right antrum. **B.** Tomograms. **C.** Waters' view. **D.** Caldwell view. (Figure 16–34 courtesy of Dr. Stanley Lovestedt, Rochester, MN.)

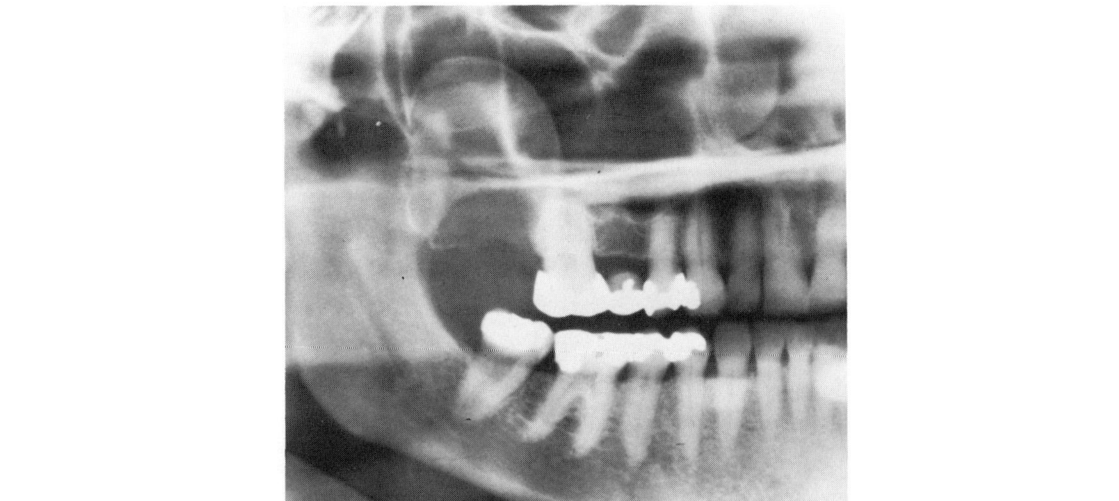

Figure 16–35. Ameloblastoma. **A.** Note the discontinuity of the sinus floor in its usual location as it bulges inward to form a superior cortical outline. Although these findings are not particularly characteristic of the ameloblastoma, they virtually rule out mucous retention cyst. (Courtesy of Dr. Stanley Lovestedt, Rochester, MN.) **B.** Note the characteristic multilocular pattern, which persists into the maxillary sinus. Courtesy of Dr. Chris Nortjé, University of Stellenbosch, Tygerberg, South Africa.

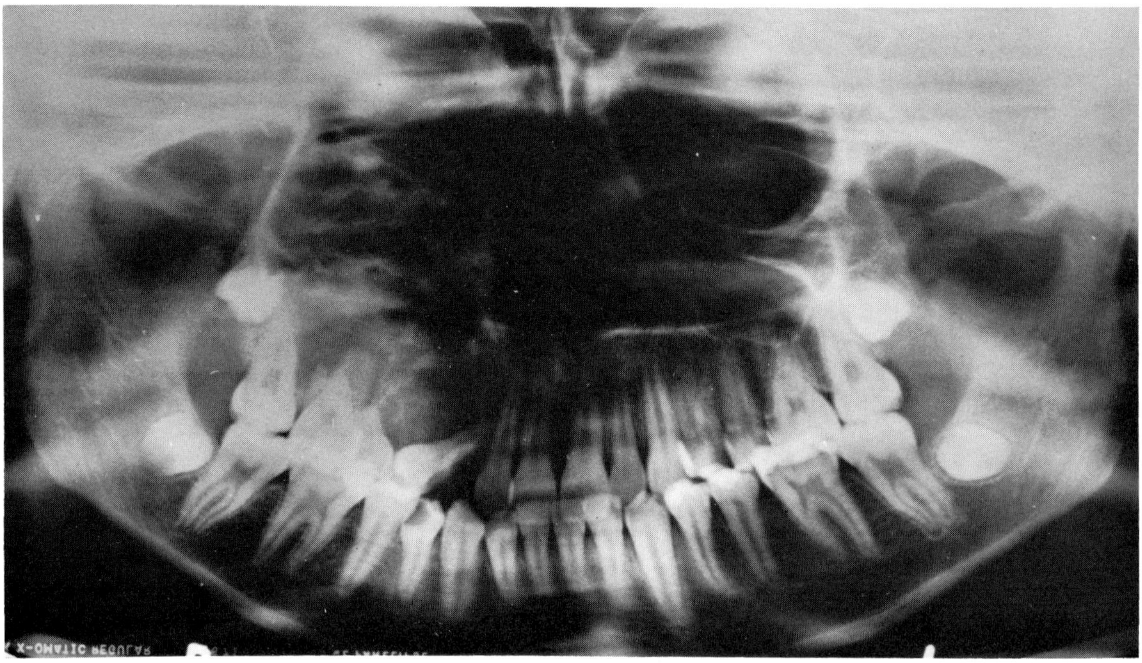

Figure 16–36. Odontogenic myxoma. (Courtesy of Dr. Chris Nortjé, University of Stellenbosch, Tygerberg, South Africa.)

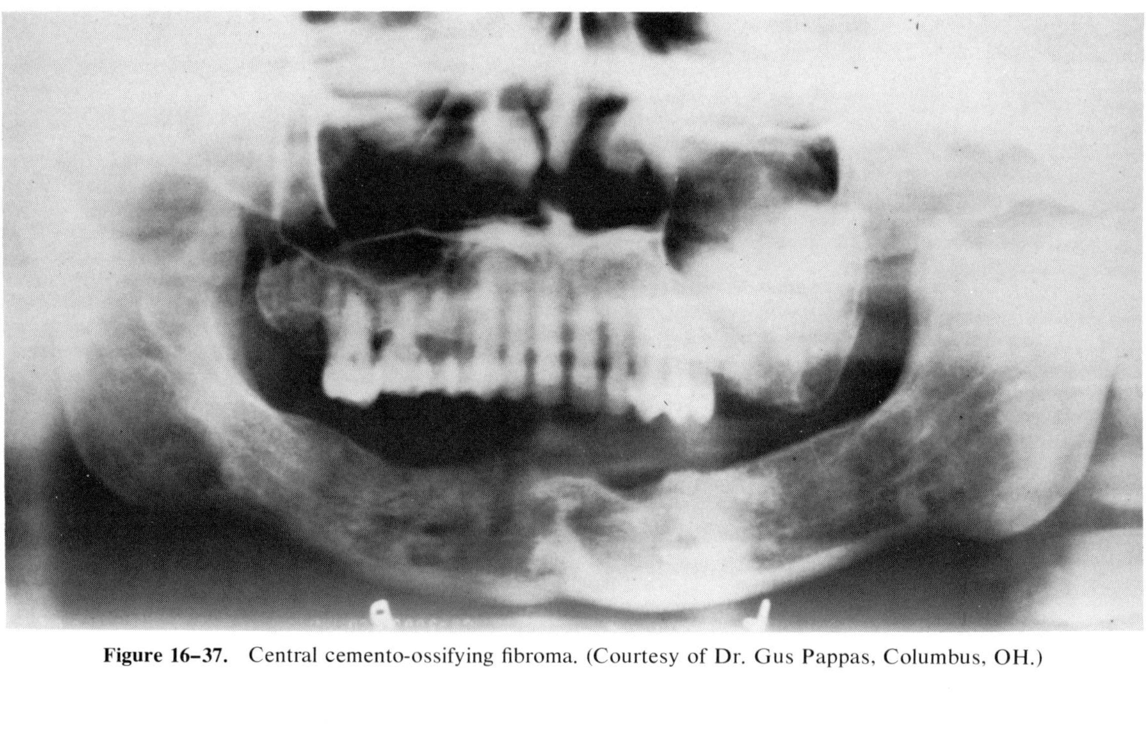

Figure 16–37. Central cemento-ossifying fibroma. (Courtesy of Dr. Gus Pappas, Columbus, OH.)

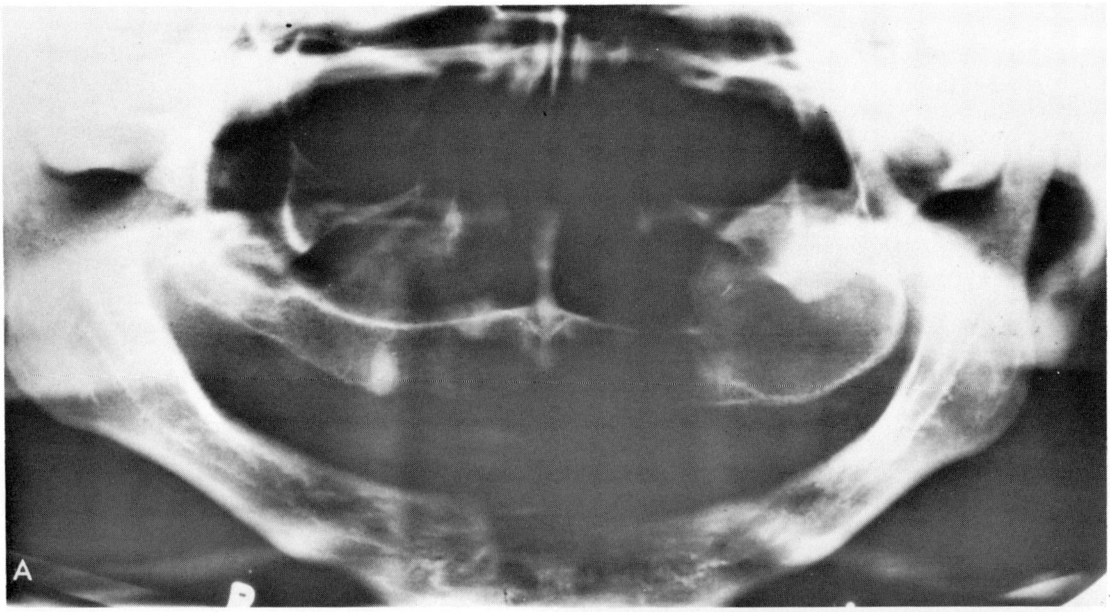

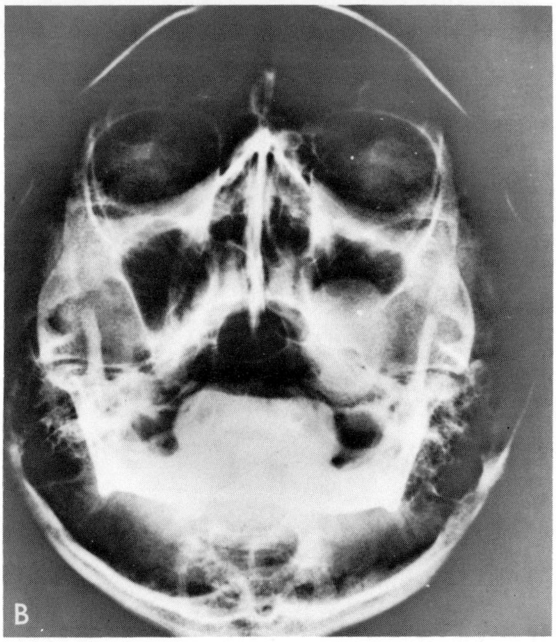

Figure 16–38. Central ossifying fibroma. **A.** Panoramic view, left sinus. **B.** Waters' view, left sinus. (Figure 16–38 courtesy of Dr. Chris Nortjé, University of Stellenbosch, Tygerberg, South Africa.)

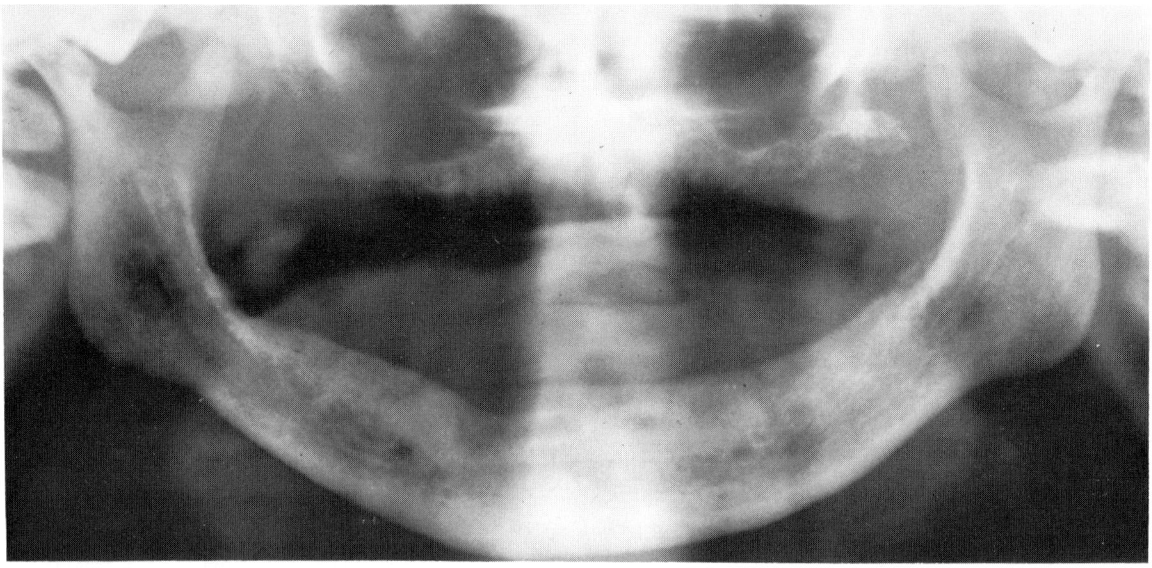

Figure 16–39. Epidermoid carcinoma. Note the destruction of the floor of the right maxillary sinus, the alveolar bone of the residual ridge, and the right maxillary tuberosity. Compare with the left side; the opacity here is artifact. (Courtesy of Dr. Gus Pappas, Columbus, OH.)

granuloma, ameloblastoma, odontogenic myxoma, central cemento-ossifying fibroma, antral carcinoma, and Ewing's sarcoma.

One condition that has not been discussed is the **nasopharyngeal angiofibroma** (juvenile nasopharyngeal fibroma). This lesion mainly affects teenage boys and clinically appears as a palatal or tonsillar mass. Additionally, there may be nasal obstruction, epistaxis, and sinusitis. Carotid angiograms are helpful in diagnosing and delineating this lesion. In panoramic films, a round, opaque, mucous-retention, cyst-like lesion may be seen to be causing an anterior bowing of the posterior wall of the maxillary sinus, an important distinction in the diagnosis of this lesion. Also, the lesion may be seen as an opacity within the airspace of the nasopharynx.

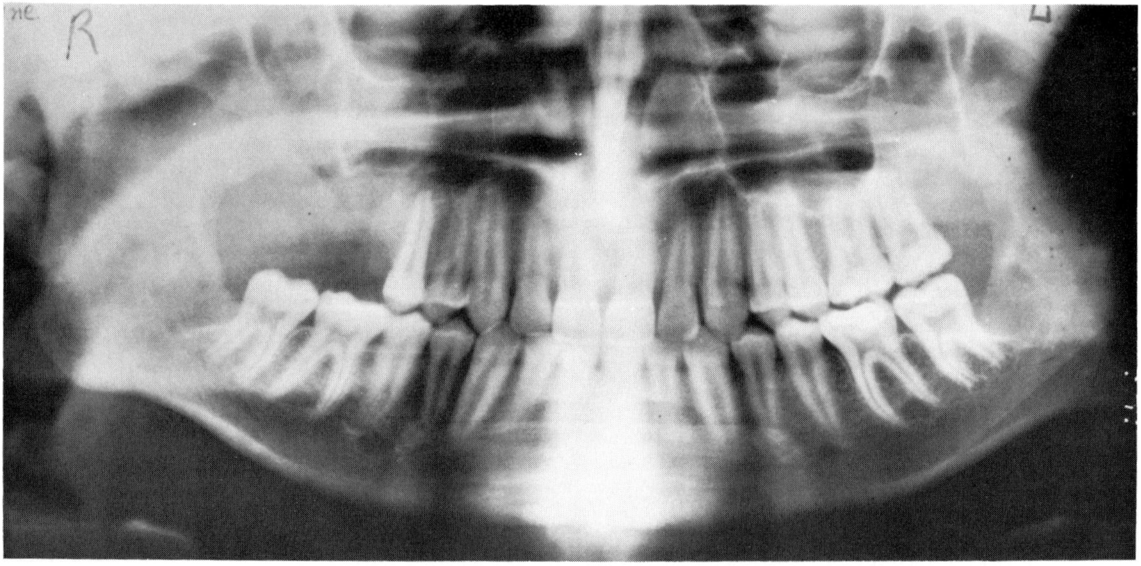

Figure 16–40. Ewing's sarcoma, right maxilla. Note the loss of definitive anatomic outlines in the affected area in this 13-year-old boy. (Courtesy of Dr. Gus Pappas, Columbus, OH.)

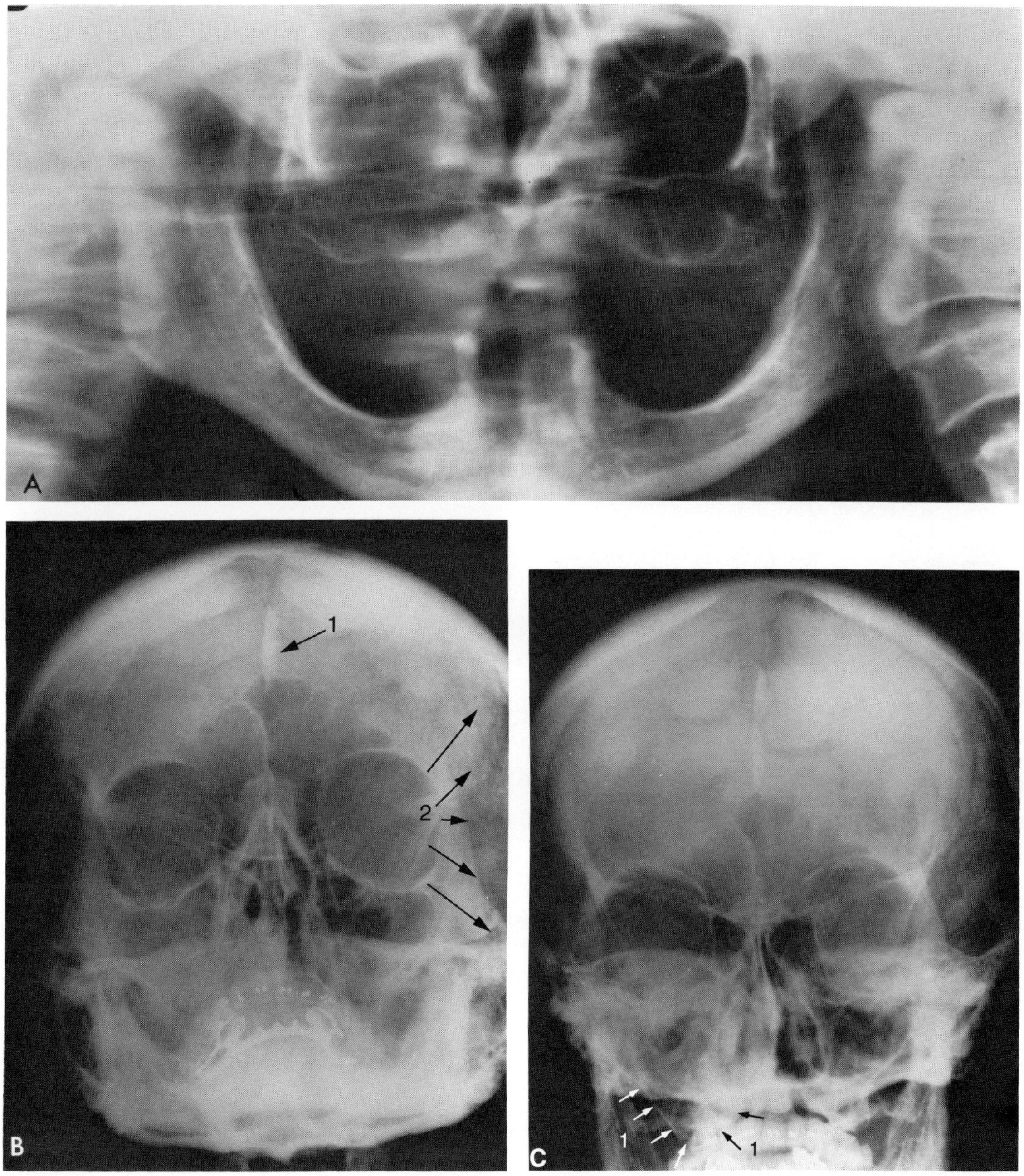

Figure 16–41. Current case: right sinus opacification, cause unknown. Case history: This 69-year-old female has Beck's sarcoid. Her sarcoidosis is generalized, with lung, kidney, adrenal, skin, and other areas of involvement. There is a long history of sinus problems, and a number of polyps were removed from the right maxillary sinus several years ago. The patient is currently asymptomatic and is taking prednisone daily. **A.** Panoramic view. Note the complete opacification of the right maxillary sinus and possibly some expansion of the medial wall, encroaching upon the right nasal cavity. **B.** Waters' view. Note the complete opacification of the right maxillary sinus, the opacification of the lower half of the right nasal fossa, the osteopetrotic thickening of the calvarium, calcification of the falx cerebri (1); and multiple soft tissue calcifications in the left side of the face (2). **C.** Caldwell view. Note that the findings are similar to those seen in the Waters' view. Note the expansion of the inferior, lateral wall of the maxillary sinus, but that the bony outline appears intact (1). Compare this area with the contralateral side. Diagnostic impression: mucocele, right maxillary sinus. Postscript: The final diagnosis was right maxillary sinus, inverted papilloma, and oroantral fistula. (Courtesy of Dr. Dale Miles, San Antonio, TX.)

REFERENCES

Reference Texts

Pernkopf, E.: **Atlas of Topographical and Applied Human Anatomy,** Vol. 1, Head and Neck. Philadelphia: W. B. Saunders, 1963, pp. 123–130.

Shafer, W. G., Hine, M. K., and Levy, B. M.: **A Textbook of Oral Pathology,** 3rd Edition. Philadelphia; W. B. Saunders, 1974.

Worth, H. M.: **Principles and Practice of Oral Radiologic Interpretation.** Chicago; Year Book Medical Publishers, 1963.

Selected References

Blashke, D., and Brady, F. A.: The maxillary antrolith. **Oral Surg. 48**:187, 1979.

Hames, R. S., and Rakoff, S. J.: Diseases of the maxillary sinus. **J. Oral. Med., 27**:90, 1972.

Hicks, J. L., and Nelson, J. F.: Juvenile násopharyngeal angiofibroma. **Oral Surg. 35**:807, 1973.

Ohba, T., and Katayama, H.: Comparison of panoramic radiography and Water's projection in the diagnosis of maxillary sinus disease. **Oral Surg. 42:**534, 1976.

Porter, J., Miller, R., and Stratigos, G. T.: Ameloblastoma of the maxilla: Report of a case. **Oral Surg. 44**:34, 1977.

Poynton, H. G.: Maxillary sinuses and the oral Radiologist. **Dental Radiogr. Photogr. 45**:43, 1972.

Worth, H. M., and Stoneman, D. W.: Radiographic interpretation of antral mucosal changes due to localized dental infection. **J. Can. Dent. Assoc. 38**:111, 1972.

Chapter 17
The Temporomandibular Joint and Upper Ramus

VISUALIZATION OF STRUCTURES

The temporomandibular joint (TMJ) remains an elusive structure to examine radiographically. In the chapter on anatomic landmarks, the authors illustrated the normal structures in the area. Note how these are fairly well visualized in Figures 17–1**A** and **B.** In Figure 17–1**B**, note the zygomaticotemporal suture of the zygomatic arch, which may mimic a fracture line. Note also the pseudocystic radiolucencies, which may be seen on the head of the condyle. These represent cupped-out anatomic depressions on the surface of the condyle. This normal variation mimics the surface erosions of degenerative joint disease, which produces similar cystlike radiolucencies (Fig. 17–2A and B). Note the bilateral radiolucencies at the sigmoid notch seen in some patients (Fig. 17–2C and D).

Virtually all of the popular panoramic machines are capable of producing excellent special TMJ views, as can be seen in Figure 17–3. For patients with TMJ pain and other suspected TMJ problems, the standard and special panoramic views are simple and excellent preliminary methods of examining this area. Most gross pathologic disorders can be visualized or ruled out using these films. In cases of myofascial pain–dysfunction (MPD) syndrome of relatively short duration, no changes may be seen, or there may be a lack of concentricity of the condyle in the fossa and a unilateral lack of translation (forward movement) upon opening. In such cases, tomographic arthrograms may

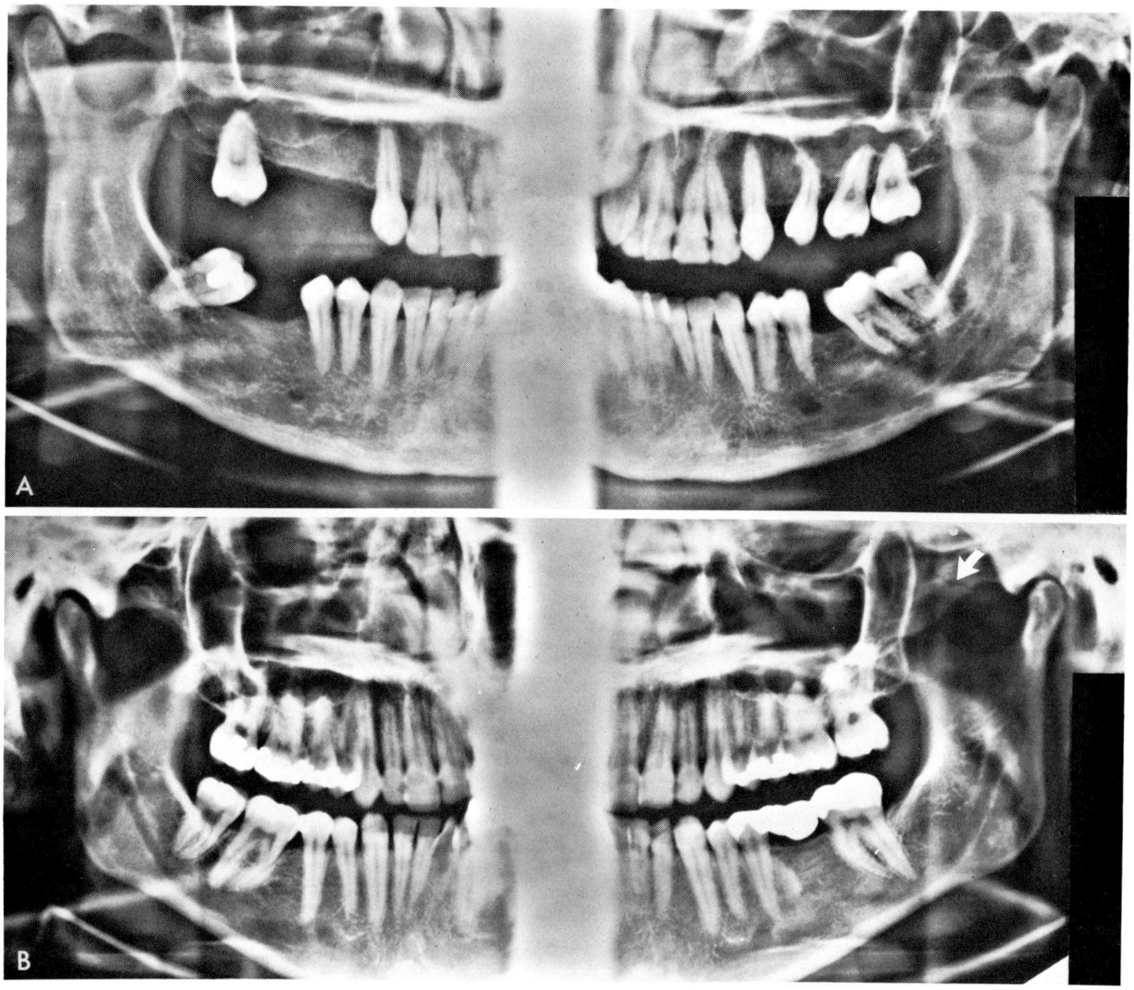

Figure 17–1. **A.** Normal panoramic TMJ area. **B.** Zygomaticotemporal suture.

show anterior displacement or perforation of the biconcave disk. In cases of MPD syndrome of long standing, the usual changes seen in degenerative joint disease may be seen. For neoplasms, ankylosis, or other conditions that are to be treated surgically, other standard examinations include the transorbital, transcranial, transpharyngeal, and submentovertex views. If available, linear tomograms are better; spiral tomograms are excellent. Computerized axial tomographic (CAT) scans may be extremely useful in determining the extent of a lesion in all directions.

In the future, better, more diagnostic visualization of the TMJ area may result from the use of nuclear magnetic resonance (NMR) scans. NMR scans may be able to produce chemical maps of internal structures, which are highly specific and may be diagnostic for a number of diseases. The system uses no x rays but rather a radiofrequency (RF) beam in a magnetic field.

Figure 17–2. **A.** Bilateral pseudocystic radiolucencies on the head of the condyles. These are variations of normal and represent a cupped-out depression on the surface of the condyles. This variation mimics arthritic change. This patient was asymptomatic. **B.** Pseudocystic radiolucency, right condyle. **C.** Bilateral anatomic radiolucencies in sigmoid notch area. These panoramic pseudoforamina have been termed medial sigmoid depressions. (**C** courtesy of Dr. Birgit Junfin Glass, San Antonio, TX.)

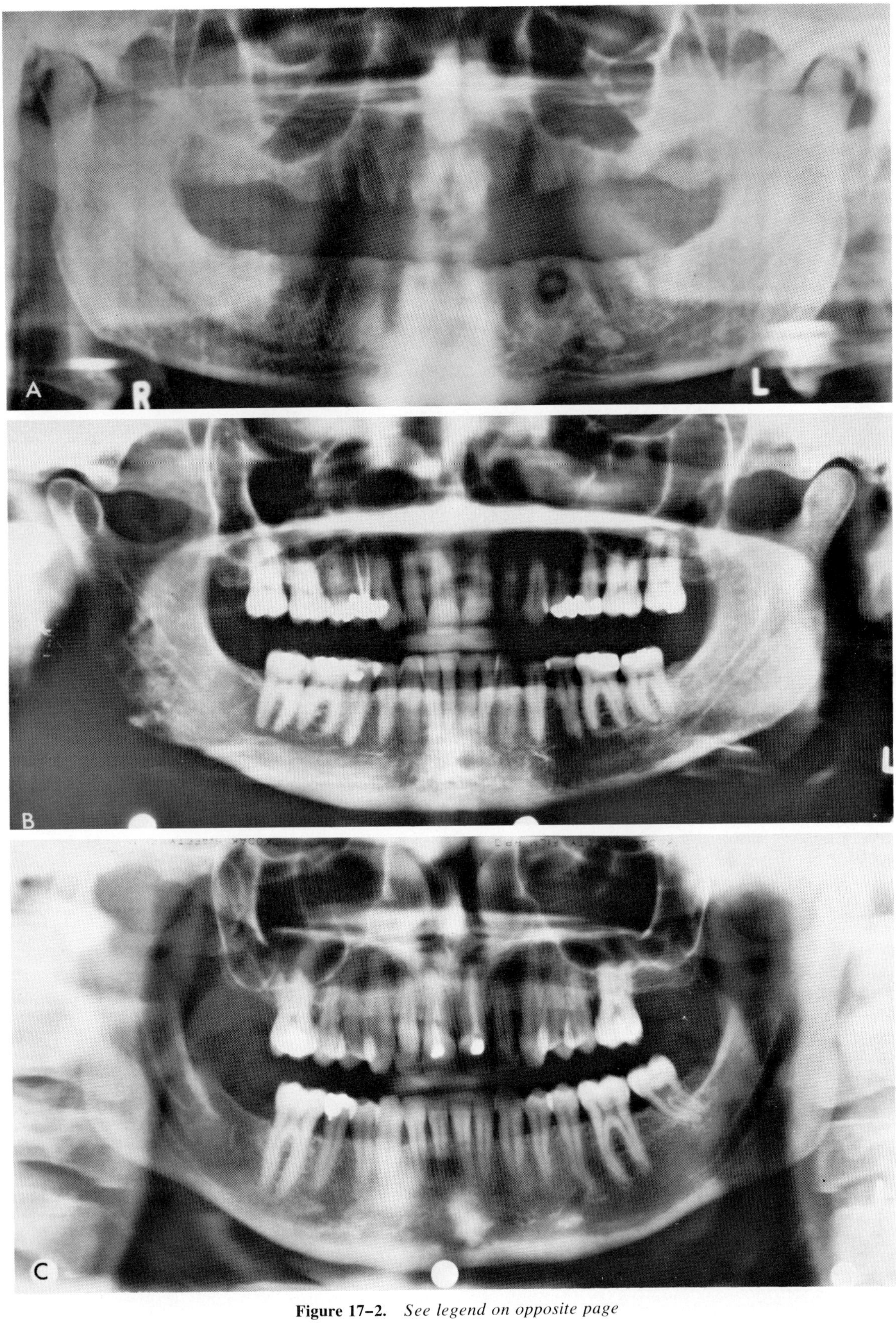

Figure 17–2. *See legend on opposite page*

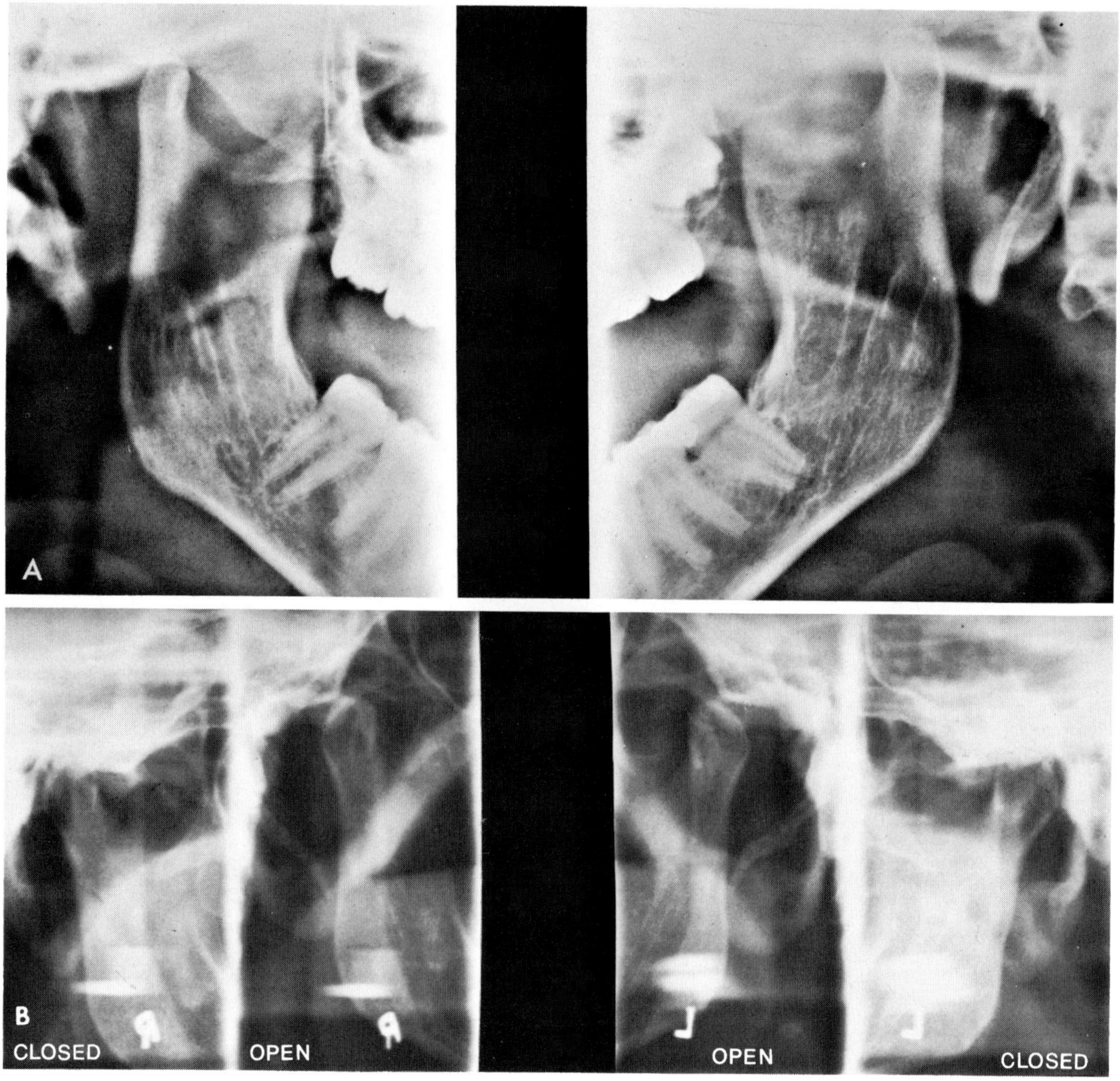

Figure 17–3. Panoramic TMJ views. **A.** Special TMJ projection. **B.** This 35-year-old female's complaint was clicking of 16 years' duration on the right side; the clicking was corrected with physiotherapy. The radiographs show no abnormality.

CONDYLAR APLASIA, HYPOPLASIA, HYPERTROPHY, AND HYPERPLASIA

BRIEF OVERVIEW AND RADIOGRAPHIC FEATURES

The term **aplasia** means lack of development of a part, and, on rare occasions, condylar aplasia occurs. This should not be confused with a surgically removed condyle, a resorbed condyle as seen in rheumatoid arthritis, a fractured condyle with displacement of the superior segment, or a compression fracture of the condylar head.

Hypoplasia means defective or incomplete development of a part. Clinically, when a hypoplastic condyle is present, the patient may exhibit facial asymmetry, with the affected side of the inferior border of the body of the mandible higher than the normal side. In comparing the right and left condyles, radiographic differences up to 3 mm are considered normal. The proximity of the sigmoid notch to the zygomatic arch may be an indication of condylar hypoplasia (Fig. 17–4). This condition is often asymptomatic and is usually idiopathic. Known causes include birth injury, radiation therapy at an early age, and trauma. Other conditions, including rheumatoid arthritis, hemifacial atrophy, scleroderma, and postsurgical defect, may

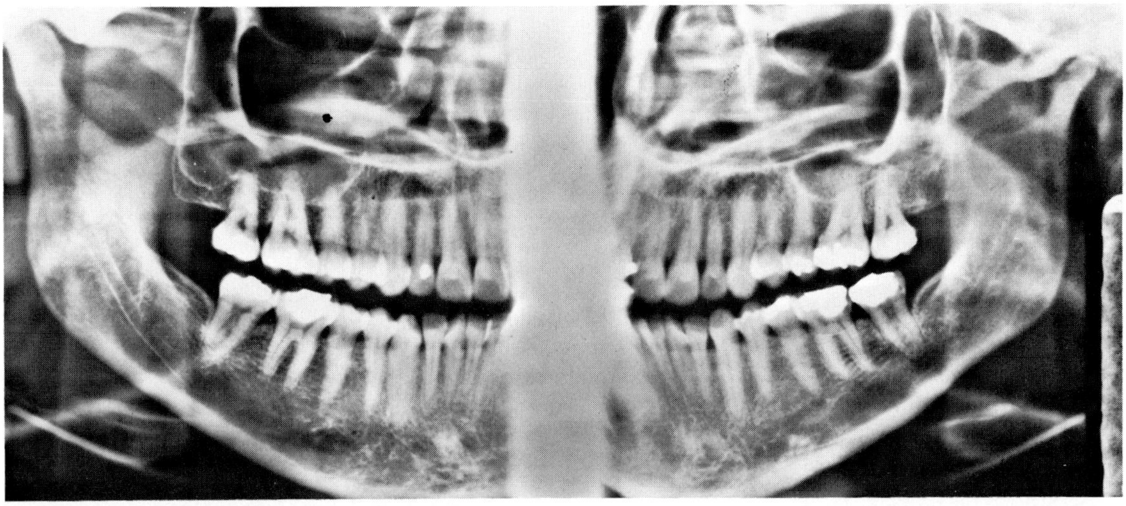

Figure 17–4. Condylar hypoplasia: left TMJ. Compare the shorter vertical distance between the base of the sigmoid notch and the zygomatic arch on the affected side with that of the normal side. A difference of 10 per cent or more indicates a size discrepancy between the contralateral condyles.

also produce a smaller than normal mandibular condyle, but the cause may not always be hypoplasia.

Hypertrophy means an increase in size of a part due to an increase in size of its constituent cells. **Hypertrophy of the condyle** may be idiopathic or may be associated with hemifacial hypertrophy (Fig. 17–5). In one reported case, condylar hypertrophy developed as a sequela to irradiation. The degree of hypertrophy may be relative owing to a projection error caused by unequal magnification of the panoramic image from one side to the other. When this projection error occurs, the ramus on the affected side, but not the body of the mandible, is usually wider. This error is important to recognize when evaluating the causes of facial asymmetry (Fig. 17–6**A** and **B**).

Hyperplasia means an abnormal increase in the number of cells. According to Worth, **hyperplasia of the condyles** may be divided into three basic types. In the first type, there are various attempts at remodeling, which produce

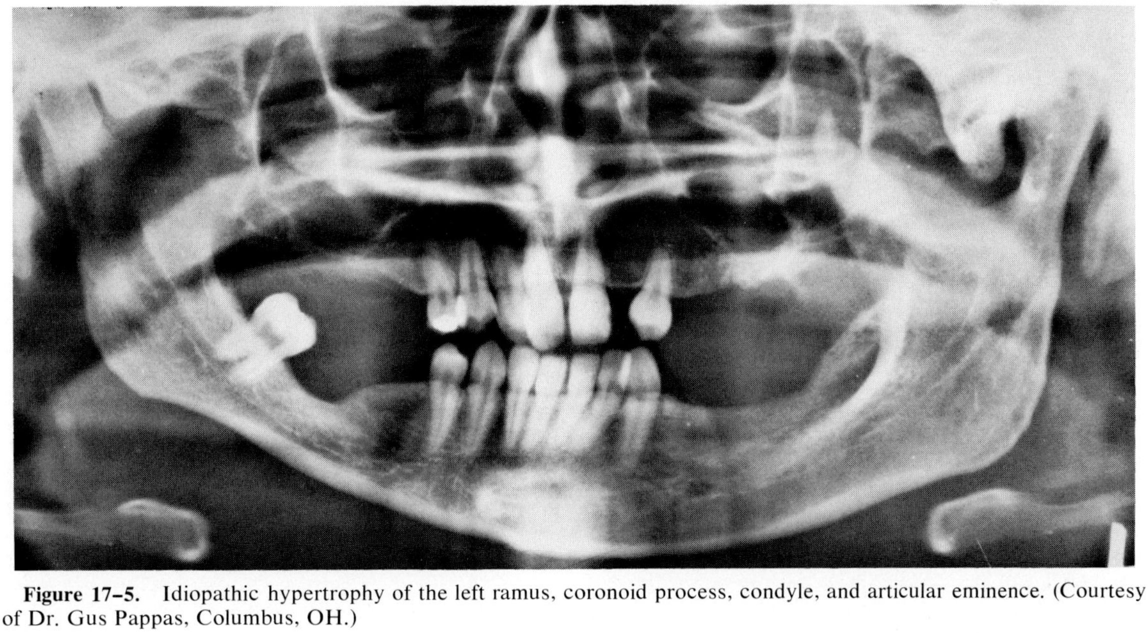

Figure 17–5. Idiopathic hypertrophy of the left ramus, coronoid process, condyle, and articular eminence. (Courtesy of Dr. Gus Pappas, Columbus, OH.)

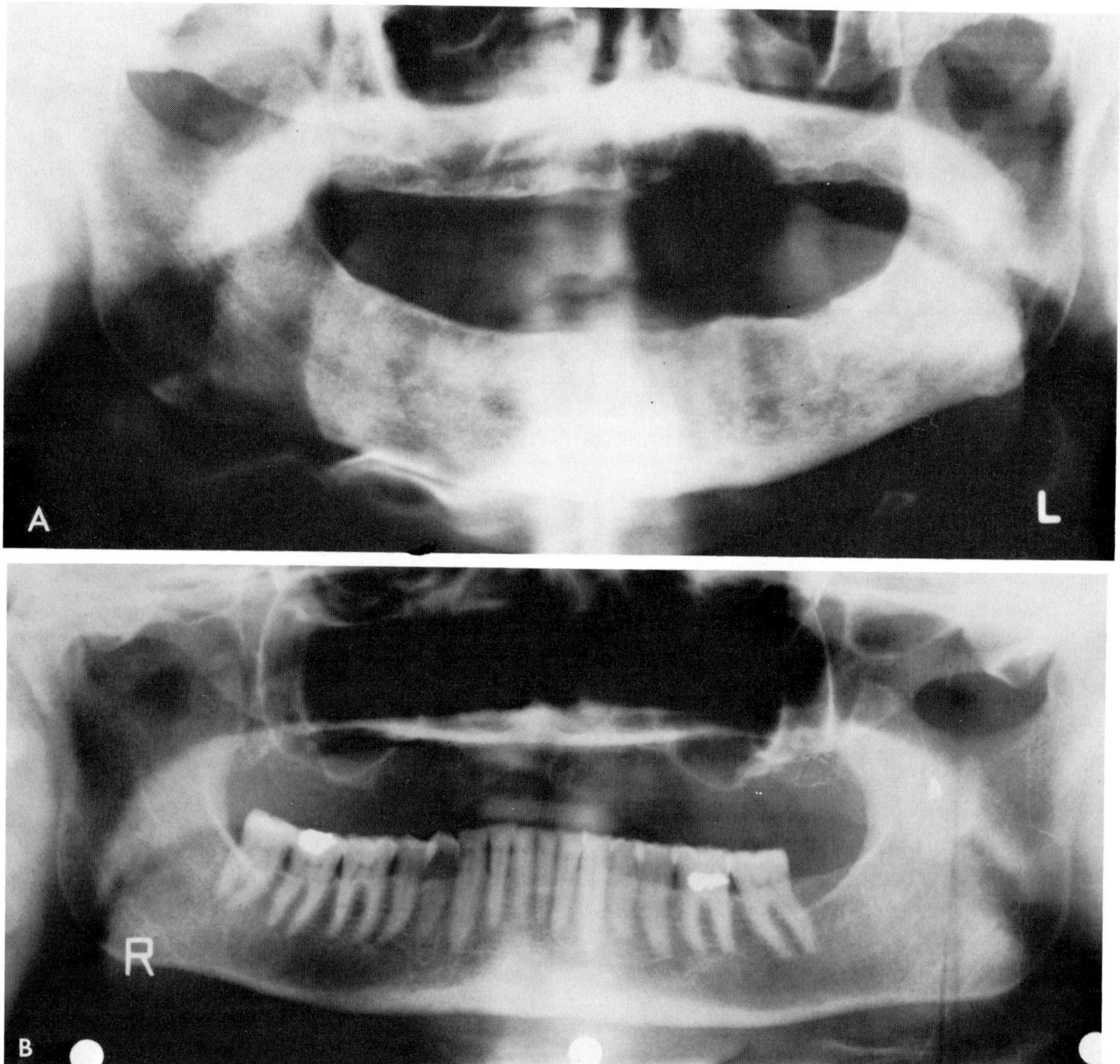

Figure 17–6. Projection hypertrophy. **A.** The right ramus and coronoid process have been magnified because the patient turned his head in the machine. **B.** Compare the left and right sides. (Figure 17–6 courtesy of Dr. Birgit Junfin Glass, San Antonio, TX.)

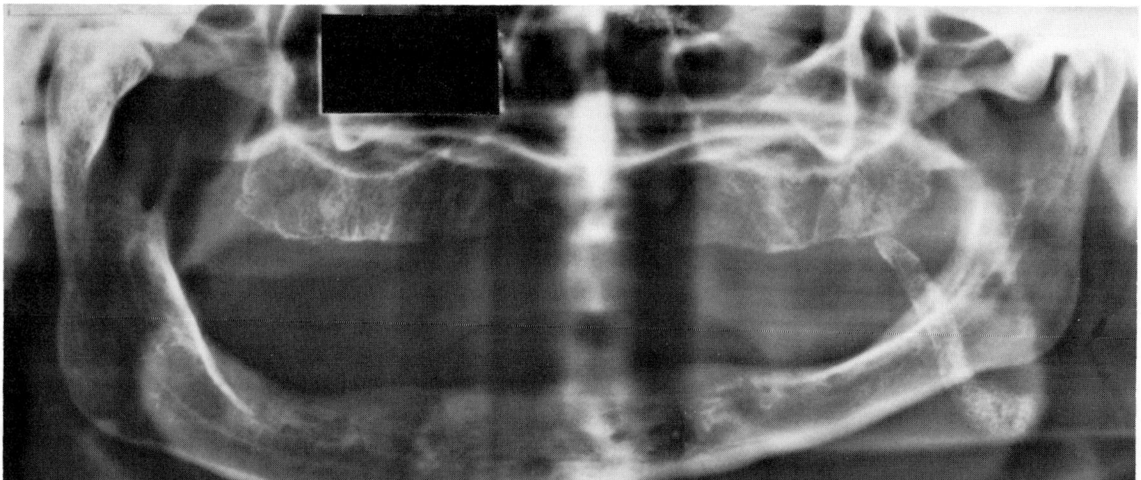

Figure 17–7. Condylar hyperplasia, Type 1. **A.** Standard panoramic view. **B.** Modified panoramic TMJ view. (Figure 17–7 courtesy of Dr. Gus Pappas, Columbus, OH.)

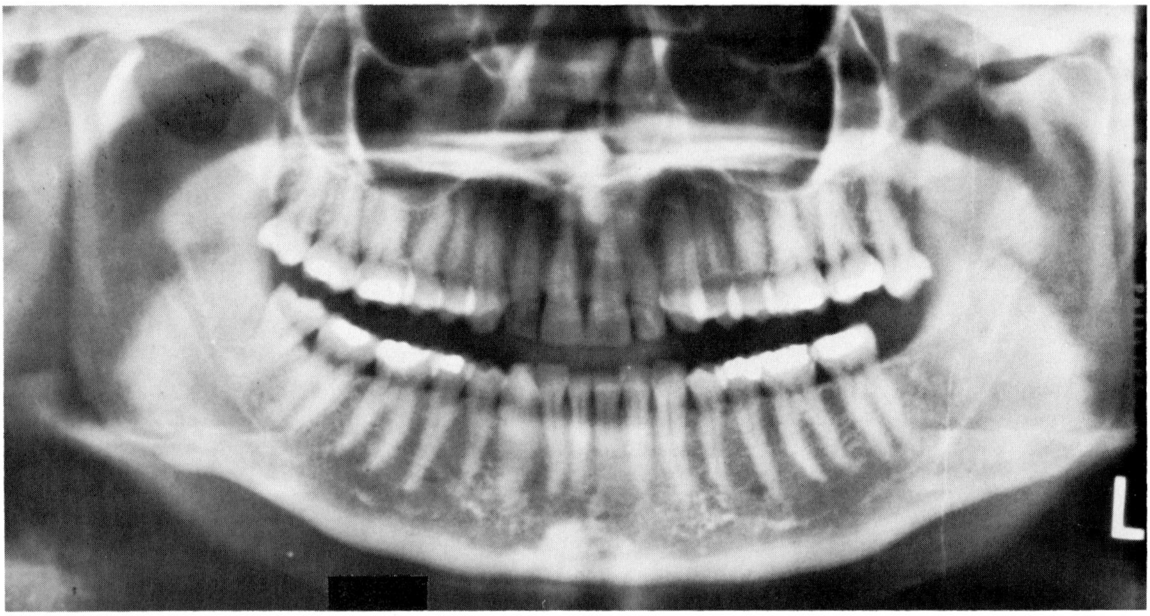

Figure 17–8. Condylar hyperplasia, Type 2. This 25-year-old female was asymptomatic with no history of trauma, pain, or other TMJ problems. (Courtesy of Dr. Richard Morse, San Antonio, TX.)

a normally shaped but much larger head of the condyle with a thickened neck area (Fig. 17–7). In the second type, no remodeling takes place, and the head of the condyle is replaced by a globular mass, which may, in some cases, resemble an inverted L (Fig. 17–8). The third type is probably an exuberant response to the inflammation of degenerative joint disease (Fig. 17–9).

Hypertrophy and hyperplasia, when unilateral, may be associated with restricted opening, facial asymmetry (which has been classified into four types by Jonck), and a progressive lack of posterior occlusion on the affected side, as was the case in Figure 17–9. Technetium^{99M} diphosphonate scans have been helpful in locating areas of overactive growth by the presence of a hot spot. This is a helpful procedure in planning interceptive surgery when the condition affects growing teenagers. Condylar hyperplasia and hypertrophy should be distinguished from the enlargement that occurs owing to the presence of an osteoma or other neoplasms and the hawk-beak appearance of the head of the

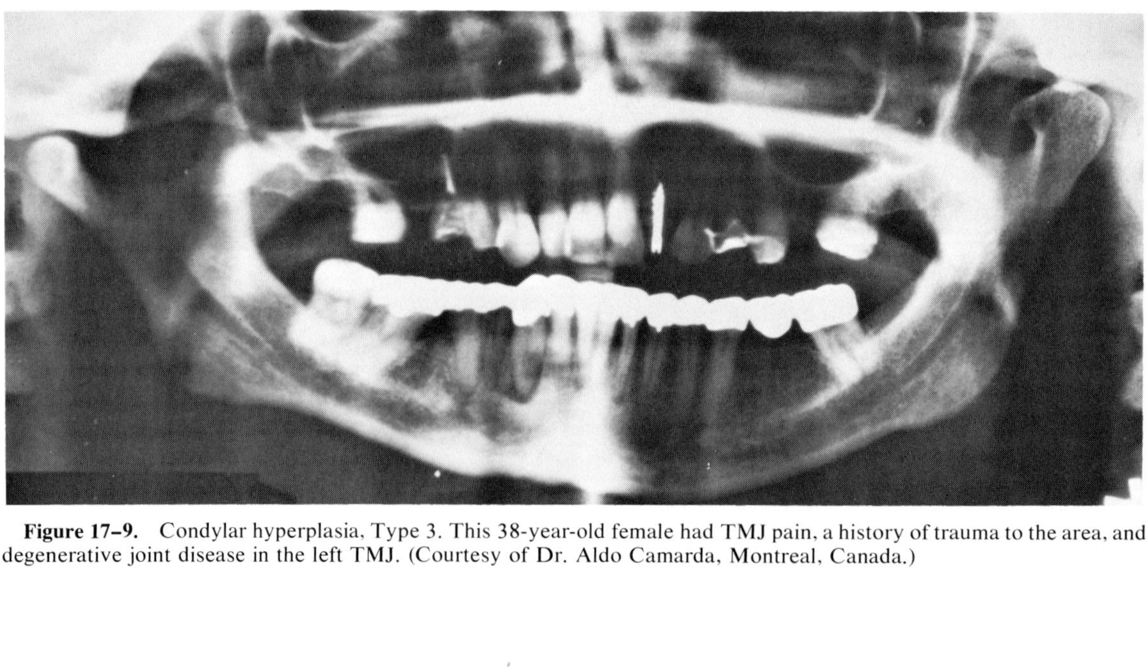

Figure 17–9. Condylar hyperplasia, Type 3. This 38-year-old female had TMJ pain, a history of trauma to the area, and degenerative joint disease in the left TMJ. (Courtesy of Dr. Aldo Camarda, Montreal, Canada.)

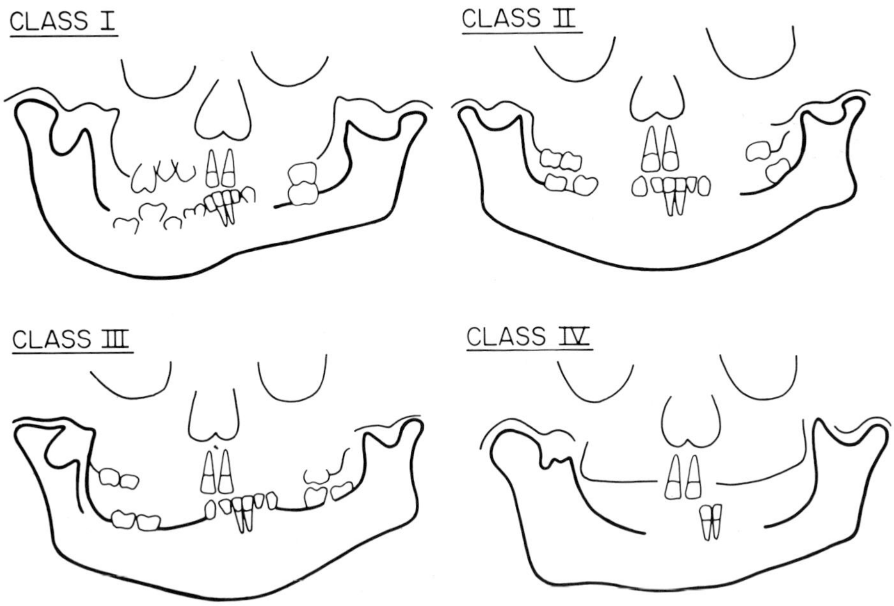

Figure 17–18. Jonck classification of facial asymmetry. (Adapted from Jonck, L. M.: Facial asymmetry and condylar hyperplasia. Oral Surg. *40*:569, 1975.)

condyle with gross osteophyte (spur) formation, seen mainly in degenerative joint disease (osteoarthritis).

In Jonck's classification of facial asymmetry (Fig. 17–10) associated with condylar enlargement, Classes I and II are developmental. In Class I there is condylar enlargement, no midline deviation, and loss of posterior occlusion on the affected side. In Class II the condyle and ramus are normal and there is midline deviation, due to an elongated mandibular body, and posterior occlusion is present on the affected side. In Class III the changes are acquired, for example, in functional or inflammatory disorders. The condyle is enlarged with the typical hawk-beak shape and spur formation and there is midline deviation and loss of posterior occlusion on the affected side. In Class IV the condylar enlargement is neoplastic and there may or may not be enlargement of the ramus and body, lack of posterior occlusion on the affected side, and midline deviation. This classification system is important, as it calls attention to TMJ disorders associated with various clinical manifestations of facial asymmetry.

CORONOID PROCESS ENLARGEMENT

BRIEF OVERVIEW

Coronoid process enlargement is an unusual occurrence but an important consideration in the diagnosis of painless limitation of mandibular opening. The limited opening is caused by impingement of the enlarged coronoid process by the inferior and medial aspects of the malar bone. Coronoid process enlargement may be unilateral or bilateral. It is most frequently unilateral, usually owing to the presence of an **osteochondroma.** Other causes of enlargement include **osteoma, exostosis, abnormal fracture healing,** and **hyperplasia.** Clinically, painless limitation of vertical opening, deviation of the mandible toward the affected side on opening, and prominence of the zygoma on the affected side will be noted.

Bilateral enlargement is much less frequently encountered and is usually due to idiopathic hyperplasia. In this instance, painless limitation of vertical opening with no mandibular deviation or facial change will be noted. Whether unilateral or bilateral, coronoid process enlargement almost exclusively affects males, usually between the ages of 12 and 30 at the time of discovery. Limitation of opening is usually less than 20 mm, and in most instances a previous history of normal opening can be elicited. Intraoral palpation of the malar bone may reveal a notch along the anterior inferior aspect. Treatment is usually by surgical excision and immediate physiotherapy until normal function is obtained.

RADIOGRAPHIC FEATURES

When the condition is unilateral, comparison of the affected side with the normal side will

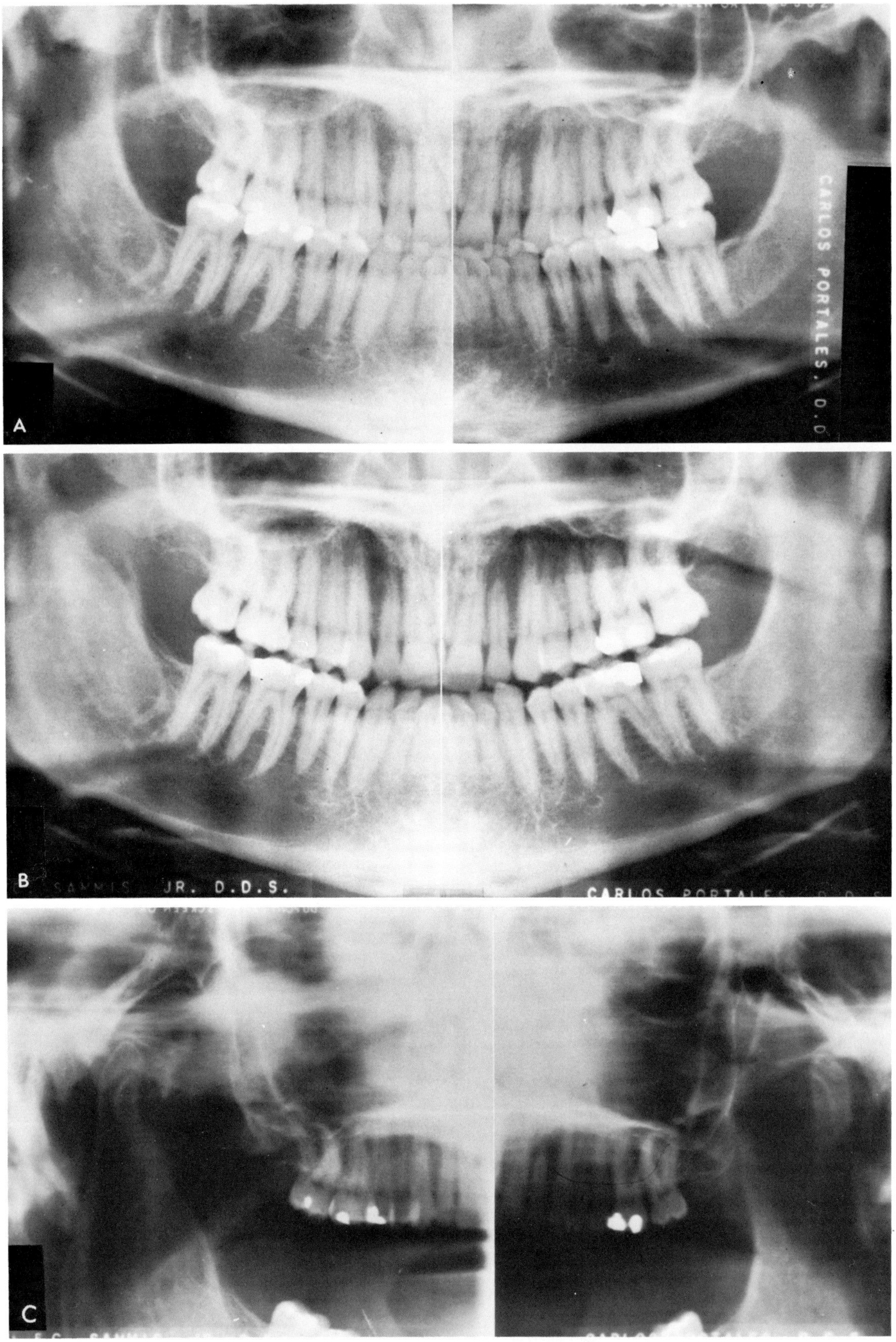

Figure 17–11. Coronoid process enlargement: osteochondroma, right coronoid process. **A.** Preoperative film in a 28-year-old female. **B.** Postoperative film, standard panoramic view. **C.** Postoperative film, panoramic TMJ view. (Figure 17–11 courtesy of Drs. Frank Sammis, Jr. and Carlos Portales, San Antonio, TX.)

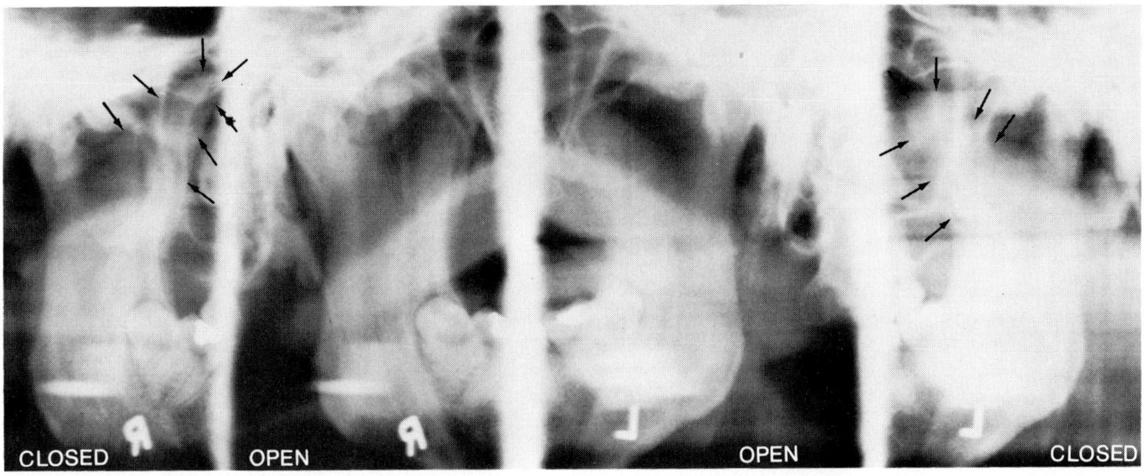

Figure 17–12. Bilateral idiopathic hyperplasia of the coronoid process. This 28-year-old male presented with limited mandibular opening. The condition was painless, there was no deviation of the mandible on opening, and the maximum interincisal distance was 20 mm. Note the lack of translation of the condyles in the open position; this is a pathognomonic radiographic sign of limited opening. (Courtesy of Dr. Dale Miles, San Antonio, TX.)

reveal an enlarged coronoid process. Additionally, when the enlargement is caused by a neoplasm, the shape of the coronoid process may be altered (Fig. 17–11). When bilateral, the enlargement is usually due to hyperplasia. In this instance, the coronoid processes will appear abnormally large but normal in shape (Fig. 17–12). In either case (unilateral or bilateral), the standard panoramic view and the special TMJ series provide excellent visualization of the coronoid process. In unilateral cases, some deformity or outward bowing of the malar bone may be noted in the basilar view.

CONDYLAR ANKYLOSIS

BRIEF OVERVIEW AND RADIOGRAPHIC FEATURES

True ankylosis of the TMJ would require bony union between the head of the condyle and the glenoid fossa. This is in fact a rare occurrence, as there is usually fibrous union between the components. The term is used when there is a complete disappearance of the joint space radiographically and an extremely limited or virtual inability to open the jaws

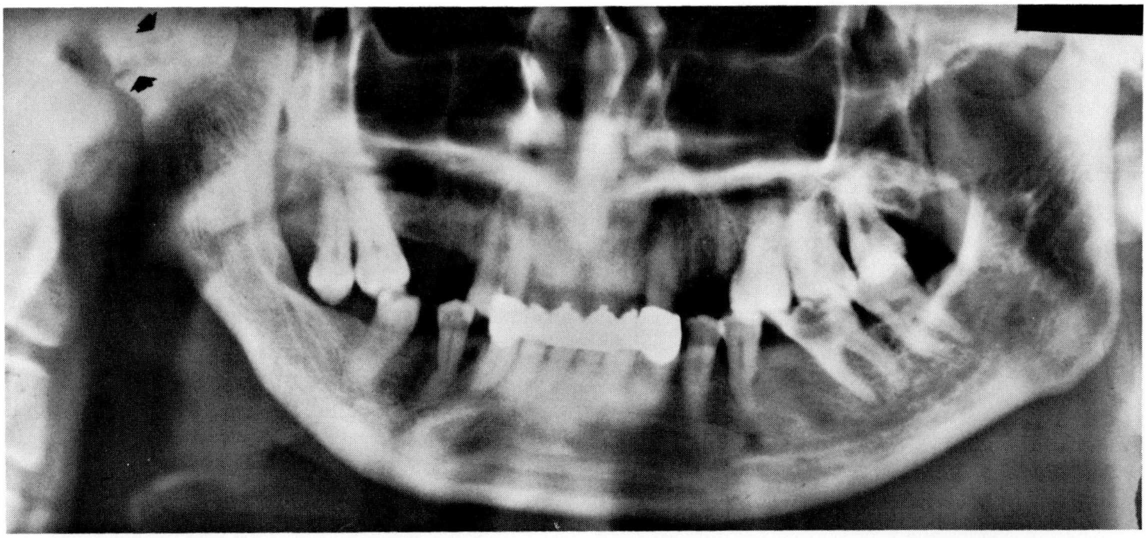

Figure 17–13. Condylar ankylosis. (Courtesy of Dr. Gus Pappas, Columbus, OH.)

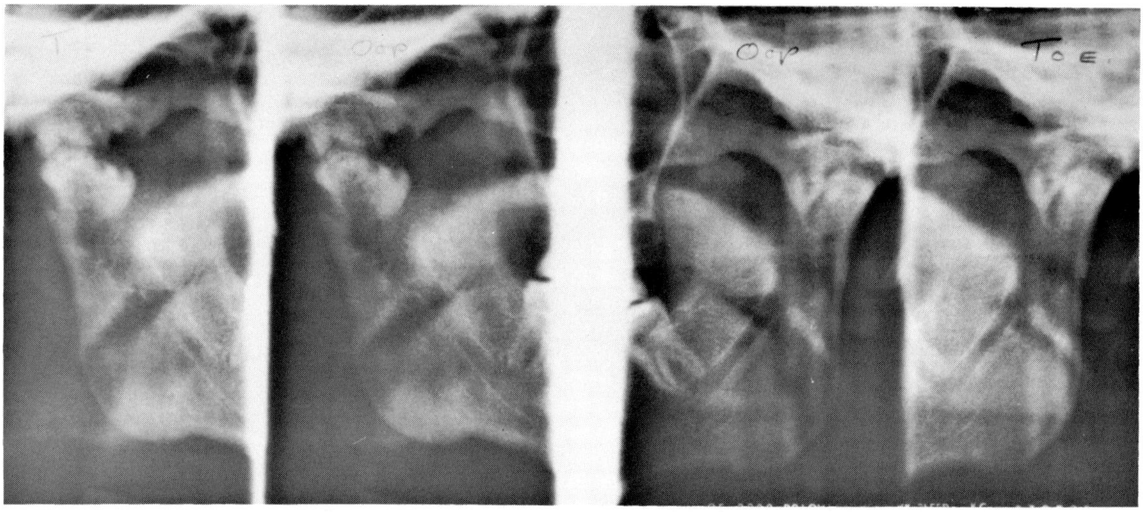

Figure 17–14. Bilateral condylar ankylosis. (Courtesy of Dr. Chris Nortjé, University of Stellenbosch, Tygerberg, South Africa.)

clinically (Figs. 17–13 and 17–14). Ankylosis may occur in children and may be a sequela of trauma or rheumatoid arthritis or may be due to the bony union of the head of the condyle to the glenoid fossa by an intervening osteoma or other neoplasm. Ankylosis, as defined here, must be clinically distinguished from trismus, muscle spasm, hypertrophy or enlargement of the coronoid process, and, in older patients, scleroderma and other collagen disorders in which there is difficulty in opening the mandible. Ankylosis is sometimes treated by osteotomy of the neck of the condyle. The subsequent formation of a fibrous union or false joint between the two bony segments of the condylar neck results in immediate postoperative jaw function with physiotherapy and no fixation.

ZYGOMATICOCORONOID ANKYLOSIS

BRIEF OVERVIEW

This is an extremely rare condition, with less than a dozen cases reported in the literature, but it remains an important consideration in the differential diagnosis of progressive painless limitation of mandibular opening. In most cases, a history of previous fracture of the zygoma will be elicited. This includes direct trauma to the zygoma, other facial fractures including the zygoma, gunshot wounds, previous surgery in the area of the pterygoid fossa, and vertical osteotomy of the rami for bilateral mandibular prognathism. Treatment is usually by surgical separation of the two bones, coronoidectomy, and immediate postoperative exercises.

RADIOGRAPHIC FEATURES

The panoramic films usually show a lack of movement of the coronoid processes when comparing the closed and open views. The submentovertex view may show a close approximation of the coronoid process and the medial aspect of the zygoma. On occasion, mineralization may be discernible between the two bones.

MYOFASCIAL PAIN–DYSFUNCTION SYNDROME (TMJ Syndrome)

BRIEF OVERVIEW AND RADIOGRAPHIC FEATURES

Myofascial pain–dysfunction (MPD) syndrome is now a well-recognized symptom complex that predominantly affects females under the age of 40. The main symptoms include pain in the TMJ, often unilateral; crepitus or popping of the TMJ; limitation of opening below 40 mm or inability to place three of the patient's fingers between the incisors; and deviation on opening. Other findings include a coexisting parafunctional habit such as bruxism, a night habit; clenching, a daytime habit; onychophagia (nail biting); gum chewing; and cheek biting (morsicatio buccarum). Psychological factors may also be present. Bizzare complaints such as vertigo, tinnitus, "worms in the jaws," cancerphobia, and the like are not uncommon. The muscles of mastication are often very tender on palpation at the points of origin and insertion. The symptomatic joint is not painful on palpation, the lateral border of the tongue may be scalloped, and the buccal mucosa may show a prominent linea alba.

Radiographically, MPD syndrome shows no degenerative alterations of the TMJ in the early stages (Fig. 17–15). There may be a unilateral lack of translation on opening (a radiographic sign of deviation), or there may be a lack of concentricity of the head of the condyle in the fossa. MPD syndrome may lead to anterior disk displacement with or without reduction or disk perforation. These conditions may be seen with arthrography, thus separating MPD syndrome and disorders of the meniscus from conditions that may give rise to any or all of the radiographic changes seen in association with degenerative joint disease.

The treatment of MPD syndrome, as advocated by the authors, should be conservative if no radiographic findings are present. The first phase should be aimed at alleviating pain and muscle spasm; the second phase involves physiotherapy to restore function and identification

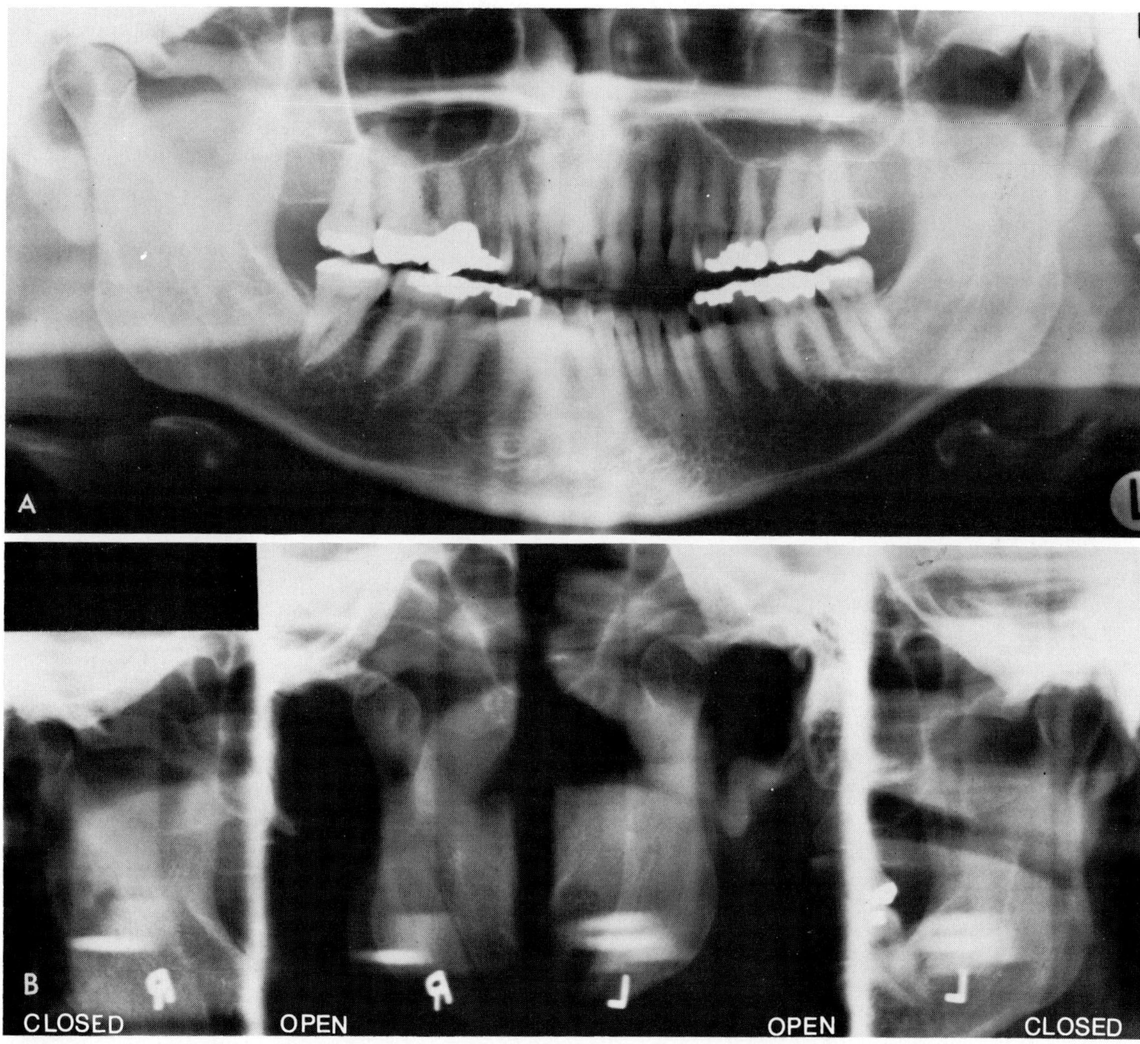

Figure 17–15. Myofascial pain–dysfunction syndrome. **A.** Normal TMJ is a typical radiographic finding. **B.** Panoramic TMJ series. This 35-year-old female with intermittent TMJ pain, tinnitus, and vertigo was diagnosed as having Meniere's syndrome and was taking Antivert ([meclizine HCl], Roerig, a division of Pfizer Pharmaceuticals, NY). There was no limitation of opening, but the right and left external and internal pterygoid muscles were exquisitely tender on palpation. The patient responded well to conservative measures and had no return of symptoms upon withdrawal of the Antivert. (Figure 17–15 courtesy of Dr. Gururaja Rao, San Antonio, TX.)

and elimination of the parafunctional habit; the third phase involves mandibular relearning. Once the patient has returned to normal function, the occlusion may now be evaluated and possibly adjusted. Throughout the treatment, supportive psychotherapy is useful and productive. Placebo muscle relaxants, placebo occlusal equilibrations, placebo nightguards, and the like are effective.

In cases that do not respond to conservative therapy, especially when there is a history of clicking or crepitus, arthrography should be performed to rule out a disorder of the meniscus.

ABNORMALITIES OF THE DISK: TMJ ARTHROGRAPHY (Internal Derangements Within the Capsule)

BRIEF OVERVIEW

With the recent renewal of interest in TMJ arthrography and arthrotomography, a number of specific disorders of the meniscus have been detected in patients whose TMJ radiographs were normal. TMJ arthrography is indicated for patients with a positive diagnosis of MPD syndrome, especially those with clicking or a history of clicking, and for those who do not respond to conservative treatment. Arthrography is also indicated for patients with a positive history of locking and for those with a limited opening of indeterminate etiology. Arthrography is contraindicated in the presence of acute infection and in patients with hypersensitivity to the contrast media.

The cycle of events leading to functional disorders of the meniscus begins with clicking on opening at about 5 mm, then at 15 mm, whence clicking occurs on opening and closing. Eventually there is intermittent locking, and vertical opening becomes limited to 15 or 20 mm. Clicking then disappears and pain is present. At this point the patient is articulating on the posterior ligament or attachment of the biconcave disk, with the disk permanently displaced in a forward position. Unlike the disk, the ligament is richly innervated and highly vascular; thus pain and inflammation may be present. Further articulation with the posterior ligament leads to eventual perforation (usually at the junction of the disk and ligament) and crepitus, as the bones articulate against each other. The three most important abnormalities of the disk are anterior displacement with reduction, anterior displacement without reduction, and disk perforation. In long-standing cases, degenerative joint disease may develop, and at this point changes in the bones become visible on the normal TMJ radiographs. Each of the three abnormalities of the disk will be discussed separately. Management should be initially conservative, consisting of muscle relaxants, analgesics, supportive psychotherapy, and muscle exercises. In the absence of a response to conservative therapy and based on the arthrographic findings, surgical repair of the disk may be helpful.

RADIOGRAPHIC FEATURES

Arthrography is accomplished by carefully locating the lower joint space with the aid of fluoroscopy and injecting water-soluble radiopaque material into the space. The same procedure is repeated to opacify the upper joint space. As soon as possible after opacification of the joint spaces, normal lateral TMJ views or TMJ tomograms are taken, usually in the closed and open positions. Figure 17–16 illustrates the normal biconcave disk between the two opacified joint spaces and its relationship to the head of the condyle, the glenoid (mandibular) fossa, and the articular eminence. Generally, the shape of the lower joint space as it alters with condylar movement provides the most diagnostic information concerning the disk. Experienced arthrographers often interpret disk abnormalities with opacification of the lower joint space only.

ANTERIOR DISK DISPLACEMENT WITH REDUCTION

BRIEF OVERVIEW

Typically, the clinical findings include TMJ pain and tenderness, otalgia, temporal headaches, muscle tenderness, TMJ clicking, and intermittent locking. Usually there is exquisite pain upon intrameatal palpation. The muscles of mastication are tender but not enough to cause the patient to pull away when the muscle attachments are palpated. Often the patient will be able to open to about 20 mm; upon pressing on the condyle, opening then increases to 40 mm or more.

RADIOGRAPHIC FEATURES

In the closed view, the posterior band is anterior to the head of the condyle. Note that

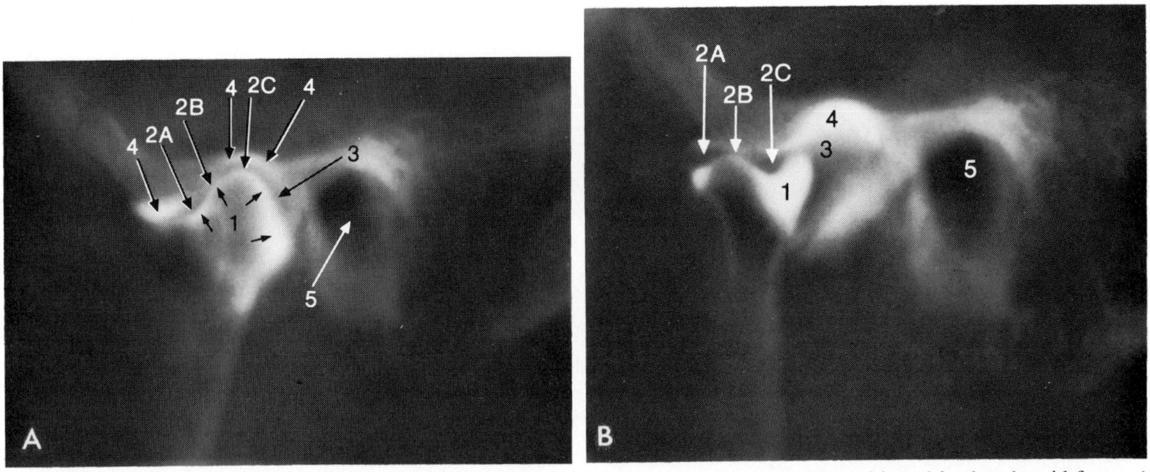

Figure 17–16. Normal TMJ arthrotomogram. **A.** Closed. The condyle is centrally positioned in the glenoid fossa, 1, Lower joint space filled. 2. Biconcave disk. 2A, Anterior band. 2B. Middle band. 2C. Posterior band. 3. Posterior ligament. 4. Upper joint space filled. 5. External auditory meatus. **B.** Open. The condyle has translated anteriorly and is at the articular eminence. 1, Lower joint space: anterior recess almost obliterated. Posterior recess filled. 2. Normal position of the disk with the mandible open. 2A, Anterior band. 2B. Middle band. 2C. Posterior band, 3. Posterior ligament, 4. Upper joint space: anterior recess obliterated. Posterior recess filled. 5. External auditory meatus. (Figure 17–16 courtesy of Dr. Frank Dolwick, San Antonio, TX,)

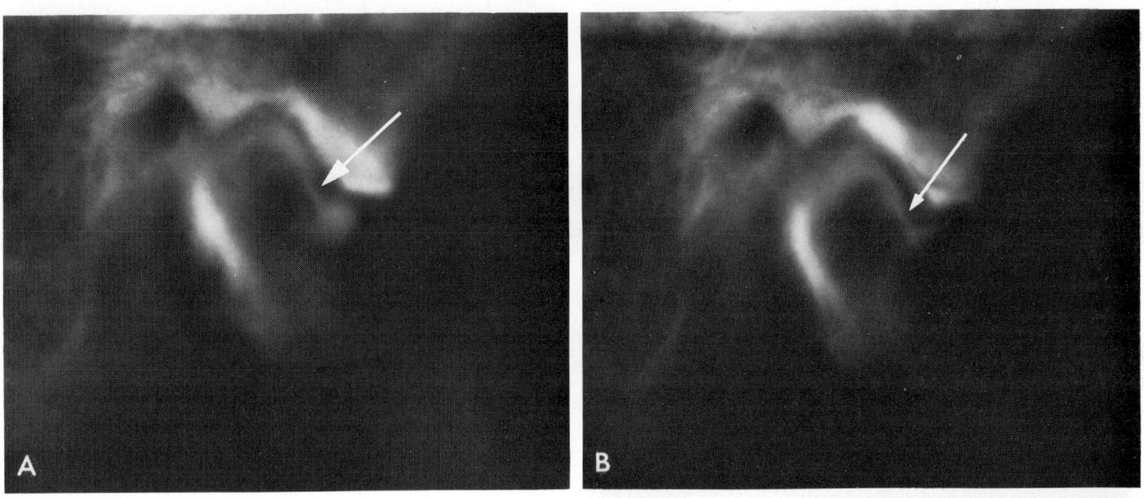

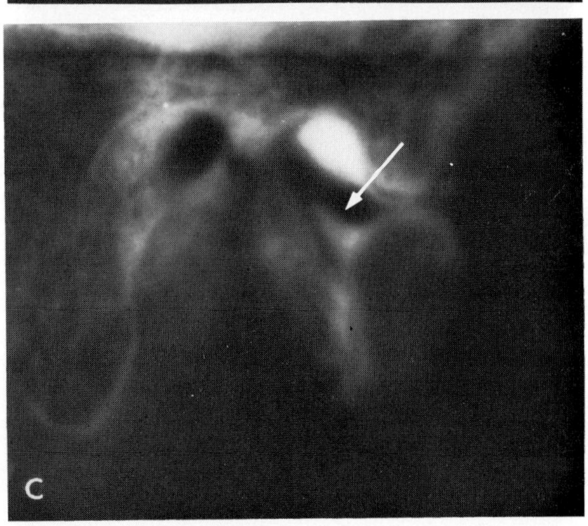

Figure 17–17. Anterior disk displacement with reduction. **A.** Closed. Arrow indicates the position of the posterior band of the biconcave disk, which is displaced anteriorly in the closed position. The head of the condyle is articulating against the posterior ligament. **B.** Just before the click. Arrow indicates a slight bunching up or thickening of the posterior band of the disk as the condyle begins to translate anteriorly. The head of the condyle is still articulating against the posterior ligament. **C.** Fully open after the click. Arrow indicates that the posterior band of the disk has now "snapped" back to the normal open position. The head of the condyle is articulating on the disk. All aspects of the arthrogram now appear normal for the open position. (Figure 17–17 courtesy of Dr. Frank Dolwick, San Antonio, TX.)

the lower joint space is larger anteriorly and more horizontally directed than normal (Fig. 17–17**A**).

The second view is taken just before the click. The disk is pushed further forward with a folding of the central articulating area (Fig. 17–17**B**).

The third view is taken after the click, in the open position. The arthrogram looks normal, as the disk has popped back into place. The posterior aspect of the biconcave disk is a little thickened (Fig. 17–17**C**).

ANTERIOR DISK DISPLACEMENT WITHOUT REDUCTION

BRIEF OVERVIEW

Typically, the clinical findings include TMJ pain and tenderness, otalgia, temporal headaches, muscle tenderness, a past history of clicking, and limited opening. The patients tend to be young adults.

RADIOGRAPHIC FEATURES

In the closed-mouth view, the posterior aspect of the disk is anterior to the head of the condyle, similar to the closed-mouth findings in anterior displacement with reduction (Fig. 17–18**A**).

In the second view the mouth is opened as wide as possible, and the typical bird-beak effect of anterior dislocation without reduction is produced. The disk remains in the anterior position, similar to the finding in anterior displacement with reduction, just before the click. The bird-beak effect is produced because both upper and lower anterior joint recesses fail to empty into the posterior recesses in the open position (Fig. 17–18**B**).

DISK PERFORATION

BRIEF OVERVIEW

Disk perforation may occur in two different situations. In degenerative joint disease, disk perforation occurs in the central depressed area of the disk; the patients are usually over the age of 40. In the second situation the patients are younger, and there is anterior disk displacement with or without reduction. The perforation is usually through the posterior ligament just at the attachment to the meniscus. In most patients, crepitus is present.

RADIOGRAPHIC FEATURES

The striking radiographic finding is a simultaneous opacification of both joint spaces upon injection into one or the other space. Anterior displacement with or without reduction is usually present. The condylar surface may show changes similar to those seen in degenerative joint disease (see Fig. 17–18).

DEGENERATIVE JOINT DISEASE (Osteoarthritis, Hypertrophic Arthritis, Arthritis Deformans)

BRIEF OVERVIEW

Degenerative joint disease occurs in about half the population over the age of 50. When the TMJ is involved, the condition is unilateral in about two-thirds of the patients. It is considered part of the aging process but may develop from a single traumatic episode, as a result of long-standing MPD syndrome, or as a sequela to functional disorders of the disk.

The clinical symptoms include crepitation, cracking, or clicking; pain or tenderness with or without function; pain on palpation; hypermobility, subluxation, or dislocation; earaches and headaches; and deviation on opening or painful limitation of opening and other excursions. The condition is usually managed with salicylates.

RADIOGRAPHIC FEATURES

Any one or a combination of the following changes may be seen radiographically: narrowing of the joint space, with or without painful or nonpainful limitation of mandibular movement; facet formation on the head of the condyle, which may be small or large with a flat or irregular surface; eburnation, which is a condensation of reactive dense bone on the surface of the condyle; surface erosions, which may look like cupped-out areas on the articular surface of the condyle or cystlike areas in the medial or lateral aspect known as osteoarthritic or Ely's cysts; osteophyte or spur formation, the latter being the better of the two terms. The spur may be small or very large, resembling a hawk beak, and is most frequently seen at the

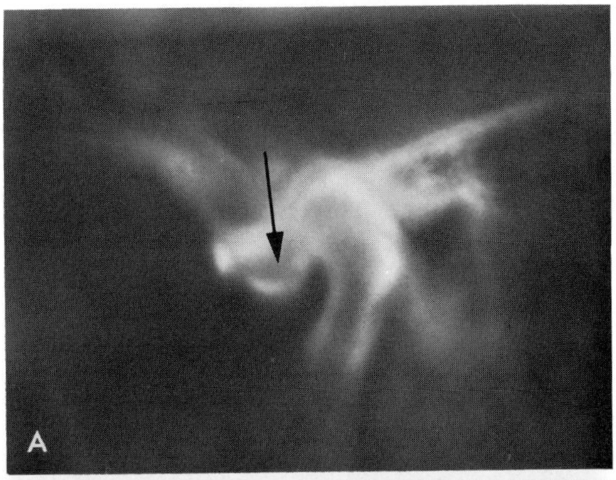

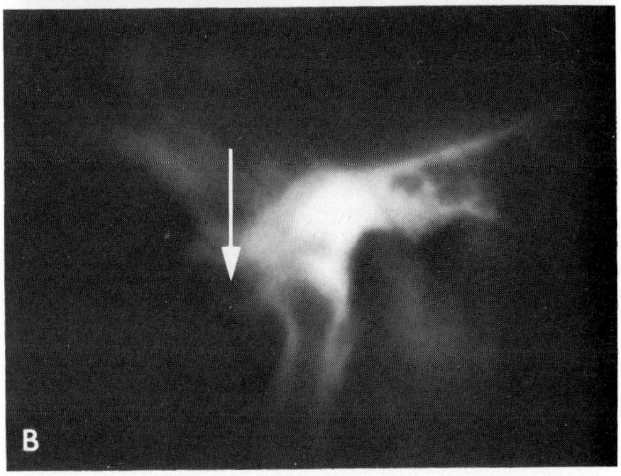

Figure 17–18. Anterior disk displacement without reduction and disk perforation. **A.** Closed. Arrow indicates the position of the posterior band of the disk displaced anteriorly in the closed position. The head of the condyle is articulating against the posterior ligament. Both joint spaces filled simultaneously upon injection of the lower space, indicating disk perforation. **B.** Open. Arrow indicates the position of the posterior band of the disk, which remains in an anteriorly displaced position. The anterior recesses retain residual pools of contrast material, forming the typical bird-beak appearance. The apparent continuity of the upper and lower posterior recesses as well as the cloudy appearance of the arthrogram indicate further evidence of extravasation of medium and disk perforation. (Figure 17–18 courtesy of Dr. Frank Dolwick, San Antonio, TX.)

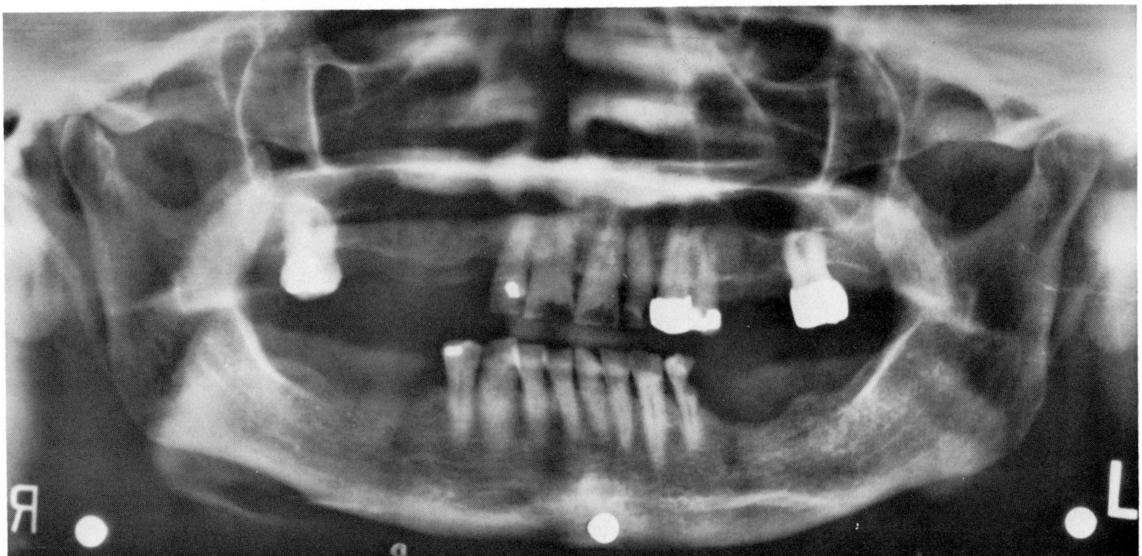

Figure 17–19. Degenerative joint disease. Right TMJ smooth facet formation. Note the flattening of the superior portion of the head of the condyle, with the loss of cortical bone and the flattening of the articular eminence. (Courtesy of Dr. Steven Bricker, San Antonio, TX.)

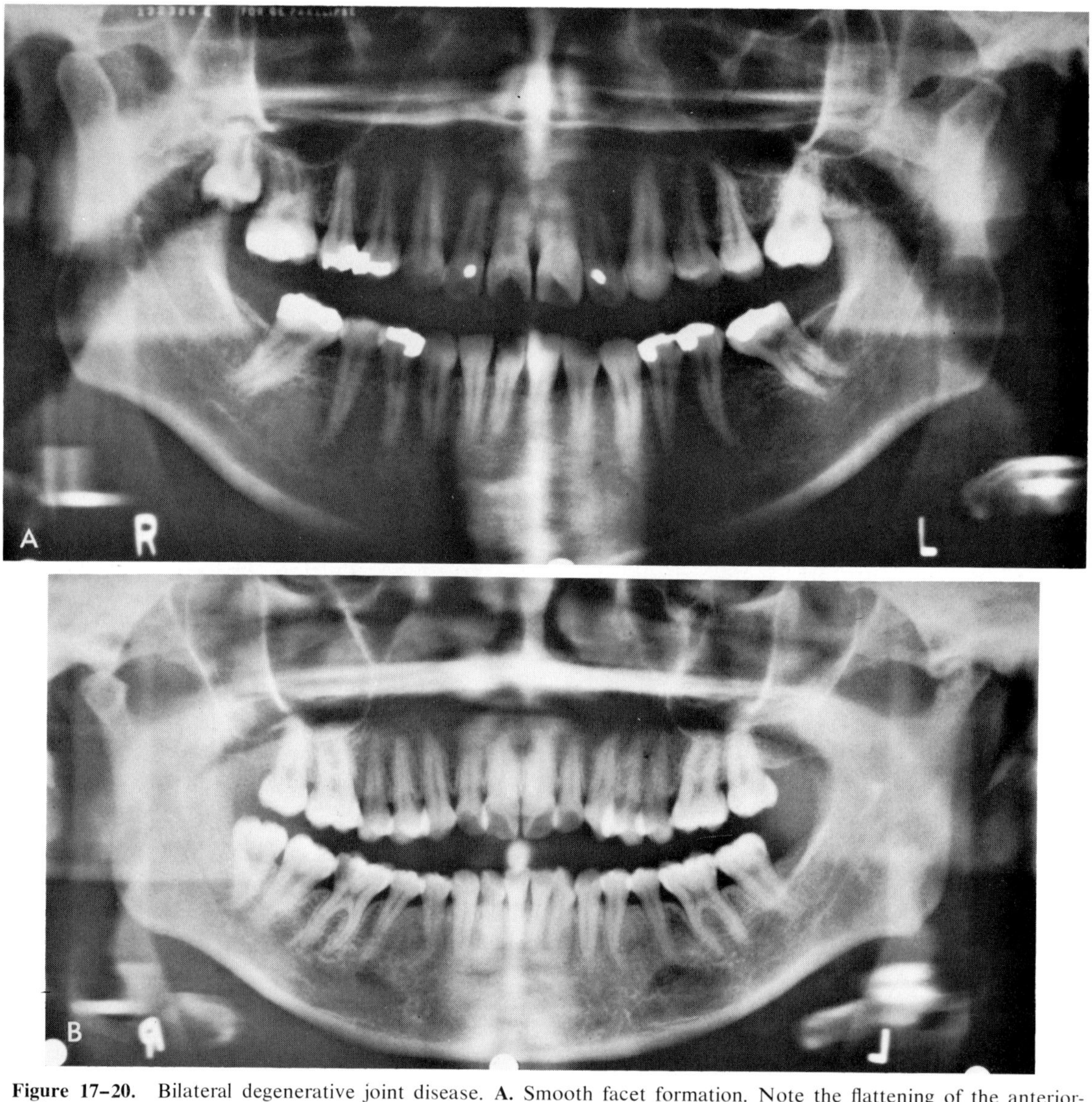

Figure 17–20. Bilateral degenerative joint disease. **A.** Smooth facet formation. Note the flattening of the anterior-superior aspect of the head of the condyles, especially on the left side. **B.** Left side: ragged facet formation. Right side: smooth facet formation with a small anterior spur. (Figure 17–20 courtesy of Dr. Steven Bricker, San Antonio, TX.)

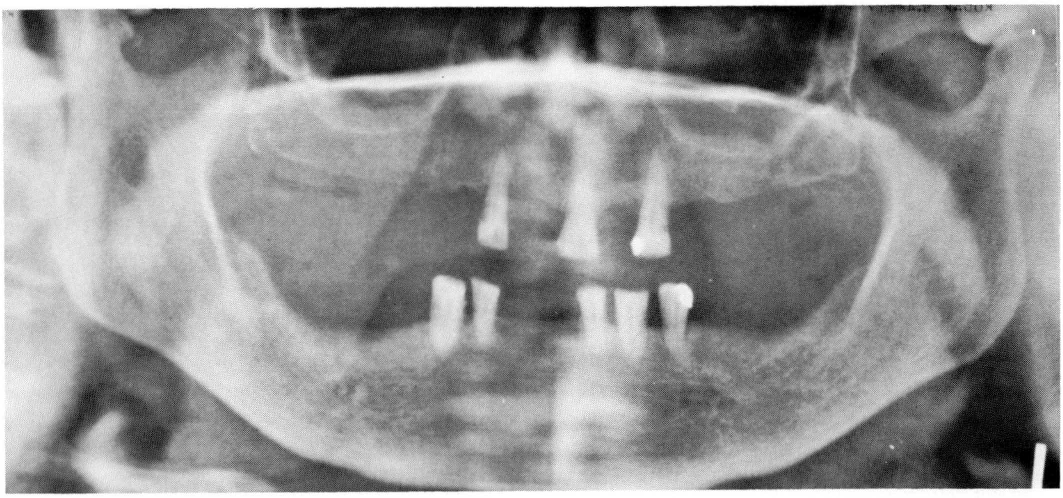

Figure 17–21. Degenerative joint disease. Right TMJ: condylar hyperplasia, Type 3 with a fractured spur (spicule). (Courtesy of Dr. Steven Bricker, San Antonio, TX.)

anterior aspect of a facet but may occur anywhere on the head of the condyle. The articular eminence may exhibit many of the same changes, with facet formation being the most common (Figs. 17–19 to 17–21). When the hands are involved, a loss of joint space may be noted at one or several terminal phalanges. Firm and sometimes tender nodules over the affected joints, clinically known as Heberden's nodes, may also be present.

This condition is separate from **ankylosing spondylitis,** which mainly affects the vertebral column but may indirectly involve the TMJ, usually as a result of muscle spasm and postural imbalance of the head and neck. In ankylosing spondylitis, radiographs are helpful in eliminating ankylosis as a direct cause of pain and inability to open the jaws. Management of TMJ pain associated with ankylosing spondylitis is similar to that for MPD syndrome.

RHEUMATOID ARTHRITIS (Still's Disease)

BRIEF OVERVIEW

As was previously stated, degenerative joint disease begins late in life and often affects one joint. When symptomatic, the pain is most severe towards the end of the day. In contrast, rheumatoid arthritis begins early in life, often in the third decade. There is a juvenile form of the disease (Still's disease) in which there may be arrested mandibular development resulting in micrognathia, with a retrognathic "Andy Gump" facial profile. Rheumatoid arthritis tends to involve multiple joints, often bilaterally. In most cases a positive rheumatoid factor is present serologically. The disease may be severe and crippling when not controlled, and, in the TMJ, partial or complete ankylosis may develop.

Management initially involves corticosteroids and salicylates, but surgical intervention for the correction of gross deformities and improvement of function may be necessary.

RADIOGRAPHIC FEATURES

The radiographic changes are similar to those seen in degenerative joint disease in the early stages (Fig. 17–22). However, rheumatoid arthritis is characterized by osteolysis, and eventually the entire condylar head is lost (Fig. 17–22C). Ankylosis and an anterior open bite are frequent sequelae. When the hands are affected, the joints of the proximal phalanges are involved as well as other joints of both hands. Clinically the affected joints may appear enlarged, and a lateral deformity of the affected digits is often present.

SCLERODERMA (Progressive Systemic Sclerosis, Acroscleroderma)

BRIEF OVERVIEW

Scleroderma is a generalized collagen disorder that causes sclerosis of the skin and connective tissues. The term scleroderma (hard

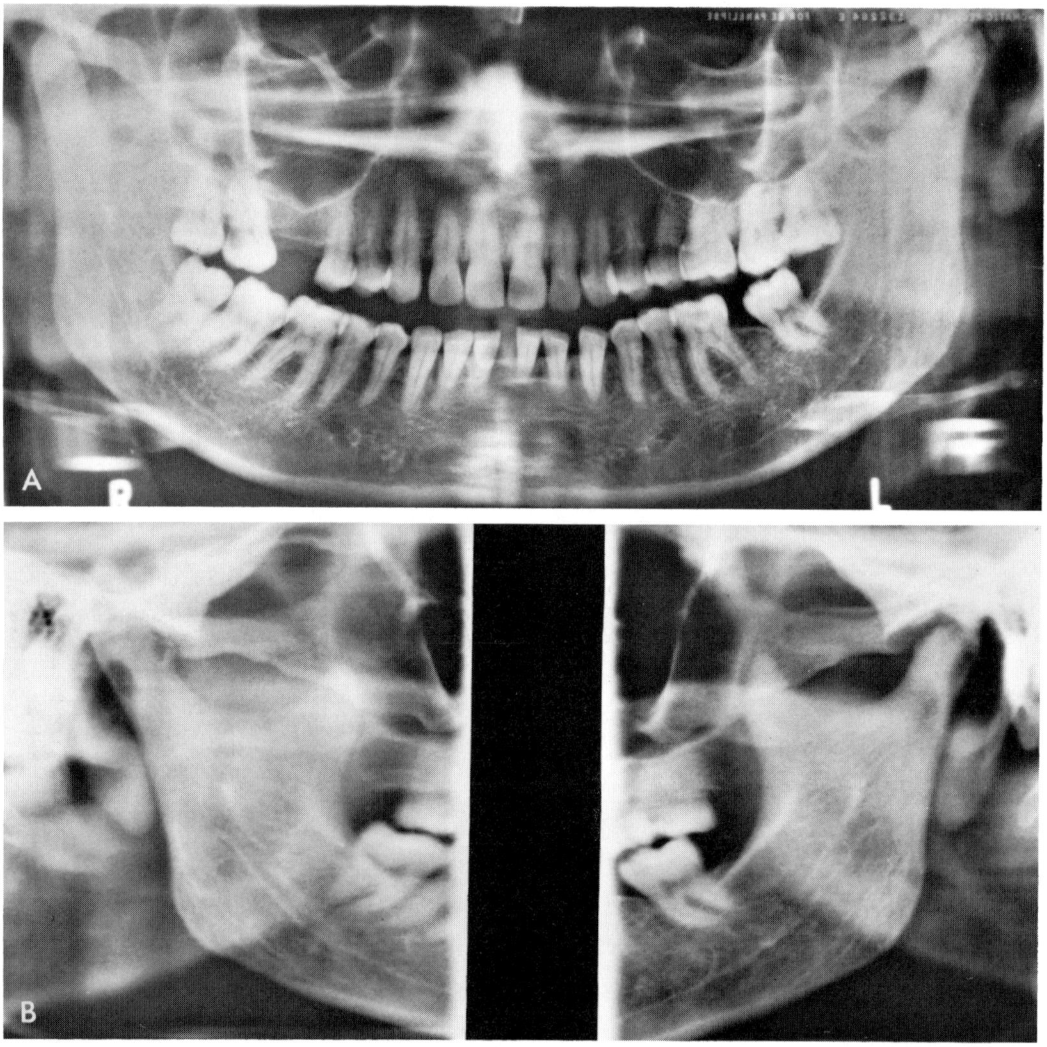

Figure 17–22. Rheumatoid arthritis. **A** and **B.** 42-year-old female. **A.** Note the ragged facet formation on the left side. Compare the right side seen in **A** with the right side in **B,** which was taken on the same day. **B.** Right side: Note the loss of joint space, the ragged facet formation, and the cystlike eroded area on the posterior aspect of the condyle.

Illustration continued on opposite page

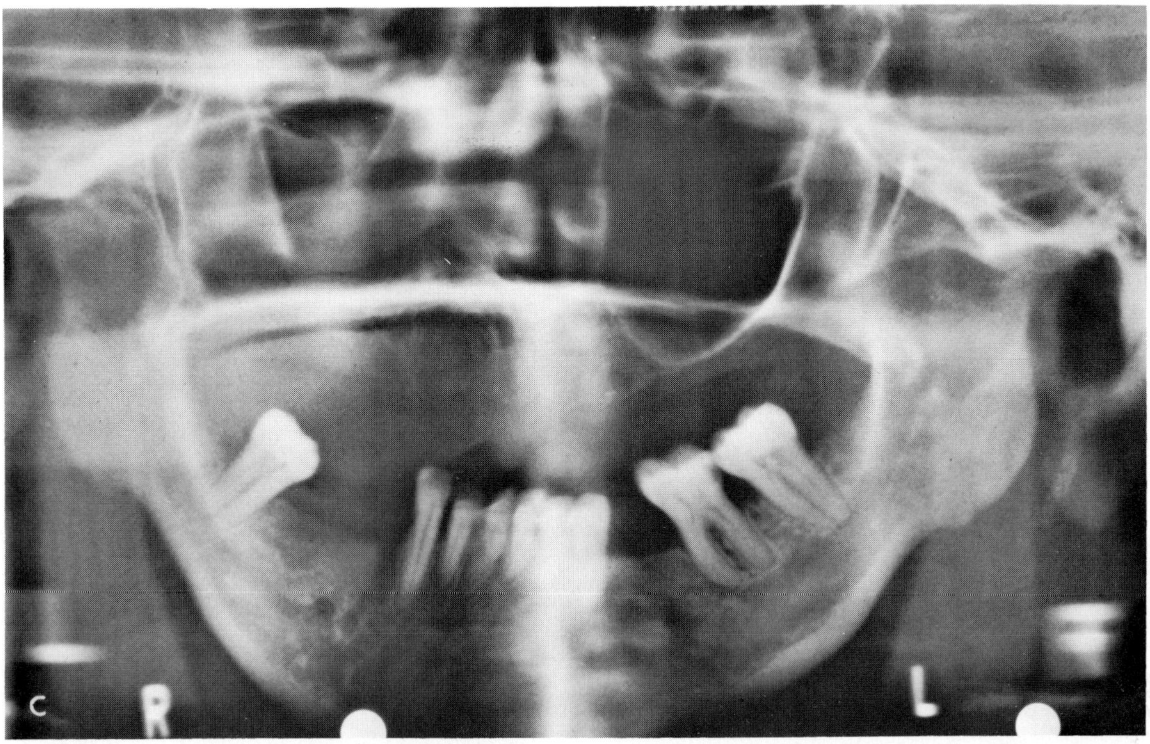

Figure 17–22 *Continued* **C.** 51-year-old-female with complete erosion of the head and neck of the condyle bilaterally. (**C** courtesy of Dr. Steven Bricker, San Antonio, TX.)

skin) describes the hidebound or waxlike quality of the affected skin. In more severe cases the disease may involve the gastrointestinal tract, leading to malabsorption and cachexia; the heart, which may lead to heart failure and arrhythmias; the lungs, in which there may be pulmonary failure; and the kidneys, leading to uremia and possibly malignant hypertension. Scleroderma has a predilection for females between the ages of 30 and 50.

In some patients the first symptom is a pitting edema of the face and extremities. Other features include dysphagia; progressive microstomia, which may be problematic in terms of eating and in the removal and placement of prostheses; telangiectasia; TMJ symptoms, including arthralgia, stiffness, and a possible positive rheumatoid factor; and the sicca syndrome (Sjögren's syndrome), which is present in as many as 12 per cent of all patients. The "scleroderma bark," an involuntary sound occurring about once every two hours during the day due to aerophagia and the subsequent expulsion of the air through the cricopharyngeal sphincter, may be heard. The etiology of scleroderma is unknown, and no specific drug has produced a consistent or prolonged benefit. When the microstomia is severe, surgical enlargement has been helpful.

RADIOGRAPHIC FEATURES

The most common oral radiographic finding is a generalized symmetric widening of the periodontal membrane space, which is most pronounced around the posterior teeth. The lamina dura remains normal. The widening of the periodontal membrane space occurs independent of periodontal disease and occlusal traumatism. A second striking feature, which is seen more commonly since the advent of panoramic radiography, is resorption of the mandibular angle, the posterior aspect of the ramus, the coronoid process, and, in some instances, the mandibular condyle (Fig. 17–23**A**). In the latter instance the patient becomes retrognathic with a typical Andy Gump appearance (Fig. 17–23**B**). When the resorption of the angle and posterior ramus is severe, pathologic fracture may occur. Other radiographic findings include resorption of the tufts of the terminal phalanges (an early finding) and eventual resorption of the terminal and middle phalanges of the hands and feet; calcareous deposits in the skin and subcutaneous layer; resorption of portions of the distal radius and ulna; and resorption of the acromion process at the acromioclavicular joint. Other findings present as the disease progresses.

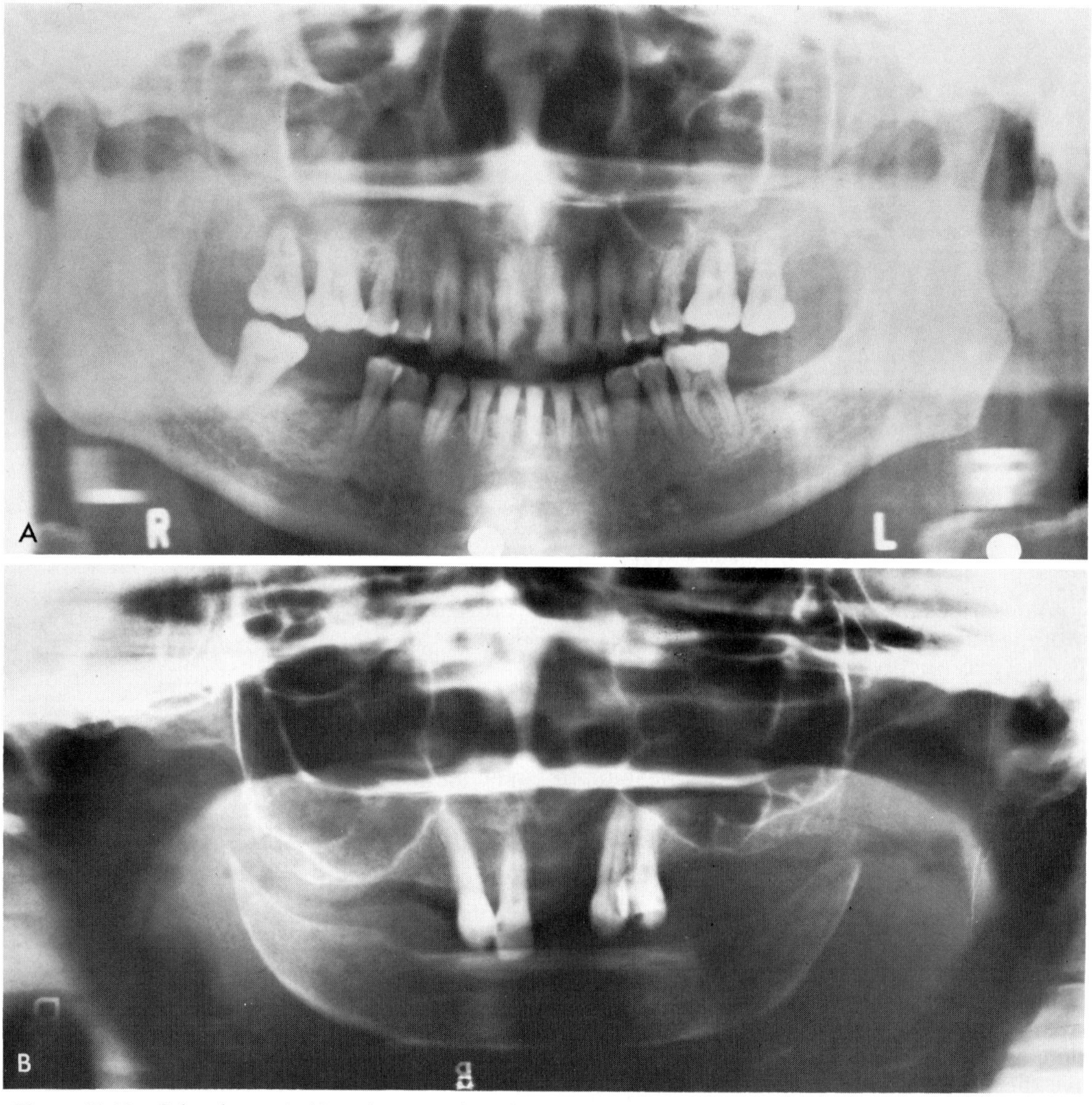

Figure 17–23. Scleroderma. **A.** Note the resorption of the left angle and possibly of the right coronoid process. Note the symmetrical generalized widening of the periodontal membrane spaces in the mandible. Note the periodontal disease in the maxilla and the associated antral changes. The patient was taking systemic corticosteroids. **B.** Note the complete bilateral resorption of the upper ramus and articulating elements in this 32-year-old female with a six-year history of the disease.

SYNOVIAL CHONDROMETAPLASIA (Synovial Chondromatosis, Osteochondromatosis)

BRIEF OVERVIEW

Chondrometaplasia is a rare joint disorder and is most frequently seen in the knee, hip, and elbow joints in that order. The condition is reported to develop as a result of active proliferation of metaplastic foci of mesenchymal cell nests located within the sublining connective tissue of the synovial membrane. These nests differentiate into cartilage cells and usually perforate the synovial membrane into the joint space either as free structures within the joint space or, less frequently, as a single mass, which in the TMJ may appear to be attached to the condylar head. As the cartilaginous bodies mature, they may ossify or calcify, whence the condition is sometimes referred to as synovial osteochondromatosis.

Chondrometaplasia involving the TMJ is a rare occurrence, with less than 20 reported cases in the literature. There is a marked predilection for females, whereas other joints have a 2:1 predominance for men. The age range of involvement is from 30 to 60 years for all joints. The major clinical signs and symptoms commonly include pain, preauricular swelling, painful limitation of mandibular movements, and tenderness on palpation. To a lesser degree, clicking, otalgia, and chronic subluxation may be seen. Facial asymmetry may be present. The treatment of choice is surgical removal, and since recurrence is possible, long-term radiographic follow-up is recommended.

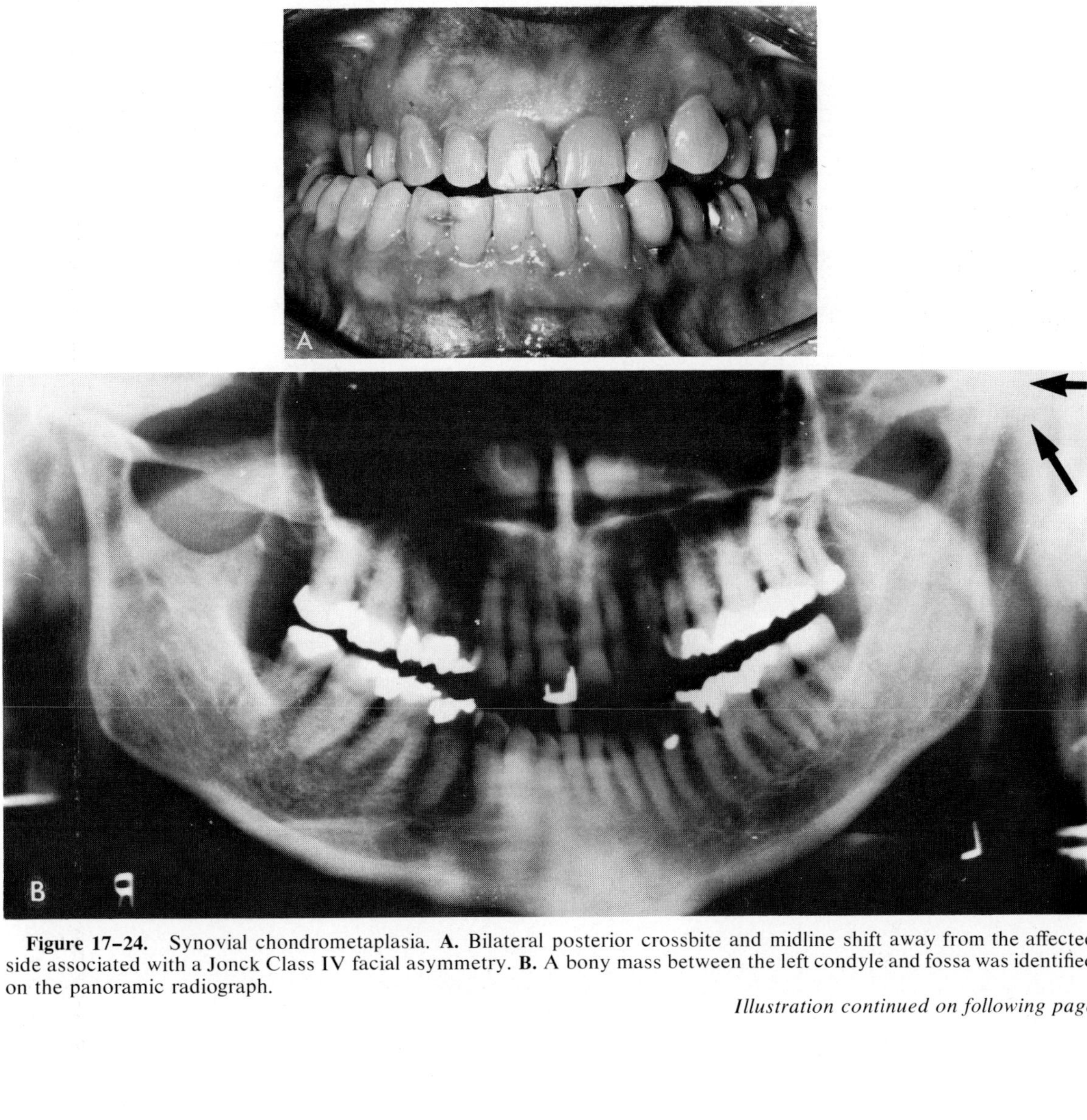

Figure 17–24. Synovial chondrometaplasia. **A.** Bilateral posterior crossbite and midline shift away from the affected side associated with a Jonck Class IV facial asymmetry. **B.** A bony mass between the left condyle and fossa was identified on the panoramic radiograph.

Illustration continued on following page

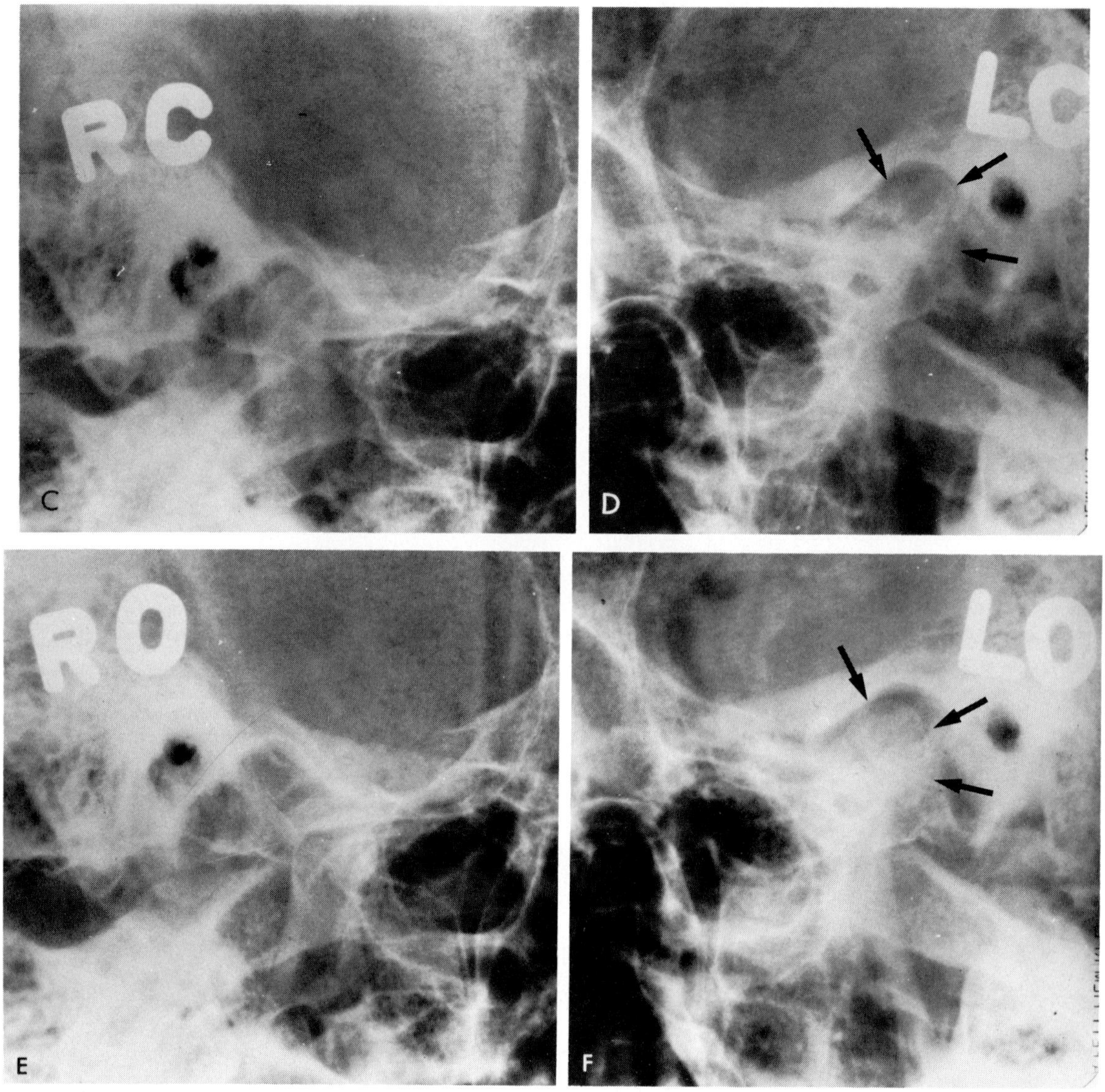

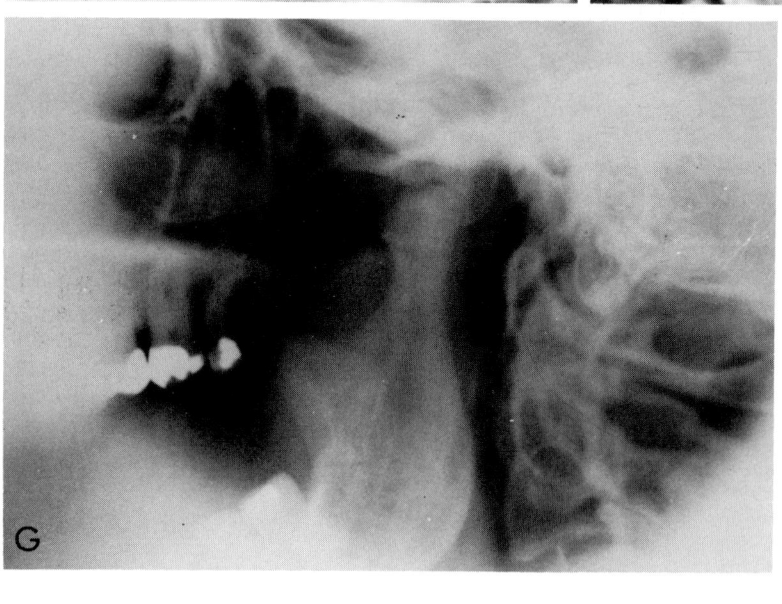

Figure 17–24 *Continued* **C, D, E,** and **F.** Right closed (**C**), left closed (**D**), right open (**E**), and right closed (**F**) transcranial views demonstrating anterior displacement of the left condylar head, enlargement of the left fossa, and almost complete lack of translation of the left condyle and bony mass upon opening, which was still a healthy 40 mm in this 68-year-old female. **G.** The mass on the surface of the left condyle is clearly visualized in the transpharyngeal (Parma) projection.

Illustration continued on opposite page

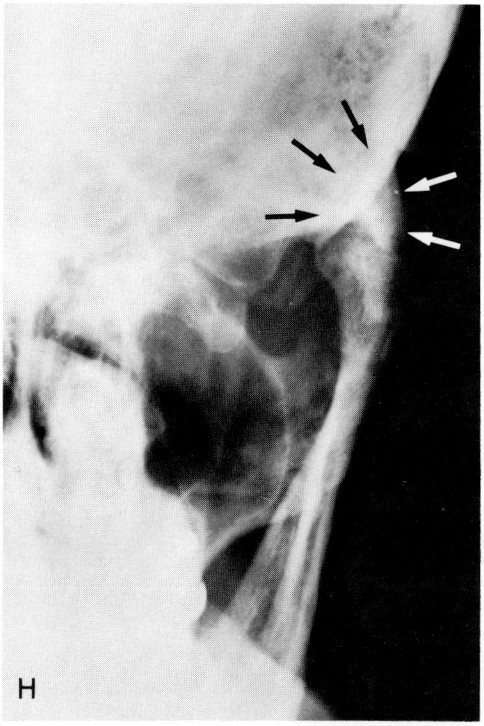

Figure 17–24 *Continued* **H.** In the periorbital view, the bony lesion resembles a bishop's mitre sitting atop the condylar head. (**B** from Stoneman, D. W.: Chondrometaplasia involving the temporomandibular joint. Oral Surg. *49*:556, 1980.)

RADIOGRAPHIC FEATURES

The radiographic features depend on the degree of mineralization of the cartilaginous bodies or mass. Most notable is the finding of numerous small bodies in and about the joint, which show varying degrees of radiopacity. Other conditions that may present loose joint bodies include osteochondritis dissecans, osteoarthritis, and tangential osteocartilaginous fracture. Less frequently, a single mass may be seen to be intimately associated with the condylar head and may resemble a typical osteophyte, an osteoma on the head of the condyle, or even condylar hyperplasia (Fig. 17–24). Additional findings include a loss of joint space, pseudocystic development, and cortical irregularities of the head of the condyle or of the glenoid (mandibular) fossa.

EVERY'S SYNDROME (Pericoronitis, Operculitis)

BRIEF OVERVIEW

Every's syndrome occurs only in association with buccally erupting maxillary third molars. The cause is postulated to be trauma to the internal pterygoid muscle from lying on the affected side at night. Additionally, operculitis and cellulitis may be contributing factors. The onset of symptoms is usually sudden, often first noticed upon awakening in the morning. The symptoms include moderate to severe TMJ pain, often unilateral; trismus with almost complete inability to open the mouth; tenderness on palpation at the points of insertion and/or origin

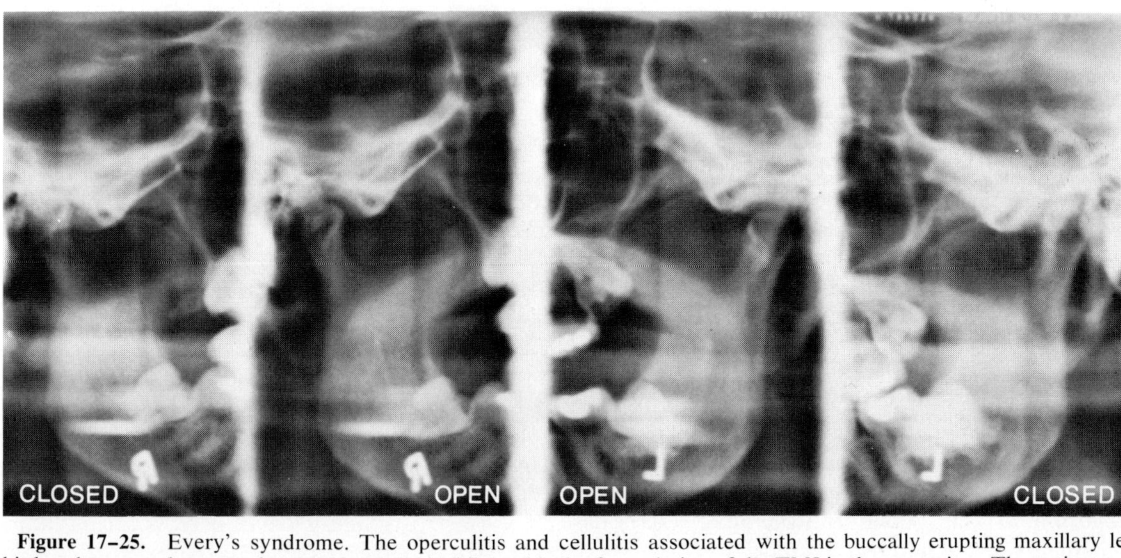

Figure 17–25. Every's syndrome. The operculitis and cellulitis associated with the buccally erupting maxillary left third molar were the causative agents. Note the bilateral lack of translation of the TMJ in the open view. The patient was almost completely unable to open his mouth.

of the muscles of mastication, especially the internal pterygoid muscle; fever; and malaise.

RADIOGRAPHIC FEATURES

Panoramic radiography is very helpful in evaluating this condition because of the inability of the patient to open the mouth. The radiographic finding of an apparently buccally erupting third molar and an absence of TMJ disease are characteristic. The condition is treated with local measures and antibiotics, followed by eventual removal of the maxillary third molar. Every's syndrome must be distinguished from MPD syndrome, disorders of the meniscus, dislocation of the TMJ, and referred pain and trismus of pulpal origin (Fig. 17–25).

TMJ TRAUMA AND FRACTURES

BRIEF OVERVIEW AND RADIOGRAPHIC FEATURES

The three most common traumatic conditions affecting the TMJ are subluxation, dislocation, and condylar fracture. **Subluxation** exists when the head of the condyle translates to a position anterior and superior to the articular eminence. **Dislocation** is identical. The distinction between these two conditions is based on the fact that, in subluxation, the patient can reduce the mandible without professional treatment. Subluxation is often chronic and may be associated with MPD syndrome or the hypermobility of Ehlers-Danlos syndrome.

In dislocation, the patient cannot reduce the TMJ. The condition is usually bilateral, and the patient is often very excited and upset. Dislocation is often caused by an acute traumatic episode such as a blow to the mandible. In chronic subluxation, eminectomy (removal of the articular eminence), shortening of the temporalis tendon, and intramaxillary fixation may be desirable treatments for some patients, whereas vertical osteotomy of the articular eminence and subsequent depression of the zygomatic arch have been successful in other cases. The dislocated jaw is treated with downward and posterior pressure, keeping the fingers away from the occlusal surfaces of the teeth. Intravenous Valium (diazepam) may be a helpful adjunct to the procedure, to calm the patient and for muscle relaxation.

Cranial dislocation of the mandibular condyle through the fractured glenoid fossa into the middle cranial cavity is a rare sequela of mandibular trauma (Fig. 17–26). The condition may remain undiagnosed and may lead to ankylosis. Mandibular movements may be limited, with premature occlusal contacts on the affected side. **Fractures of the condylar head and neck** are easily visualized on appropriate panoramic views and represent one-third of all mandibular fractures. The fracture may or may not involve dislocation of the head of the condyle. When dislocated, the superior segment may be displaced anteriorly or medially and, rarely, laterally or posteriorly (Figs. 17–27 and 17–28). If the condylar fracture is unilateral, there may be an additional fracture of the contralateral body of the mandible (Fig. 17–29). If the condylar fracture is bilateral, there may be a further fracture in the symphysial area, the so-called flailed mandible. In the latter case, the lower face has been pushed in, and the angle of the mandible may be level with the mastoids in the PA view.

A rare fracture-dislocation involves an intact dislocated condyle due to ipsilateral fracture of the ramus, angle, or body of the mandible. In children up to the age of 14, condylar fractures usually heal with remodeling and uprighting of the superior dislocated segment; within two years there may be no sign of the previous fracture. In children, the jaws should function during the day, with elastic-band fixation at night. A stable occlusion is a sign of progress, whereas the development of an anterior open bite is an indication of abnormal healing. Children are more prone to develop ankylosis than adults. In older adolescents and adults, there are lesser degrees of remodeling, and a deformity may result.

The head of the condyle may heal in a rotated or a tilted position, so that the neck of the condyle appears deformed. When the superior segment is dislocated, the inferior segment may become the new articular surface, and the displaced superior segment may graft itself to an area on the neck below the level of articulation. Fractures usually produce ragged margins, and shortly thereafter there may be a reactive osteosclerosis at the margins. Rounding off of fracture margins and equalization of the bone density at the fracture site may be early evidence of nonunion. Bullet wounds and impact by other foreign objects are further sources of trauma and fracture (Fig. 17–30). In adults, condylar fractures are usually treated by intermaxillary arch fixation for a period of about six weeks followed by exercises and physiotherapy.

Text continued on page 441

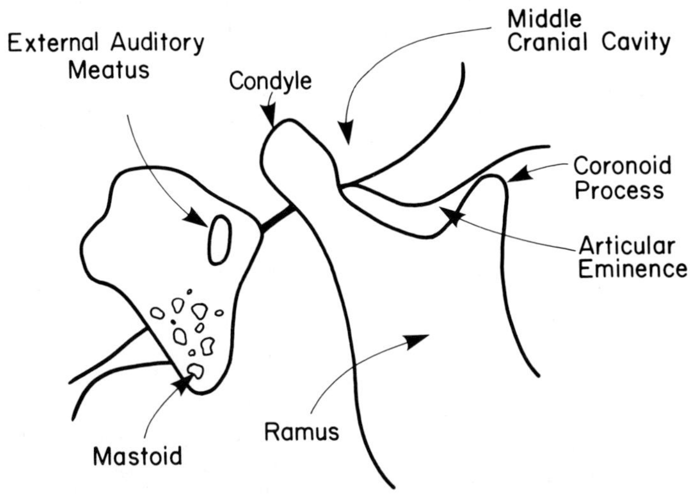

Figure 17–26. Cranial dislocation of the condyle. (Courtesy of Dr. H. M. Worth, Vancouver, Canada.)

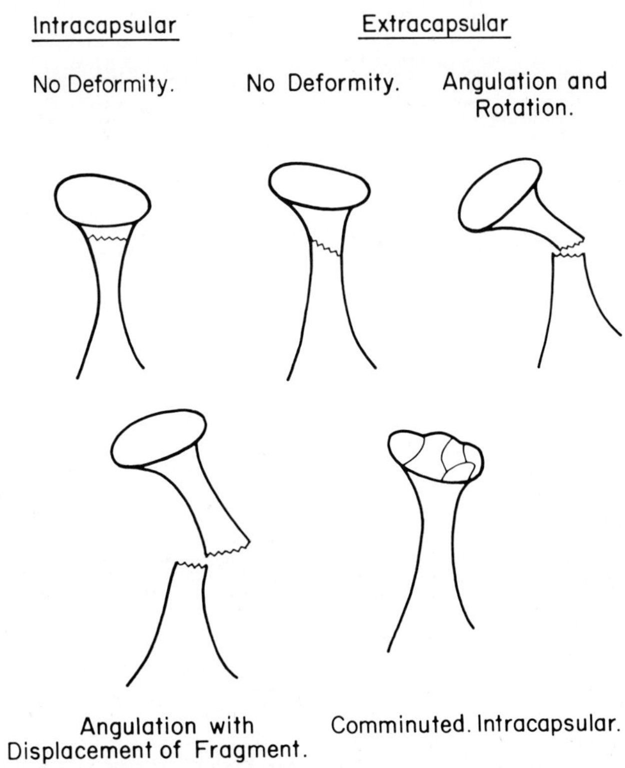

Figure 17–27. Classification of condylar fractures. (Courtesy of Dr. H. M. Worth, Vancouver, Canada.)

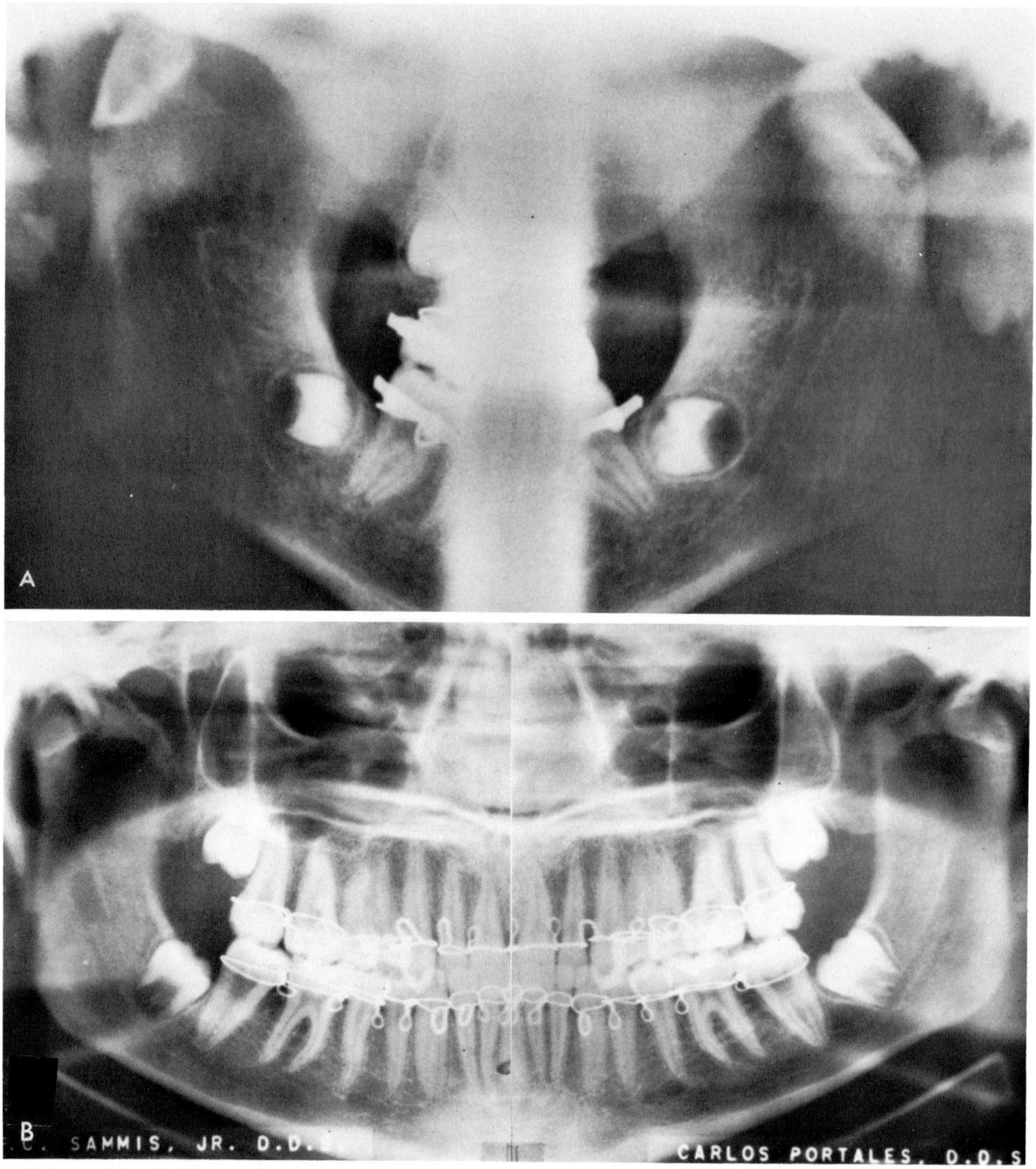

Figure 17–28. Bilateral condylar fractures. **A.** Anterior dislocation of the superior segment. **B.** Anterior dislocation of the superior segment on the left side and medial dislocation of the superior segment on the right side.

Illustration continued on opposite page

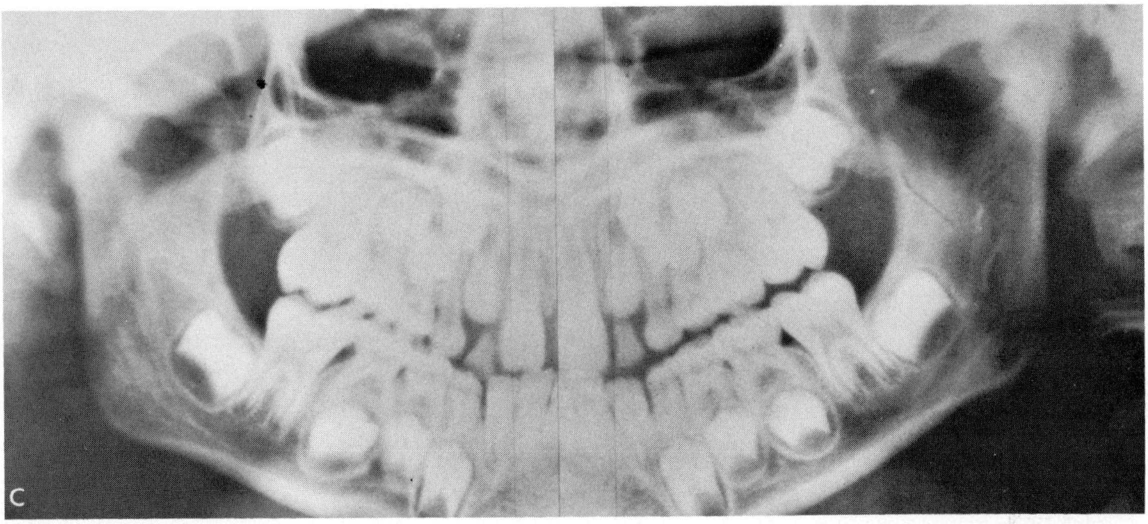

Figure 17–28 *Continued* **C.** Anterior dislocation of the superior fragment on the left side and compression of the condylar head on the right side. (**A** and **B** courtesy of Drs. Frank Sammis, Jr. and Carlos Portales, San Antonio, TX. **C** courtesy of A. Brugeman, St. Louis, MO.)

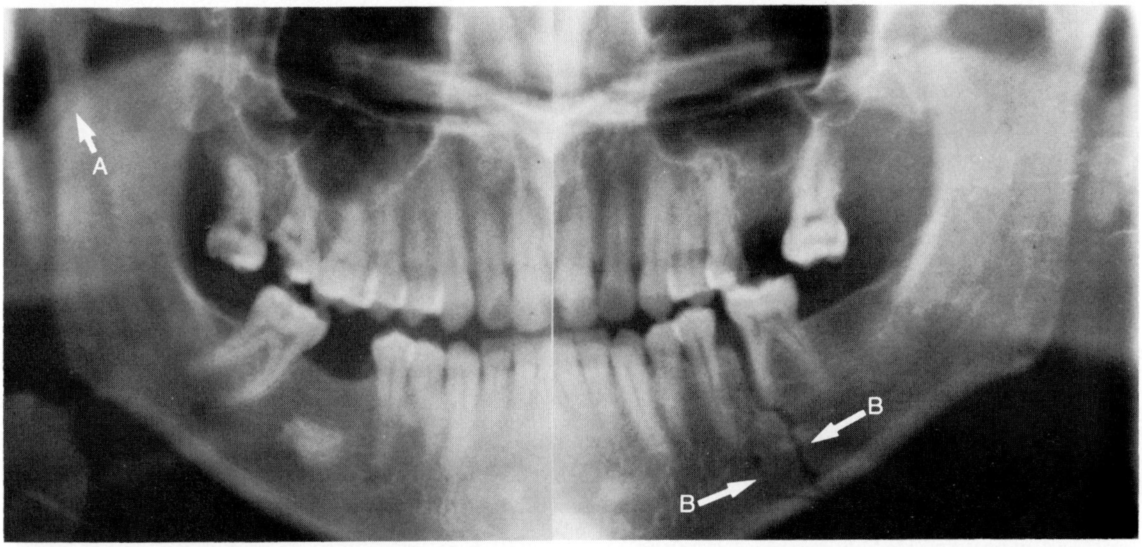

Figure 17–29. Mandibular fractures. A. Nondislocated fracture of the right condylar neck. B. Contralateral compound fracture of the left body of the mandible. (Courtesy of Drs. Frank Sammis, Jr. and Carlos Portales, San Antonio, TX.)

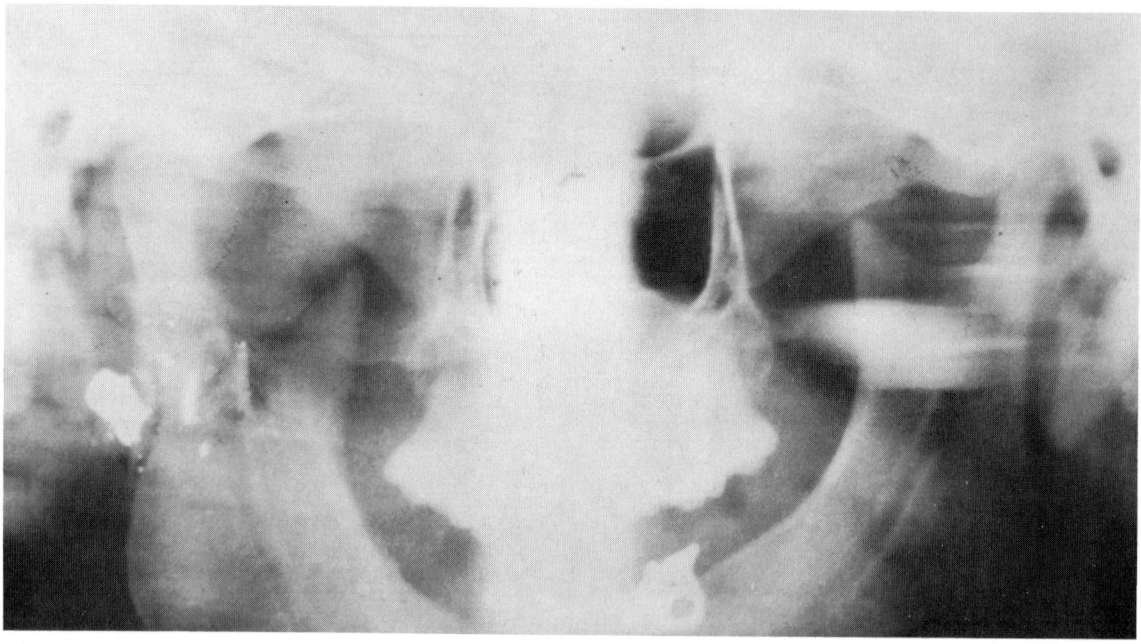

Figure 17–30. Bullet wound in the right TMJ area. Note the ghost images of the metallic fragments on the contralateral side. (Courtesy of Drs. Frank Sammis, Jr. and Carlos Portales, San Antonio, TX.)

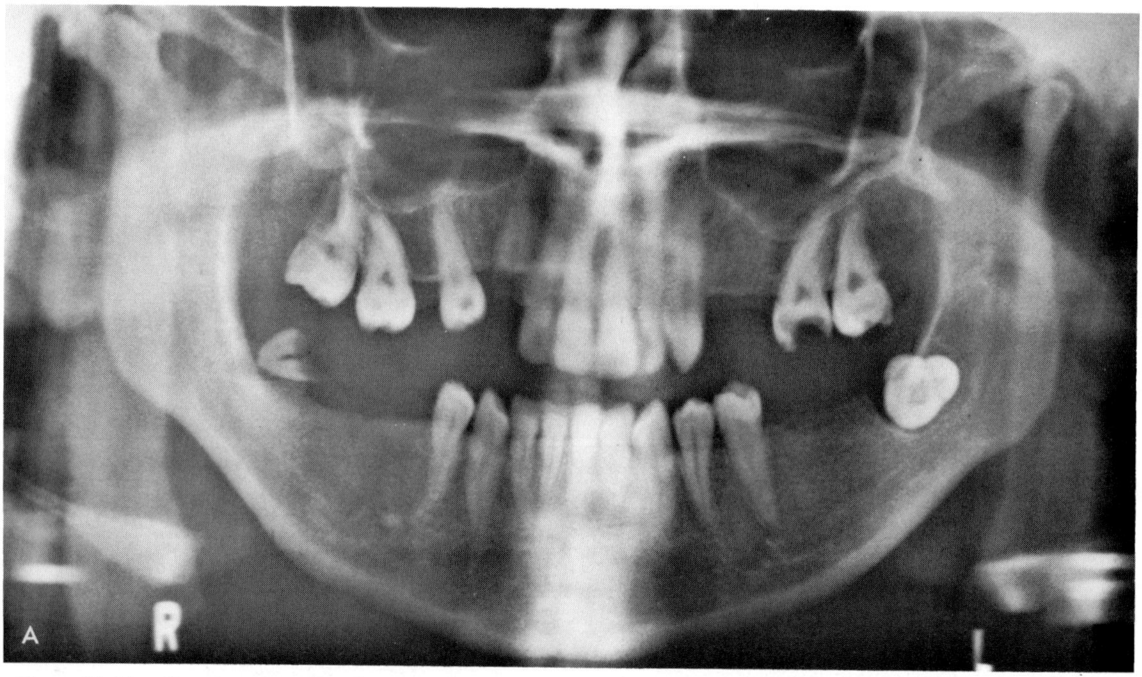

Figure 17–31. Osteoma. **A** and **B.** The lesion is located on the right condyle. (**B** courtesy of Dr. Stephen Ahing, Indianapolis, IN.)

Illustration continued on opposite page

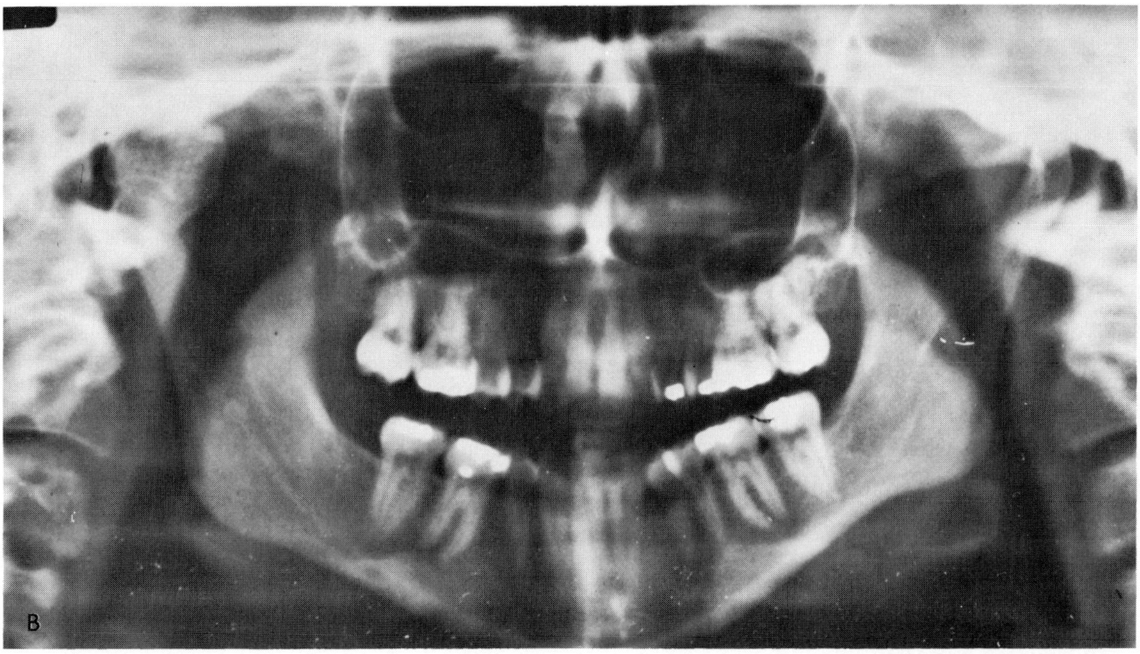

Figure 17–31 *Continued*

TMJ OSTEOMA

BRIEF OVERVIEW AND RADIOGRAPHIC FEATURES

Osteomas are benign neoplasms of normal bone and occur on the head and neck of the condyle and the upper portions of the ramus (Figs. 17–31 and 17–32). When osteomas are detected, Gardner's syndrome should be ruled out. If the osteoma interferes with function or if it causes an undesirable facial deformity, it should be removed. Osteomas do not tend to recur. They are discussed in some detail in Chapters 6 and 13.

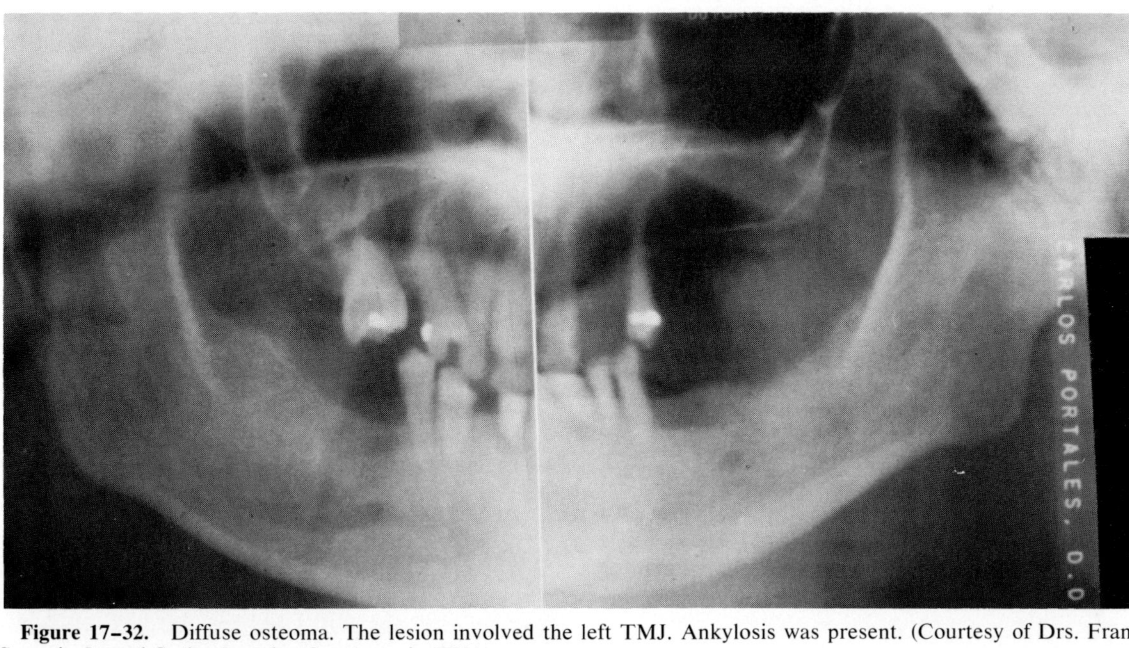

Figure 17–32. Diffuse osteoma. The lesion involved the left TMJ. Ankylosis was present. (Courtesy of Drs. Frank Sammis, Jr. and Carlos Portales, San Antonio, TX.)

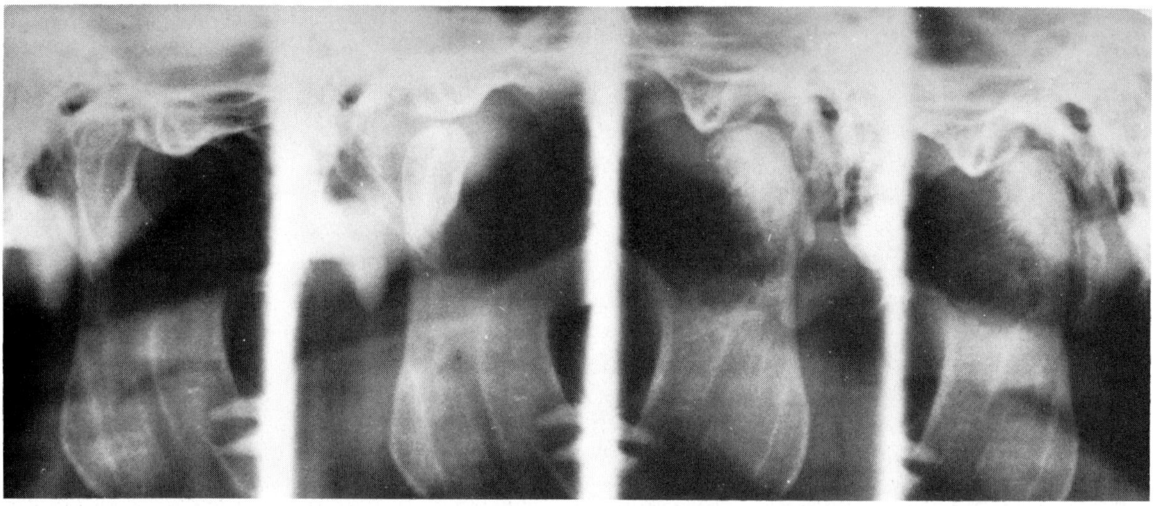

Figure 17–33. Condylar chondrosarcoma. Note the sunray pattern of the anterior aspect of the lesion, which involves the left coronoid process. (Courtesy of Dr. Chris Nortjé, University of Stellenbosch, Tygerberg, South Africa.)

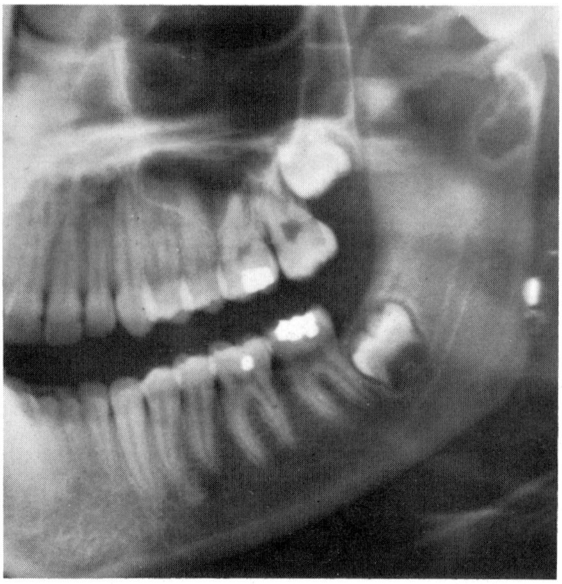

Figure 17–34. Central giant cell granuloma, left condyle. (Courtesy of Dr. James Duncan, San Antonio, TX.)

Figure 17–35. Odontogenic myxoma, right condyle. (Courtesy of Dr. William J. Updegrave, Fort Lauderdale, FL.)

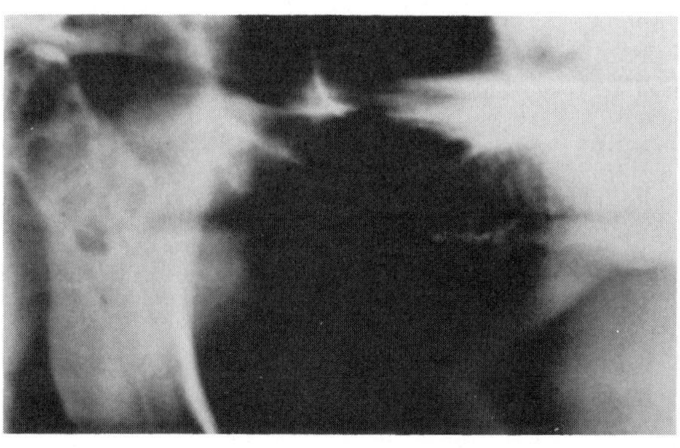

CONDYLAR CHONDROMA AND OSTEOCHONDROMA

BRIEF OVERVIEW

In the jaws, the chondroma is a rare benign neoplasm of mature cartilage, which sometimes ossifies to some degree, whence it may be referred to as osteochondroma. The osteochondroma is the most common of all benign tumors of bone but remains very rare in the jaws. Since vestigial cartilage remnants appear in the mandibular condyle and coronoid process, they are thought to give rise to these lesions. Clinically, there may be facial asymmetry, with elongation on the affected side and limitation of vertical opening. In extremely rare instances, **chondrosarcomas** may develop in these lesions (Fig. 17–33). Surgical excision is the treatment of choice.

RADIOGRAPHIC FEATURES

Owing to the scarcity of lesions in the TMJ area, no specific radiographic features can be ascribed to them. The chondroma most certainly begins as a radiolucency, as the neoplastic proliferation of cartilage replaces bone. As ossification occurs, opacity in varying degrees may result, with an eventual enlargement of the head of the condyle, resembling an osteoma or hyperplasia.

OTHER TMJ LESIONS

Any number of lesions may occur in the upper portion of the ramus or condylar area including **benign chondroblastoma** (Codman's tumor). The authors have illustrated a **central giant cell granuloma,** which is said by some not to occur beyond the tooth-bearing area, and an **odontogenic myxoma.** The characteristic features of these two lesions are discussed in detail in Chapter 11 (Figs. 17–34 and 17–35).

Aside from the causes of restricted mandibular opening previously discussed, **masses originating in the zygomatic arch** may affect TMJ function. In rare instances, **metastatic disease** has been reported in the mandibular condyle. In a review by Mizukawa and associates, nine of the eleven reported cases found in the literature involved females, and seven of these consisted of metastatic breast carcinoma of varying histologic type.

REFERENCES

Reference Texts

Morgan, D. A., Hall, W. P., and Vamvas, S. J.: **Diseases of the Temporomandibular Apparatus, A Multidisciplinary Approach.** St. Louis, C. V. Mosby, 1977.

Schwartz, C., and Chayes, C. M.: **Facial Pain and Mandibular Dysfunction.** Philadelphia: W. B. Saunders, 1969.

Worth, H. M.: **Principles and Practice of Oral Radiologic Interpretation.** Chicago: Year Book Medical Publishers, 1963.

Selected References

Baddour, H. M., McAnear, J. T., and Tilson, H. B.: Eagle's syndrome: Report of a case. **Oral Surg. 46**:486, 1978.

Beirne, O. R., and Leake, D. L.: Technetium 99m pyrophosphate uptake in a case of unilateral condylar hyperplasia. **J. Oral Surg. 38**:385, 1980.

Blashke, D. D., Solbey, W. K., and Sanders, B.: Arthrography of the temporomandibular joint: Review of current status. **J.A.D.A. 100**:388, 1980.

Boudreau, R. G., and Tideman, H.: Treatment of chronic mandibular dislocation: Report of a case. **Oral Surg. 41**:169, 1976.

Brady, F. A., and Leake, D. L.: Remodeling of the fractured mandibular condyle in a child: Review of the literature and report of a case. **J. Oral Med. 33**:57, 1978.

Campailla, E., and Tagliapietra, E. A.: Note on skeletal lesions in scleroderma with three case reports. **Bull. Hosp. Joint Dis. 32**:100, 1971.

Caplan, H. I., and Benny, R. A.: Total osteolysis of the mandibular condyle in progressive systemic sclerosis. **Oral Surg. 46**:362, 1978.

Cherry, C. Q., and Trew, A.: High condylectomy for treatment of arthritis of the temporomandibular joint. **J. Oral Surg. 35**:285, 1977.

Correll, R. W., Jensen, J. L., Taylor, J. B., and Rhyne, R. R.: Mineralization of the stylohyoid-stylomandibular ligament complex: A radiographic incidence study. **Oral Surg. 48**:287, 1979.

Cramin, A. N.: A second coronoid process. **Oral Surg. 48**:571, 1979.

Crum, R. J., and Loiselle, R. J.: Temporomandibular joint symptoms and ankylosing spondylitis. **J.A.D.A., 83**:630, 1971.

Dolwick, M. F., Katzberg, R. W., Helms, C. A., and Bales, D. J.: Arthrotomographic evaluation of the temporomandibular joint. **J. Oral Surg. 37**:793, 1979.

Domnitz, J. M., Swintak, E. F., Schriner, W. R., and Shereff, R. H.: Myofascial pain syndrome masquerading as temporomandibular joint pain. **Oral Surg. 43**:11, 1977.

Eagle, W. W.: Elongated styloid process: Report of two cases. **Arch. Otolaryngol. 25**:584, 1937.

Eagle, W. W.: Elongated styloid process: Symptoms and treatment. **Arch. Otolaryngol. 47**:630, 1948.

Eller, D. J., Blakemore, J. R., Stein, M., and Byers, S.: Transoral resection of a condylar osteochondroma: Report of a case. **J. Oral Surg. 35**:409, 1977.

Fitzpatrick, B. N.: Bilateral hyperplasia of the mandibular coronoid process. **Oral Surg. 29**:184, 1970.

Franks, A. S. T.: Temporomandibular joint arthrosis associated with psoriasis: Report of a case. **Oral Surg. 19**:301, 1965.

Frommer, J.: Anatomic variations in the stylohyoid chain and their possible clinical signficance. **Oral Surg. 38**:659, 1974.

Goode, R. L., Linehan, J. W., and Shorago, G.: Recurrent mandibular dislocation: Relieved by removal of articular eminence. **Arch. Otolaryngol. 98**:97, 1973.

Gould J. F.: Shortening of the temporalis tendon for hypermobility of the temporomandibular joint. **J. Oral Surg. 36**:781, 1978.

Iannetti, G., and Martucci, E.: Fracture of the glenoid fossa following mandibular trauma. **Oral Surg. 49**:405, 1980.

Jonck, L. M.: Facial asymmetry and condylar hyperplasia. **Oral Surg. 40**:567, 1975.

Kallal, R. H., Gans, B. J., and Lagrotteria, L. B.: Cranial dislocation of the mandibular condyle. **Oral Surg. 43**:2, 1977.

Katzberg, R. W., Dolwick, M. F., Bales, D. J., and Helms, C. A.: Arthrotomography of the temporomandibular joint: New technique and preliminary observations. **A.J.R. 132**:949, 1979.

Katzberg, R. W., Dolwick, M. F., Helms, C. A., Hopens, T., Bales, D. J., and Coggs, G. C.: Arthrotomography of the temporomandibular joint. **A.J.R. 134**:995, 1980.

Keen, R. R., and Callahan, G. R.: Osteochondroma of the mandibular condyle: Report of a case. **Oral Surg. 35**:140, 1977.

Kellner, M. J., Sher, M., and Stoopack, J. C.: Extracapsular fibrous ankylosis of the mandible after open reduction of a zygomatic arch fracture: Report of a case. **J. Oral Surg. 37**:665, 1979.

Koehl, G. L., and Tilson, H. B.: Osteochondroma associated with facial asymmetry and masticatory dysfunction: Report of two cases. **J. Oral Surg. 35**:934, 1977.

Lomba, J. A., Cabañas, R., Marrero, I.: Synovial chondrometaplasia of the temporomandibular joint: Report of a case. **J. Oral Surg. 35**:675, 1977.

Marciani, R. D.: Fracture-dislocation of the mandibular condyle: Report of a case. **J. Oral Surg. 35**:209, 1977.

Maurer, R. M., and Wildin, R. E.: Hypertrophy of the coronoid process of the mandible: A cause of restricted opening of the mouth. **Radiology 83**:1060, 1964.

Miller, A. S., Harwick, R. D., and Daley, D. J.: Temporomandibular joint synovial chondromatosis: Report of a case. **J. Oral Surg. 36**:467, 1978.

Mizukawa, J. H., Dolwick, M. F., Johnson, R. P., and Miller, R. I.: Metastatic breast adenocarcinoma of the mandibular condyle: Report of a case. **J. Oral Surg. 38**:448, 1980.

Nickerson, J. W., Grafft, M. L., Sazima, H. J.: Bilateral coronoid process enlargement: Report of a case. **J. Oral Surg. 27**:885, 1969.

Ostrofsky, M. K., and Lownie, J. F.: Zygomatico-coronoid ankylosis. **J. Oral Surg. 35**:752, 1977.

Parel, S. M.: Scleroderma: A prosthetic problem. **J. Prosthet. Dent. 27**:560, 1972.

Rao, P., and Prodesh, A.: Conservative treatment of bilateral persistent anterior dislocation of the mandible. **J. Oral Surg. 38**:51, 1980.

Rivas, P. H.: Reduction of mouth opening due to mandibular coronoid process enlargement: Report of a case. **Oral Surg. 47**:131, 1979.

Ronald, J. B., Keller, E. E., and Weiland, L. H.: Synovial chondromatosis of the temporomandibular joint. **J. Oral Surg. 36**:13, 1978.

Sanders, B., McKelvy, B., and Cruickshank, G.: Correction of microstomia secondary to sclerodermatomyositis. **J. Oral Surg. 35**:57, 1977.

Sanders, B., and Halliday, R.: Psoriasis and rheumatoid arthritis: Their relationship in TMJ ankylosis. **J. Oral Med. 34**:4, 1979.

Seifert, M. H., Steigerwald, J. C., and Cliff, M. M.: Bone resorption of the mandible in progressive systemic sclerosis. **Arthritis Rheum. 18**:507, 1975.

Sharav, Y., and Feinsod, M.: Nasopharyngeal tumor initially manifested as myofascial pain dysfunction syndrome. **Oral Surg. 44**:54, 1977.

Shelton, D. W.: Late effects of condylar irradiation in a child: Review of the literature and report of a case. **J. Oral. Surg. 35**:478, 1977.

Shensa, D. R., and Nasseri, S.: Central giant cell reparative granuloma of the mandibular condyle. **J. Oral Surg. 36**:642, 1978.

Sheppard, I. M., and Sheppard, S. M.: Subluxation of the temporomandibular joint. **Oral Surg. 44**:821, 1977.

Shira, R. B., and Lister, R. L.: Limited mandibular movements due to enlargement of the coronoid process. **J. Oral Surg. 16**:183, 1958.

Silver, T. M., Farber, S. J., Bole, G. G., and Martel, W.: Radiological features of mixed connective tissue disease and scleroderma — Systemic lupus erythematosus overlap. **Radiology 120**:269, 1976.

Simon, G. T., Kendrick, R. W., and Whitlock, R. H.: Osteochondroma of the mandibular condyle: Case report and its management. **Oral Surg. 43**:18, 1977.

Stafne, E. C., and Austin, L. T.: A characteristic dental finding in acrosclerosis and diffuse scleroderma. **Am. J. Orthod. 30**:25, 1944.

Stoneman, D. W., Speck, J. E., Weinberg, S., and Mock, D.: Chondrometaplasia involving the temporomandibular joint. **Oral Surg. 49**:556, 1980.

Updegrave, W. J.: Visualizing the mandibular ramus in panoramic radiography. **Oral Surg. 31**:422, 1971.

Webber, D. D., Blunt, M. H., and Caldwell, J. B.: Fracture of mandibular rami complicated by scleroderma: Report of a case. **J. Oral Surg. 28**:860, 1970.

Weinberg, S.: Osteoma of the mandibular condyle: Report of a case. **J. Oral Surg. 35**:929, 1977.

Weisman, R. A., and Calcaterra, T. E.: Head and neck manifestations of scleroderma. **Ann. Otol. Rhinol. Laryngol. 87**:332, 1978.

White, S. C., Frey, N. W., Blashke, D. D., Ross, M. D., Clements, P. J., Furst, D. E., and Paulus, H. E.: Oral radiographic changes in patients with progressive systemic sclerosis (scleroderma). **J.A.D.A. 94**:1178, 1977.

Winkelmann, R. K.: Classification and pathogenesis of scleroderma. **Mayo Clin. Proc. 46**:83, 1971.

Worth, H. M.: The role of radiological interpretation in disease of the temporomandibular joint. **Oral Sci. Rev. 6**:3, 1974.

Yune, H. Y., Vix, V. A., and Klatte, E. C.: Early fingertip changes in scleroderma. **J.A.M.A. 25**:1113, 1971.

Index

Note: Page numbers in *italics* represent illustrations; page numbers followed by t represent tables.